Handbook
of
Gerontological Nursing

Handbook
of
Gerontological Nursing

Edited by

Bernita M. Steffl, R.N., M.P.H.

College of Nursing
Arizona State University

VNR VAN NOSTRAND REINHOLD COMPANY

Manufactured in the United States of America

Published by Van Nostrand Reinhold Company Inc.
135 West 50th Street
New York, New York 10020

Van Nostrand Reinhold Company Limited
Molly Millars Lane
Wokingham, Berkshire RG11 2PY, England

Van Nostrand Reinhold
480 Latrobe Street
Melbourne, Victoria 3000, Australia

Macmillan of Canada
Division of Gage Publishing Limited
164 Commander Boulevard
Agincourt, Ontario M1S 3C7, Canada

15 14 13 12 11 10 9 8 7 6 5 4 3 2 1

Library of Congress Cataloging in Publication Data

Main entry under title:

Handbook of gerontological nursing.

    Includes index.
    1. Geriatric nursing.   I. Steffl, Bernita, M.
[DNLM: 1. Geriatric nursing—Handbooks. WY 152 H236]
RC954.H35   1983   618.97'0024'613   83-10478
ISBN 0-442-27845-4

to my students and patients

Contributors

Marjorie Vander Linden Albert, R.N., M.S.N.
Associate Professor
Samaritan College of Nursing
Grand Canyon College
Phoenix, Arizona

Irene Mortenson Burnside, R.N., M.S., F.A.A.N.
Assistant Professor, School of Nursing
San Jose State University
San Jose, California

Marianna Cadigan, R.D., M.S.
Chief Nutritionist, Bureau of Nutrition
Maricopa County Dept. of Health Services
Phoenix, Arizona

Imogene G. Eide, R.N., B.S.N.
Administrator, Home Health Care
Department of Health Services
Division of Public Health
Maricopa County
Phoenix, Arizona

Veronica Evaneshko, R.N., Ph.D., F.A.A.N.
Former Assoc. Prof. College of Nursing
Arizona State University
Tempe, Arizona

Marilyn S. Giss, R.N., M.S.
Director, Older Adult Program
Phoenix South Community Mental
    Health Center
Phoenix, Arizona

Linda Ellison Jessup, R.N., M.P.H.
Family Nurse Practitioner
Silver Springs, Maryland

Frances S. Knudsen, R.N., Ph.D.
Associate Professor, College of Nursing
Arizona State University
Tempe, Arizona

Gloria Rowell, R.N., M.S.N.
Instructor, California State College
Hayward, California

Eleanor Sidor Sheridan, R.N., B.S.N., M.S.N.
Assistant Professor, College of Nursing
Arizona State University
Tempe, Arizona

Lida F. Thompson, R.N., M.S.N.
Former Assistant Professor, College of Nursing
Arizona State University
Tempe, Arizona

Nancy E. White, R.N., M.S.N.
Doctoral Student, College of Nursing
University of Arizona
Tucson, Arizona

Mary Opal Wolanin, R.N., M.P.A., F.A.A.N.
Associate Professor Emeritus
University of Arizona
Tucson, Arizona

Preface

The *Handbook of Gerontological Nursing* has come about as a result of personal experience in working with older individuals and groups and experience encountered in preparing and developing core content for elective courses in gerontological nursing, as well as in helping nursing educators and students to identify and integrate essential gerontological content into various levels of nursing curricula and nursing practice. Many of us believe that practicing nurses and nursing students need more specialized knowledge and skills to care for older individuals effectively, just as they need specialized content to be therapeutically effective with pregnant women or sick infants.

Though older individuals have for some time occupied the greatest percentage of hospital beds and are the greatest consumers of health services, we have not planned well to meet the special nursing needs of this group. Attitudes toward aging, the aged, and gerontological nursing are still relatively negative (compared to critical care nursing, for example). Yet when nurses are enthusiastically exposed to the exciting biopsychosocial research, education, and creative service programs in gerontology, they do become interested in career possibilities in the field of aging. They also learn that caring for and about older persons is very rewarding. Many have been contributors to the research and professional literature in gerontological nursing.

Therefore, this book attempts to bring together essential and useful gerontological nursing information in the biopsychosocial aspects of aging. There is considerable emphasis on psychosocial and geropsychiatric aspects because of my firm belief that we must be able to understand and deal with the feelings and behaviors of older persons in order to be therapeutic helping professionals. Recognizing and dealing with feelings and behaviors are prerequisites for implementing technical care such as intrusive procedures. The content has been based on scientific rationale and on the philosophy that the research and basic information available at this time must be organized into a theoretical framework for teaching and learning about the health and sick care of older adults. The role of the nurse is seen as that of advocate, assessor, and intervenor.

Since the need for geriatric physical assessment skills continues to surface in long term care facilities and in the community, and since the ability to assess is crucial to planning and intervention in caring for the elderly, another major thrust of this book is physical assessment, which is dealt with in a substantial section written by a nurse practitioner.

Because rehabilitation is a constant theme in the care of the frail elderly and because of the scarcity of literature on geriatric rehabilitation, considerable space is also allocated to rehabilitation and maintenance of activities of daily living.

The term "gerontological" rather than "geriatric" nursing is used because we are talking about "health care" as well as "illness care," emphasizing the holistic and comprehensive approach to care. In order to do this, we draw on more than medical knowledge — we draw on gerontological content from many disciplines. In gerontological nursing we assess the total person, not just his disease or what is gone: we emphasize what is left and how we can maximize the potential for high level wellness.

The authors make the assumption that the readers will have some basic preparation in the sciences and in the fundamentals of nursing. As editor and contributor, I am painfully aware of gaps and overlapping of topics. For this I apologize and rationalize that the content herein has evolved from that which contributors believe to be essential to gerontological nursing practice in many settings. A special effort has been made to include current theory, practice, and research so that the book may serve as a handy reference as well as a textbook.

In summary, this book aims (1) to identify essential theoretical content for gerontological nursing practice, (2) to provide basic physical assessment skills, (3) to describe assessment and implementation of rehabilitation needs, (4) to emphasize and encourage gerontological nursing research, (5) to provide knowledge and skills for clinical practice, and (6) to supply a handy reference for the practitioner in the field as well as textbook for the student in the classroom.

This is first and foremost a handbook on gerontological nursing; however, comprehensive health care of the elderly requires a variety of professional knowledge and skills, and a multidisciplinary team approach. So, as we draw on many disciplines for comprehensive, coordinated continuity of nursing care, we hope that professionals in these disciplines too will find this book useful and helpful. Readers are encouraged to peruse the appendix material for professionally approved standards of care and additional resources.

Bernita M. Steffl

Acknowledgments

I am most grateful to the many older patients and friends who have so willingly shared their feelings and beliefs about aging and the care of the frail aged.

Above all, I am forever indebted to Irene Mortenson Burnside, friend, teacher, scholar, for what she has taught me, her generous assistance and support in this endeavor and her chapters. She remains an outstanding leader and guiding light for gerontological nurses and an enduring advocate for the aged. She is loved and respected by her students of all ages.

I have also been privileged to have the encouragement and contributions from Mary Opal Wolanin, another well known and loved nurse advocate for the elderly.

I wish to thank each of my contributors for putting forth their best efforts in making this a reputable piece of work. I wish to acknowledge the many readers who have helped from time to time, with special thanks to LoAnn Bell, Gerri Ellison, and Sarah Jane Tobiason.

I sincerely appreciate and wish to thank Susan Munger, my editor, who has remained patient and encouraging for many months; and Alberta Gordon who has been extremely helpful in copy editing.

Last, but certainly not least, a heartfelt thanks to Jody Dean for all her typing and assisting me with editorial work over a three year period.

Contents

Handbook
of
Gerontological Nursing

Part I
Foundations

1
Why Gerontological Nursing?

Bernita M. Steffl

The teaching nursing home will emerge and with the affiliation of students may well become a prototype for research practice, education, and administration in nursing.

Vernice Fergeson (1981)*

Gerontological nursing is young in the United States. Educationally prepared gerontological nurses are still rare. The shortage is both quantitative and qualitative; even the term gerontology is still uncommon in nursing vocabulary and nursing literature.

It is estimated that 60% of hospital beds in our country are occupied by the elderly and that they consume at least 60% of health services. In 1975 one-third of all acute hospital beds were used for old people, and there were 1.2 million patients in 23,000 nursing homes (Butler, 1979). We have not and are not preparing nurses to keep up with the trend. Why? Perhaps it is for the following reasons. First, nurses are as guilty as the rest of American society in their negative attitudes toward aging and the aged. Studies indicate that they simply do not want to work with old people (Brower, 1980, 1981; Steffl, 1982; see Chapter 2). Second, nurses who care for the aged in this country have not always enjoyed a reputable professional status. Working in a nursing home is not popular and has often been a last resort. Also, the usual avenues of continuing education for nurses involved in the care of the aged have not always been available as they are now. Though the science of gerontology had its origins in the 1940s, research in geriatric nursing has been almost nonexistent till very recently, and a variety of textbooks on the subject are just beginning to appear.

*Vernice Fergeson, M.S., F.A.A.N., Director, Nursing Service, Veterans Administration, Department of Medicine and Surgery, Washington, D.C.

Also, it is only recently (1975) that the American Nurses' Association Division of Geriatric Nursing has expanded its thinking and horizons, and resolved to change the word geriatric to gerontological (Davis, 1975). The use of the term gerontological nursing is broader. It implies that we care for and treat the whole person, not only his disease: that is, we give health care instead of sick care. Unfortunately, there still seems to be considerable concentration in nursing on the disease rather than on the person and his total health. This is understandable. Holistic care is not intuitive and it is not always easy. One needs to be educated to do it and do it by design. Teaching and supervising health maintenance and maximizing all of an older person's biopsychosocial resources take special skills; they are as important, probably more important, than simply caring for his medically diagnosed need.

One can easily collect reasons for developing better preparation in gerontological nursing. The older population is growing faster than provider programs in nursing for chronic disease and long term care. For example, it is estimated that 10% of the population over age 55 has a drug or alcohol problem (Community Advisory Committee, 1979). The aging alcoholic/addict is the least visible among sufferers of addictive problems, and society and nursing seem unprepared to help him. All helping professionals need to prepare for this, but our appeal is directed toward nurses because they have a great deal of direct contact with the infirm elderly and tremendous potential as change agents. Moreover the older population is getting older which will mean more dependency problems related to mental health and mental functioning.

Alvin Goldfarb pointed out years ago that as longevity increases, so will the rates of psychosocial and mental health problems of the elderly

(Goldfarb, 1970). Hopefully, geropsychiatric nurses will emerge within the decade. If not, others in psychology, theology, and psychiatric social work may well carry the load of mental health care of the aged, or a new discipline may be formed to work in mental health and aging (Burnside, 1976).

Despite the pessimistic overtones of this introduction, there are positive and encouraging transitions toward gerontological nursing and gerontological nursing education. When nurses do get "tuned in" and "turned on" to gerontological nursing, they find it very interesting, rewarding, and satisfying. Why is it so interesting and exciting? First, it involves us very personally. Aging is a universal experience; we know we will age, yet nobody wants to grow old and everybody wants to live a long time. In spite of our negative attitudes toward aging and the aged, we want life and, if we are lucky, will live to be old. Second, the scientific research — particularly in cellular biology and cognitive functioning — holds personal fascination because it may affect us as individuals. Also, bringing this kind of research into our practice and to the bedside is a very interesting challenge. In addition, there is opportunity for creativity. Indeed, there is a need for every bit as much, and maybe more, ingenuity and creativity as in any other branch of nursing. For example, the research findings about cognitive functioning in the aged are voluminous, but getting them to the bedside is difficult. Even a small part of these findings, such as understanding memory loss and what happens to short term memory, has tremendous application to nursing care and can make it more interesting and more scientific. Third, caring for and about the aged is a multidisciplinary affair. Not only is it stimulating and interesting to mix with other disciplines, it is a necessity. Professionals need to recognize, accept, share, and utilize each other's interests, skills, and resources. Nurses have to do more of this. Conversely, our role also needs to be more recognized and accepted by other disciplines. Perhaps nurses themselves are to blame for not selling their skills at full scale. Nonprofessionals may deliver most of the personal care at this time, but of the professional team, the nurse still has the most

contact potential with the institutionalized patient and even with the patient in the community (i.e., more than the doctor, social worker, psychologist, or other therapists). Professional nurses now receive quite extensive background in the social and behavioral sciences and should be more visible on mental health teams and in community mental health centers.

GERONTOLOGICAL NURSING ROLES

What are some of the special roles of gerontological nursing?

Advocacy

Nurses need to be advocates both as individual citizens and as professionals. They have a unique opportunity to be "liaison advocates" between patient and doctor, between patient and other health professionals, and between patient and family. Every nurse should be aware of, and familiar with, the patient's bill of rights and see that these rights are respected. In this way, the nurse becomes a role model for other staff and for students (see Appendix A for patient's rights). Advocacy is the key to assessing the older client (Rogers, 1980).

Assessment

Skilled assessment is the essential ingredient for developing and implementing any kind of health care. Physical and psychosocial assessment skills are vital and basic. In the writer's opinion, understanding the feelings and behaviors of old people is most important. For example, it is terribly important for the nurse to be able to assess and to differentiate between a functional and an organic disorder. In other words, she needs to know if the patient really has organic brain syndrome or if he is sinking into oblivion because of a well-founded depression. When assessing for psychosocial needs, loss is a constant theme. Losses increase and resources decline as we age. Included in Chapter 5 is a guide listing the kinds of losses common to the elderly.

Intervention

In *Gerontological Nursing,* Jessie Mantle, a Canadian nurse, describe nurses' contribution to quality care by describing four classes of intervention (see Table 1-1). She prefaces these with a list of developmental and situational stressful events faced by the elderly, such as ability to cope with the tasks of late maturity, coping strategies, institutionalization, illnesses leading to loss of mobility and decreased independence, pain, confusion, losses, retirement, and hostile environments (Mantle, 1978). These forces must be considered in intervention, and will greatly affect patient outcomes . They will differ for each patient.

THE PATIENT'S EXPECTATIONS

What do older patients want from the nurse? Take a moment to mentally isolate yourself, close your eyes, and try to visualize yourself ten years older. Where will you be? What will you be doing? Will you be well? Now move ahead another ten years and another and another. Now you are really old, more likely to be the woman with a new hip fracture or a man who wakes up to the tune of a cardiac monitor. Both will need nursing care. What do you expect from that nurse who comes to your bedside whether at home or in the hospital? Interestingly, most people of a variety of ages first express wishes for someone who is kind, who will listen to and hear them — hear their interpretation of what is going on in their bodies — and who will care about their feelings.

Each of us wants that and more. We all want the nurse to understand and accept our feelings and behavior, but we also want the broken hip to be comfortable, we want to feel safe, and we hope that the nurse knows what

Table 1-1. Nursing's Contribution to Health Care of the Elderly.

GOALS OF HEALTH CARE

To facilitate adequate functioning and adaptation in a stated environment which has taken into consideration the stressful *developmental forces* and *situational forces* faced by each elderly person.

CLASSES OF INTERVENTION	NURSING STRATEGIES
1. Caring for and maintaining the biological organism	1. Personal care with activities of daily living 2. Empathic understanding
2. Modifying the response	1. Health teaching 2. Rehabilitation, i.e., activation programs 3. Preventive care, i.e., skin care, exercises, sensory stimulation, mouth care 4. Listening/counseling 5. Activating resources — referrals

3. Modifying the forces	1. Modifying the physical environment, i.e., ramps, bellcords, side rails, color coding
	2. Modifying the psychosocial world, i.e.,
	  • community action
	  • attitude training
	  • family counseling

4. Facilitating the medical management of disease processes	1. Case finding 2. Monitoring illness states 3. Implementing the medical treatment plan 4. Teaching the patient how to care for himself using the medical plan as the guideline 5. Planning for and implementing continuity of care to the home

NOTE: Adapted with permission from "Nurse's Contribution to Quality Care." J. Mantle, *Gerontological Nursing* 4(2): 36 (1978).

the cardiac monitor is saying and how important its proper mechanical function and monitoring is for each individual (for us!). The implication, of course, is that professional gerontological nurses need to be well prepared in the psychosocial aspects of aging as well as in technical nursing skills. Despite our increased preparation in social sciences, however, nurses are apt to have more knowledge and skill about the fracture and the monitor than about the behaviors and feelings of the old people involved.

More than a decade ago, it was pointed out that Medicare would bring nursing educators face-to-face with the health care needs of the aged and with the lack of health professionals and paraprofessionals prepared to respond to those needs. Nursing education has not progressed nearly fast enough to keep pace with the increasing numbers of the elderly, but there is now a considerable and increasing body of scientific knowledge about aging available to nurses for application in training and education. Early research produced characteristics of groups of aged congregated in poor farms, nursing homes, and state mental hospitals, which lead to a general picture of impairment that resulted in negative stereotypes of the elderly. Now the profession must aid in dispelling those myths and must convince itself that most older people are capable, valuable, self-sustaining, significant, and necessary segments of society, and that they do respond to medical treatment, nursing intervention, and social services.

SUMMARY

The emergence of gerontological nursing is genuine and encouraging. Clinicians, educators, and researchers are increasingly visible in their advocacy, development of programs, and publications. The American Nurses' Association initiated a certification program in clinical gerontological nursing in January 1976. Thus far, 785 (1983) nurses in the United States have passed its rigorous qualifications. There is a rapidly increasing cadre of nursing educators advocating and implementing more gerontological content in nursing curricula. Nursing leaders from all over the world came together for the first International Conference in Gerontological Nursing in Los Angeles in June 1981. Many of them are referred to frequently in this book. The gerontological nursing needs discussed were universal. The greatest need, identified over and over, was the need for more gerontological nursing education to facilitate delivery of quality care to older adults (Abdellah, 1981; Bryan, 1981; Burnside, 1981, Mantle, 1981; Reid, 1981, Van Maanen, 1981). (These proceedings of this conference have been published by C.B. Slack Publishing Company of Thorofare, New Jersey.) Finally, a recent review of gerontological nursing research indicates that we've come a long way in a relatively short period of time (Brimmer, 1979; Burnside, 1981).

REFERENCES

Abdellah, F. *Nursing care of the aged in the U.S.A.* Keynote address given at the International Conference on Nursing Care of the Aged, Los Angeles, California, June 25–26, 1981.

Arizona State Nurses' Association. Communication with executive director (August 1980).

Brimmer, P.F. Past, present, and future in gerontological nursing research. *Journal of Gerontological Nursing* 5(6): 27–34 (1979).

Brower, H.T. *The effect of the social organization on nurse's attitudes towards the aged.* Paper presented at the National Gerontological Society's 33rd Annual Scientific Meeting, San Diego, California, November 22, 1980.

Brower, H.T. Advocacy, what is it? *Journal of Gerontological Nursing* 8(3): 141–143 (1982).

Bryan, N.E. *Nursing care of the aged in Australia.* Address given at the International Conference on Nursing Care of the Aged, Los Angeles, California, June 25–26, 1981.

Burnside, I.M. Training and education of psychiatric nurses in mental health of the aging. Unpublished report, 1976.

Burnside, I.M. *Nursing and the Aged* (2nd ed.). New York: McGraw-Hill, 1981, pp. 654–677.

Burnside, I.M. *Psychosocial issues in nursing care of the aged.* Address given at the International Conference on Nursing Care of the Aged, Los Angeles, California, June 25–26, 1981.

Butler, R.N. *Medicine and Aging: An Assessment of Opportunities and Neglect.* Testimony before U.S. Senate Special Committee on Aging, October 13, 1976 (NIH Publication No. 79-1699). Washington, D.C.: U.S. Department of Health, Education, and Welfare, September 1979, p. 3.

Community Advisory Committee. *Aging and Addiction in Arizona.* Phoenix, Ariz.: St. Luke's Medical Center, 1979, pp. 4-10.

Davis, B.A. Gerontological nursing comes of age. *Journal of Gerontological Nursing* 1(1): 6 (1975).

Goldfarb, A. Harmful psychosocial effects of life expectancy. *Geriatric Focus* 9(6): 5-6 (1970).

Mantle, J. Nursing's contribution to quality care. *Gerontological Nursing* 4(2): 34-37 (1978).

Mantle, J. *The nursing care of older persons in Canada.* Address given at the International Conference on Nursing Care of the Aged, Los Angeles, California, June 25-26, 1981.

Moses, D.V. Nursing advocacy for the frail elderly. *Journal of Gerontological Nursing* 8(4): 144-145 (1982).

Namerow, M.J. Integrating advocacy into the gerontological nursing major. *Journal of Gerontological Nursing* 8(4): 149-151 (1982).

Reid, E. *Nursing care of the aged: an overview of the nursing issues concerned with education, research, and practice.* Address given at the International Conference on Nursing Care of the Aged, Los Angeles, California, June 25-26, 1981.

Rogers, J.C. Advocacy is the key to addressing the older client. *Journal of Gerontological Nursing* 6(1): 33-39 (1980).

Steffl, B.M. Nurse's choice of clinical interest area for practice and factors influencing interest and choice. Research study in progress, College of Nursing, Arizona State University, 1982.

Van Maanen, H. *Nursing care of the aged in the Netherlands.* Address given at the International Conference on Nursing Care of the Aged, Los Angeles, California, June 25-26, 1981.

2
Facts about Old People and Health Manpower

Bernita M. Steffl

It's a worldwide demographic revolution. Clearly we're headed for a profoundly different society. The changes cross all boundaries of race, sex, and nationality because aging is a life-long process that affects all of us.

Robert Butler (1980)*

The facts and figures about our older population leave no doubt about directions for nursing education and delivery of nursing service. By the year 2000 more than 12% of our population, about 32 million, will be over age 65. The U.S. population is living longer, and more people are surviving to the upper age brackets than ever before in our nation's history. These increases are primarily a reflection of decreased mortality rates for younger age categories rather than increased longevity after age 65 (U.S. Department of Health, Education and Welfare, 1978).

Therefore, we can expect the need for more health care, especially long term care. Multiple chronic conditions are common among the elderly. Approximately 86% of the population over age 65 have one or more chronic conditions. The treatment of these chronic conditions constitutes the major health care problem of the older population and the professionals who give the care. The problems encompass the quality and quantity of nursing care available, the cost of care, and the preparation and attitudes of nurses (Harris, 1978). Only 5% of the aged population are in institutions. Residents of nursing homes are largely the very elderly, females, white, and widowed. Ninety-five percent of the elderly reside in the community, with the majority of them functioning independently and owning their own homes. See Figure 2-1 for the national distribution of the elderly population.

Most older individuals do not consider themselves to be seriously handicapped in pursuing their ordinary daily activities. When asked to compare their health with others their own age, the overwhelming majority rate their health as "good" or "excellent."

The limitation of activities is a major consequence of both the chronic and the acute health problems of the aged. Though most older persons have no serious limitations, the percentage of persons with some degree of limitation is substantial. In 1972 about 18% had an interference with mobility, 6% had trouble getting around alone, 7% needed a mechanical aid to get around, and 5% were homebound (U.S. Department of Health, Education and Welfare, 1978).

The five most prevalent chronic conditions which affect the physical health of older persons are arthritis (38%), hearing impairments (29%), vision impairments (20%), hypertension (20%), and heart conditions (20%). The prevalence of chronic disorders differs between the sexes, with older females displaying considerably higher rates of arthritis and hypertension, slightly higher rates of visual disorders, and lower rates of hearing difficulties. Heart conditions are more similar for both sexes. The prevalence of all chronic conditions except ulcers is higher among the poor.

Though the older population has higher rates of chronic conditions than the younger population, it has relatively low rates of reported acute conditions. The most prevalent types of acute illness reported by the elderly are respiratory conditions (see Table 2-1), and females

---

*Robert N. Butler, Director of the National Institute on Aging, in a speech at NARP Convention, Phoenix, Arizona, June 11, 1980.

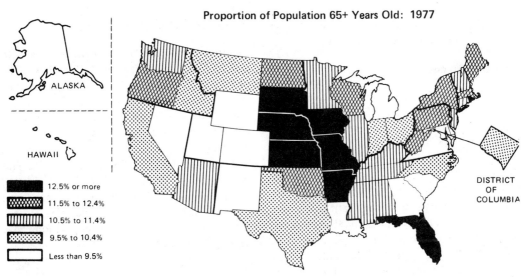

Proportion of Population 65+ Years Old: 1977

12.5% or more
11.5% to 12.4%
10.5% to 11.4%
9.5% to 10.4%
Less than 9.5%

U.S.: 10.9%

Figure 2-1. Distribution of population 65+ years old: 1977. [Source: U.S. Department of Health, Education and Welfare. *Facts about Older Americans 1978.* Office of Human Development Services, Administration on Aging, National Clearinghouse on Aging. DHEW Publication No. (OHDS) 79-20006.]

Table 2-1. Incidence of All Acute Conditions and Acute Respiratory Conditions per 100 Persons Per Quarter, by Sex and Age.

SEX AND AGE	ALL ACUTE CONDITIONS				ACUTE RESPIRATORY CONDITIONS			
	JAN.-MAR.	APR.-JUNE	JULY-SEPT.	OCT.-DEC.	JAN.-MAR.	APR.-JUNE	JULY-SEPT.	OCT.-DEC.
	NUMBER OF CONDITIONS PER 100 PERSONS PER QUARTER							
BOTH SEXES, ALL AGES	68.7	44.4	43.3	3361.8	43.6	19.0	17.0	36.2
Under 6 years	114.9	83.3	79.2	109.8	70.7	35.9	33.4	66.2
6–16 years	97.4	53.3	47.0	75.2	65.6	23.4	19.7	44.1
17–44 years	66.7	44.5	49.2	64.2	41.1	19.4	18.8	37.3
45 years and over	40.8	27.9	23.3	37.1	25.8	11.2	8.2	21.5
MALE, ALL AGES	65.1	42.6	41.8	57.6	42.2	18.8	15.5	33.3
Under 6 years	120.1	86.1	80.2	116.5	73.9	36.3	34.6	69.7
6–16 years	94.9	51.2	45.0	70.5	62.4	22.5	16.8	38.8
17–44 years	60.1	41.1	44.6	57.0	39.8	18.3	16.1	33.5
45 years and over	34.2	25.5	23.5	31.1	21.5	11.5	7.7	17.7
FEMALE, ALL AGES	72.1	46.0	44.7	65.7	45.0	19.2	18.3	38.9
Under 6 years	109.3	80.5	78.2	102.7	67.4	35.5	32.0	62.5
6–16 years	100.0	55.5	49.0	80.0	68.9	24.4	22.7	49.5
17–44 years	72.9	47.7	53.5	70.9	42.4	20.3	21.4	41.0
45 years and over	46.3	29.9	23.1	42.1	29.4	10.9	8.7	24.7

Source: U.S. Department of Health, Education and Welfare, Vital and Health Statistics, data from the National Health Survey Series 10, #130. *Current Estimates from the Health Interview Survey: U.S. 1978,* Office of Health Research, Statistics, and Technology, National Center for Health Statistics, Hyattsville, Md., November 1979. NOTES: Excluded from these statistics are all conditions involving neither restricted activity nor medical attention.

show slightly higher rates of acute illnesses for all major illness categories.

Mortality Trends

Whites and females show greater life expectancy and lower mortality rates. There are presently 105 male babies born for every 100 female babies. By age 65, there are 70 males per 100 females, and by the age of 85, there are only 50 males per 100 females. At age 65, a male can expect to live 14 years and a female 18 years. This discrepancy of age in the death rate creates many problems of loneliness and living arrangements for older women. In 1977 most older men (77%) were married; most older women (52%) were widows. There were five times as many widows as widowers. What's more, to compound the dyad of old age and loneliness for women, most older men (35%) had wives under age 65. Some gerontologists have said that old age is a feminist problem (see Figure 2-2).

The leading causes of death are well known, but a few tables will be included here to reinforce the rationale for increased attention to chronic and long term conditions. It should be noted that general demographic data do not reflect the impact of mental illness problems. Other chapters in this book point out the medical and psychosocial economic significance of mental and emotional problems in the elderly (see Table 2-2, 2-2A and Figure 2-3).

Visual and Auditory Impairments

Figure 2-4 illustrates the dramatic increase with age in visual and auditory dysfunctions. The prevalence of defective visual acuity (less than 20/40 vision) increases dramatically with age. Within the 75-79 age group, only 15 persons per hundred have 20/20 vision even with correction.

From about age 30 there is a sharp increase in hearing problems. Among the 45-54 age group, 19% of the population evidence some hearing difficulty. Among the 75-79 age group, about 75% of the population have hearing impairments.

Dental Morbidity

The incidence of periodontal disease and the prevalence of tooth loss increase steadily with age. In fact, periodontal disease is the leading cause of tooth loss among the elderly, and tooth loss (see Table 2-3) is the most prevalent dental problem of persons over age 65 (Harris, 1978). (See Chapters 22, 33 and 38 for further information and implications for gerontological nursing.)

Older Populations at Risk

An epidemiological approach to determine the needs of the elderly and the elderly population

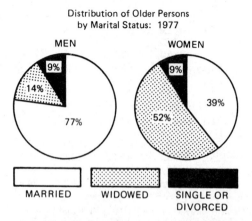

Distribution of Older Persons
by Marital Status: 1977

MEN   WOMEN

MARRIED   WIDOWED   SINGLE OR DIVORCED

Figure 2-2. Distribution of older persons by marital status: 1977. [Source: U.S. Department of Health, Education and Welfare. *Facts about Older Americans 1978.* Office of Human Development Services, Administration on Aging, National Clearinghouse on Aging. DHEW Publication No. (OHDS) 79-20006.]

Table 2-2. Deaths and Death Rates for the Ten Leading Causes of Death in Specified Age and Sex Groups: 1976.

RANK	AGE, SEX, CAUSE OF DEATH, AND CATEGORY NUMBERS OF THE EIGHTH REVISION INTERNATIONAL CLASSIFICATION OF DISEASES, ADAPTED 1965	NUMBER	RATE PER 100,000 POPULATION IN SPECIFIED GROUP
	65 YEARS AND OVER, BOTH SEXES		
	All causes	1,245,118	5,428.9
1	Diseases of heart 390–398, 402, 404, 410–429	548,956	2,393.5
2	Malignant neoplasms, including neoplasms of lymphatic and hematopoietic tissues 140–209	224,543	979.0
3	Cerebrovascular diseases 430–438	149,304	694.6
4	Influenza and pneumonia 470–474, 480–486	48,405	211.1
5	Arteriosclerosis 440	28,032	122.2
6	Diabetes mellitus 250	24,797	108.1
7	Accidents E800–E949	23,961	104.5
8	Bronchitis, emphysema, and asthma 490–493	17,623	76.8
9	Cirrhosis of liver 571	8,378	36.5
10	Nephritis and nephrosis 580–584	5,732	25.0
	65 YEARS AND OVER, MALE		
	All causes	624,778	6,672.1
1	Diseases of heart 390–298, 402, 404, 410–429	272,205	2,906.9
2	Malignant neoplasms, including neoplasms of lymphatic and hematopoietic tissues 140–209	123,983	1,324.0
3	Cerebrovascular diseases 430–438	65,052	694.7
4	Influenza and pneumonia 470–474, 480–486	24,307	259.6
5	Bronchitis, emphysema, and asthma 490–493	13,315	142.2
6	Accidents E800–E949	12,527	133.8
7	Arteriosclerosis 440	10,963	117.1
8	Diabetes mellitus 250	9,273	99.0
9	Cirrhosis of liver 571	5,297	56.6
10	Suicide E950–E959	3,489	37.3
	65 YEARS AND OVER, FEMALE		
	All causes	620,340	4,571.1
1	Diseases of heart 390–398, 402, 404, 410–429	276,751	2,039.3
2	Malignant neoplasms, including neoplasms of lymphatic and hematopoietic tissues 140–209	100,560	741.0
3	Cerebrovascular diseases 430–438	94,252	694.5
4	Influenza and pneumonia 470–474, 480–486	24,098	177.6
5	Arteriosclerosis 440	17,069	125.8
6	Diabetes mellitus 250	15,524	114.4
7	Accidents E800–E949	11,434	84.3
8	Bronchitis, emphysema, and asthma 490–493	4,308	31.7
9	Cirrhosis of liver 571	3,081	22.7
10	Nephritis and nephrosis 580–584	2,763	20.4

SOURCE: U.S. Department of Health, Education and Welfare, Public Health Service, National Center for Health Statistics, *Facts of Life and Death*, Hyattsville, MD 20782, November 1978.

Table 2-2A. Leading causes of Death among the U.S. Population, 65 Years of Age and Over (Rates per 100,000 Population) 1975.

	ALL AGES	65–74	75–84	85+
Diseases of heart	339.0	1339.9	3333.8	7258.4
Cerebrovascular diseases (stroke)	91.8	300.8	1096.5	2701.1
Malignant neoplasms (cancer)	174.4	798.0	1243.9	1431.0
Influenza and pneumonia	27.0	70.6	273.8	818.9

SOURCE: U.S. Department of Health, Education and Welfare, Public Health Service, Health Resources Administration, National Center for Health Statistics, *Monthly Vital Statistics Report,* "Provisional Statistics, Annual Summary for the U.S., 1975, Births, Deaths, Marriages, Divorces."

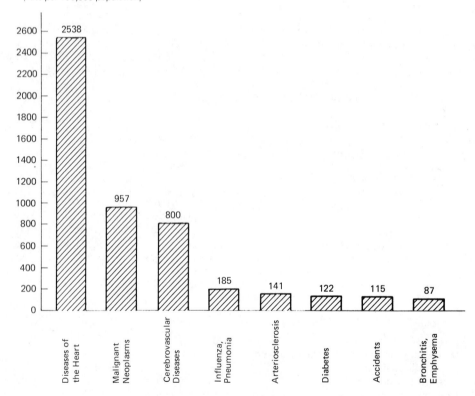

Figure 2-3. Major causes of death for persons 65 years and over, 1974.

at risk is more encompassing and less limiting than mere mortality and morbidity reports. Epidemiology is defined as the study of diseases, health problems, and their distribution in a population group. In the epidemiological (epi) approach, the focus is not only on who and what, but also on how, why, when, and where — in a systematic examination of all these inter-relationships (Hayner and Feinleib 1980). The epi approach allows professionals to go beyond merely presenting facts and symptoms (which occurs if we simply rely on morbidity and mortality rates): it allows for specific inferences for prevention, treatment, control, and rehabilitation. Presently, epidemiological data about older people indicate that chronic conditions

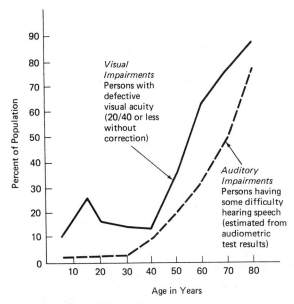

Figure 2-4. Percentage of persons in the U.S. with visual and auditory impairments, age 6–79 years, 1960–1970.

Table 2-3. Tooth Loss in the United States.

AGE GROUP	PERCENT EDENTULOUS
Total population	11.2
Ages 45–64	23.2
Ages 65 and older	50.2

SOURCE: Yellowitz, J., Portnoy, R., and Smith, B. *Pilot Dental Care Program for Senior Citizens,* Minnesota Department of Public Welfare, Minnesota Board on Aging, 204 Metro Square, St. Paul, MN 55101, 1979.

have replaced infectious diseases as the major risk over the life span (Hickey, 1980), and as stated earlier, there is increasing incidence of chronic diseases requiring long term care in the older population.

It is important to note that long term care is not limited to institutions. We are seeing an increase in home health care services. The advantages relate to psychosocial and socioeconomic benefits for the patient, family, and community. Patients who can remain in their own home have more autonomy and responsibility in their own health maintenance (Hickey, 1980). Early studies testing cost effectiveness of home health services compared to nursing homes and hospitals suggested considerable savings in alternatives to institutionalization

(Hammond 1979). More detailed studies which followed indicated that alternatives may produce positive health outcomes but at increased cost (Weissert 1979). However, the results of a still more recent study suggests that community-based services targeted to those most at risk of institutionalization may be cost effective (Skellie, Mobley and Coan 1982). Care in the home should be considered before all other alternatives (Eide, 1980; Steffl and Eide, 1978). The expansion of home health services in the community has implications for the educational focus in public health nursing, for the use of community resources, and for the preparation and implementation of discharge planning (see Chapter 39).

In 1975 almost 30% of the national health care expenditures went to health care for the elderly, although they comprise only 10% of the population. More frequent illnesses, the greater expense of treating chronic conditions, and the required hospitalization for much of the treatment — all account for the disproportionate amount spent on this segment of the population (Harris, 1978).

The national trend toward public financing of health care has been more pronounced for the elderly than for the general population. About two-thirds of the health care expenditures of the older population are covered by public funds; less than one-third is paid directly by the elderly themselves.

Since its initiation in July 1966, Medicare has had a profound impact on the quantity and the quality of health care received by the elderly. Nevertheless, Medicare's greatest problem is that it is oriented toward short term acute illnesses and accidents; therefore, it fails to cover the greatest medical need of the elderly: chronic care for long term illnesses and accidents (Harris, 1978).

Accidental injuries become more frequent and serious in later life. Factors which make the elderly more prone to accidents are poor eyesight and hearing, arthritis, neurological diseases, impaired coordination, medications, alcohol, and preoccupation with personal problems. Injuries tend to be greater even for minor accidents and they heal more slowly. Falls are the most common cause of fatal injury in the elderly. Motor vehicle accidents are the most common cause of accidental death among the 65–74 age group and the second most common cause among older persons in general (NIA Age Page, 1980). See Table 2-4 for a comparison of automobile and home accidents. The long range consequences of accidents among the aged have a socioeconomic impact on the cost of health care, as well as obvious implications for nursing and other health care professionals and for the community at large.

MEDICAL AND NURSING MANPOWER

A Rand study (Kane, Solomon, Beck, Kuler, and Kane, 1980) designed to assess the need for geriatric manpower in the United States in the next 50 years states that medical care for the aged is often indifferent and that the problem will probably get worse before it gets better. The authors say that a 1977 profile of physicians compiled by the American Medical Association showed that only 0.6% of the physicians that responded indicated any interest at all in geriatric patient care. For that 0.6%, geriatric care was one of three possible areas of interest, and members of this group were more likely to be older men and less likely to be members of professional societies. This study reports that from 7,000 to 10,300 physicians committed to geriatric practice will be needed in the United States by 1990 (Kane et al., 1980).

Statistical data of concern to all health professionals also indicate that those aged 65 and over spend almost twice as many days in bed as people 45–64 years old, three times as many days in acute care hospitals, and nearly 30 times as many days in nursing homes. They account for roughly 30% of the health care dollars spent today (Kane et al., 1980).

The National Institute of Aging is committed to beefing up the curricula of medical schools with regard to geriatric medicine. It is supporting a number of biomedical research and educational programs in medical schools, and specific content for geriatrics has been defined (Besdine, 1979; Butler, 1979). In 1978, only about half of the nation's 126 medical schools offered courses in geriatric medicine.

However, with a steadily growing number of Americans aged 65 and older, 81 medical schools are now providing some form of geriatric medicine and training in their curricula (*Information on Aging*, 1982).

Gerontological Nursing Manpower

In 1975 the American Nurses' Association conducted a survey of 1374 basic nursing education programs to ascertain the extent of gerontological content in the curricula. Eighty-three percent of the schools responded. The responses were somewhat inconsistent and generalized, perhaps due in part to the difficulty in defining content in integrated curricula. Fourteen percent of the reporting schools indicated that they offered specialized courses in gerontological nursing; the majority of those required them of students. Earlier surveys had reported a range of from 12 to 50% of schools teaching such courses (Wells, 1979).

At the recent International Conference on Nursing Care of the Aged held in Los Angeles, California, June 25-26, 1981, gerontological nursing leaders from all over the world reported a need for increased and improved gerontological nursing education. They indicated the following: *nurses still have limited knowledge of the specific needs of older patients; the least nursing education focus is given to that age group in which dependency needs are the greatest and continually increasing; special courses must be given because integration of geriatric content into the general curriculum has failed to meet current needs; students who do receive experience in nursing homes are sent there to practice basic technical skills in learning to care for old people; and geriatric courses in nursing tend to focus more on medical aspects than on nursing care* (Abdellah, 1981; Bryan, 1981; Mantle, 1981; Van Maanen, 1981).

There are 1.4 million registered nurses in the United States who hold active license to practice. They are the largest group of professional care providers and the largest single group of professionals providing health care and health services to the elderly. About 8% (79,647) of them work in nursing homes. Of that group, almost 50% are in administrative or supervisory posi-

Table 2-4. Number of Persons Injured and Number of Persons Injured per 100 Persons per Year, by Class of Accident, Sex, and Age: United States, 1978.

SEX AND AGE	TOTAL	CLASS OF ACCIDENT				
		MOVING MOTOR VEHICLE		WHILE AT WORK	HOME	OTHER
		TOTAL	TRAFFIC			
NUMBER OF PERSONS INJURED IN THOUSANDS						
BOTH SEXES, ALL AGES	67,519	4,575	3,827	10,511	25,413	29,747
Under 6 years	6,110	44	–	–	3,939	2,312
6–16 years	15,542	604	424	–	5,942	9,224
17–44 years	30,861	2,874	2,454	8,252	8,637	12,980
45–64 years	10,011	607	503	2,140	3,960	3,635
65 years and over	4,996	446	446	119	2,935	1,595
MALE, ALL AGES	38,102	2,656	2,060	8,359	12,484	16,714
Under 6 years	3,333	44	–	–	2,208	1,219
6–16 years	9,700	311	175	–	3,918	5,606
17–44 years	18,408	1,647	1,276	6,627	4,154	7,483
45–64 years	5,245	409	364	1,732	1,454	1,836
65 years and over	1,515	245	245	–	751	570
FEMALE, ALL AGES	29,417	1,919	1,767	2,152	12,928	18,033
Under 6 years	2,777	–	–	–	1,731	1,093
6–16 years	5,841	293	249	–	2,024	3,618
17–44 years	12,453	1,227	1,179	1,625	4,482	5,497
45–64 years	4,865	198	139	408	2,506	1,800
65 years and over	3,481	201	201	119	2,184	1,025
NUMBER OF PERSONS INJURED PER 100 PERSONS PER YEAR						
BOTH SEXES, ALL AGES	31.6	2.1	1.8	4.9	11.9	13.9
Under 6 years	33.2	0.2	–	–	21.4	12.6
6–16 years	38.3	1.5	1.0	–	14.6	22.7
17–44 years	34.8	3.2	2.8	9.3	9.7	14.6
45–64 years	23.1	1.4	1.2	4.9	9.1	8.4
65 years and over	21.9	2.0	2.0	0.5	12.9	7.0
MALE, ALL AGES	36.9	2.6	2.0	8.1	12.1	16.2
Under 6 years	35.3	0.5	–	–	23.4	12.9
6–16 years	47.0	1.5	0.8	–	19.0	27.1
17–44 years	42.9	3.8	3.0	15.4	9.7	17.4
45–64 years	24.8	2.0	1.8	8.4	7.0	8.9
65 years and over	16.1	2.6	2.6	–	8.0	6.1
FEMALE, ALL AGES	26.6	1.7	1.6	1.9	11.7	11.8
Under 6 years	31.0	–	–	–	19.3	12.2
6–16 years	29.3	1.5	1.2	–	10.1	18.1
17–44 years	27.3	2.7	2.6	3.6	9.8	12.0
45–64 years	21.5	0.9	0.6	1.8	11.1	7.9
65 years and over	26.0	1.5	1.5	0.9	16.3	7.7

SOURCE: U.S. Department of Health, Education and Welfare, Vital and Health Statistics, data from the National Health Survey Series 10, #130. *Current Estimates from the Health Interview Survey: U.S. 1978,* Office of Health Research, Statistics, and Technology, National Center for Health Statistics, Hyattsville, MD., November, 1979.

NOTES: Data are based on household interviews of the civilian noninstitutionalized population.
Excluded from these statistics are all conditions involving neither restricted activity nor medical attention.
The sum of data for the four classes of accidents may be greater than the total because the classes are not mutually exclusive.

tions. Less than 1% (207) of all clinical nursing specialists work in nursing homes (Moses and Roth, 1979; Newswatch, 1980).

Gerontological nursing is young and, in this writer's biased opinion, has not moved as positively or rapidly as it could (and should) to provide the quantity and quality of care needed by much of the elderly population. It would seem that a great deal more commitment is required from educators, service providers, and legislators to support training programs proportionate to others that have been funded over the years to meet the needs of special populations (e.g., maternal and child health). However, increasing interest in this field is evidenced by the appearance of a few graduate practitioner programs in gerontology, by the many new references and textbooks on gerontological nursing, by two new journals devoted to this specialty, and by notable beginnings in gerontological nursing research on the part of a growing cadre of nurses who have become advocates of gerontological nursing. These books, journals, and researchers will be referred to throughout this book.

REFERENCES

Abdellah, F. *Nursing care of the aged in the U.S.A.* Keynote address given at the International Conference on Nursing Care of the Aged, Los Angeles, California, June 25–26, 1981.

Besdine, R.W. *Observations on Geriatric Medicine* (DHEW Publication No. NIH 79-162). Washington, D.C.: 1979.

Bryan, N.E. *Nursing care of the aged in Australia.* Address given at the International Conference on Nursing Care of the Aged, Los Angeles, California, June 25–26, 1981.

Butler, R.N. *Medicine and Aging: An Assessment of Opportunities and Neglect* (NIH Publication No. 79-1699). Washington, D.C.: September 1979.

Eide, G. Home care for the elderly. In Burnside, I.M. (Ed.) *Psychosocial Nursing Care of the Aged* (2nd ed.). New York: McGraw-Hill, 1980, p. 90.

Federal Statistical System. *A Monthly Chartbook of Social and Economic Trends.* September 1976 (using National Center for Health Statistics data).

Harris, C.S. *Fact Book on Aging: A Profile of America's Older Population.* Washington, D.C.: National Council on Aging, 1978, pp. 103–140.

Haynes, S.G. and Feinleib, M. *Second Conference on the Epidemiology of Aging,* National Institute on Aging Bethesda, Md, Pub. no. 80-969, 1980, pp. 1–13.

Hickey, T. *Health Aging.* Monterey, Calif.: Brooke/Cale, 1980, pp. 33–52.

Information on Aging, No. 25. Detroit, Mich.: Institute of Gerontology, Wayne State University, April 1982.

Kane, R.L., Solomon, D.H., Beck, J.C., Kuler, E., and Kane, R. *Geriatrics in the United States: Manpower Projections and Training Considerations* (Rand Publication No. R-2543-HJK 1980). Santa Monica, Calif.: Rand Corporation, 1980, pp. 7–48.

Mantle, J. *The nursing care of older persons in Canada.* Address given at the International Conference on Nursing Care of the Aged, Los Angeles, California, June 25–26, 1981.

Moses, E. and Roth, A. Nursepower. *American Journal of Nursing* 79(10): 1745–1752 (1979).

Newswatch. *Geriatric Nursing* 1(4): 219 (1980).

NIA Age Page. *Accidents and the Elderly.* Bethesda, Md.: National Institute on Aging, August 1980.

Skellie, F.A., Mobley, G. M., and Coan, R. E., Cost Effectiveness of Community-Based Long Term Care: Current Findings of Georgia's Alternatives Health Services Project, *American Journal of Public Health,* 72(4) April 1982 pp. 353–357.

Steffl, B.M. and Eide, G. *Handbook on Discharge Planning.* Thorofare, N.J.: C.B. Slack, 1978, pp. 21–22.

U.S. Department of Health, Education and Welfare, Public Health Service, Health Resources Administration, National Center for Health Statistics. Provisional statistics, annual summary for the U.S., 1975, births, deaths, marriages, divorces. *Monthly Vital Statistics Report.* Hyattsville, Md. 1975.

U.S. Department of Health, Education and Welfare, Public Health Service, National Center for Health Statistics. *Facts of Life and Death.* Hyattsville, Md.: November 1978.

U.S. Department of Health, Education and Welfare, Office of Human Development Services, Administration on Aging, National Clearinghouse on Aging. *Facts about Older Americans 1978* (Publication No. OHDS 79-20006). Washington, D.C. 1979.

U.S. Department of Health, Education and Welfare, Vital and Health Statistics. *Current Estimates from the Health Interview Survey: U.S. 1978* (Data from the National Health Survey Series 10, #130). Hyattsville, Md.: Office of Health Research, Statistics and Technology, National Center for Health Statistics, November 1979.

Van Maanen, H. *Nursing care of the aged in the Netherlands.* Address given at the International Conference on Nursing Care of the Aged, Los Angeles, California, June 25–26, 1981.

Wells, T.J. Nursing committed to the elderly. In Reinhart, A.M. and Quinn, M.D. (Eds.) *Current Practice in Gerontological Nursing.* St. Louis: C.V. Mosby, 1979, pp. 187–196.

Yellowitz, J., Portnoy, R., and Smith, B. *Pilot Dental Care Program for Senior Citizens.* St. Paul, Minn.: Minnesota Department of Public Welfare, Minnesota Board on Aging, 1979.

3
Attitudes toward Aging and Gerontological Nursing

Bernita M. Steffl

Everybody wants to live a long time but nobody wants to grow old.

Anonymous

Professionals, as well as lay people have tended to depersonalize, dehumanize, categorize, and devalue the worth of the retiree. Younger people expect old people to "step down and step aside." We live in a youth-oriented society in America, where individual worth is stressed yet valued mostly in terms of production. Your identity and your place in society are largely determined by the work you do and the money you earn.

The elderly themselves have negative attitudes toward aging. Two themes tend to permeate a large segment of our population. One is a sort of self-fulfilling prophecy. That is, many elderly held negative attitudes toward aging and the aged in their early years. Then suddenly, one day, when their 65th birthday arrived, they seemed to place themselves in a "worthless, useless, *finito* category." It behooves the youth of today to consider this attitude because their mature years will probably number twice as many as their youthful years.

A second strong and well-diffused negative attitude is analogous to the procrustean Greek mythology, where Procrustes ("the stretcher") made all travelers fit into a bed of a certain length by either stretching their bodies or cutting off their feet. In other words, the attitude of many toward the old is, "You made your bed, now lie in it," which implies that old people themselves are responsible for their situations.

Teaching and learning about attitudes are important because attitudes do determine actions toward the aged and the problems of

aging in our society. It is not impossible to change attitudes, but this is a delicate proposition because it involves individual and very personal values, as well as an examination of our own beliefs and anxieties.

The contemporary views of society on aging and attitudes toward aging may be changing because of the sheer increase in numbers of old people, but the following quote is still too often true:

The American attitudes towards older people emerge forcefully in our language. We scorn them ("old coot," "old fool"); find them rigid and useless ("you can't teach an old dog new tricks"); think they are silly ("old biddy"); and, in a revealing phrase, perceive in them a sexual threat ("dirty old man"). At the same time, language also reveals the euphemistic attitudes which cover the underlying hostility ("golden years," "senior citizens"). Other myths and stereotypes abound. We believe that old people are serene; that their children usually abandon them; that older people's behavior can be attributed to senility as the brain degenerates. None of these stereotypes is accurate, yet this childlike portrait influences the way the young behave toward the old. We humor old people, visit them dutifully, care for them if necessary, and keep them out of sight. (Manney, 1975)

Though the older population is becoming more visible, particularly through the efforts of advocates such as the Gray Panthers, they are largely invisible in offices, schools, and the mainstream of society. When they do appear, a curious thing happens: we don't see them. The French novelist Benoite Groult captured this well when she described a young woman accidentally coming face-to-face with an old man on a bus. The woman turned her eyes away "to avoid catching the disease" (Curtin, 1973).

The American author Sharon Curtin noticed something similar in rigidly enforced age segregation between old and young within a small park near a nursing home. The old people sat on one side; young mothers supervised their children's play on the other. Whenever a child ran over to the old people's side of the park, a mother would follow anxiously, hustle the child away, and murmur an apology to the oldsters. Curtin comments: "Now, it seemed to me that the children didn't feel any particular fear, and the old people didn't seem to be threatened by the children. The division of space was drawn by the mothers. And the mothers never looked at the old people who lined the other side of the park like so many pigeons perched on the benches. These well-dressed young matrons had a way of sliding their eyes over, around, through, the old people; they never looked at them directly. The old people might as well have been invisible; they had no reality for the youngsters, who were not permitted to speak to them, and they offended the aesthetic eye of the mothers" (Curtin, 1973).

Expectations based on chronological age are pervasive. What is the age of my boss, my mayor, my spouse, the TV performer, the people I shall meet with tomorrow? How old am I? We want to know the answer in terms of a quite specific number of years. It makes a subtle difference in response and expectation if one's boss is 46 or 55, if one's spouse is 29 or 37. Even if the chronological age can make no conceivable difference, we simply need to know it. In a newspaper or magazine profile of a public personality, the individual's exact chronological age is usually among the first facts offered. To establish people in our minds, we tend to believe we must know their age.

Such age stereotyping is destructive for older people because it allows our casual attitudes toward age to merge with our more formal conceptions of age. Beneath all the euphemisms and unscientific prejudices, Americans view aging as an irreversible biological process which systematically degrades the individual. The very word "aging" conjures up physical and biological images: gray hair, wrinkles, weakness, fatigue, bent spine, shuffling walk, sickness, pain, physical dependency. At the end of aging is death, our universal fate.

Michel Philibert, a French gerontologist and philosopher, sums up the Western perspective on aging in four main points: (1) aging is a biological rather than a spiritual, social, and cultural process; (2) aging is unfavorable; (3) aging is universal and eternal, rather than differential and variable; and (4) aging is unmanageable (Philibert, 1979).

NURSES' ATTITUDES TOWARD AGING AND THE AGED

There have been a multitude of studies by social scientists on attitudes toward aging and the aged. Many have revealed negative attitudes toward aging and the aged, as well as a prevailing ageism. These studies are well reported and easily available for review. This chapter will concentrate on a review of literature and research on nurses' attitudes toward working with the aged. Unfortunately, nurses are no exception to the general societal values and attitudes. In this writer's opinion, these negative attitudes of nurses are a current barrier to meeting the needs of gerontological nursing.

Burnside, in all of her work, points out the existence of negative attitudes, their implications, and significance in the care of older patients, particularly the frail elderly. Her writing and teaching are often experiential and can be very helpful in examining and changing attitudes (Burnside, 1980; also see Chapters 9, 10, and 11 by Burnside).

Attitudes and behaviors in the environment of the aged are discussed in terms of (1) the source of these attitudes, (2) the tenuous link between attitudes and behavior, (3) a comparison of nurses to other professionals, and (4) personal preparation for aging [in a comprehensive chapter in an excellent text on aging (Yurick, Robb, Spier, and Magnussen, 1980)]. Religious, ethnic, and cultural differences are significant in forming attitudes, developing myths, and stereotyping the elderly (Murray,

Huelskoetter, Wilson, and O'Driscoll, 1980; also see Chapter 35). Studies and articles linking attitude and behaviors have suggested that experience with specific patients may be more responsible for the negative attitudes of nurses toward older patients than age per se (Hatton, 1977; White, 1977).

In a study of 162 senior nursing students, Gunter (1971) found that the lowest preference was for working in institutions for the aged and that after a course in gerontological nursing, fewer students expressed strong interest in work with the aged. Her findings highlighted important questions relating to the preparation of health professionals for work with aged patients such as, How can this preparation be included in a curriculum for young students, most of whom are not interested in working with geriatric patients? She has since developed guidelines for education in gerontological nursing (Gunter, 1977).

A study by Kayser and Minnigrode (1975) supported Gunter's findings that baccalaureate nursing students at all levels and registered nurse students showed minimal interest in working in nursing homes compared with other fields of specialization. Those who had previously worked in convalescent hospitals and nursing homes reported that these experiences were satisfying, but they generally preferred not to continue in that field. These authors strongly suggested that professional nurses become more concerned and interested in long term care, that schools of nursing include theoretical content and clinical experience in geriatrics in the curriculum, and that educators act as influential role models.

Another survey (Campbell, 1971) of 165 subjects — all registered nurses, licensed practical nurses, and nursing assistants who were on duty over a 24-hour period — was conducted utilizing the Tuckman and Lorge Attitude Scale. The results indicated that (1) no one (from all the categories tested) demonstrated a lack of stereotyped attitudes concerning the elderly; (2) registered nurses were the least willing to accept the stereotyped statements but preferred not to work with old people; (3) the licensed practical nurses and nursing assistants preferred working with the elderly more

than did the registered nurses; (4) salary increases or shift preference did not greatly increase willingness to work with the nonpreferred group (elderly). Campbell also seems to believe that in "recognizing the importance of work with the geriatric patient, nursing education and in-service should be structured to attempt to modify or to change the stereotyped attitudes held concerning old people" (Campbell, 1971).

Two hundred and four nursing students at San Diego State University were surveyed to determine specialty preference within the nursing profession and to develop criteria predictive of their choices. Less than 3% listed gerontological nursing as a first or second choice. Those who did express such a preference entered nursing with a general interest or fulfillment orientation. In contrast to those who prefer medial-surgical nursing, they do not seek sociability, adventure, or advancement in their field. Almost 30% described geriatric nursing as depressing (De Lora and Moses, 1969).

A comparative survey study of attitudes toward the aged held by professional nurses working directly with the elderly and those who did not, revealed that those ($N = 28$) who worked in pediatrics had a significantly more positive attitude toward old people than those ($N = 36$) employed in geriatric settings. Significant group differences in characteristics were considered as a possible factor. Nurses working in pediatric settings were white, younger, unmarried, and more educated; had attended fewer geriatric workshops; and had higher salaries than those working in gerontological settings. Nurses working with the elderly were defined as being older and as having spent more time living and working with the "old old" elderly (Meyers, 1978).

To determine the place of geriatric nursing in the baccalaureate curriculum, a survey was conducted of 150 National League for Nursing accredited baccalaureate programs in the United States. Ninety-two percent completed the survey. Of these, only 12% offered courses in which the emphasis was on geriatric nursing, while 72% indicated that it was integrated into the curriculum when questioned as to whether more specialized teaching in geriatric nursing is needed in nursing programs across the nation, 71 schools (51%) said yes and 45 schools (33%) said no. The researchers felt that "if the nursing profession is to meet the challenge of providing quality care and supplying the number of nurses needed to staff the rapidly increasing numbers of extended-care bedside services, nursing educators must face their responsibilities in this area. More attention to the gerontological aspect of nursing is obviously needed at all levels. Basic education programs must investigate creative approaches toward motivating students to see the challenge in geriatric care" (Moses and Lake, 1968). This writer believes that this study needs to be replicated to document progress (or lack of it) in the past decade.

In spite of their well-publicized needs, the aging have drawn commitments from relatively few professionals. A far larger number have remained aloof, and the proportions of this detachment from a major population at risk suggest a major problem. The shortage of personnel equipped to work with old people is widely recognized. It has been attributed to lack of funds, to the use of resources for more emergent conditions, or − in moments of candor − to straightforward dislike of working with older people (Putnam, 1974).

Putnam suggests a developmental approach to produce resilient professionals oriented toward care of the elderly: that is, preparing persons and presenting problem of aging in a way that would enable young adult students to manage their negative reactions. She says, "No living creature can reasonably be expected to face a daily preview of their own decay." She suggests (1) more utilization of the elderly themselves and (2) protecting the learner from the subliminal panic which may develop from visions of himself becoming old − when these difficulties are seen as developmental problems, appropriate counseling can serve as an antidote (Putnam, 1974).

In a study to evaluate the impact of a gerontologic nursing course on the beliefs and behavioral intentions of nursing students toward the elderly, Robb (1979) reported limited support of positive course impact. She stated, "If positive attitude toward the elderly is a desired outcome of gerontologic courses, the course does not necessarily have to focus on the healthy elderly, but should involve a generous opportunity for clinical experience with the elderly to balance classroom presentations and permit development of attitudes through experiences." Since there was little evidence (found in the study) that nursing students held negative attitudes toward the elderly, the researcher raised this question, "If a positive attitude doesn't influence a student to work with elderly after graduation, what does this type of attitude mean, if anything, in terms of behavior toward the elderly?" (Robb, 1979).

In a study to ascertain if faculty preferences affect students' preferences for nursing practice, findings did not support a convergence. One hundred and seventy junior nursing students and fourteen faculty members were evaluated with three instruments over a semester. An important finding was that students' perceptions of their clinical faculty member's reputation, as well as personal contact or clinical experience, may have been as significant in students' preferences for practice (Waltz, 1978).

Wilhite and Johnson (1976) conducted a study to determine whether students' stereotyped attitudes toward old people would change during an eight-week course and whether changes in student attitudes toward the aged were related to instructor attitude toward old people. Eighty nursing students were randomly assigned to ten faculty members for experimental treatment which consisted of nursing home laboratory experience and within-group interaction and instruction. Students were pre- and post-tested using the Attitude toward Old People Questionnaire. The same instrument was used to assess instructors' attitudes at the beginning of the course. Results revealed that students' stereotypic attitudes decreased during the course and that the amount of change in student attitude was functionally related to faculty attitude toward the aged.

Futrell and Jones (1977), in a study of attitudes using the Kogan Scale, surveyed nurses (75), social workers (33), and physicians (42). Findings indicated that all had slightly positive attitudes toward the elderly. Nurses ranked behind social workers and ahead of physicians. The older, better educated, and more experienced registered nurse tended to have the most positive attitudes.

An unpublished study by Christensen in 1963, reported by Carnevali and Patrick (1980), noted that nurses reflected the following attitudes when treating patients over age 65. They raised their voices when speaking, assisted them with eating without asking if they wanted help (e.g., cut meat, cracked eggs, buttered toast), provided less privacy (e.g., less attention to pulling screens and closing doors), avoided explaining details of diagnostic tests, and taught the family — not the old person. More studies of this type are needed. Miller (1976) states that nurses have a pressing responsibility to develop and maintain a positive attitude in seeking and utilizing appropriate knowledge and skills.

There are a few reports of positive attitudes of nurses or nursing students. In several of these the students' first exposure to gerontological nursing was to the well, or relatively well, mobile older person in the community (Safier, 1974; Tobiason, Knudsen, Stengel, and Giss, 1979). In a study using the Kogan Scale with workshop participants, 71 nurses in the group demonstrated attitudes ranging from positive to neutral (Taylor and Harned, 1978).

Brower (1977, 1979, 1981) is emphatic in her advocacy of specialty education in gerontological nursing, which is needed. She states, "to change the way nurses behave or assume responsibility in the long term care facility." She also emphasizes the need for nurse-teachers in gerontology: "The need becomes even more cogent in the light of past studies and experiences which indicate that negative attitudes of nurses toward the elderly were passed down to students from their nursing teachers who were ill prepared to teach courses concerning the older adult. Perhaps the most pressing need to stimulate young nursing students into service for the elderly is a nucleus of enthusiastic, informed teachers. While more schools are currently offering content in gerontological nursing, it is most often provided by faculty who have a medical surgical acute care orientation" (Brower, 1980).

In a survey by this author of 280 baccalaureate nursing students from three different nursing programs, now in progress, the findings also reveal some negative attitudes. The purpose of the study is to learn about students' preferred area of clinical practice and factors which influence their choice. Tables 3-1 through 3-4 summarize data which seem to corroborate the review of nursing literature on attitudes; however, further statistical analysis is needed and is underway.

In this survey of 280 nurses (28.6% registered nurses and 71.4% basic baccalaureate students) to examine preference for area of practice and factors that influenced the preference, clinical practice was chosen as the most influential factor by 59% of the sample, while about 17% indicated that role models and teachers were most influential. In other questions, 19% indicated that they considered working with old people to be frustrating, frightening, and depressing, and 8% checked the uninteresting, tedious, and boring category (Steffl, 1982).

Table 3-1. Clinical Area of Choice.*

AREA OF CLINICAL NURSING	ADJUSTED FREQUENCY
Medical-surgical	32.4%
Obstetrics	21.9%
Community health	20.8%
Pediatrics	13.8%
Mental health	13.8%
Gerontological	8.8%
Total	100.0%

NOTE: This table summarizes responses to the question asked of nursing students, What clinical area of nursing are you most interested in now? ($N = 280$; Steffl, 1982).

Table 3-2. Ranked Choice of Setting for Clinical Practice.

SETTING	ADJUSTED FREQUENCY
Critical care	28.6%
Community health nursing	26.3%
Acute care setting	18.4%
Education	11.6%
Supervision and consultation	7.2%
Nursing administration	4.3%
Long term care	3.6%
Total	100.0%

NOTE: This table illustrates which setting subjects ranked as their first choice for practice ($N = 280$; Steffl, 1982).

Table 3-3. Preference for Work with Gerontological Patients.

INTERESTED	ADJUSTED FREQUENCY
Yes, by choice	12.2%
Yes, if necessary, for a job	11.5%
Maybe, undecided	49.4%
No, definitely	26.9%
Total	100.0%

NOTE: This table illustrates answers to the question, Do you ever consider working specifically in gerontological nursing? (N = 280; Steffl, 1982).

Table 3-4. Reasons for Avoiding Gerontological Nursing.

REASON FOR AVOIDING GERONTOLOGICAL NURSING	ADJUSTED FREQUENCY (ROUNDED OUT)
Too much hard physical labor in bedside care, e.g., lifting patients	33.0%
Physically ill, old, decubitus, incontinent patients who can only go downhill	32.0%
Mentally ill, depressed, confused, or disoriented old people	20.0%
Low status of gerontological nursing	15.0%
Total	100.0%

NOTE: This table indicates how subjects ranked reasons for avoiding gerontological nursing (N = 280; Steffl, 1982).

Table 3-5. Factors Influencing Choice of Clinical Area of Practice.

FACTORS	RELATIVE FREQUENCY
Clinical experience	59.1%
Factors outside professional education, e.g., family and need to earn a living	9.3%
Role models in clinical settings	10.0%
Literature, theory, and research	7.2%
Enthusiasm and expertise of teacher	6.7%
Job opportunities	6.1%
Unknown	1.6%
Total	100.0%

NOTE: This table presents results obtained when subjects were asked to rank the above factors in terms of influencing their choice of clinical practice. The percentages indicate the number who rated each of the above most influential (N = 280; Steffl, 1982).

Table 3-6. Preparation for Gerontological Nursing

	ADJUSTED FREQUENCY	
	YES	NO
Is there a need for more and better prepared gerontological nurses?	98.2%	1.8%
Do nurses need more preparation in theory and practice for working with older people in long term care?	84.6%	15.4%
Would you like to see a required course in gerontological nursing in your present program?	57.8%	42.2%

NOTE: This table presents summary responses to three questions in the survey by Steffl (1982; N = 280).

The researcher was interested also in learning how influential faculty might be in influencing students and other nurses to choose work in gerontological nursing. Tables 3-5 through 3-8 should be of special interest to nursing educators (Steffl, 1982). It is of special interest and concern to note in Table 3-6 that although most nurses see a need for more preparation in gerontological nursing, many do not want a required course.

Brower (1981) conducted a survey of 581 registered nurses in south Florida which revealed widespread prejudice against the aged, very little training in geriatric nursing, and little interest in obtaining further training. Her study concluded that frustration, lack of knowledge about aging, negative stereotypes, and fear contributed to the problem.

This review of the literature indicates (1) that there has been concern for more than a decade among gerontological nurse leaders about nurses' negative attitudes toward, and lack of interest in, caring for the aged; (2) that not much if any progress has been made in increasing interest in long term care; and (3) that nursing schools and nursing educators must take responsibility for devising means to prepare professional nurses to meet manpower needs in this field. Whether or not faculty members influence students, preferences is questionable, but clinical practice does seem to have some influence according to the research reviewed.

Table 3-7. Opinions about Preparation.

Yes		58.9%
No		41.1%
	Total	100.0%

NOTE: This table illustrates responses to the statement: My nursing program (thus far) has prepared me well in theory and practice for working with the elderly ($N = 280$; Steffl, 1982).

Table 3-8. Influence of Faculty.

Not at all	7.1%
Very little	12.7%
Some	36.0%
Much in some courses	37.8%
Much in most courses	6.4%
Total	100.0%

NOTE: This table illustrates responses to the question, Do you believe faculty interest has had influence on your interests? ($N = 280$; Steffl, 1982).

REFERENCES

Arizona State Board of Nursing. *Annual Statistical Report.* Phoenix, Az. April 1979.

Brower, H.T. A study of graduate programs in gerontological nursing. *Journal of Gerontological Nursing* 3(6): 40–46 (1977).

Brower, H.T. A study of content needs in graduate gerontological nursing curricula. *Journal of Gerontological Nursing* 5(5): 21-31 (1979).

Brower, H.T. Editorial. *Journal of Gerontological Nursing* 6(5): 251 (1980).

Brower, H.T. Survey of registered nurses' preference to work with certain age groups. Unpublished report, University of Miami, 1981.

Burnside, I.M. *Psychosocial Nursing Care of the Aged.* 2nd Ed New York: McGraw-Hill, 1980.

Campbell M.E. Study of the attitudes of nursing personnel toward the geriatric patient. *Nursing Research* 20(2): 147-151 (1971).

Carnevali, D.L. and Patrick, M. *Nursing Management for the Elderly.* Philadelphia: J.B. Lippincott, 1979, pp. 45–46.

Chamberland, G., Rawls, B., Powell, C., and Roberts, M.J. Improving students' attitudes toward aging. *Journal of Gerontological Nursing* 4: 44–45 (January–February 1978).

Curtin, S. *Nobody Ever Died of Old Age.* Boston: Little, Brown, 1973.

De Lora, J.R. and Moses, D.V. Specialty preferences and characteristics of nursing students in baccalaureate programs. *Nursing Research* 18(2): 137-144 (1969).

Futrell, M. and Jones, W. Attitudes of physicians, nurses, and social workers toward the elderly and health maintenance services for the aged: implications for health manpower policy. *Journal of Gerontological Nursing* 3: 42-46 (May–June 1977).

Gunter, L.M. Students' attitudes toward geriatric nursing. *Nursing Outlook* 19(7): 466–469 (1971).

Gunter, L.M. and Miller, J.C. Toward a nursing curriculum – gerontology. *Nursing Research* 26: 208-221 (May–June 1977).

Hatton, J. Nurse's attitude toward the aged: relationship to nursing care. *Journal of Gerontological Nursing* 3: 21-26 (May–June 1977).

Iverson, D. and Portnoy, B. Reassessment of the knowledge/attitude/behavior triad. *Health Education* 3(6): 31-34 (November–December 1977).

Kayser, J.S. and Minnigerode, F.A. Increasing nursing students' interest in working with aged patients. *Nursing Research* 24: 23-26 (January–February 1975).

Manney, J.D., Jr. *Aging in American Society.* The University of Michigan–Wayne State University Institute of Gerontology, Detroit 1975.

Meyers, M.H. A comparison of attitudes toward the aged held by professional nurses working directly with the elderly and those who do not work directly with the elderly. Unpublished master's thesis, University of Kansas, School of Nursing, College of Health Sciences, 1978.

Miller, Sr. P. Rx for the aging person: attitudes. *Journal of Gerontological Nursing* 2(2): 22-26 (1976).

Moses, D.V. and Lake, C.S. Geriatrics in the Baccalaureate Curriculum Nursing Outlook 16: 41-43 July 1968.

Murray, R.B., Huelskoetter, H., Wilson, M., and O'Driscoll, D.L. *The Nursing Process in Later Maturity.* Englewood Cliffs, N.J.: Prentice-Hall, 1980, pp. 121-128.

National League for Nursing, Division of Research. *National League for Nursing Data Book* (Publication No. 19.1751). New York: 1978, p. 75.

Philibert, M. Philosophical approach to gerontology. In Hendricks, J. and Hendricks, C. (Eds.) *Dimensions of Aging: Readings.* Cambridge, Mass.: Winthrop, 1979, pp. 384-388.

Putnam, P. Orienting the young to old age. *Nursing Outlook* 22(8): 519-521 (1974).

Robb, S.S. Attitudes and intentions of baccalaureate nursing students toward the elderly. *Nursing Research* 28(1): 43-50 (1979).

Safier, G. Nursing students and their learning experiences in geriatrics. *Journal of Psychiatric Nursing and Mental Health Services* 12: 34-41 (May–June 1974).

Steffl, B.M. Nurses' choice of clinical interest area for practice and factors influencing interest and choice. Research study in progress, College of Nursing, Arizona State University, 1982.

Taylor, K.H. and Harned, T.L. Attitudes toward old people: a study of nurses who care for the elderly. *Journal of Gerontological Nursing* 4(5): 43-47 (1978).

Tobiason, S.J., Knudsen, F., Stengel, J., and Giss, M. Positive attitudes toward aging: the young teach the old. *Journal of Gerontological Nursing* 5(3): 34-39 (1979).

Waltz, C.F. Faculty influence on nursing students' preference for practice. *Nursing Research* 27(2): 89-97 (1978).

White, C.M. The nurse-patient encounter: attitudes and behavior in action. *Journal of Gerontological Nursing* 3: 16-20 (May–June 1977).

Wilhite, M.J. and Johnson, D.M. Changes in nursing students' stereotypic attitudes toward old people. *Nursing Research* 25(6): 430-432 (1976).

Yurick, A.G., Robb, S.S., Spier, B.E., and Magnussen, M.H. *The Aged Person and the Nursing Process.* New York: Appleton-Century-Crofts, 1980, pp. 81-121.

4
Theories of Aging: Biological, Psychological, and Sociological

Bernita M. Steffl

Now King David was old and stricken in years; and they covered him with clothes but he gat no heat. Wherefore his servants said unto him, Let there be sought for my lord the king a young virgin: and let her stand before the king, and let her cherish, and let her lie in thy bosom, that my lord the king may get heat. . . .And the damsel was very fair, and cherished the king, and ministered to him: but the king knew her not.

King James Version, 1 Kings 1:1-4

Human aging is a complex and still mysterious process. Attempts to push back the clock have existed since biblical times. While we do not yet have a universally accepted definition of aging, we do have increasing scientific information which makes the study of gerontology interesting and exciting. More scientific data need to reach the bedside. That is, the results of biological and sociological research must be converted into theoretical foundations for nursing practice and must serve as the rationale for action in nursing.

Definitions

Though there are no universally accepted definitions of aging, students of gerontological nursing should speculate and contemplate theoretical definitions for their own scientific operation. Birren (1977) points out that "investigators can become overly concerned with definitions, a tendency that is more likely to appear in the absence of data. Refined definitions sharpen our discourse but cannot substitute for clarification resulting from research information."

"Two conflicting views are held today by students of aging in man. One considers aging as an involuntary process which operates cumulatively with the passage of time and is revealed in different organ systems as inevitable modifications of cells, tissues, and fluids. The other view interprets the changes found in aged organs as structural alterations due to infections, toxins, traumas, nutritional disturbances or inadequacies giving rise to what are called degenerative changes and impairments" (Cowdry, 1942). These conflicts are still present today. The following are a few definitions by noted contemporary gerontologists:

Senescence is a change in the behavior of the organism with age, which leads to a decreased power of survival and adjustment. (Comfort, 1970)

Aging is the deterioration of a mature organism resulting from time dependent, essentially irreversible changes intrinsic to all members of a species, such that, with the passage of time, they become increasingly unable to cope with the stresses of environment, thereby increasing the probability of death. (Handler, 1960)

Aging refers to the regular changes that occur in mature genetically representative organisms living under representative environmental conditions as they advance in chronological age. (Birrin and Renner, 1977)

Aging is the loss of temporal organization. (Samis, 1968)

This writer prefers the short definition by Samis because it seems in keeping with nature's rhythmic, time-dependent cycles. Just as the sun, stars, moon, and tides control the universe, so do the timed mechanisms of the cells and organs, which affect various body rhythms such as respirations and pulse, control our bodies. Many of the theories of aging relate to some interruption and/or deterioration of the timing mechanisms of the cells of the body and the brain. The definition becomes meaningful when one conceptualizes that interruptions of these intricate rhythms and the molecular "lock and key" operation of cellular systems cause disorganization and mutations which affect physical functions, complicate mental functions such as memory, and eventually lead to deterioration. The remainder of this chapter will focus on the most common, most accepted, and most clearly defined biological, psychological, and sociological theories of aging.

BIOLOGICAL THEORIES OF AGING

Most biologists agree on the following principles: (1) all organs in any one organism do not age at the same rate; and (2) any one organ does not necessarily age at the same rate in different individuals of the same species (Rockstein and Sussman, 1979).

The basic assumptions and concepts which guide current research and clinical practice (Rockstein, Chesky, and Sussman, 1977; Rockstein and Sussman, 1979; Sinex, 1977) are:

- Human aging as a total process begins at conception.
- The course of aging varies from individual to individual, depending on various genetic, social, psychological, and economic factors.
- Senescence, the final biological stage in any organism, is a period when breakdown is not balanced by repair mechanisms.
- Traumatic experiences (stress) may weaken an individual.
- No one really dies from old age.

Any theory of aging must meet the following three criteria: (1) the aging phenomenon under consideration must be evident universally in all members of a given species; (2) the process must be progressive with time; (3) the process must be deleterious in nature, leading ultimately to the failure of the organ or system.

Universal Manifestations

The universal anatomical and physiological manifestations of aging observed in vertebrates and invertebrates are:

- *Hair.* The graying and thinning of hair is not unique to humans, it occurs in horses, dogs, and sheep; insects and bees lose fine hairs with age.
- *Teeth.* When not preserved by modern dental care, teeth are worn, decayed, broken, or missing. Such conditions are also commonly observed in old animals like mice, deer, elephants, horses, dogs, cats, and camels. An animal's age is often estimated by observing the teeth.
- *Body weight.* Mammals generally tend to gain weight until they reach maturity. During their finals years, old people tend to undergo a loss of weight. This also occurs in old animals.
- *Nervous system.* A general decline in the number of nerve cells occurs with advancing age in many species.
- *Muscle mass.* Skeletal muscle tissue decreases in mass due to a reduction in the number and/or volume of muscle fibers. Skeletal muscle is not capable of replacing fibers that have been destroyed by environmental stresses. Similar changes have been observed in several strains of rat.
- *Aging pigments.* The accumulation of aging pigment granules (particularly in cardiac muscle cells and nerve cells) is a widely demonstrated phenomenon in many species. These pigments are generally termed lipofuscin, although their composition may vary from one species to another.
- *Motor activity.* An age-related decrease in motor activity occurs in almost all animal species, most notably humans, dogs, rats, mice, bees, and flies.

- *Reproductive senescence.* A decline in reproductive activity and fertility occurs in all animals at advanced ages. Only the human female undergoes menopause (sometime during the fifth decade of life), but other animals do undergo reproductive senescence with advancing age, which results in fewer offspring per litter and decreased egg production, for example.
- *Adaptability to stress.* Perhaps the most universal characteristic of aging is the progressively decreasing ability to adapt to environmental stresses.

Problems and Difficulties in Studying Human Aging

Obtaining accurate scientific data on human aging is complicated by the length of the life span itself. Longitudinal studies are required, but it becomes very difficult to maintain rigorous techniques when the scientist's work must be passed on from generation to generation; keeping track of subjects over a period of years in the human life span is very difficult. The few longitudinal studies that have survived have had a prevailing influence on the study of gerontology. One of these is the Baltimore Longitudinal Study of the National Institute on Aging which was developed more than 20 years ago. (Granick and Patterson, 1971) The reader is also referred to longitudinal studies of the Center for the Study of Aging and Human Development at Duke University (Palmore, 1970).

It is even difficult for one researcher or one research group to maintain continuity of study with domestic animals such as dogs, cats, and horses because of their life spans. Rats and mice are used because of their relatively short lives. Rotifers and fruit flies lend themselves to genetic studies because of their short lifetimes. In most cases, it is desirable for the researcher to observe many, or at least several, cycles in the life span of the subjects of his research.

The cost of healthy research animals and the necessary governmental protective control procedures for humans and animals all add to the difficulty and the high cost of research (Rockstein and Sussman, 1979).

Genetic Theories

If we believe that the life span of animal species is determined by a genetic program, then ultimately all biological theories of aging have a genetic basis. Shock (1977) divides the biological theories of aging into two primary categories: (1) those that focus on how information is transferred from DNA molecules to form critical enzymes and (2) those that concentrate on nongenetic changes which may occur, with the passage of time, in cellular proteins after they have been formed.

Leonard Hayflick, when at Stanford University, demonstrated that man's biological (genetic) time clock is wound up for no more than 110–120 years. That is the estimated time it would take for cells to divide to the maximum of 50 times. He has proved that unlimited cell division does not happen and that immortality of cells is more abnormal than normal. Diploid cell division of humans goes through about 50 divisions and then deteriorates. Given a culture of normal human cells, it can be determined at what age they were taken. Cells taken from young adults divide about 30 times. Cells taken from mature adults divide about 20 times. Hayflick also found that freezing cells halted the biological clock, but when the cells were thawed, activity resumed where it left off (Hayflick, 1974b).

Somatic Mutation Theory. According to the theory of somatic mutation, radiation accelerates aging. Early experimentation indicated that by exposure of guinea pigs to x-ray or by direct application of certain chemicals like carbon tetrachloride to the liver, a considerable number of liver cells were destroyed and subsequent cells which replaced them produced a high rate of abnormal chromosomes (Rockstein and Sussman, 1979). This theory is passing from the scene because (1) the effects of radiation occur primarily in dividing cells, (2) the rate at which mutations occur in the absence of exposure to radiation indicates that in mammals the number of cells apt to go through mutation is too small to account for the overall age changes, and (3) recent studies show that most cells contain mechanism for the repair of damaged DNA molecules (Sinex, 1977).

However, we do know that exposure to sublethal doses of radiation will shorten life. Takashi Makinodan is now researching the effects of radiation on the survivors of Hiroshima. A problem for basic research in this area has been finding radiation-free subjects because everyone is exposed to sunlight; however, studies of bats living in caves have been attempted.

The Error Theory. The popular, but relatively unsubstantiated, error theory proposes that as cells continue to function, random errors may occur in the synthesis of new proteins (Rockstein and Sussman, 1979). According to this theory, aging and death of the cell are the result of errors which may occur at any step in the sequence of information transfer, resulting in the formation of a protein or enzyme which is not an exact copy of the original and is therefore, unable to carry out its function. In other words, the genetic code is not transferred accurately (Shock, 1977).

Many enzymes grow less active with age; others increase in activity. There are myriads of these changes, some not well understood, but just about all of them controlled by the genes. The roles of DNA and RNA are very significant in the genetic theories. The DNA molecules are located in the nucleus of the cells. The RNA is a messenger formed on the DNA which migrates to the ribosomes of cells where protein is synthesized.

Nongenetic Theories

Study of the changes occurring in specific molecules has resulted in the "cross-linkage" and "free-radical" theories. Molecules accidently become entangled with each other, which reduces their functioning; or pieces of molecules eagerly seek other molecules to latch onto which also clogs or interferes with normal function.

The cross-linkage theory was proposed over 25 years ago by Johan Bjorksten, an industrial chemist working with nylon and polyesters. He observed that the protein gelatin used in the Ditto machine was irreversibly altered, or denatured, by chemicals such as formaldehyde.

Therefore, he proposed that the irreversible aging of proteins such as collagen is responsible for the ultimate failure of tissues and organs in old age. This results in the disturbance of normal cell functioning, the cross-linked network impeding intracellular transport or producing changes in the DNA responsible for normal immunological function and protein synthesis in general (Rockstein and Sussman, 1979).

Free radicals are chemical components of the cell which are by-products of normal cell processes resulting from the action of oxygen. They last for very brief periods (a second or less) and are highly reactive chemically with other substances, especially unsaturated fats. The cell membrane envelope is made up in part of such fatty or lipid substances; it can easily be damaged and then become "leaky" if subjected to excessive accumulation of free radicals. Free radicals may also cause mutations of chromosomes and damage the genetic machinery. They are self-propagating and capable of releasing new free radicals while reacting with a molecule. Because naturally occurring antioxidants like vitamins C and E can reduce or inhibit the production of new free radicals, there is popular argument that these vitamins can extend the life span. BHT (butylated hydroxytoluene), a common food preservative, is an antioxidant and free-radical inhibitor. Fed to mice, it has been shown to extend their life span significantly. Further studies are required before such antioxidants can be promoted as having life-prolonging properties for humans (Rockstein and Sussman, 1979).

Alex Comfort says, "A free radical is like a convention delegate away from his wife....a highly reactive chemical agent that will combine with anything that's around and...can have damaging results" (Comfort, 1974).

The Wear and Tear Theory. Proponents of the wear and tear theory maintain that aging is a programmed process, that organisms behave like machines, and that cells are constantly wearing out. The supposition is that the process is aggravated by harmful stress factors and an accumulation of injurious by-products. The processes of aging in the striated skeletal tissues, heart muscles, and all the nerve cells lend support to this theory (Rockstein and Sussman, 1979, p. 42).

Researchers have reported a direct relationship between oxygen uptake and life span in various animals. Increasing the environmental temperature significantly shortens the life span of cold-blooded animals. At lower temperatures, life spans have been lengthened. These experiments seem to support the wear and tear theory; however, they also support all other theories (Shock, 1977).

The Autoimmune Theory. The autoimmune theory states that aging is simply a consequence of autoimmunity. It suggests that as a person ages, his antibodies, which are produced by the body's specialized white blood cells, either become weak and almost useless or else in a bizarre kind of betrayal turn against the very body they were supposed to protect. We know that older people are more prone to secondary infections, that antibodies are often less effective, and that fever is a less reliable indicator of infection in old age.

We also know that the immunological system is composed of several different parts (lymphocytes, immunoglobulins, macrophages, etc.), that its effectiveness depends on the interactions of several different types of cells, and that the system is diffused throughout the body. This is necessary to its role of finding, identifying, and inactivating foreign molecules.

Recent literature reports that the two great arms of the immunological system are the B and T cells. Both originate from stem cells in bone marrow (in vertebrates). After contact with antigens, B cells become plasma cells from which emerge five classes of immunoglobulins. The proteins, because of their ability to react with the antigens, are called antibodies. The role of T cells (lymphocytes) is more complex. Some help B cells in synthesizing antibodies; some suppress antibody synthesis; some are directly involved in cellular responses (in contrast to antibody responses), that is, cell-mediated versus antibody-mediated immunity. Cell-mediated immunity apparently involves more physiological responses, whereas antibody-mediated immunity is involved in protection.

The crux of the matter is that there are changes in T and B cells with age. What these changes signify is uncertain, but there is speculation that as the cell activity declines, the immunological changes are double edged: not only resulting in a decline in the body's defenses but also increasing the likelihood that parts of the immunological system, in a bizarre way, may attack the body itself and cause autoimmune diseases (Rockstein and Sussman, 1979; Shock, 1977; U.S. Department of Health, Education and Welfare, 1978).

Takashi Makinodan, an eminent biologist who has done a great deal of research in autoimmunity, says, "Autoimmunity is all a lock and key mechanism that has to function smoothly." He injected old mice with white cells from young mice. Their disease resistance shot up, and they survived what should have been lethal doses of bacteria. He speculates about the future when young people may freeze their still-efficient white blood cells and use them later on for old age (Cherry and Cherry, 1974).

Physiological Theories of Aging

Physiological theories are generally linked to the breakdown in performance of a single organ system. Some gerontologists believe that the hypothalamus, a small part of the brain which acts as an overseer of all the body's endocrine glands, may trigger many of the changes of old age. After menopause, for example, a woman's tissues lose their youthful shape and resiliency, but the ovaries themselves may not be entirely at fault. If a barely functioning ovary from an old female rat is transplanted to a young one, it will resume manufacturing hormones and the fertilized eggs can produce healthy offspring. In rats, at least, the culprit seems to be the hypothalamus, which alters the signals it first began sending the ovaries at puberty (Cherry and Cherry, 1974). In the past, the thyroid, pituitary, and sex glands have been implicated but at this time research does not substantiate their specific incrimination.

Physiological Controls. It is becoming apparent that the overall performance of an animal is closely related to the effectiveness of a variety of control mechanisms which regulate the interplay of different organs and tissues. For example, many metabolic processes are regulated by the endocrine control system and nervous control mechanisms. Some researchers believe that theories relating to these control mechanisms offer promise for the future because they take into consideration the interrelationships between cells, tissues, and organs (Shock, 1977).

Stress Theory. The stress theory of aging holds that aging is the result of the accumulation over time of the effects of the stresses of living. The basic assumption of this theory, namely that there is residual damage which persists and accumulates, is not supported by experimental data (Shock, 1977).

Environmental Temperature. A number of studies covering quite a span of years have proved that lowered temperature has a marked influence on the life span of animals. Reducing temperature by 14°F has doubled the life of fruit flies. The main obstacle in applying this research to humans is that human body temperature is regulated by the hypothalamus, which we have not learned to control. Dangerous fever or chills occur when body temperature is changed too radically.

Using tiny amounts of calcium ions (inserted into the hypothalamus), Robert D. Myers of Purdue University has lowered the body temperature of monkeys by 10 to 12°F with no ill effects so far (Cherry and Cherry, 1974). This type of research is in its infancy and results are still in question.

Starvation Theory. There has been classic research on the starvation theory since 1952. When rats are fed half the ration they normally eat, there is a marked increase in life span (Kent, 1978).

It is significant that nutrition and temperature affect different periods of the life span. For example, experiments on rotifers with undernutrition resulted in an expanded period of egg laying. By contrast, increase in environmental temperature shortened the life span, and all reduction concentrated on the *postmenopausal* period (Shock, 1968).

The starvation theory is important because we have a great deal of evidence that obesity and overeating shorten the life span. It is also known that as we age, we require less calories. Therefore, the middle-aged years are a time when we should cut down calories and keep up physical activity. This has proved very difficult in our present culture in affluent America. Moreover the deciding factor is that we are dealing with something that requires behavioral change and man does not change his behaviors very easily!

The Eternal Search

The search for the fountain of youth has persisted through the ages and has been documented in ancient history and in the Bible, as indicated by the quote at the beginning of this chapter. The quest for a means to turning back the time clock of age is evidenced today by the number of dollars spent on potions, medications, foods, and treatments, such as face-lifts and wrinkle removers, to ward off or reverse the aging process. If a truly effective formula were found, not only would the discoverer become wealthy overnight, but it would change the world population pyramid drastically and result in some frightening consequences. The main goal of research, however, is not necessarily to prolong life (the life span has changed very little, but life expectancy has changed a great deal since 1900) but to improve the quality of life in old age (Bylinsky, 1976; Comfort, 1974).

An example of current efforts is research with the drug Gerovital H3 which originated in Romania with Dr. Anna Aslan. Gerovital is a procaine derivative, a monoamine oxidase (MAO) inhibitor which has been reported to curb depression, increase mental vigor and alertness, lower blood pressure, and improve the appearance of aged skin. This drug is not yet available in the United States except for clinical trials. Research findings are still controversial (Jones, 1978).

PSYCHOLOGICAL THEORIES OF AGING

Research on the psychological theories of aging covers a broad spectrum of behavioral and developmental changes in personality development and adaptation, cognitive functioning, motivation, and sensory and perceptual areas. There is an overlapping or interrelatedness with biological and sociological theories. Baltes and Willis (1977) state, "All existing theories (psychological) are of the proto-theoretical kind and are incomplete or insufficient in precision, scope, and deployability."

There is a move toward the development of a psychosocial theory of change in adulthood and old age, and of the processes of change across the adult life course. The shortcomings have been a lack of conceptualization about the points of articulation between the individual and his society (Lowenthal, 1977).

Psychological research findings about aging are especially pertinent to nursing. Information about developmental tasks, personality development, and role changes can improve nursing assessment skills and enhance intervention and care (see Chapter 5).

Intelligence

Does intelligence decline with age? The results of intelligence tests have frequently been contradictory. Scores on most intelligence tests in the past have indicated a decline with age, while others have shown that intelligence stays the same or increases. Most researchers in the field, when asked this question, say no with qualifications, such as the consideration of generation differences. There seems to be a consensus that differences are more quantitative than qualitative (Botwinick, 1977; Elias, Elias, and Elias, 1977).

Memory and Learning

There are literally volumes of research on memory and learning. They are important in the study of gerontology and essential to nursing care, health education, and health maintenance. The two mechanisms are so interrelated that it is impossible to study one without considering the other. Research findings indicate that old people are able to learn as well as the young, but it takes longer. The factors involved are stress and environmental forces, neuronal influences, and physiological insults.

Memory loss and loss of cognitive function are perhaps the greatest fears of the aging person and constitute the greatest problem in health care of the frail elderly. Nurses will be able to give better care and manage problems better if they understand what is happening to the memory process. The locus of most memory problems of the aged is in short term memory and involves the processes of acquisition, retention, and retrieval. The difference between short term and long term memory is not the difference between yesterday and many years ago. Short term memory is much more immediate. It is the memory process we use in all daily activities — the sorting out, registering, and holding of information for use from moment to moment. It is being able to read a telephone number, register it in the memory just long enough to get to the telephone, and then retrieve it for immediate use. This has special relevance to nursing because we give many directions to patients, and often ask and answer questions rather hurriedly, when in fact, slower, deliberate, and repeated reinforcement may be necessary (Elias and Elias, 1977, pp. 357-383; Wolf, 1971).

Motivation

Motivation is part of the choice-making mechanism that helps us decide among a number of alternatives. We are continually working to maintain that balance (homeostasis) within our total life sphere which sustains our present status and moves us toward what we want to become (Kennedy, 1978).

Research on human motivation has demonstrated that while older persons may show more caution in a laboratory setting, they are not necessarily less motivated than younger people (Elias and Elias, 1977). There is some evidence that the need to achieve is slightly weaker in older people but that age differences are not great (Chown, 1977).

Sensory and perceptual changes and cognitive function, which are discussed quite extensively elsewhere in this book, will not be covered here.

SOCIOLOGICAL THEORIES OF AGING

Sociological theories of aging have tended to focus on roles, relationships, and social adaptations in later life. Again, the interrelatedness with biological and psychological theories and concepts cannot be ignored. Knowledge and understanding of these theories are reflected in professional attitudes toward the elderly and in the quality of human services for the elderly.

The Disengagement Theory

The disengagement theory has provoked a flurry of controversy, criticism, and counterresearch for several decades.

The disengagement theory was first formulated by Elaine Cumming and William Henry. It maintains that both society and the individual prepare for the ultimate "disengagement" of death by an inevitable, gradual, and mutually satisfying process of withdrawal from each other. Society wants to disengage its older members so it can avoid the disruption that their deaths would cause if they died while fully engaged in a variety of social roles. Therefore, society institutionalizes retirement and reduces the number of options available to older people. In their turn, older people are most successful if they can accommodate themselves to this process, and gradually relinquish one social role for another. As this process goes on, the older person is released from the constraints of social norms, becomes more centered on himself, and is freer to review and integrate his life in preparation for death. Thus, disengagement theory views old age as a developmental stage in itself, with its own norms and appropriate patterns of behavior; it is not a continuation of middle age. According to disengagement theory, aging is a process which transforms the individual from a middle aged person centered on society to an elderly person centered on himself. (Manney, 1975)

The value judgment embraced in the disengagement theory is that it is better to achieve a state of psychological and social equilibrium than to fight forces that hem in the social world of old age. Freedom and happiness are said to be the acceptance of old age as an integral state of life. These presumptions put the disengagement theory at odds with the activity theory, and challenge the work ethic and certain other widely held American values. Most younger people cannot respond positively to this theory on an emotional level. Those who are deeply engaged tend to feel that involvement and activity are the very fuel of life. They find it hard to accept the possibility that withdrawal and passive self-centeredness may someday actually be attractive.

It is important to distinguish between disengagement as a description of a social-psychological process and disengagement as a theory of successful aging. Most gerontologists seem to believe that "disengagement" appears to be an accurate term to describe what actually happens as people grow older. With age, people reduce their social and psychological engagement with others. There is little doubt that society does in fact disengage from the older person, but disengagement seems to be a deficient explanation for the full complex reality of personal adjustment to aging. Some older people are happy when they are active; some are happy when they are "disengaged."

Disengagement is by no means inevitable. Society appears to be becoming less insistent that older people move to the social sidelines, and older people now have more resources, more opportunities, and a greater inclination to sustain a high level of activity for a longer period of time (Back, 1977; Butler and Lewis, 1977; Maddox and Wiley, 1977; Manney, 1975).

The Activity Theory

The activity theory contends that older people have the same social and psychological needs as middle-aged people and that the person who ages successfully resists the circumstances of aging and fights to stay young. It holds that the older person should maintain the interests and activities of middle age as long as possible. When he retires, he finds new productive activities. When his friends and spouse die, he finds new friends, perhaps younger ones. When illness and frailty limit his physical activity, he substitutes intellectual pursuits. According to the activity theory, aging is a continuous struggle to remain middle aged.

The activity theory presumes that it is better to be active than inactive, that it is better to be happy than unhappy, and that the aging individual, rather than the observer, is the best judge of his success. In all these presumptions, this theory is congenial with modern American values. That is, most older people try to maintain their usual level of activity as long as they can, and it seems that older Americans prefer to think of themselves as middle aged rather than old and would like others to do so as well (Atchley, 1980, 1983).

Both the disengagement theory and the activity theory are based more upon value perspectives than empirical data. The evidence supporting the activity theory as a general theory of aging is mixed. "As men and women move beyond age 70. . .they regret the drop in role activity that occurs in their lives. At the same time, most older persons accept this drop as an inevitable accomplishment of growing old; and they succeed in maintaining a sense of self-worth and a sense of satisfaction with past and present life as a whole. Others are less successful in resolving these conflicting elements . . . .not only do they have strong negative affect regarding losses in activity, but the present losses weigh heavily and are accompanied by dissatisfaction with past and present life" (Havighurst, Neugarten, and Tobin, 1968).

Older People as a Subculture

The view of the elderly as a subculture holds that society's negative response to older people forces them to interact with each other across class and other social barriers. It views older people as a subculture, much as urban adolescents, drug addicts, college students, street people, and other groups can be viewed as subcultures. This theory is more a prediction

of a possible social trend than a description of what is actually happening among the elderly.

Older People as a Minority Group

Another theory holds that older people, by showing a visible biological trait which society dislikes, undergo discrimination as racial minorities do and that they constitute a minority group in their own right. Minority group status for the elderly has been discredited on definitional grounds and because of evidence indicating that they are less disadvantaged than was once assumed. Membership in the aged group is not exclusive or permanent: anyone who lives long enough will become a part of this group. Neither is physical appearance exclusively negative: the appearance of certain old people such as judges is revered. The concept of the elderly as a minority is not a useful framework for describing their status in society. The idea lacks conceptual clarity and is not supported by empirical facts and research (Manney, 1975; Streib, 1968; Yurick, Robb, Spier, and Ebert, 1980).

The Interactionist Theory

The interactionist theory has not been widely publicized or researched, but it is of interest. "Interactionists believe that the individual changes role or career involvements in the later years, disposing of major ones and taking on new ones of his choosing. Whether he assumes new careers or not, the significance of his middle year 'career set' remains. He remains engaged with society, in which he may or may not experience isolation, alienation, acceptance or joy" (Yurick et al., 1980).

The Continuity or Developmental Theory

The most acceptable theory at this time seems to be the continuity or developmental theory, which attempts to explain something that anyone with a reasonably broad acquaintance with older people probably suspects: neither activity nor inactivity necessarily brings happiness. Engaged or disengaged older people can be either happy or unhappy, depending upon forces more mysterious, or at least less evident, than the simple level of activity in their lives. This impressionistic suspicion has been documented in most personality studies. Their overall conclusion is that active and involved older people are more likely to be satisfied with their lives than disengaged individuals. However, disengaged old people can be happy too, and both active and inactive people can be miserable (Manney, 1975).

The developmental theory holds simply that as a person ages, he tries to maintain continuity of his habits, commitments, preferences, and all factors that have contributed to his personality. This theory is favored because it takes into consideration situational factors that may necessitate adjustment and variable styles of adaptation to aging. It evaluates factors within the individual's history that might determine adaptive patterns. Generally, when older people fail to remain engaged with their social environment, the source of the failure lies in the social environment not in their age. Such factors as work status, health, financial resources, and marital status affect the older person's capacity to lead a satisfying life much more strongly than age does (Atchley, 1980; Manney, 1975; Yurick et al., 1980).

In summary, the continuity theory holds that old age, to be properly understood, should be viewed as an integral part of the life cycle, not as a terminal period apart from earlier life. As such, the individual old person's life-style and personality will be reflected in old age, as in younger years.

The continuity theory has several important implications for gerontological nursing practice, education, and research. In terms of practice, it emphasizes the importance of planning for the aged in diversified and individualized ways, and of consulting the older person in the planning. Nurses must reject stereotyping the elderly and basing needs assessments on that stereotype (Vander Zyl, 1979).

To date, the theoretical bases of social gerontology are not all they should or could be, but the growth of explanatory models witnessed in the last decade has definitely laid the groundwork for significant advances. No theory can ever be completely rejected, only disregarded in

favor of those that offer a greater utility in the real world of the elderly (Hendricks and Hendricks, 1979). Linda George uses a social stress model to provide a useful framework to look at and study role transitions in old age (George, 1980).

REFERENCES

Atchley, R.D. *Aging: Continuity and Change.* Belmont, Calif.: Wadsworth, 1983, pp. 77-80, 249-269.

Atchley, R.C. *The Social Forces in Later Life* (3rd ed.). Belmont, Calif.: Wadsworth, 1980.

Back, K.W. Personal characteristics and social behavior, theory and method. In Binstock, R.H. and Shanas, E. (Eds.) *Handbook of Aging and the Social Sciences.* New York: Van Nostrand Reinhold, 1977, pp. 411-412.

Baltes, P. and Willis, S.L. Toward psychological theories of aging and development. In Birren, J.E. and Schaie, W. (Eds.) *Handbook of the Psychology of Aging.* New York: Van Nostrand Reinhold, 1977, pp. 128-154.

Birren, J.E. and Renner, V.J. Research on the psychology of aging: principles and experimentation. In Birren, J.E. and Schaie, W. (Eds.) *Handbook of the Psychology of Aging.* New York: Van Nostrand Reinhold, 1977, p. 4.

Botwinick, J. Intellectual abilities. In Birren, J.E. and Schaie, W. (Eds.) *Handbook of the Psychology of Aging.* New York: Van Nostrand Reinhold, 1977.

Butler, R.N. and Lewis, M. *Aging and Mental Health.* St. Louis: C.V. Mosby, 1977, pp. 26-27.

Bylinsky, G. Science is on the trail of the fountain of youth. *Fortune* pp. 134-140 (July 1976).

Cherry, R. and Cherry, L. Uncovering the secrets of a longer life. *New York Times* (May 12, 1974).

Chown, S.M. Morale, careers, and personal potentials. In Birren, J.E. and Schaie, W. (Eds.) *Handbook of the Psychology of Aging.* New York: Van Nostrand Reinhold, 1977, pp. 675-676.

Comfort, A. Biological theories of aging. *Human Development* 13: 127-139 (1970).

Comfort, A. *We Know the Aging Process Can Be Slowed Down.* Santa Barbara, Calif.: Center for the Study of Democratic Institutions, 1974.

Cowdry, E.V. *Problems of Aging.* Baltimore: Williams and Wilkins, 1942, p. xvi.

Elias, M.F. and Elias, P.K. Motivation and activity. In Birren, J.E. and Schaie, W. (Eds.) *Handbook of the Psychology of Aging.* New York: Van Nostrand Reinhold, 1977, pp. 359-382.

Elias, M.F., Elias, P.K., and Elias, J.W. *Basic Processes in Developmental Psychology.* St. Louis: C.V. Mosby, 1977, pp. 48-199.

George, Linda K. *Role Transitions in Later Life.* Monterey, Calif: Brooks/Cole Publishing Co., 1980, pp. 127-137.

Granick, S. and Patterson, R.D. *Human Aging II, An Eleven-year Follow Biomedical and Behavioral Study*. National Institute of Mental Health, Rockville, Md. 1971, pp. 1-136.

Handler, P. Radiation and aging. In Shock, N.W. (Ed.) *Aging*. Washington, D.C.: American Association for the Advancement of Science, 1960, p. 200.

Havighurst, R.J., Neugarten, B.L., and Tobin, S.S. *Disengagement and Patterns of Aging*. Chicago: University of Chicago Press, 1968, p. 6.

Hayflick, L. Longer vigorous life span is gerontologists' goal. Paper presented at Western Gerontological Society Meeting. Tucson, Az. March 25, 1974.

Hayflick, L. The longevity of cultured human cells. *Journal of the American Geriatrics Society* 22(1): 1-12 (January 1974).

Hayflick, L. The cellular basis for biological aging. In Finch, C. E. and Hayflick, L. (Eds.) *Handbook of the Biology of Aging*. New York: Van Nostrand Reinhold, 1977, pp. 159-179.

Hendricks, J. and Hendricks, C.D. *Dimensions of Aging: Readings*. Cambridge, Mass.: Winthrop, 1979, p. 205.

Jones, L. Review of literature on Gerovital. Unpublished paper, College of Nursing, Arizona State University, 1978.

Kennedy, C.E. *Human development: The Adult Years and Aging*. New York: MacMillan, 1978, pp. 40-41.

Kent, S. Can dietary manipulation prolong life? *Geriatrics* 33(4): 102-108 (1978).

Kimmel, D.C. *Adulthood and Aging*. New York: Wiley, 1980, pp. 357-365.

Lowenthal, M.F. Toward a sociopsychological theory of change in adulthood and old age. In Birren, J.E. and Schaie, W. (Eds.) *Handbook of the Psychology of Aging*. New York: Van Nostrand Reinhold, 1977.

Maddox, G.L. and Wiley, J. Scope, concepts, and methods in the study of aging. In Binstock, R.H. and Shanas, E. (Eds.) *Handbook of Aging and the Social Sciences*. New York: Van Nostrand Reinhold, 1977, p. 6.

Makinodan, T. Immunity and aging. In Finch, C.E. and Hayflick, L. (Eds.) *Handbook of the Biology of Aging*. New York: Van Nostrand Reinhold, 1977, pp. 379-402.

Manney, J.D., Jr. *Aging in American Society*. Detroit: The University of Michigan–Wayne State University Institute of Gerontology, 1975, pp. 15-21.

Old Testament, King James Version. 1 Kings 1:1-4.

Palmore, E. (Ed.). *Normal Aging: Reports from the Duke Longitudinal Study 1955-1969*. Durham, N.C.: Duke University Press, 1970.

Rockstein, M., Chesky, J., and Sussman, M. Comparative Biology and Evaluation of Aging. *Handbook of the Biology of Aging*. New York: Van Nostrand Reinhold, 1977, pp. 3-31.

Rockstein, M. and Sussman, M. *Biology of Aging*. Belmont, Calif.: Wadsworth, 1979, pp. 3-45.

Samis, H.V. The loss of temporal organization. *Perspectives in Biology and Medicine* 12: 95-105 (1968).

Shock N. Biologic concepts of aging. In Simon, A. and Epstein, L. (Eds.) *Aging in Modern Society*. Washington, D.C.: American Psychiatric Association, 1968, pp. 18-19.

Shock, N. Systems integration. In Finch, C.E. and Hayflick, L. (Eds.) *Handbook of the Biology of Aging*. New York: Van Nostrand Reinhold, 1977, pp. 639-665.

Sinex, F.M. The molecular genetics of aging. In Finch, C.E. and Hayflick, L. (Eds.) *Handbook of the Biology of Aging*. New York: Van Nostrand Reinhold, 1977, pp. 37-62.

Streib, G. Are the Aged a Minority Group? In Middle Age and Aging, Edited by B. Neugarten, Chicago University of Chicago Press 1968, pp. 35-46.

U.S. Department of Health, Education and Welfare. *Changes – Research on Aging and the Aged* (DHEW Publication No. NIH-78-85). Washington, D.C.: U.S. Government Printing Office, 1978, pp. 13-14.

Vander Zyl, S. Psychosocial theories of aging. *Journal of Gerontological Nursing* 5(3): 47 (1979).

Wolf, V.C. Some implications of short-term, long-term memory theory. *Nursing Forum* 10(2): 151-165 (1971).

Yurick, A.G., Robb, S.S., Spier, B.E., and Ebert, N.J. *The Aged Person and the Nursing Process*. New York: Appleton-Century-Crofts, 1980, pp. 56-64.

Part II
Psychological Aspects of
Gerontological Nursing

5
Basic Human Needs and Developmental Tasks of Aging

WHAT IT MEANS TO BE OLD

It means stepping down and stepping aside.
It means more time alone.
It means neglect.
It means a back seat.
It means less money.
It means giving up many things.
It means loss.
It means accepting help from others.
It means the threat of illness or disability.
It means being frightened.
It means accepting past failures and realizing that much of the record of one's life is in.
It means trying to figure out what one's life has meant.
It means figuring out what you want to get done before you die.
It means facing death.

Anonymous

Gerontologists have tended to approach research and the study of gerontology from three main perspectives — biological, psychological, and sociological. These aspects cannot be completely separated, nor can it be assumed that one is more important than the other. However, for empirical reasons, it is necessary to separate the concepts of each and then put together pieces of information which can provide a theoretical framework for nursing practice, such as the psychosocial aspects of aging defined and described in this part of the book. This and the following two chapters attempts to describe the feelings and behaviors of older individuals which lead into, and directly relate the areas of mental health and geropsychiatry discussed in Part III.

A person's feelings, actions, and attitudes will determine his health needs, his health care of himself, and his well-being. The ability of

the nurse to recognize, understand, and deal with feelings and behaviors will determine the quality and efficacy of the nursing assessment and intervention. Caring is so tied to feelings and behaviors that it is tempting to say that these are more important than physiological aspects and if we really pay attention to behaviors and feelings, the other kind of nursing care (such as intrusive procedures) will be easier for the nurse as well as for the patient. We may even go so far as to say that for a patient of any age, the feelings and behaviors will decide whether a special diet, medical regime, or intrusive procedure works. We take great pains to provide student nurses with the special knowledge and skills required to work with the feelings and behaviors of children and pregnant women. There is also special knowledge (developmental acquired) about the feelings and behaviors of older individuals that is essential for truly therapeutic, quality care.

The task then is to develop a workable theoretical framework for identifying and assessing the feelings and behaviors of older persons. This chapter does so by describing two major concepts: (1) the basic human needs and (2) the developmental tasks of aging.

BASIC HUMAN NEEDS

Most psychological theories of basic human needs use a hierarchical framework such as Maslow's hierarchy of basic human needs (see Figure 5-1). A fundamental premise is that the way in which these basic human needs are met, beginning with the physiological needs, will influence and affect emotional growth and maturity. For example, one is not apt to feel security, love, and trust if he has always had to

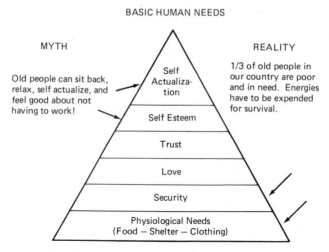

Figure 5-1. Basic human needs (adopted from Maslow, 1948). This figure implies that the needs at each level must be met in satisfactory succession to reach self-actualization; it points out that, unfortunately, old people expend tremendous energy just managing their physiological needs when, indeed, they are expected to be self-actualizing or satisfied with themselves, their lifestyle, and their environment.

The behavior and personality characteristics of all of us have been influenced by the way our basic human needs are met. What we as "helping people" do and say depends on our basic human needs and how they were met in our personality development. The way in which patients respond to nurses and the actions they take depend on their basic human needs. In order to understand these needs and help people to help themselves, we need to recognize this so that we can perhaps fill some losses and gaps, and provide a much needed lifeline.

Basically, we all want to be effective "helping people" and can do a lot intuitively; however, since we are committed professionals, we need to understand the process and prepare to do this by design when intuition is not there. Helping by plan and design enables us to offer the best possible care more consistently than if we depend on intuition alone.

battle for, and worry about, food, clothing, and shelter. Basic human needs persist throughout life. It takes psychic energy as well as physical energy to meet these needs, and different age groups expend different amounts of energy at different levels of the hierarchy. For example, a 2 year old does not worry about his clothing and appearance, whereas teenagers may expend a tremendous amount of energy on how their hair looks or how their jeans fit, as well as in belonging. Where do old people expend their energy? Are they self-actualizing with a healthy degree of self-esteem?

There are a great many misconceptions about where older people are expending their energies. All too often we may expect old people to be self-actualizing when, in fact, their self-esteem is being shattered and they are devoting all their energy to worrying about the first rung on the ladder, that is, how to keep body and soul together. If we can assess the older persons' needs in these terms, we might be more realistic in our expectations of them and better able to help.

Maslow, though he postulates a need for self-actualization, has pointed out in his writings that this is rarely totally experienced. In other words, most of us will not be completely satisfied with what we have done with our lives (Maslow, 1948, 1968). The following are some obvious implication of Maslow's work. First, physical needs almost always have priority over all other needs; that is, the person in pain cannot participate in activities to bring him recognition and companionship. Second, attention must be given to security needs; it is very important not to downgrade the patient's fears — he needs allowance to express them openly and should be helped to examine them objectively. Third, every attempt should be made to acquaint the patient with the structure of his environment, i.e., "the rules of the game" (Hulicka, 1972).

There is a considerable amount of research being done at this time on specific physiological changes in the aging process and old age with regard to hunger, thirst, sex, and sleep. These findings will, of course, have application to the concepts discussed here (Butler, 1982; Elias, Elias, and Elias, 1977).

Another framework for assessing basic human needs which can serve as a guideline for working with the elderly is the beautiful description by Erich Fromm (1955) of the following universal needs:

Identity	I need to be me.
Rootedness	Everyone needs a place in time and space. Rerooting is difficult and high risk for older people.
Relatedness	Our society depends on a relatedness to somebody or something.
Transcendence	Man is the only animal that has awareness of his own finiteness and speculates about it, about his passing on. He has a need to leave something behind.
A frame of reference	Man needs a set of beliefs to fall back on, whether religious or nonreligious. There are great changes in society — times of crisis when old truths don't hold anymore and a frame of reference is needed. These crises are very hard on old people.

Sister Michael Sibille (1976), who has had extensive experience in working with the psychosocial needs of the elderly, says old people have:

The need for love and understanding
The need to feel useful
The need for recognition
The need for social involvement

Maintaining Identity

Wolanin (1981) describes four basic elements in maintaining self-identity which are profound in their implication for nursing:

Family	Self-identity begins and ends with the family. It comes slowly. It is a lifetime process, but we can lose it in a minute! When the infirm body cannot be restored, humans still strive for identity. For the very old, family is often gone, but there is still a "ghost" family in memory. Professionals should tap in on this; see Figure 5-2.
Name	Our name has great meaning. We should help keep that identity for old people, perhaps even maintaining more formality than is customary. Names and nicknames with family and lovers are important and should be respected, but loving names used out of context are contemptuous.
Body	It is our inescapable identity. It changes in length and size and appearance, but we are "stuck" with it. There is no escape for even a minute. Nurses' assessment and feedback about the body are crucial to help preserve, maintain, and cope with destruction or deterioration of body image. Wolanin also describes the difficulty in accepting and coping when the body begins to give misinformation, i.e. information that does not fit with our body image. For example, the pain in the knee that causes a limp is a message that affects our self-image and identity.
Life history	Every person has an individual and different history, and becomes more individualistic with age. We are what we were and have been all our lives. "Life history is left behind or outside when we go into a nursing home. We are who we were, but family and friends who knew us as we

were are no longer there or all those who knew us as we were are buried. Then they see us only as we are — sick and old" (Wolanin, 1981).

The following is a poignant vignette from the nursing experience of Mary Opal Wolanin (1980) which describes basic human needs without further interpretation:

Mrs. Doe had not been at the center for a while. The nurse knew why and went to visit her in her home. Mrs. Doe's husband had died recently after a long illness. She had taken very good care of him. When the nurse arrived, she noticed that Mrs. Doe was wearing one of her deceased husband's old and threadbare shirts. After a few minutes as they spoke of her husband's death, Mrs. Doe gestured toward the shirt. The nurse nodded and said, "And, yes, you're wearing his shirt because it reminds you of him and feels like his arms around you." Mrs. Doe, after an emotional pause, said in a confident tone, "Yesss—and—these too...." Without further words, she lifted up the shirt to reveal she was also wearing an old pair of men's valentine shorts covered with red hearts.

Restoring Identify

My concern has been with the older person as a thinking, feeling person with all the needs common to mankind, but with drastically limited opportunities for meeting these needs.

Hulicka (1972)

Professionals are often faced with the challenge of restoring identity to socially depersonalized older individuals, particularly those in institutions. How they become depersonalized will be left to the reader's speculation; unfortunately, it is sad but truly documented that professionals also often contribute to or cause depersonalization of the elderly, especially the frail and institutionalized elderly (Butler, 1975; Townsend, 1971).

Three critical social-psychological needs of elderly individuals, described by the sociologist Vern Bengston, are identity, connectedness, and effectance (ICE). Identity is self-explanatory; connectedness is defined in terms of the social situation in which we all live and die; effectance means having some sort of influence on your environment, that is, being able to effect change (Bengston, 1978).

Restoring identity in a long term care setting necessitates dealing with interrelated social needs that form a complex whole which is the self, living and acting in a social context with integrity, individuality, and significance for oneself and others (Gossett, 1966). Table 5-1 describes the needs which should be considered

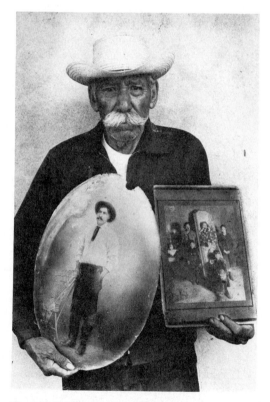

Figure 5-2. This man's heritage is very important to him. At age 85 he holds photographs of his father as a young man and his mother in the coffin. He is the smallest child in the photo of his mother. The revolution in 1914 disrupted his family. He has lived in the United States most of his life, maintaining close ties with his homeland.

Table 5-1. Maintaining and Restoring Identity.

BASIC NEED	IMPLICATIONS FOR INTERVENTION
Continuity of life experience	This is maintaining a thread to the past, a living present, and a future to move toward.
Identity	The most important element of identity is who one is – surname, title (Doctor, Reverend, Mr., Mrs., or Miss). When moving from one town to another or into an institution, one becomes a nonentity and has to make oneself known, sometimes aggressively. This may be very difficult for an old person who is perhaps sick, sensorily deprived, and emotionally tired of reconstructing identity in a receding environment.
Independence	This includes freedom of movement and basic rights guaranteed by the Constitution.
Privacy	In congregate living this is difficult, but professional care givers are often negligent in providing what is possible, e.g., using bed screens, closing doors, and allowing some personal space.
Stability	Everyone needs a nucleus of certainty, an anchorage of security, and things to count on such as a home base.
Meaningful living	Institutional residents, especially, have nothing expected of them – no responsibilities.
Reason for being	There is a need to mean something to someone else.

NOTE: Adapted from Gossett (1966).

in planning for the long term care of older individuals, particularly the frail elderly.

Need for a Confidant or Significant Other

Communication and interaction with other human beings are basic human needs which are as important and vital as food and shelter. Maintaining a "lifeline" of interaction with others becomes harder and harder in old age when family and friends die off. An elderly neighbor once said to me, "Steffie, I'm tired of you telling me to find new friends and new bridge partners – all my good friends are gone. Don't you know that when you get old, your environment recedes from you?"

The research has demonstrated that the frail elderly have higher life satisfaction levels if they have a confidant or "significant other" with whom to communicate. In the very old, when all family and friends are gone, some helping professional such as the nurse or social worker often becomes the significant other and the only confidant (Kimmel, 1980). Though face-to-face personal contact is most desirable, a telephone can be a lifesaver, a reassurance, and the most feasible and satisfying channel to social interaction for some elderly folks.

Space

Personal space, territorial domain, and spatial arrangements are crucial elements in basic human needs. Personal space is carried around with us. It is the space we need to speak, to eat, and to sleep. It is psychological. That is, we set individually determined spatial distances for our conversation and social interactions. The need for personal space is directly related to a sense of well-being and can contribute to stress. Stress tolerance lowers when personal space is compromised (Gioella, 1978; Pastalan, 1970; Trienweiler, 1978).

Nurses do not generally perceive themselves as change agents for manipulating the environment in care settings, but in fact, they may be fostering a deprivation of basic human needs when they insist on such things as "chairs all neat in a row around the dayroom." Institutional depersonalization can be minimized by allowing as many options as possible, and as much personal space and privacy as possible.

These are usually more possible than the care-taker has observed, perceived, or acknowledged.

Pets

Pets play an important role in the social inter-action of many older persons. Indeed, they may be the main source of socializing and the only link to social interaction and visibility in the neighborhood or community. Not infre-quently, an older person's need for someone to talk to, take care of, or touch is met by a pet (see Figure 5-3) sometimes even plants are pets to older people. Pets have many therapeutic roles; some, such as dogs, also serve a protective role (Butler and Lewis, 1977; Corson and O'Leary, 1977). If space permitted, this writer could document pages of stories of older people whose lives revolve around pets. When asked why she liked Cleo the cat, Mrs. D., aged 91, replied, "I like her because she's cuddly. I like to cuddle — I'm a cuddle bug."

Even when many basic human needs are being met, anxiety is common in old age. Irene Burnside speaks of the need for us to recognize and be able to deal with anxiety, loneliness, grief, and depression in the elderly: "Anxiety is common in old age and may be present intermittently or chronically" (Burnside, 1981). Assessing how the basic human needs are being met may help us to identify and alleviate some of this anxiety. All of the basic human needs mentioned have been presented with the intention of serving as a guide for nursing assessment and as a theoretical framework for the development of nursing care plans.

Table 5-2 lists losses which should be con-sidered when assessing basic human needs and the ability to cope with the developmental tasks of old age. Table 5-3 provides specific terms for recording behaviors in order to obtain a meaningful client profile.

The psychosocial aspects of aging which relate to basic human needs have been well described with helpful and practical intervention strategies by Burnside (1980, 1981); Carnevali and Patrick (1979); Murray, Huelskoetter, and O'Driscoll (1980); Yurick, Robb, Spier, and Ebert (1980); and many others. *Aging and Mental Health* by Butler and Lewis (1982) has very positive approaches to the psychosocial aspects of caring for the aged; it — along with *Psychosocial Care of the Aged* by Burnside (1980) — is highly recommended as a multidisciplinary text on this topic.

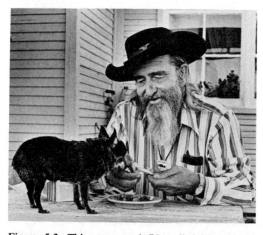

Figure 5-3. This man, aged 75, called himself the "Arizona Kid." He was a severe cardiac case yet man-aged to walk several blocks every day to a "Kentucky Fried" to get a piece of chicken which he skinned and fed to his toothless, blind, aged dog. His pet was 15 years old and completely dependent on him. They helped each other survive to a ripe old age. (Photo by Jeff Stanton.)

DEVELOPMENTAL TASKS OF AGING

A developmental task is a task which arises at or about certain periods in the life of an individual, successful achievement of which leads to happiness, good adjustment to society and self and to success with later tasks. On the other hand, failure leads to unhappiness, maladjustment, disapproval by society and difficulty with later develop-mental problems.

Barrett (1972)

The knowledge and skill to deal with crises in the later stages of life are necessary if nurses intend to aid patients and families in the attainment of developmental tasks. The follow-ing pages contain a brief historical summary of theories about developmental tasks of aging which have direct application to the advocacy, assessment, and intervention roles of nursing.

Table 5-2. Losses Accompanying Progressive Aging.

I. Biological Losses
   Global function
   Health
   Vigor, strength, power
   Motility, mobility
   Organ system
   Perceptual apparatus: sensory decrements
   Nervous system
   Organs surgically removed
   Control of one's destiny — dependency and independence

II. Psychological Losses Linked to Biology
   Short-term memory, immediate recall ability
   Motor skills linked with reaction time
   Virility, libido
   "Looks," body image

III. Psychological Losses Centering on Esteem (these focus on the need for self-respect and other's respect, and anxiety about being neglected, forgotten, needed, by-passed, retired out of usefulness)
   Self-esteem
   Regard of others
   Influence, power
   Prestige positions, status, role confusion, rites of passage

IV. Personal Losses (these focus on a need for affection from those who care out of love, duty, respect)
   Parents
   Spouse
   Children
   Siblings
   Extended family
   Friends ("I see strange faces now")

V. Social Losses (these focus on the need for recognition and approval)
   Friends
   The circle, group (evening card game group)
   Memberships
   Leader, advice giver in community

VI. Losses of Identity (these focus on the need for security, stability)
   Job, position
   Productivity
   Familiar place, home
   Familiar place of employment
   Familiar surroundings: faces, places, landmarks
   Familiar routines
   Territorial loss or change

VII. Philosophical Losses (these focus on the need to have one's life count for something, add up, make some kind of sense)
   Purpose in living
   Joy of living
   Will to live

VIII. Religious Losses (these focus on the need to believe that one's life has meaning, purpose, and a future since religion deals with one's total orientation to life and death; the quality of relationships one develops with others and with God is of primary importance)
   I-thou vs I-it relationship
   Physically unable to attend church
   Architecture of church or environment makes it impossible to attend church
   Lack of transportation
   Financially unable to attend church
   Attends alone: spouse ill or dead
   Change of worship, scripture, language
   Absence of pastor decreases symbolic presence and power of God
   Composition of church membership changes
   Church — like society — builds programs around couples, families (singles?)
   Belief that one is religious when attending church and less religious when one stays away: "Will God love me less now?"

NOTE: Reprinted with permission from Donald Sanner, Chaplain, Bethany Home, Fargo, N.D., 1980.

Table 5-3. Specific Feelings and Behaviors to Record in Psychosocial Assessment of the Elderly.

BEHAVIORAL DISABILITIES TO LOOK FOR AND RECORD	POSITIVE BEHAVIORS TO LOOK FOR AND RECORD
Forgetful	Communicates easily
Communicates with difficulty	Seems satisfied with self
Periods of agitation	Finds things to keep busy
Periods of depression	Wants to do for others
Wanders off	Likes to reminisce about good things of the past
Nuisance to neighbors	Talks about self and family
Drinking problem (social setting upset)	Curious — wants to know what is going on
Panics readily	Sometimes critical of younger generation
Loses personal belongings (money, glasses)	Well groomed
Fire and burn hazard	Has a routine
Severe and specific fears	Enjoys eating
Hallucinations and delusions	Makes plans for the future
Spends time in bed	Creative
Signs of deterioration in personal habits:	Strives to maintain leadership/responsibility
1. Incontinence of bladder	Interested, active — a doer
2. Incontinence of bowels	Friendly — outgoing
3. Perspiration odor	Smiles a lot
4. Clothing soiled	Jokes with workers
5. Hair uncombed	Responds to friendly approach
6. Fingernails long and dirty	Shares freely
Short tempered and irritable	Reads the paper
Withdrawn from surroundings — passive	Interested in mail
Dependent — repeatedly asks for help	Writes letters and cards
Submissive — excessive capitulation to suggestion	Sometimes sings and/or whistles
Hostile, challenging	Good appetite — enjoys eating
Nervous, tense, "jumpy," anxious	Reaches out for touch and has warm personal touch
Ashamed of, and tries to hide, disability	Concerned about governmental affairs
Indecisive, uncertain, hesitant	Copes with limitations
Demanding — constantly seeks attention	
Overly affectionate	
Domineering, dogmatic	
Nagging dissenter; objects, complains	
Unrealistic, immature	
Lonely	
Negative, rejecting	
Suspicious, distrustful of others	

NOTE: A goal that students can be assigned is to add to the list of positive behaviors seen.

One of the first researchers to gather data on developmental tasks was the Viennese psychologist Charlotte Buhler. She contended that mental abilities such as intelligence do not decline as rapidly as physical capacities and that old age may be a time for continued goal development and concerns about self-fulfillment. Her work included interviews with old people which showed that fulfillment in old age often involved the following four major considerations: (1) the aspect of luck, (2) feelings about the realization of one's potentialities, (3) the aspect

of accomplishment, and (4) moral evaluation (Weiner, Brok, and Snadowsky, 1978).

Psychiatrist C. G. Jung postulated changes in the process of psychic organization of the self. He believed that changes in late life involved a tendency for the personality to change in the direction of the opposite sex. Cross-cultural research concerned with age changes seems to uphold Jung's early notions. Jung considered the natural end in life to be wisdom not senility, but he believed that this wisdom could only be achieved by not competing with youth. He deplored pseudo-youthful images. He suggested that as individuals age, they go through a continual process of interiorization, that is, that life contracts, but with an inner exploration that adds meaning to life (Weiner et al. 1978).

Erik Erikson's work on developmental tasks is classical, and he states so much when he says that the developmental task of old age is "maintaining integrity versus despair — to be through having been and to face not being" (Erikson, 1963). Because his descriptive work on later life was rather global, Robert Peck attempted to further delineate and specify issues crucial to old age by expanding on Erikson's theory. His additions included four issues in the middle-age stage of life and three in old age. The three in old age (Peck, 1956) are:

Ego differentiation versus role preoccupation	Stresses establishment of a variety of valued activities and new roles to modify loss of occupation and parental role.
Body transcendence	Stresses ability to focus on comforts, enjoyments, and mental tasks while de-emphasizing body aches and pains and losses.
Ego transcendence versus ego preoccupation	Stresses living usefully and placing more value on what has been accomplished and what will be left behind for children or society, rather than concentrating on personal death.

Robert Butler describes the main tasks for the aged person as (1) learning to live with his infirmities, (2) coming to some kind of peace or satisfaction with himself in terms of what he has done with his life, and (3) preparing for his demise (Butler and Lewis, 1982).

If one looks at developmental tasks in a continuum from early age to old age and assesses for progressive growth versus progressive loss, it soon becomes apparent that the tasks of old age add up to many losses and few gains. It also becomes apparent that we expect a great deal of "coping" despite multiple losses and diminishing resources, and that old age is not for sissies (see Table 5-4).

Another meaningful and relevant way to assess developmental tasks has been described by Barrett (1972); see Table 5-5. He differentiates between regressive and compensatory tasks. Regressive tasks have been studied in relation to disengagement theories. Compensatory tasks have not been well defined or researched.

Table 5-4. Old Age Is Not for Sissies ("Aging Gracefully" Takes a Great Deal of Strength in a Time of Diminishing Resources).

AGE	PHYSIOLOGICAL	PSYCHOLOGICAL	SOCIOLOGICAL
2	Needs about 12 hrs sleep Sphincter control developing Weight gain is steady Molars coming in (Gains)	Ceaseless activity Easily frustrated Learns power of "no" Learning new words (Gains)	Likes company Uncooperative Claims friends, toys Learning games (Gains
68–70	Gray hair Loss of muscle strength Loss of teeth Decrease in endocrine function Thinning of vertebral disks (Loss)	Sensory losses: Hearing-vision Taste-smell Depression Loneliness (Loss)	Loss of productive roles Loss of income Loss of mobility Loss of loved ones Decreased social activity (Loss)

NOTE: The developmental tasks of aging clearly spell "loss" in all biopsychosocial aspects. We tend to expect older individuals to cope with and accept these overwhelming changes as their due expectations, perhaps unconscious of, or insensitive to, the tremendous amount of stamina it takes to sustain ongoing and accumulating losses.

Table 5-5. Barrett's Developmental Tasks.

REGRESSIVE DEVELOPMENTAL TASKS	COMPENSATORY DEVELOPMENTAL TASKS
1. Accepting and adjusting to a debilitating body	1. Developing new leisure time activities to meet changing abilities
2. Adjustment to reduction of sexuality	2. Learning new work skills
3. Readjustment in dependence-independence patterns	3. Making necessary dietary adjustments
4. Accepting a different role in the family circle	4. Adjusting to changing environments
5. Learning to accept more than one is capable of giving	5. Adjusting to the changing mores of society
6. Reorientation to primary social groups	6. Initiating a new search for status
	7. Modifying individual self-concepts

NOTE: Clearly, the developmental tasks of aging consistently involve the theme of learning to give up some tasks, replace others, and make new adjustments (Barrett, 1972).

Doing so may prove very helpful to professionals and older people.

Priscilla Ebersole describes receptive tasks, expressive tasks, and dynamic tasks of later life. The receptive tasks reflect relinquishing power and capacity. Expressive tasks reflect developing a self-transcending philosophy. Dynamic tasks of late life are dying and teaching others how to die (Ebersole, 1976).

Hendricks and Hendricks (1979) list and describe in detail three major developmental tasks for later life similar to those gleaned from Butler and Lewis. They are: (1) redirection of energy to new roles and activities, (2) acceptance of one's life, and (3) developing a point of view about death.

Current concepts and models for the study of the developmental tasks of aging all tend to imply that there is a necessity for (1) some "giving up or giving in" (i.e. some regression must be accepted; for example, at age 60 one has to learn to accept that he cannot suddenly and swiftly run across the street to beat oncoming traffic or easily hop over the tennis net after a game) and (2) some compensating for ever-increasing losses (conpensatory mechanisms need to be studied further to learn more about how and why some individuals compensate, while others allow devastating regression to occur).

Losses in every aspect of late life compel the elderly to spend enormous amounts of physical and emotional energy in grieving and resolving grief, adapting to the changes that result from loss, and recovering from the stresses inherent in these processes (Butler and Lewis, 1982).

In summary, when assessing for basic human needs and attempting to assist patients in meeting these needs and accepting the hard work of the developmental tasks of aging, the first step is to look at what is left, not what is gone.

REFERENCES

Barrett, J.H. *Gerontological Psychology*. Springfield, Ill.: Thomas, 1972, p. 9.
Bengston, V.L. The institutionalized aged and their social needs. In Seymour, E. (Ed.) *Psychosocial Needs of the Aged: A Health Care Perspective* (rev. ed.). Los Angeles University of Southern California Press, 1978, p. 36.
Burnside, I.M. *Psychosocial Care of the Aged*. New York: McGraw-Hill, 1980.
Burnside, I.M. *Nursing and the Aged* (2nd ed.). New York: McGraw-Hill, 1981, pp. 54–157.
Butler, R.N. *Why Survive Being Old in America?* New York: Harper & Row, 1975.
Butler, R.N. and Lewis, M.I. 3rd Ed *Aging and Mental Health*. St. Louis: C.V. Mosby, 1982, pp. 142, 376–379.
Carnevali, D.L. and Patrick, M. Editors *Nursing Management for the Elderly*. Philadelphia, J.B. Lippincott Co., 1979.
Corson, S.A. and O'Leary, E. *The role of pet animals as non-verbal communication links in mental health programs*. Paper presented at American Public Health Association Annual Meeting, Chicago, November 2, 1977.
Ebersole, P. Developmental tasks in later life. In Burnside, I. M. (Ed.) *Nursing and the Aged*. New York: McGraw-Hill, 1976, pp. 69–71.
Elias, M.F., Elias, P.K., and Elias, J.W. *Basic Processes in Adult Developmental Psychology*. St. Louis: C.V. Mosby, 1977, pp. 95–114.
Erikson, E. *Childhood and Society* (2nd ed.). New York: W.W. Norton, 1963.

Fromm, E. *The Sane Society.* New York: Rinehart, 1955.

Gioella, E.C. The relationship between slowness of response, state anxiety, social isolation, and self esteem and preferred personal space in the elderly. *Journal of Gerontological Nursing* 4(1): 40–43 (1978).

Gossett, H.M. *Restoring identity to socially deprived and depersonalized older people.* Paper presented at meeting of Community Council's Citizen Committee on Aging, Phoenix, Arizona, October 20, 1966.

Hendricks, J. and Hendricks, C.D. *Aging in Mass Society: Myths and Realities.* Cambridge, Mass, Winthrop Publishers Inc. 1977, pp. 10–50.

Hulicka, I.M. Understanding our client, the geriatric patient. *Journal of the American Geriatrics Society* 20(9): 438–448 (1972).

Kennedy, C. *Human Development: The Adult Years and Aging.* New York: Macmillan, 1978, pp. 142–146.

Kimmel, D.C. *Adulthood and Aging* (2nd ed.). New York: Wiley, 1980, p. 406.

Maslow, A.H. Higher and Lower Needs. *Journal of Psychology* 25: 433–436 (1948).

Maslow, A.H. *Toward a Psychology of Being.* New York: Van Nostrand, 1968.

Murray, R.B., Huelskoetter, M.W., and O'Driscoll, D.L. *The Nursing Process in Later Maturity.* Englewood Cliffs, N.J.: Prentice-Hall, 1980, pp. 278–280.

Murray, R.B. and Zentner, J.P. *Nursing Assessment and Health Promotion through the Life Span* (2nd ed.). Englewood Cliffs, N.J.: Prentice-Hall, 1979, pp. 379–382.

Newman, B.M. and Newman, R.R. Later adulthood: a developmental stage. In Hendricks, J. and Hendricks, C.D. (Eds.) *Dimensions of Aging: Readings.* Cambridge, Mass.: Winthrop, 1979, p. 141.

Pastalan, L. *Spatial Behavior of Older People.* Ann Arbor: University of Michigan, 1970, pp. 212–213.

Peck, R.C. Psychological developments in the second half of late life. In Anderson, J.E. (Ed.) *Psychological Aspects of Aging.* Washington, D.C.: American Psychological Association, 1956.

Sanner, D. Chaplain, Bethany Homes, Fargo, ND 58103.

Sibille, Sr. Michael. The Sociopsychological Aspects of Patient Care. Address given at Workshop on Care Needs of the Elderly. Phoenix, Arizona – Sponsored by Assn. of Nursing Home Administrators, Feb 12, 1976.

Townsend, C. *Old Age: The Last Segregation.* New York: Bantam Books, 1971.

Trienweiler, R. Personal space and its effect on an elderly individual in a long term care institution. *Journal of Gerontological Nursing* 4(5): 21-23 (1978).

Weiner, M.B., Brok, A.J., and Snadowsky, A.M. *Working with the Aged.* Englewood Cliffs, N.J.: Prentice-Hall, 1978, pp. 3–30.

Wolanin, Mary Opal. Adjustments to Chronic Conditions in Aging. Speech at Workshop Sponsored by College of Nursing Arizona State University, Tempe, Az. May 8, 1981.

Yurick, A.G., Robb, S.S., Spier, B.E., Ebert, N.J. *The Aged Person and the Nursing Process.* New York: Appleton-Century-Crofts, 1980.

6
Sensory Deprivation in the Elderly

Bernita M. Steffl

When you grow old your environment recedes from you.

Elsa Krouch (1960)

The term sensory deprivation as used in this chapter means a loss or denial of input or stimulation to the sense organs. In one sense, the term is a misnomer because to deprive means to divert or take away and in most cases the sensory process is not completely taken away (Jones, 1976). The literature describes the subject by at least 25 terms (Zubek, 1969). Bolin (1974) suggests that it would be more accurate to use the term sensory alteration.

SENSORY ALTERATIONS

The exact mechanism through which we receive and organize patterns of stimulation is not known, but there is increasing evidence that it is through the reticular activating system. Anatomically, the reticular activating system (RAS) is composed of a dense network of neurons, the reticular formation, which forms a core from the medulla of the lower brain to the thalamus in the forebrain. Functionally, it controls the overall degree of central nervous system activity, including the control of wakefulness and sleep, and monitors, at least in part, the ability to direct attention toward specific parts of our environment. In other words, the monitoring system reacts to patterned and changing environments. It responds to arousal in varying degrees and to cues from the environment (Bolin, 1974).

The prevailing characteristics of sensory deprivation are (1) lessened sensory input or sensory underload, (2) decrease of meaningful activity or lack of stimuli, and (3) alteration in the reticular activating system (Chodil, 1970). As indicated exactly what happens to the RAS

is unknown, but the implication is that it is functionally dependent on stimuli, and when sensory input (stimuli) is decreased, the RAS is no longer able to project a normal level of activation to the cortex. The sensorially deprived individual's thoughts and perceptions may then become dominated by residual stimuli, and he may even hallucinate in an attempt to maintain an optimal level of arousal (Bolin, 1974).

A study of 180 young, healthy adults who were put in moderate social isolation for only 2 3/4 hours showed unmistakably distorted auditory, visual, olfactory, kinesthetic, and tactile sensations experienced by at least 20% of the subjects (Downs, 1974). What must happen to the elderly debilitated and isolated patient who lies in bed day after day?

GENERAL SENSORY LOSSES IN THE ELDERLY

Sensory losses and changes in the elderly are gradual, and rarely occur suddenly except in the case of accidents or serious illness. Multiple losses, such as combined visual and auditory loss, are more difficult to cope with than a single loss. Older people have a capacity to cope, and they consciously or unconsciously develop various compensatory mechanisms to adapt to their sensory changes and physical declines. Even though sensorial changes are present in most older people, they vary in degree and do not necessarily imply dysfunction; nor do all old people sense and perceive their environment in a dysfunctional manner.

Acute medical conditions such as high fever, dehydration, and shock often cause reversible sensory alteration at any age, but most commonly in the elderly because their metabolic processes are altered and, thus, their responses and recovery are slower. This is important for nurses to note so that the elderly patient is not misdiagnosed as senile while treatment is delayed.

In one study of 74 patients who had undergone open and closed heart surgery, data collected from their charts, and from pre- and postoperative interviews, indicated that 67% had experienced one or more indeterminate stimulus experience (Ellis, 1972).

Irene Burnside defined four types of deprivation in the elderly: sensory, emotional, physical, and spiritual. She was concerned primarily with the first two in her work with deprived nursing home patients and successfully used sensory stimulation as an adjunct to group work with a small group of disabled patients. Much of the deprivation was believed to be due to institutionalization. She utilized food, flowers, newspapers, and touch freely. She found that the concept of future – a belief in tomorrow – was necessary to give point and meaning to what was done today (Burnside, 1973).

Tables 6-1 and 6-2 describe the causes, signs, and symptoms of sensory deprivation. Therapeutic intervention can be performed to assist and support older persons, to modify the environment spatially, and to provide necessary accoutrements and stimuli. Caretakers need to be aware of their power and potential in such matters as providing clocks, calendars, and newspapers. Most older people depended a great deal on a newspaper in early life, and it is still a significant lifeline to things and people of importance to them.

VISION LOSS IN THE ELDERLY

There are 1.7 million people in the United States today with severe vision impairment, and 65% of these are over age 65. About two-thirds are women (see Table 6-3).

The three most common disorders of vision which occur with increasing incidence in old age are: (1) retinal disease which includes senile macular degeneration and diabetic retinopathy, (2) glaucoma, and (3) cataracts. These disorders cause impairments which are responsible for most of the sensory deprivation due to vision loss.

The condition that occurs almost universally with aging is presbyopia – farsightedness. This usually becomes obvious when individuals can no longer read the telephone directory or newspaper with ease. It generally begins in the mid-forties and is easily alleviated with corrective lenses.

Normal physiological changes in the eye which affect all older individuals to some degree are the loss of accommodation, senile miosis, increased lens opacity, decreased peripheral vision, and yellowing of the lens (Buseck, 1976). (For more detail, see Chapter 18; only the three most common conditions causing vision loss and sensory deprivation will be described here.)

Retinal Disease

Retinal disease includes macular degeneration and diabetic retinopathy. About 25-30% of the older population is afflicted (Colenbrander, 1978).

Macular degeneration is a condition in which the macula, the small retinal area responsible for distinct central vision, no longer functions well enough to read a newspaper. The person sees only a gray shadow in the center of the visual field. Macular degeneration does not lead to total blindness, but it is devastatingly incapacitating in regard to mobility and sensorial comfort. Peripheral vision remains, so there is the potential for maximizing what remains and limited rehabilitation. The etiology is unknown, but it is believed to be due to decreased blood supply (from many causes) to the sensitive nerve endings in that area (Carnevali and Patrick, 1979; Yurick, Robb, Spier, and Ebert, 1980).

There is an increasing incidence of diabetic retinopathy, perhaps because diabetics are living longer. In this condition, the retina displays microaneurysms, and small hemorrhages occur in or on the retina. The broken blood vessels prevent light from getting through to the retina and cause vision loss. Diabetic retinopathy is the leading cause of new blindness in the United States today. Physicians are not sure of the cause of retinopathy, but it is known that the longer a person has had diabetes, the more

Table 6-1. Sensory Deprivation.

CAUSES	SIGNS AND SYMPTOMS
Physical injury and trauma to the sense organ Disease processes Deterioration due to unknown phenomenon of aging process Lack of stimulation Isolation Alienation Emotional starvation Nutritional starvation	Drowsy, sleepy feelings Anxiety and tensions apparent Inability to concentrate and organize thoughts Increased suggestibility Vivid sensory imagery – visual and auditory Body illusions Somatic complaints Intense subjective emotions Many preoccupations Depression and anger

Table 6-2. Sensory Deprivation in Aging.

SENSORY LOSS	COMMENTS	INTERVENTION
Auditory	Most problematic of losses. Leads to social isolation, depression, suspiciousness, paranoia, subjection to ridicule, and irrational thinking because of missing stimuli. About 30% of older population have significant hearing loss. More loss in men than women. Becomes noticeable at about age 50. Others tell us before we realize it or admit it.	Audiological examination. Communications skills: 1. Face person. 2. Place hand on arm gently for attention. 3. Speak slowly, distinctly. Do not shout (loss of high frequency). 4. Use body language. 5. No groups. 6. Use stethescope at ears of older person and speak in cone (temporary measure).
Visual	1.7 million people in the United States have severely impaired vision; 65% are over age 65. However, 80% of older people have adequate vision. Women have more problems than men. Causes decreased mobility, poor orientation, frightening visual images. Size of pupil decreases, lens thickens, less light reaches retina, and accommodation decreases. Individual may appear disarrayed; social interaction decreases.	Large print, large numbers on clocks, hand magnifier, etc. Support, assurance of staff regarding cataract surgery.
Gustatory (taste)	After age 50, ability to taste declines (e.g., salty-sweet, bitter-sour). Women are more sensitive to taste then men. Most persons 60 years and over lose 50% of taste buds. Taste buds at front of tongue atrophy first (salty-sweet area). Larger taste buds at back of tongue function well into old age (bitter-sour). Salivation declines, gums recede, etc.	Educate people to understand declining taste buds. Find substitutes for salt and sugar. Caution persons on salt-free diets. Do not assume that all old people need bland diets. Realize reason for behaviors. Enhance food with spices and seasonings.
Olfactory	Sense of smell best at puberty; begins to decline about age 45. People over 70 show pronounced atrophy of olfactory bulb. Smell contributes almost as much as taste to food enjoyment. Hazards are failure to detect smoke and dangerous odors.	Educate for preventive measures. Encourage use of smoke detectors.
Kinesthetic	Physiological changes cause decrease in proprioception; person feels less secure in spatial orientation especially in the dark. Complains of dizziness, buzzing in ear, nystagmus.	Provide adequate light, handrails in corridors, benches for resting. Understand patient's perception if coming from wheelchair level. Use eye contact; verbalize before pushing.
Tactile	Though there is some decline in sensory receptors, the need for the intimacy of touch is so strong it transcends most other needs and never leaves us completely.	Many very old and ill hunger for touch. Be generous with handshakes. Provide touch with familiar objects. Provide pets.

Table 6-3. Estimates of Persons with Selected Impairments by Age and Sex, United States, 1977 (Thousands of Persons).

TYPE OF IMPAIRMENT BY SEX	AGE				
	TOTAL	<17	17–44	45–64	65 +
Blind and visually impaired					
Total*	11,415	678	2,877	2,959	4,902
Male	5,910	436	1,891	1,702	1,881
Female	5,505	241	986	1,257	3,021
Deaf and hearing impaired					
Total*	16,219	856	3,480	5,365	6,518
Male	8,925	489	2,093	3,233	3,110
Female	7,294	366	1,387	2,133	3,408
Speech impaired					
Total*	1,995	913	555	315	212
Male	1,306	606	366	208	127
Female	688	307	189	107	86
Paralysis					
Total*	1,532	121	353	470	588
Male	803	67	188	270	279
Female	729	55	165	200	309
Orthopedic handicap – upper extremities					
Total*	2,500	105	934	827	634
Male	1,486	69	671	479	268
Female	1,014	36	264	348	366
Orthopedic handicap – lower extremities					
Total*	7,147	1,124	2,491	1,914	1,618
Male	3,643	634	1,466	951	592
Female	3,503	490	1,025	963	1,025
Absence of major extremities					
Total*	358	13	70	136	138
Male	252	8	53	109	82
Female	106	6	17	27	56

*In 1976, the total U.S. population was 216,745,000. This includes 2,142,000 people in the armed forces, 469,000 of whom were overseas, and 1,550,100 people in institutions. The civilian, noninstitutionalized population, to which this table refers, numbered 213,053,000 people in 1976.

Source: Digest of Data on Persons with Disabilities U.S., O.H.O.S., D.H.E.W., 1979.

likely is retinopathy to occur (American Foundation for the Blind, 1979; Yurick et al., 1980).

Glaucoma

Glaucoma is a disease of the eye characterized by increased intraocular pressure, resulting in hardness of the eye, degenerative changes in the retina, optic atrophy, and blindness. It may be "secondary" to a variety of ocular conditions such as iritis, tumor, or massive vitreous hemorrhage, but in the vast majority of cases, glaucoma is "primary" and of unknown etiology. The incidence is highest in the over-40 age group. See Table 6-4 for facts about glaucoma.

Table 6-4. Glaucoma.

Glaucoma is an eye disease usually found in those over 40.

Glaucoma can lead to blindness if not detected and treated.

Glaucoma occurs frequently – in one out of every 50 persons over 40 years of age.

If found and treated, the progression of glaucoma can usually be arrested.

People over 40 should have their eyes checked for glaucoma every two years.

Family history of glaucoma is significant.

NOTE: Nurses and other professionals need to teach these facts to all ages for self-health maintenance, but especially to the middle aged.

The intraocular tension represents a balance between the amount of aqueous humor that is produced and the amount that is drained away. Normally the aqueous humor produced in the posterior chamber passes through the pupil into the anterior chamber and drains through the angle of the anterior chamber at an even rate of flow. In glaucoma, for reasons not at all well understood, the fluid does not drain away as rapidly as it is formed and the pressure within the eyeball increases.

The angle through which the aqueous humor drains from the eye may be either shallow or wide in glaucoma. Shallow-angle glaucoma, which accounts for approximately 15% of all cases, is usually acute in onset and symptomatic in nature, causing considerable pain, nausea, and vomiting. Wide-angle glaucoma, the more common type (85% of all cases), most often is insidious in onset and asymptomatic for varying periods of time, but eventually produces bilateral loss of vision unless properly treated.

Diagnosis. The symptoms that suggest glaucoma are headaches, blurred or smoky vision, halos or rainbows around lights, and aching in the eye. Frequently, there will have been several recent changes in glasses, and sometimes the person will mention having been uncommonly clumsy (from inadequate vision) in the recent past. Diagnostic procedures include tonometry, visual field testing, and provocative tests. Normal tension limits are 17 to 22 units.

The Management of Glaucoma. If diagnosed early, most chronic simple glaucoma can be prevented from progressing by instilling into each eye daily an effective miotic. Pilocarpine hydrochloride is the miotic most commonly employed. The evening and first morning instillations are the most important because of the physiological increase in pressure that occurs during the night. Treatment usually includes a well-balanced diet, some fluid restriction, and avoidance of medications containing caffeine, such as Anacin and APC, and of preparations containing atropine-like substances. When a diuretic such as Diamox is given, there may be need for increased potassium intake.

Patients with glaucoma should have checks on intraocular tension at least every three months; visual fields and fundi should be checked as recommended by a physician. If there is progression despite the use of miotics, surgery may be needed to prevent blindness. Iridectomy (for shallow-angle glaucoma) and the so-called filtering operations are the most common surgical procedures.

The most important factors for the person with glaucoma are early detection and staying on medication under a physician's orders. There is no cure for glaucoma, but it can be controlled. Many older people discontinue medications when there is no pain. This can be disastrous, since medication is the critical variable in preventing blindness from glaucoma (Carnevali and Patrick, 1979; Soll, 1974).

Cataracts

Everyone would acquire cataracts if he lived long enough. The age of onset varies greatly in individuals and families. The lenses thicken, yellow, become less permeable, and diffuse light, causing distressing glare for the afflicted individual. About 61% of older individuals (up to 95% after age 70) have cataracts but only 8–9% of these ever reach the stage of needing surgery. The extent to which a cataract affects vision depends on its position and density. Advances in surgical techniques have made cataract removal and lens implantation relatively uncomplicated and more than 95% successful (American Foundation for the Blind, 1979; Buseck, 1976). For further information and details on eye surgery, see Chapter 26.

Perhaps most important and most helpful to the patient is planned nursing care to assist with adjustment to daily living after surgery, i.e., adjustment to glasses, contact lenses, and sensory distortions. The removal of a cataract creates aphakia, and thus inability to focus. For example, the nausea, dizziness, and wavy, jerky appearance of objects viewed through the edges of the thick glasses which are necessary postoperatively can be reduced if the nurse reminds patient to look through the center of the lens and consciously turn the head to see objects to the side. It is also helpful to have the patient wear his new glasses initially when sitting and then gradually start walking around on safe, flat levels because there is a 33% size increase which makes everything appear closer than it is and causes poor depth perception (Carnevali and Patrick, 1979).

Since cataracts develop at various rates, there is usually a period of time leading up to surgery when those with developing cataracts have frightening and devastating reactions to bright lights, glare, and sudden darkness (e.g., entering a theater). It is this kind of sensory alteration which calls for support systems and careful education of both patient and family.

Interventions for Vision Deprivation

Doctor August Colenbrander stated in testimony to the U.S. Senate Committee on Aging that a major problem and task in the definition of blindness is to determine "how blind is blind"

(Colenbrander, 1978). Some years ago (1965), the World Health Organization found that 65 different countries used 65 different definitions of blindness. In this confusion of definitions, more people are blinded by definition than by any other cause. There is a large gray area between normal vision and blindness.

For more precise reporting and more realistic classification and intervention, the World Health Organization has adopted the terminology and classifications given in Tables 6-5 through 6-8. Tables 6-5 and 6-6 illustrate the current World Health Organization definitions of vision loss which promote concentration on what is left rather than what is gone. Tables 6-7 and 6-8 point out that in sensory rehabilitation the focus should be on the handicap rather than the disorder. These tables illustrate a useful way of looking at visual loss and its impact on the individual by concentrating on the handicap and disability which can be altered even if the disorder cannot.

Table 6-5.

Normal Vision
Low Vision
Blindness

Table 6-6.

Legally seeing	Normal vision	Normal Near-normal
Legally blind	Low vision	Moderate Severe Profound
	Blindness	Near-blind Blind

Tables 6-5 and 6-6 are current World Health Organization definitions.

Table 6-7.

VISUAL DISORDER	VISUAL IMPAIRMENT	DISABILITY	VISUAL HANDICAP
Pathology Media Retina Brain	Organ Function Acuity Field	Visual skills Reading Mobility Living	Effort Dependence Physical Economic Social

←—Medical Care —→
←— Visual Aids —→
←— Education —→

Table 6.8.

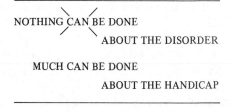

NOTHING CAN BE DONE
        ABOUT THE DISORDER

MUCH CAN BE DONE
        ABOUT THE HANDICAP

Tables 6-7 and 6-8 illustrate how to define and focus on handicap versus disorder.

NOTE: Reprinted with permission from *Vision Impairment among Older Americans,* prepared for the Senate hearing before the Special Committee on Aging, United States Senate, Ninety-fifth Congress, Second Session, Washington, D.C., August 3, 1978 by August Colenbrander, M.D., Pacific Medical Center, San Francisco, California.

The most common age-related visual disorders cause visual loss that should be classified as low vision rather than total blindness. Visual impairment is only one factor that determines disability. Rehabilitation of a person depends on nonvisual as well as visual skills. Deficiencies in one of these can be compensated by extra concentration on the other via two avenues: vision enhancement and vision substitution. Vision enhancement involves the use of aids such as optical aids, large print, and writing with felt pens. Vision substitution is the use of other senses to replace or supplement vision, e.g., raised dots on a thermostat, talking books, and radio rather than newspapers. The use of the term visual handicap widens the perspective of care for the patient because we are forced to define his specific handicap. For example, providing an environment free of steps does not reduce the disability but does reduce the handicap (Colenbrander, 1978).

Guidelines for Assisting the Older Person with Vision Loss

The best guide, in this writer's opinion, for aiding the visually impaired is *An Introduction to Working with the Aging Person Who Is Visually Handicapped,* published in 1972 by the American Foundation for the Blind, 15 West 16th Street, New York, NY 10011. It describes and illustrates the following skills:

Shaking hands	Locating and inserting a key
Walking	
Negotiating passageways	Clothing selection
Negotiating doorways	Locating dropped
Stairs	objects
Trailing and exploring	Bed making
Room familiarization	Threading a needle
Car travel	Sewing on a four-hole
Seating	button
Audience seating	Shaving (face, for
Phone dialing	men)
Smoking	Brushing teeth
Identifying money	Cleaning dentures
Eating	Tying ties
Telling time	

Caretakers should remember that many older people who have low vision or are blind

have had sight most of their lives, so they can easily be oriented to the environment. Other senses are often very sharp: unless there is a hearing problem, the ears of the blind are very sensitive to sounds, and loudness can be distressing. When an older individual has both a vision and a hearing problem, sensory deprivation may be severe.

Some general guidelines for working with the blind older person are presented here:

- Always introduce yourself. Let the blind person know whom he is talking to so he doesn't have to try to figure out who you are while trying to listen.
- When you leave a blind person, tell him that you are going.
- Do not worry about using words such as "look" and "see" when you are talking to someone who is blind.
- Speak directly to the blind person. If he is with a friend, do not use his companion as an interpreter.
- Unless he is deaf, there is no need to speak more loudly to the blind person than you would to others.
- Do not pet a dog guide or otherwise distract him from his job.
- Use the same common sense and sensitivity toward the elderly blind person that you would with anyone else.
- Certain things have to be explained. For example, a nurse who is about to give an injection should tell the blind patient so that he is aware of what will happen to him.
- When teaching a blind person, explain the procedures fully and, wherever you can, let the sense of touch replace the sense of sight.
- Allow the blind person the time he needs to learn a new skill. If the skill is complicated, break it down into steps and teach one step at a time.
- Remember that the person who is older may not have a good memory.
- Refer to the numbering on a clock when telling a blind person where things are placed in front of him. This is especially useful for placement of food

at mealtime. For example, certain foods are always placed at 6 o'clock and milk is always above the plate at about 10 o'clock.

The American Foundation for the Blind recommends the following essentials in teaching skills for daily living: (1) orientation to position and relationship to significant objects in the environment to maximize utilization of the remaining senses, (2) establishing mobility aptitude and patterns, (3) teaching the use of trailing — the art of using the backs of fingers to follow lightly over surfaces to determine location, find objects, and determine line of travel (American Foundation for the Blind, 1972).

HEARING LOSS IN THE ELDERLY

Aging of auditory function begins at adolescence and becomes evident around age 50 (Timiris, 1972). Auditory function decreases steadily throughout life in both men and women, but more so in men. Almost twice as many men as women over age 65 have hearing impairments (Table 6-3) does not reflect this because of an obviously more liberal diagnosis of impairment. Presbycusis is the term used to describe hearing impairment in old age. Contrary to the self-discovery of presbyopia, in presbycusis the individual has to be told that he is not hearing. Admission of hearing loss is traumatic. The following situation describes what often occurs:

Junior: "Dad, Dad, DAD!" When he gets dad's attention, "Gee, Dad, you can't hear anymore!"

Dad: "There's nothing wrong with my hearing; if you kids would just shut up, we could all hear."

How do we hear? In order to understand the kinds of hearing loss and interventions, one must recall how hearing takes place. Sound vibrations are funneled to the eardrum through the ear canal. As the eardrum vibrates in tune with the sound waves that strike it, this same movement is transmitted to the three tiny bones in the middle ear. Th carry the sound vibrations delicate inner ear. The vibrati bones causes waves in the fluid, which stimulate thousands of microscopic hair cells in the inner ear. The stimulation of these hair cells produces electrical signals corresponding to the sound vibrations that entered the ear. These electrical impulses pass through a bundle of nerves and travel to the brain for interpretation.

Most Common Hearing Losses

Conduction Hearing Losses. Conduction hearing losses are due to a variety of causes which interfere with the conduction process described above, for example, infections and otosclerosis. The hearing impairment in conductive losses is usually amenable to improvement with surgery, medical treatment, or hearing aids. Convincing the older person of his loss and of the possibilities for improvement is a problem.

Sensorineural Hearing Loss. Sensorineural hearing loss implies a dysfunction in the transmission of nerve impulses to the brain. It can be caused by changes in the inner ear, the auditory nerve, or the brain. Exposure to loud noises over a long period of time is believed to be a contributing factor. Presbycusis is usually the result of neural changes. Sensory presbycusis may be caused by atrophy to the organ of Corti, where the microscopic hair cells described earlier respond to and transmit sound waves on the way to the brain. Neural presbycusis results from degenerative changes in the nerve fibers of the cochlea. Metabolic presbycusis is caused by atrophy of blood vessels and vascular changes. Mechanical presbycusis results from atrophic changes in structures involved in the vibration of the cochlea partition (Yurick et al., 1980). Sensorineural losses are more difficult to deal with and do not respond as well to amplification devices (hearing aids) as conduction losses do.

Mixed Hearing Losses. Mixed hearing losses involving both conductive and sensorineural loss are not uncommon and are especially difficult to deal with because of many cause and effect relationships in the aging process.

Another hearing difficulty, tinnitus, is essentially "biological noise" which is actually generated within the auditory system. It is characterized by ringing in the ears. About 9% of people aged 55–64 experience this affliction. About 11% of persons 65–74 years of age complain of tinnitus. There is good evidence that this condition is generally more common in women than in men (Rockstein and Sussman, 1979).

Cerumen. Occlusion of the ear canal by cerumen is a common problem in old age, particularly among the frail elderly living alone or in long term care facilities. It should not be allowed to occur and is inexcusable if the affected individual is under professional care. The sad fact is that health professionals may forget to examine for cerumen because they are not surprised when an old person does not hear. The removal of cerumen is simple and very rewarding if it was the cause of the hearing loss. Though procedures for removal are relatively simple, they should not be attempted by nonprofessionals. Hearing loss caused by cerumen is completely reversible.

Interventions for Hearing Losses

Thorough assessment and evaluation are essential for any kind of therapeutic treatment or rehabilitation. Adults, especially those who work in noisy environments, are advised to have a hearing test as part of a regular physical examination. The examination should be done by qualified professionals who have no connection with the sale or rental of hearing aids. Hearing aids are very effective and many older persons could benefit from them, but it is important to realize that the different losses described above may vary greatly in their response to a hearing aid. The use of a hearing aid is a very selective procedure. In some instances, certain aids are a waste of money, and there are many cases on record of an older person being persuaded to purchase an aid or device without thorough audiological evaluation.

A relatively new device which seems to have great potential in certain situations is the infrared hearing system. Under conditions in which the conventional hearing aid has been found to provide limited assistance, the infrared (IR) hearing system has proved beneficial: e.g., attending church, going to the theater, participating in normal classroom activities, and listening to television. The IR system eliminates background noise. Incorporating the principles of light wave communications, the IR hearing system transmits sound directly to the listener over an invisible and silent light beam uncontaminated by the noise and reverberation which normally distroy the sound message. The device consists of two components: a transmitter and a receiver. The desired sound message is converted by the transmitter into the modulated light beam by use of light-emitting diodes. The receiver, worn inconspicuously by the listener, then takes the beam and converts it back into sound. Power is provided by rechargeable batteries. A portable transmitter, about the size of a hand-held calculator, is now available (Leshowitz, 1979, 1982). [Further information can be obtained from Audio Devices, Inc., 4702 East Calle Del Medio, Phoenix, AZ 85018; (602) 959-6927.]

Advocates for the deaf should also watch for new information and progress in cochlear implants. Research in the implantation of electrodes into the cochlea of the profoundly deaf has been in existence in the United States and France since 1954. It is progressing slowly but surely with the support of the Deafness Research Foundation, 342 Madison Avenue, New York, NY 10017.

Hearing loss limits the enjoyment of social interaction in gatherings and causes many older persons to isolate themselves from society. Helping professionals are not always able to motivate the hard-of-hearing person to get assistance and are frequently unable to help persons cope successfully with a hearing aid. The fact that most hearing aids amplify all sounds makes adjustment to them difficult and annoying. Imagine trying to sort out your spouses's conversation in a busy airport terminal with a hearing aid amplifying all sounds several hundred decibels! A hearing aid, in some cases, may help the family as much as the person who is hard-of-hearing (see Figure 6-1).

Simple Courtesies for the Hard of Hearing

- Speech should be paced slowly enough to clearly enunciate syllables and give the person time to comprehend.
- Keep your voice at about the same volume throughout each sentence; do not drop the voice at the end of the sentence.

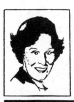

Dear Abby
Abigail Van Buren

Selfish sister won't hear of wearing aid

DEAR ABBY: My older sister has a hearing problem, and she's driving us all crazy because she won't admit it. Several years ago you had a letter in your column from Nanette Fabray, who pointed out the selfishness of such people. If you can find it, please run it again.
Florida fan

DEAR FAN: I had to go back into my 1971 files, but here it is:

DEAR ABBY: There are some 20 million people in this country with hearing problems. Most of them could and should wear aids.

Some say, "I'll wait until I need one." But if you have even a slight problem, you need one now! It is important first to have your hearing checked by a doctor to see if your loss is one that can be corrected. Many people wait until it is too late to correct what might have been a simple medical problem in the beginning. If nothing can be done to restore your loss, and if the tests show an aid can help you, then by all means get one.

The woman who feels that wearing a hearing aid will attract attention to her hearing loss fools only herself, and she's usually a pain in the neck to everyone she comes in contact with.

There are many ways of letting others know one can't hear: cupping a hand behind the ear, asking people repeatedly to speak up or repeat things, etc. Everyone knows you have a problem, and everyone wonders why you aren't doing something about it.

I have worn hearing aids for years, so I know the problems of vanity, despair, adjustment, irritation ... the list goes on and on. But I do not try to hide my aids, and interesting enough, most people do not notice I wear one and sometimes two, even on television.

A dear friend opened my eyes about wearing an aid. Many years ago she told me I was being very selfish by making others cope with what was my problem alone. She was right. I had to do something about my hearing and not expect my family and friends to speak louder than was comfortable for them, or repeat things I had missed, turn up the volume on the TV, etc.

If you suspect you have a problem, see an audiologist or a doctor, or even a reputable hearing aid dealer. Take all the necessary tests. No reputable dealer will try to sell you an aid without first making sure there is no way to correct your loss and that an aid will really help you. And if he is honest, he'll put it in writing.

Thank you, Abby. Please print this as a favor to people with a hearing loss as well as people who have to live with them.

Figure 6-1. (Reprinted with permission from Abigail Van Buren and the Universal Press Syndicate, 1980.)

A lower voice range is often easier to hear.

- Always speak as clearly as possible. Distinctness does not mean shouting.
- Make the change to a new subject, a new name, a number, or unual word at a slower rate.
- Watch the expression on the listener's face and note when your words are not caught. Do not repeat the whole sentence. Usually one word or name was not clear.
- Remember that the hard-of-hearing may depend to a considerable extent on reading your lips. Face them so they can see your lips as you speak.
- Don't speak to hard-of-hearing persons abruptly. Attract their attention first by facing them and looking straight into their eyes, or by touching their hands or shoulders lightly.
- If persons have one good ear, stand or sit on that side when talking. Be sure their hearing aid is in place and turned on, and check to see that the batteries are working. (Every nurse in gerontological nursing should know how to change a hearing aid battery.)
- Facial expressions are important clues to meaning. Remember that an affectionate or amused tone of voice may be lost on a hard-of-hearing person.
- Many hard-of-hearing persons are unduly sensitive about their handicap and will pretend to understand you when they don't. When you detect this situation, tactfully repeat your meaning in different words until it gets across.
- When you're in a group that includes a hard-of-hearing person, try to carry on your conversation with others in such a way that he can watch your lips. Let him know what is being discussed. *Never* take advantage of his handicap by carrying on private conversations in his presence in low tones he cannot hear.
- Use synonyms. Words with sibilant sounds (*sh* and *s* sounds in words such as fish and juice) are harder for older people to understand. (NAHSA, 1977)

CHANGES IN TASTE AND SMELL

Very little is known about how food tastes and smells to old people; however, most of the literature and studies available indicate a decline in both gustatory and olfactory sensitivities. Some studies have been contradictory.

Taste

A decline or lack of taste is called hypogeusia. The number of taste buds is fairly constant through adolescence, but in maturity and into early old age (up to the age of 70), there is a slight decrease in the number of these taste receptors. In advanced old age, however, the number of taste buds is drastically reduced. Other factors which contribute to the reduction in taste sensation are the lowered secretion of saliva, and the fissuring and furrowing of the tongue known to occur in older persons (Rockstein and Sussman, 1979).

It has been established that in older individuals sensitivity to sweet, sour, and salt does change. Some studies indicate that the decline in sensitivity to salt may be greatest. Shiffman found that, blindfolded, elderly subjects are less able to recognize blended foods than are young college students. This study suggests that the loss in ability to identify food is predominantly due to sensory loss (Shiffman, 1977).

The loss of taste sensibility probably explains the increased use of condiments or spices observed in the elderly. This has significance for the helping professions and caretakers in long term care facilities. The tendency is to coddle old people with bland food because of the assumption that spicy food is not good for them or that they can't tolerate it. Actually, adding spices such as curry, cinnamon, cloves, as well as other flavoring, may be more in order. Most old people can tolerate spices quite well and have fairly healthy digestive tracts.

Smell

In general, it can be said that the sense of smell becomes best developed at puberty and appears to begin to decrease only after age 45, continuing to decline gradually thereafter. Microscopic examination of tissue from the lining of the nasal epithelium of people over age 70 shows pronounced atrophy of the olfactory bulbs. This is accompanied by a reduction in the number of olfactory nerve elements. It has been estimated that there is an 8% loss of olfactory fibers from birth to age 15, which increases to 73% from 76 to 91 years of age. However, such summary figures are deceptive because the rate of loss of such fibers averages only 0.9% per year up to age 37, rising to 1.6% per year between ages 37 and 52. Thereafter, however, the rate of loss actually decreases to 0.7% per year from ages 52 to 67, and later to as low as 0.3% per year. In general, then, it is accepted that the loss in olfaction with advancing age is related to this cumulative loss in the number of nerve endings in the olfactory nasal epithelium (Rockstein and Sussman, 1979).
nasal epithelium (Rockstein and Sussman, 1979).

In two research studies, Schiffman demonstrated a loss in the accuracy of food recognition based on cues from the taste and smell of blended foods. She found that amplification of odors in foods with artificial flavors greatly improves the ability of elderly subjects to recognize blended food (Schiffman, 1977). A subsequent study using commerical food flavoring also indicated that the ability to discriminate food odors was considerably diminished in the elderly (Schiffman and Pasternak, 1979).

It is very difficult to differentiate smell from taste. If one is affected, it seems to affect the other. The reasons for professional interest and concern are twofold. First, the inability to enjoy taste and smell contributes to poor appetite, followed by malnutrition, decreased alertness, depression, and altered functional abilities — a vicious cycle. Second, cooking and housekeeping are more hazardous. Burning food and gas fumes are not as apt to be recognized, and judging from the frequent deaths due to fires in long term care facilities and residences for the elderly, one can suspect that the inability to detect smoke may have been a contributing factor.

TOUCH DEPRIVATION

Rockstein and Sussman state that sensitivity to touch decreases through the sixth decade of life and that this is probably due to a decrease with age in the number and sensitivity of the neuronal receptors in the skin. This seems to reverse in the seventh and eighth decades, and touch sensitivity appears to increase, due perhaps to increased thinning of the skin (Rockstein and Sussman, 1979).

There is also a decrease in sensitivity to pain associated with the changes in sensory receptors mentioned earlier (Rockstein and Sussman, 1979). This has serious implications because bruises, scratches, cuts, burns, and infections not perceived by the older person, may therefore remain untreated, and can lead to such serious conditions as skin breakdown and decubitus; see Table 6-9.

The skin is the largest organ of the body, and the tactile functions of the skin have a very large representation in the brain. We do not understand all of the mysteries of the tactile sense, but experiments with animals suggest that stimulation of the body sends messages that stimulate the brain which in turn activates critical responses throughout the organism (Montagu, 1971).

"As we grow older we begin to discover qualities of the skin, firmness, elasticity,

Table 6-9. Definitions Related to Touch.

Esthesia	Capacity for sensation or feeling sensitivity.
Esthesio-	Combining form of the word; e.g. esthesiometry is a technique to measure the degree of tactile sensibility.
Anesthesia	General or local insensibility to sensation; also loss of the sensation of pain, due to drugs.
Paresthesia	Abnormal sensation such as prickling and itching (e.g., itching due to organic changes such as lack of blood supply or nerve impairment), as well as numbness in hands resulting from arthritic changes in cervical vertebrae which interfere with nerve function.
Paralgesia	Sense of pain – any condition marked by abnormal and painful sensations.

texture, we had failed to notice at all until we began to lose them. With the accumulation of years we are apt to regard our aging skin as a rather dirty trick, a depressing public evidence of aging, and a somewhat unwelcome reminder of the passage of time. No longer the good fit it once was, it grows loose and baggy, and is often wrinkled, dry and leathery, sallow, splotched, or otherwise disfigured" (Montagu, 1971). It is then that people begin to touch less and be touched less. It is then that professionals make less touch and sensory stimulation available. No one seems to want to touch an older person intuitively as they reach out to touch a baby. Physical encounters with them are often perfunctory, with no warmth or conviction behind them, and old age becomes a lonely fortress (Verwoerdt, 1966).

Touch and the meaning of touch transcend all the other senses. Harry Stack Sullivan, a noted psychiatrist, says, "The need for intimacy and physical as well as interpersonal closeness exists and develops throughout our lives." The greatest need, he says, is experienced in preadolescence, but that need never leaves us completely (Sullivan, 1953).

The kind of touch the old yearn for is the intimate hug received in childhood and as lovers — a warm hug, firm and close enough to blot out worries, troubles, and fears about what is happening to them (Hollander, 1970).

There is a strange dyad between touch, which is a form of contact, and loneliness, a form of noncontact that creates feelings and longing for the presence of others and for the rituals and routines of the past, such as the longing for the warmth and love of an animal or the feel of things familiar. The pleasure bond of touch includes familiar things held and touched with our hands: pets, plants, flowers, a piano, familiar household objects, and ritual objects such as prayer beads.

How and where to touch? Irene Burnside says that touching is talking. She always greets older persons with a warm and gentle handshake. She also points out that a great deal of physical and psychosocial assessment is possible during a handshake and greeting. A handshake conveys messages of anxiety; different kinds of tremors;

the condition, color, and temperature of the skin; and something about the physical condition of the individual and the kind of care he is receiving (Burnside, 1973; Burnside, Ebersole, and Monea, 1979). There are also, of course, messages of anger, aggression, repulsion, hunger, pleasure, and desire which come from both the sender and the receiver. This writer has heard patients say, "I didn't like the way that nurse shoved me around" or "She is rough" or "I didn't like being treated like a sack of potatoes!"

Touch is an important element of sensory stimulation, which professionals may not think about, in so many activities of daily living with family, friends, pets, and personal surroundings such as favorite chairs or a special cup. When these are no longer available to the elderly, nursing intervention with touch becomes increasingly important. Touching is nuturing. To touch is to feel and to be felt. Touch is especially meaningful during pain and with the dying person (Moustakas, 1975).

Touch seems to be helpful in caring for the confused person. Nurse researcher Ruth McCorkle found that patients who were touched responded more positively than patients who were not touched during conversations (McCorkle, 1974). Elderly patients who have to be fed take more fluid and eat better if the nurse sits close by and touches them (see Figure 6-2).

Stereognosis is the ability to recognize the form of an object. Closely related is the ability to tactically recognize figures imbedded in a more geometrical form. This capacity seems to decline with age (Kenshalo, 1977). This needs to be carefully assessed when there is difficulty in implementing certain therapeutic rehabilitation tasks. The condition is believed to be connected with impairments of the central nervous system processes (Kenshalo, 1977).

For the elderly who are well — and there are many of them who are deprived of the warmth of human touch, such as widows and widowers

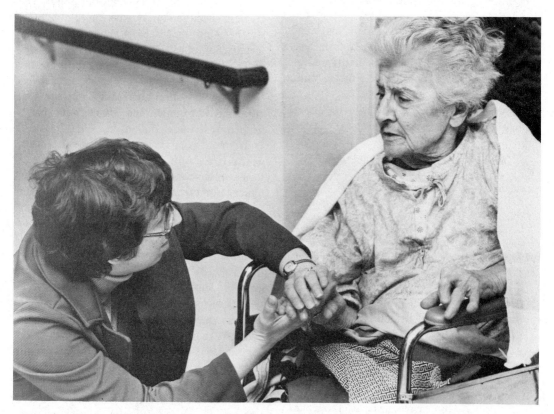

Figure 6-2. The patient calms down and is less anxious when the nurse holds her hand and speaks to her at eye level. (Photo by Jeff Stanton.)

— activities which promote touch with other human beings should be encouraged. Even games and activities like cards and bingo provide more sensory stimulation than purely spectator recreation such as television.

Dancing is physical therapy as well as socialization. Through dance we can promote and provide opportunity for the expression of sexuality. In dance, body touch — even with strangers — is appropriate. These activities that promote touch also help build and maintain self-esteem because they are an incentive to keep up personal appearance. Touch also sustains human sexuality (Steffl, 1981).

Dr. Ann Cain a family therapist at the University of Maryland conducted a survey of pet owners after she noticed that people talk about their pets as family members. She asked 60 people in the survey to tell her who got the most strokes. She described strokes as any form of recognition such as physical touch, a look, a word, a smile, or a gesture that conveys, "I know you are there." Forty-four percent of those surveyed said their pets got the most strokes (Cain, 1978).

Dr. Duncan Halbert, age 65, contracted poliomyelitis many years ago and became paralyzed from the neck down. For 25 years he has been practicing medicine from an iron lung. He states that what he misses most is touch. "I'm deprived of man's basic need — the sense of touch. Tactile contact is vitally important. People are so unconscious about touching. They touch something or someone every day, wherever they go. I finally realized why I had felt so lonely. It was because of my need to touch. I used to burst into tears over this. When someone touches me, it's like an electric shock that brings me out of that unusual lonely state" (*Hospital Tribune*, 1977).

Just as touch is rooted in antiquity so are many taboos regarding touch (De Thomaso, 1971). In cultures other than middle class America, one may find religious or historical reasons for non-touch. For example, some Eastern religions forbid the touching of food with the hand that takes care of body hygiene. A hearty handshake is not proper in all cultures. Strong eye contact which is often advocated by the helping professionals is not acceptable to certain native Americans. Therefore, professionals should be careful to assess for individual and cultural differences, and should take the opportunities to respect those differences in regard to the many ways we touch.

This writer believes that professionals are more likely to fall short on touching rather than to overdo it. Don't wait to be asked. Old people may hesitate to ask for touch because asking to be touched would cause suspicion or disapproval. An 84-year-old woman said, "I am lonely at times but still reach out and I guess forgetting just how wrinkled I am and how untouched. So what! Don't expect it." To be touched is to be reached. To hold and to be held are opportunities we should promote and provide for the elderly (Steffl, 1979).

KINESTHESIA

Kinesthesia is the sensation of movement in muscles, tendons, and joints. It is muscle and joint sense. In other words, knowing where your foot is. Increased susceptibility to falls and altered gait may conceivably be due to increased input or to the failure of input from kinesthetic receptors; however, this is still a matter of debate. Originally it was assumed that both muscle stretch receptors and the Golgi tendon organs, together with those receptors in and around the joints, were responsible for relaying information to the nervous system concerning limb position. More recently, strong evidence has been reported that muscle afferents also participate in kinesthesia. These findings have been reported by numerous researchers (Kenshalo, 1977).

Awareness of, and assessment for, kinesthesia and difficulty in proprioception are nursing responsibilities with tremendous preventive potential for care givers in planning care, providing a protective environment, and educating the patient. Older people may need to be educated to accept the fact that at some point they may not be as surefooted and agile in going up and down stairs or judging curbs as they were in their younger years. Whether the cause is neurological or otherwise the fact is that in old age knowing exactly where the foot lands appears to be more difficult.

ADJUNCT THERAPIES FOR SENSORY STIMULATION

Music

Music is a universal method of communication. It transcends race, culture, color, age, and sex. Music puts people in touch with their feelings. It is sensory input. It brings back happy and sometimes sad memories of the past. Music excites and energizes us, and it also lulls and soothes the mind and the body to dream and sleep. Its healing properties have long been known by professionals and nonprofessionals. Not only is the reaction to music sensorial, but music stimulates reactions in the entire body. Everyone to whom the succession of tones means anything responds by exhibiting very slight but characteristic changes of muscular tonicity. It is the listener and not the performer alone who creates the melody. In the act of response to the successive tones that strike upon the ear, he binds them together" (Bingham, 1968).

Nurses may find it very rewarding to confer with music therapists in planning care for the elderly. The work of Hennessey (1978) and Moore (1976) is beautiful and effective. Their writing not only is informative but also offers strategies for nurses when a music therapist is not available.

Pets

Pets, especially dogs and cats, offer love and tactile reassurance without criticism (see Figure 6-3). Dogs also offer protection. The need to be needed and the need for meaningful activities can be met for many older individuals by pets. Pets are totally dependent, and they give unconditioned love and affection. Studies have shown that older individuals who were depressed and withdrawn responded very positively to pets (Corson et al., 1975). In some instances, a pet is the most significant other an individual has.

Elsie is 80 years old, in poor health, and very allergic to the sun. Her little black poodle rules her life. Her activities outside her home are increasingly limited, but she does not seem to be as upset about giving up her freedom as she is when she has to leave "Oney." She cut short a visit to her relative in another state because she was afraid "Oney" would get away from the house sitter. Elsie is out every morning at daybreak, bundled up and covered with a big hat and gloves to keep off the sun as she walks "Oney."

Mr. William Henry Thomas made an unforgettable impression on this writer. He had taken a bus to the emergency room of the county hospital. He had many medical problems and had been there often. This day he was very short of breath and uncomfortable, but he was most upset about his legs, "They just won't work." He had fallen frequently. Placement in a long term care facility was in progress. Mr. Thomas' main concern was that he be able to bring his dog. "I gotta find a place for my little dog, there's nary a body to take care of him."

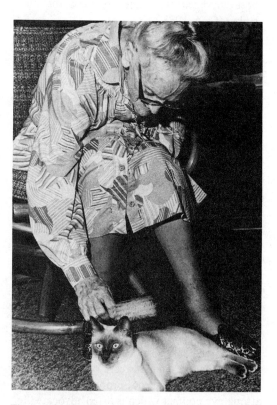

Figure 6-3. The pleasure bond of touch is not limited to humans. (Photo by Jeff Stanton.)

As tears slowly rolled down his cheeks, I asked, "And where is he today?" Mr. Thomas responded, "Oh, I carried him to the vet before I came." Mr. Thomas was admitted and died within 48 hours.

Telephones, Radios, Clocks, and Calendars

A telephone is often literally the lifeline of an elderly person. It offers reassurance, service, and security. Butler reports a study in England indicating that the mortality rate was higher among people without a telephone (Butler and Lewis, 1982).

A big, old, ticking alarm clock has an element of comfort for almost any age person, but it may have special significance to an elderly person whose working life began long before electric clocks were popular. There is also a routine tactile task involved because old fashioned clocks need daily winding.

Clocks and calendars seem to be scarce in long term care facilities and so are newspapers — all items which have lifetime significance as sensory input (Burnside, 1970). There are situations in which it is difficult to maintain these at bedside with confused persons; however, in this writer's opinion, the bigger problem may be with staff not being committed to providing and using them in their interactions with patients and families.

Radios often provide religious programs and music which is not available on television. Radio programs, news, and weather reports not only assist in reality orientation but often provide a "feeling" level link with the past. This can apply, for example, to hymns that were sung as a child. A registered nurse from a long term care facility said, "When I'm in a room when the radio is tuned to a church program, I sing the hymns with the patients while I'm working in the room." Today radios are inexpensive, small, and durable so they are truly not prohibitive.

SUMMARY

Sensory deprivation is perhaps the most devastating loss in old age. Most sensory loss can be categorized in the five areas discussed in this chapter: vision, hearing, taste, smell, and touch. Professional staff should be able to make organic and functional assessments, and to intervene therapeutically. Most professional staff need education or orientation to these conditions, as well as some clinical skills, in order to do the best job. A number of trainers have developed simulated situations, empathic models, and experiential teaching-learning suggestions such as blind walks and simulation of hearing loss for students in classes and for staff in-service education.

REFERENCES

American Foundation for the Blind. *An Introduction to Working with the Aging Person Who Is Visually Handicapped.* New York: 1972.

American Foundation for the Blind. *Facts about Aging and Blindness.* New York: 1979, pp. 1–2.

Bingham, W.V. Introduction to the Effects of Music. In *The Effects of Music* Edited by Schoen, M., Freeport, N.Y., Books for Libraries Press 1968, p. 6.

Bolin, R.H. Sensory Deprivation: An Overview, *Nursing Forum* 13(3): (1974) 241–257.

Burnside, I.M. Clocks and Calendars. *American Journal of Nursing* 70(1): 117–119 (1970).

Burnside, I.M. Touching is talking. *American Journal of Nursing* 73(12): 2060–2063 (1973).

Burnside, I.M., Ebersole, P., and Monea, H.E. *Psychosocial Caring throughout the Life Span.* New York: McGraw-Hill, 1979, pp. 582–592.

Buseck, S.A. Visual status of the elderly. *Journal of Gerontological Nursing* 2(5): 34–37 (1976).

Butler, R.N. and Lewis, M. *Aging and Mental Health.* 3rd Ed. St. Louis: C.V. Mosby, 1982, pp. 223–224.

Cain, A. Pets get loving strokes. *Arizona Republic* (March 20, 1978).

Carnevali, D.L. and Patrick, M. *Nursing Management for the Elderly.* Philadelphia: J.B. Lippincott, 1979, pp. 490–493.

Chodil, J. and Williams, B. The Concept of Sensory Deprivation. *Nursing Clinics of North America* 5: 453–465, 1970.

Colenbrander, A. Aging and Vision Loss. *Vision Impairment Among Older Americans.* Hearing before the Special Committee on Aging, United States Senate, Ninty-Fifth Congress, Second Session, Washington, D.C. August 3, 1978, p. 5–11. U.S. Govt. Printing Office Washington, D.C. 1979.

Corson, S.A., Corson, E., Gwyne, P.A., and Arnold, L.E. Pet facilitated psychotherapy in a hospital setting. *Current Psychiatric Therapies* 15: 277–286 (1975).

De Thomaso, M.T. Touch power and the screen of loneliness. *Perspectives in Psychiatric Care* 9(3): 112–118 (1971).

Downs, R.S. Bed rest and sensory disturbances. *American Journal of Nursing* 74(3): 434–438 (1974).

Dunn, C.A. Hands that help — but how? *Nursing Forum* 392–400 (October 1971).

Ellis, R. Unusual Sensory and Thought Disturbances After Cardiac Surgery. *American Journal of Nursing* 72: 2021 (1972).

Ernst, P. and Shaw, J. Touching is not taboo. *Geriatric Nursing* 1(3): 193–195 (1980).

Hall, E.T. *The Silent Language.* New York: Doubleday, 1956, p. 26.

Hennessey, M.J. Music and music therapy groups. In Burnside, I.M. (Ed.) *Working with the Elderly.* North Scituate, Mass.: Duxbury Press, 1978, pp. 255–270.

Hollander, M.H. The need or wish to be held. *Archives of General Psychiatry* 22: 445–453 (May 1970).

Hospital Tribune. Practice from a procrustean bed. Los Angeles, California (December 5, 1977; newspaper story about Dr. Duncan Halbert of Santa Cruz).

Kenshalo, D.R. Age changes in touch vibration, temperature, kinesthesia, and pain sensitivity. In Birren, J.E. and Schaie, K.W. *Handbook of the Psychology of Aging.* New York: Van Nostrand Reinhold, 1977.

Krauch, E. Personal conversation (1962). Ms. Krauch, translator of languages, writer, neighbor, and friend. Deceased.

Krizinotski, M.T. Human sexuality and nursing practice. *Nursing Clinics of North America* 8: 673–681 (December 1973).

Leshowitz, B. The infrared light transmission hearing aid. *Bulletin of Prosthetic Research.* BPR 10-32: 177–189 (1979).

Leshowitz, B. Lecture and personal consultation. Department of Psychology, Arizona State University, May 6, 1982.

McCorkle, R. Effects of touch on seriously ill patients. *Nursing Research* 23: 125–132 (March–April 1974).

Montagu, A. *Touching: The human Significance of the Skin.* New York: Columbia University Press, 1971, pp. 5–7, 102–103.

Moore, E.C. Using music with groups of geriatric patients. In Burnside, I.M. (Ed.) *Working with the Elderly: Group Processes and Techniques.* North Scituate, Mass.: Duxbury Press, 1978.

Moustakas, C.E. *The Touch of Loneliness.* Englewood Cliffs, N.J.: Prentice-Hall, 1975.

NAHSA, National Association of Hearing and Speech Agencies. *Simple Courtesies for the Hard of Hearing.* Washington D.C.: 1977 (reprint).

Pearson, J. Sensory deprivation. *Image* 10(2): 49–55 (1978).

Rockstein, M. and Sussman, M. *Biology of Aging.* Belmont, Calif.: Wadsworth, 1979, pp. 64–69.

Schiffman, S. Food Recognition by the Elderly, *Journal of Gerontology* 32(5): 586–592 (1977).

Shiffman, S. and Pasternak, M. Decreased Discrimination of Food Odor in the Elderly, *Journal of Gerontology* 34(1): 73–79 (1979).

Soll, D.B. Glaucoma. *American Family Physician* 9(1): 125–132 (1974).

Steffl, B. *The Meaning of Touch.* Slide cassette program, 1979 (copyright 1981).

Steffl, B.M. Touch and Human sexuality in later life, *Generations. Journal of the Western Gerontological Society* 6(1): 27–28 (1981).

Storlie, F. The human touch. *American Journal of Nursing* 111–112 (December 1962).

Sullivan, H.S. *The Interpersonal Theory of Psychiatry.* New York: Norton, 1953.

Timiras, P.S. *Developmental Physiology and Aging.* New York: Macmillan, 1972.

Verwoerdt, A. *Clinical Geropsychiatry.* Baltimore: Williams and Wilkins, 1976, pp. 255–265.

Weinberg, J. Sexual expression in late life. *American Journal of Psychiatry* 715 (November 1969).

White, M.A. Communication through touch! Report on innovative programs at Philadelphia Geriatric Center. *Concern* 19–21 (December–January 1977).

Yurick, A.G., Robb, S.S., Spier, B.E., and Ebert, N.J. *The Aged Person and the Nursing Process.* New York: Appleton-Century-Crofts, 1980, pp. 293–300, 318–327, 349–372.

7
Communication with the Elderly

Bernita M. Steffl

One must also listen to silences.
                    R.N. Butler and M. I. Lewis (1977)

The outstanding characteristic of lack of communication with the elderly (and indeed all ages) is not the generation gap or ageism, it is simply the almost universal inability to listen, let alone listen actively and effectively. This is readily demonstrated in everyday conversations between people of all ages:

Mother: "You like school, don't you dear?"
Son: "Johnie wouldn't play with me."
Mother: "School is not the place to play ....What did you learn in school today?"
Son: "Do you think I could have a dog like Johnie?"
                                    Epstein (1977)

Nurse: "Here's your medicine, Minnie, it will make you feel better."
Patient: "I used to get two little yellow pills that helped me so much."
Nurse: "It is important that you drink a lot of water with this medicine."
Patient: "I don't believe much in medicine; my condition doesn't change."
Nurse: "You should drink a full glass of water with this medicine. It's good for your kidneys."

(Conversation overheard in a hospital)

It is obvious in both conversations that neither the senders nor the receivers of messages were listening. (See also Figure 7-1.)

Talk to the Elderly

Conversation is the social interchange of life and living. The very old and sick old are often deprived of meaningful conversations for days on end. It becomes very easy for nurses to simply perform the nursing care and not make an effort to communicate, especially when the patient is confused, disoriented, or hard-of-hearing.

Old people who live alone also go for days with only minimal communication which takes place at the store or post office. They become a so-called nuisance if they slow down the line in the supermarket by their personal conversation with the cashier. They are often hungry for meaningful conversation.

The following exerpt taken from the letter of a middle-aged daughter whose mother died in a nursing home clearly indicates some directions and goals for professionals.

My mother spent fifteen of her last seventeen months on this earth in your nursing home. There she died. To my knowledge no one ever talked to my mother, even when she mentioned death. She was able to talk intelligently many times. Have you ever considered having an active, sensitive, trained person to help patients and families communicate, share feelings, show support? [Abstracted from a much longer and moving letter (Alpaugh and Haney, 1979)]

Stop, Look, and Listen

A brief review of communication theory and process seems in order here because professionals involved in the delivery of health care consistently report that communication problems are always present — with staff, community agencies, and the government. Some years ago a master teacher of communication skills opened the eyes and ears of this writer. She taught everyone to stop, look, and listen in this way:

'Is Anybody Listening?'

The following letter was forwarded to The Times by the author's niece. Neither woman identified herself "because we are fearful." Although The Times ordinarily will not accept anonymous articles for publication, the editors believe that this woman's message is exceptional.

Hello! Is there anyone out there who will listen to me?

How can I convince you that I am a prisoner?

For the past five years, I have not seen a park or the ocean or even just a few feet of grass.

I am an 84-year-old woman, and the only crime which I have committed is that I have an illness which is called chronic. I have severe arthritis and about five years ago I broke my hip. While I was recuperating in the hospital, I realized that I would need extra help at home. But there was no one. My son died 35 years ago, my husband, 25 years ago. I have a few nieces and nephews who come by to visit once in a while, but I couldn't ask them to take me in, and the few friends I still have are just getting by, themselves. So I wound up at a convalescent hospital in the middle of Los Angeles.

All kinds of people are thrown together here. I sit and watch, day after day. As I look around this room, I see the pathetic ones (maybe the lucky ones—who knows?) who have lost their minds, and the poor souls who should be out but nobody comes to get them, and the sick ones

who are in pain. We are all locked up together.

I have been keeping in touch with the world through the newspaper, my one great luxury. For the last few years I have been reading about the changes in Medicare regulations. All I can see from these improvements is that nurses spend more time writing. For, after all, how do you regulate caring?

Most of the nurse's aides who work here are from other countries. Even those who can speak English don't have much in common with us. So they hurry to get their work done as quickly as possible. There are a few caring people who work here, but there are so many of us who are needy for that kind of honest attention.

A doctor comes to see me once a month. He spends approximately three to five seconds with me and then a few more minutes writing in the chart or joking with the nurses. (My own doctor doesn't come to convalescent hospitals, so I had to take this one.) I sometimes wonder about how the nurses' aides feel when they work so hard for so little money and then see that the person who spends so little time is the one who is paid the most.

I notice that most of the physicians who come here don't even pay attention to things like whether their patient's fingernails are trimmed or whether their body is foul-smelling. Last week when the doctor came to see me, I hadn't had a bath in 10 days because the nurse's aide took too long on her coffee break. She wrote in the

chart that she gave me a shower—anyway, who would check or care? I would be labeled as a complainer or losing my memory, and that would be worse.

It is now 8 o'clock. Time to be in bed. I live through each night—and it is a long night—with memories of my childhood. I lived on an apple farm in Washington.

I remember how I used to bake, pies and cakes and cookies for friends and neighbors and their children. In the five years I have been here, I have had no choice—no choice of when I want to eat or what I want to eat. It has been so long since I have tasted fruit like mango or cherries.

As I write this, I keep wishing I were exaggerating.

These last five years feel like the last five hundred of my life.

Last year, one of the volunteers here read us a poem. It was by Robert Browning. I think it was called "Rabbi Ben Ezra." It went something like this: "Grow old along with me, the best of life is yet to be." How can I begin to tell you that growing old in America is for me an unbelievable, lonely nightmare?

I am writing this because many of you may live to be old like me, and by then it will be too late. You, too, will be stuck here and wonder why nothing is being done, and you, too, will wonder if there is any justice in life. Right now, I pray every night that I may die in my sleep and get this nightmare of what someone has called life over with, if it means living in this prison day after day.   □

Figure 7-1.

When you go into a room to see a patient or knock on the door for a home visit, stop. Stop and put yourself in a state of no mind. Put everything out of your mind except what you are about to do. Don't let distractions like all the work you have to do or the quart of milk you must pick up on the way home creep into your mind while you are talking with your client. You can't do it now anyway. LOOK, look with all of your senses and assessment skills, at the person, the affect, and the environment. LISTEN, listen actively and with the third ear to hear what the person did not say. (Madore, 1970)

This lesson is very applicable in working with older individuals and groups, and is a helpful guide to avoid the common pitfall of not listening. One must also listen to silences (Butler and Lewis, 1977) and strive to hear what the person did not say.

Space does not permit us, and it would be impossible, to do justice to even basic communication theory here. The intent is to suggest that professionals always examine their communication skills in terms of (1) the intent, purpose, and motivation they have for communicating; (2) the clarity, level, amount, and completeness of the message; (3) their voice, body language, position, space, and motion; (4) the climate or atmosphere of interest, trust, support, and openness; (5) the effect on the receiver; and (6) feedback exchange.

By allowing ourselves to be affected in the region of our solar plexus by another person's posture, facial expression, or tone of voice, we

Table 7-1. Communicating with the Elderly.

INFLUENCING FACTORS	BARRIERS	TECHNIQUES AND STRATEGIES

Culture
Anxiety
Illness
Somatic concerns
Sensory orientation
Cautiousness
Losses and loss reaction
Fear of loss of control
Fear of death
Unrealistic expectations of self,
physician, and nurse
Education – understanding
Attitudes
Socioeconomic status
Past history
	Non-listening
	Sensory deprivation: hearing,
	vision, touch, taste, smell
	Environmental setting
	  Noise
	  Degree of privacy
	Time
	  Amount of time
	  Time of day
	Tone of voice
	  Condescending
	  Encouraging
	Language of sender and receiver
		Identify yourself – clearly and often
		Speak clearly and slowly
		Use appropriate terminology
		Pace conversation or interview for
		comprehension and response
		Pay attention to nonverbal communi-
		cation
		Use touch
		Maintain continuity
		Use redundancy cues
		Prepare person for discussion of
		specific topic: "We will be discussing
		the news for one half hour."
		Be realistic, but hopeful

NOTE: The items listed in this table have direct implications for developing care plans for older individuals at home or in institutions (adapted from Burnside, 1980; Epstein, 1977; Pfeiffer, 1980).

can usually tell immediately whether that other person is sad or cheerful, or whether he is pretending to be cheerful while attempting to hide the fact that he is sad. Professionals must try to gain an impression by the way in which a person expresses himself in relation to the world around him and in relation to his past and future self. It is not an easy task to allow another person to unfold his message in front of us, to acknowledge that message, and to respond to it in a way that will be meaningful to the sender (Ujhely, 1972); see Table 7-1.

Touch is generally perceived positively by patients and conveys many messages. It is an especially important part of communication with elderly widows and widowers (see Figure 7-2; also see Chapter 6 for discussion of sensory needs and touch).

Interviewing the Elderly

Irene Burnside defines three distinct factors which can assist helping professionals to communicate effectively during interviews (Burnside, 1980):

1. *Assessment of distance.* The immediate task is to establish comfortable physical distance in a sphere or bubble of space which is conducive to communication

(usually 1 1/2–2 1/2 feet). The interviewer's placement of self for face-to-face and eye-to-eye contact is necessary. The placement of the elderly interviewee is even more important in terms of physical comfort in the seating arrangement, and the elderly often have territorial imperatives that must be respected. Burnside points out from her own work and the research of others that it is only recently that nurses have begun to acknowledge "patient territory." This physical and psychological distancing by patients

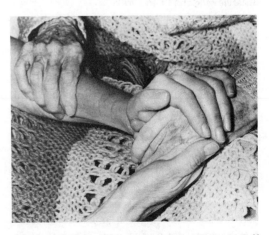

Figure 7-2. Communication by touch. (Photo by Jeff Stanton.)

is affected by: (1) diminished attention span, (2) physical exhaustion, (3) poor interpersonal relationships, and frequently, (4) a recent dose of medication.

2. *Assessment of hearing.* Almost all older people have some hearing loss and usually hear better from one ear than the other. The interviewer should ask about this and position himself accordingly.

3. *Assessment of comprehension.* Two common barriers to comprehension are dementia and aphasia. Both have many dimensions and variations. Disorientation may come and go, so it is possible that a patient who was lucid and coherent one day may be confused or disoriented the next. Confusional states may arise from acute illness or medication and, in turn, be quickly alleviated. Assessment tools for this are described in Chapter 12. Aphasia is depressing and frustrating to the patient and to the caretaker. The interviewer needs to determine whether the aphasia is motor, sensory, or global, and then to design appropriate communication techniques. Cultural background, language, and education strengths and limitations are also major factors in comprehension.

Interviewing the "Old Old"

There is a rapidly increasing number of "old old" (over age 75) in our population and an increasing need for an interest in research in this cohort group. Schmidt (1975), in a study of residents of two homes for the aged, demonstrated that the very old who are impaired can be interviewed successfully if extra time is spent and if instruments and approaches are honed to meet their needs. She lists six special challenges commonly encountered in interviewing the "old old": intermittent confusion, chronic confusion, dysphagia, problems of sight and hearing, unwillingness, and overprotective nurses and relatives. The cardinal rule throughout is: go slow (Schmidt, 1975).

Cognitive Function and Sensory Alterations

The nurse must be prepared to assess for cognitive function and ability. This is a prerequisite to effective communication with the frail elderly. Patients in the age group over 65 are at high risk for cognitive impairment. There are many methods of assessing cognitive functioning; some are discussed in Chapter 12. A number of helpful, reasonably reliable, and valid assessment tools have been developed by Kahn, Goldfarb, Pollack, and Peck (1960) and by Pfeiffer (1974). The Kahn-Goldfarb et al. Mental Status Questionnaire and Pfeiffer's Short Mental Status Questionnaire are reproduced in Chapter 12. Both use a scale to measure the degree of intellectual functioning, orientation to time, place, and person, and intellectual impairment.

The impact of sensory losses and sensory alterations, with their ensuing deprivation, on communications with the elderly is second only to the failure of people to listen and hear what is being said. Assessment for sensory deficits and intervention strategies are discussed in detail in Chapter 6.

Communicating with a Stroke Victim

Each stroke patient is an individual, and though the affliction shows itself in common signs, each person responds uniquely. When communicating for professional reasons or visiting, sit on the "good side" because of the possible damage to vision and hearing capabilities on the other side. The following are guidelines for communicating with a stroke victim with communication deficits (Carnevali and Patrick, 1979; *Healing with Time and Love,* 1979):

- Talk to them in normal volume, one person at a time.
- Use short sentences; don't change the subject abruptly.
- Let the patient struggle to get the word out. Try not to supply the word until it is absolutely necessary. Do not correct mistakes.
- Assure patients that you want them to try talking.

- Phrase your questions so that the aphasic person can respond with a yes or no, or with a movement of the head.
- Start a sentence and let the patient finish.
- Allow time to finish conversation.
- Writing the word is sometimes helpful — bring a large pad.
- If the stroke patient cannot write, use pictures of common things to which he can point.
- Give the patient choices. This facilitates independence and helps supply the missing vocabulary. (Do you want candy? Do you want fruit?)
- Explore the possibility of singing (this may come automatically).
- Instead of correcting errors, restate what you think the person is trying to say.
- Remember that the wrong words come out sometimes, so "no" may not mean "no."
- Ignore profanity.
- Be honest and realistic, but always give hope, encouragement, and touch.

Nonverbal Communication

A great deal has been said elsewhere in this book about nonverbal communication such as attitudes reflected in behaviors, mannerisms, body language, music, and touch. Teaching and learning about nonverbal communication for work with patients of all ages are basic parts of nursing educations. The use of nonverbal dialogue and nonverbal therapeutic strategies by specific design, in work with the frail elderly, appears to be relatively unexplored, and is perhaps unexplored because the physically frail and mentally impaired elderly are not expected to respond to art or music therapy.

In a study of 12 brain-damaged nursing home residents, 63–89 years of age, an art therapy program demonstrated rather remarkable revitalizing results for patients with all levels of impairment. Some had lived withdrawn and in the isolation of their inner realm for years (Fischer and Fischer, 1978).

SUMMARY

Young students frequently ask for opening questions for interviewing and communicating with older individuals. There are the usual dos and don'ts and many suggested topics. This writer prefers a guideline of six questions developed by Thompson (1970) which leads us to focus on the person first as a individual:

- Who is this man?
- What has he done during his lifetime?
- How did he get to where he is now?
- What is important to him?
- What has he enjoyed doing?
- What are his expectations for the future?

The third question often leads to life history. A final suggestion is to listen to what topic the client brings up first and then use that information or clue as a starter for further conversation.

REFERENCES

Alpaugh, P. and Haney, M. *Counseling the Older Adult: A Training Manual* (2nd printing). Los Angeles: University of Southern California, The Andrus Gerontology Center, 1979.

Bakdash, D.P. Communicating with the aged patient: a systems view. *Journal of Gerontological Nursing* 3(5): (1977).

Burnside, I.M. (Ed.). *Working with the Elderly: Group Processes and Techniques.* 2nd Ed. North Scituate, Mass.: Duxbury Press, 1984.

Burnside, I.M. Interviewing the aged. In Burnside, I.M. (Ed.) *Psychosocial Nursing Care of the Aged* (2nd ed.). New York: McGraw-Hill, 1980.

Butler, R.N. and Lewis, M. *Aging and Mental Health* (3rd ed.). St. Louis: C.V. Mosby, 1982.

Carnevali, D.L. and Patrick, M. (Eds.). *Nursing Management for the Elderly.* Philadelphia: J.B. Lippincott, 1979, p. 289.

Epstein, C. *Learning to Care for the Aged.* Reston, Va: Reston Publishing-Prentice Hall, 1977. pp. 1-17, 43-105, 155-168.

Fischer, T. and Fischer, R. Nonverbal dialogue with the brain-damaged elderly. *Continia Psychiatrica* 20: 61-78 (1978).

Graney, M.J. and Graney, E.E. Communications activity substitution in aging. *Journal of Communication* 24(4): 88-96 (1974).

Healing with Time and Love. Santa Monica, Calif.: Westside Ecumenical Conference, 1979.

Kahn, R.L., Goldfarb, A.I., Pollack, M., and Peck, A. Brief objective measure for the determination of mental status in the aged. *American Journal of Psychiatry* 117: 326 (1960).

Kuzmierczak, F.G., Moser, D.H., and Russo, M.A. Communication problems encountered when caring for the elderly individual. *Journal of Gerontological Nursing* 1(1): 21-27 (1975).

Madore, E. Nursing education course materials. Unpublished material College of Nursing, Arizona State University, 1970.

Moore, E.C. Using music with groups of geriatric patients. In Burnside, I. M. (Ed.) *Working with the Elderly: Group Processes and Techniques.* North Scituate, Mass.: Duxbury Press, 1978, pp. 275–291.

Pfeiffer, E. The psychosocial evaluation of the elderly patient. In Busse, E. W. and Blazer, D.G. (Eds.) *Handbook of Geriatric Psychiatry.* New York: Van Nostrand Reinhold, 1980, pp. 275–284.

Schmidt, M.G. Interviewing the "old old." *The Gerontologist* 544–547 (December 1975).

Thompson, P.W. Mental health of the aged. In *Summary Proceedings of Workshop: The RN and the Aged Patient.* Los Angeles, Calif.: University of Southern California, The Andrus Gerontology Center, 1970, pp. 1–8.

Ujhely, G.B. Nursing assessment of psychosocial function in the aged. Unpublished paper, Adelphi University, New York, 1972.

8
Loss, Grief, and Death in Old Age

Marjorie Vander Linden Albert
Bernita M. Steffl

For the aged person, social death may be worse than physical death.

(Paraphrased by B. Buckelew, 1982)

A development of recent years is the rediscovery of the realities of death and dying. A new "death awareness" has evolved. This awareness was initially stimulated by Feifel and Engel who first identified the adjustment that any loss requires. They recognized that grief and mourning were a necessary part of the resolution of any loss. They identified three stages: the first reaction is *shock and disbelief* which can last a few minutes or several days; the second is *developing an awareness* when reality is viewed; and the third, the actual grief work or *restitution.* Normal successful grief work may require a full year to recovery (Engel, 1964; Feifel, 1959). Bereavement whether prolonged or usual has resulted in physiological changes, so that the stress of grief and later illness are related (Lindemann, 1944). The literature provided by these and other authorities refers to death as one of many losses. Death is the most crucial major loss and is, of course, most imminent for the elderly.

Kübler-Ross (1969) enlarges upon this theme and describes five possible stages of dying. She views death as the final opportunity for growth. Much of her work is based upon actual interviews with dying individuals; see Table 8-1 for Kübler-Ross' stages. The length of time or sequence of these stages can vary for the dying as well as for those who grieve. Each person may experience these phases according to individual needs. Kübler-Ross' international recognition and fame for actual work with the dying have stimulated an awakening of professional responsibility by health care givers to actively care for the dying aged (Kübler-Ross, 1969).

Quint researched the inclusion of content on death in nursing curricula and found it lacking. She questioned how nurses could care for those with terminal disease and yet deny a need for knowing how one experiences death (Quint, 1967). This denial of death has changed to a current high level of interest, with many courses available on the subject, textbooks acknowledging and suggesting interventions, experiential and media dramatizations, and even daily newspapers carrying information for the public on the resolution of death. Currently, the hospice movement is sweeping the country.

Loss and grief work and death and dying are of special interest to the gerontologist because as fewer people die of infectious disease, they live into old age. More deaths are occurring in old age. In 1900, in the United States, only 25% of all deaths involved individuals over the age of 65. This figure rose to 63% by the year 1970 and will continue as technology allows man to survive previously fatal diseases (Neugarten and Maddox, 1978).

There are some thanatologists who are concerned about this current and growing intellectualization of the subject; they fear that death talk and interest may be a fad that will fade. The elderly are conspicuously absent from writings and education about death. They are perhaps the most sorely neglected group when it comes to honest talk about death with professionals and family. See Table 8-2 for subject matter and goals for death education for elderly persons. These topics and goals do not interfere with any religious orientation; they are topics that can be covered in several sessions, and they deal with both knowledge and feelings (Wass, 1980).

Table 8-1. Kübler-Ross' Stages of Dying.

1. Denial	"No, not me." This is a typical reaction when patients learn they are terminally ill. Denial, says Doctor Ross, is important and necessary. It helps cushion the impact of the patient's awareness that death is inevitable.
2. Rage and anger	"Why me?" The patient resents the unfairness that others will remain healthy and alive while he must die. God is a special target for anger, since He is regarded as imposing, arbitrarily, the death sentence. To those who are shocked at her claim that such anger is not only permissible but inevitable, Doctor Ross replies succinctly, "God can take it."
3. Bargaining	"Yes, me, but . . . ." Patients accept the fact of death but strike bargains for more time. Mostly they bargain with God — "even people who never talked with God before." They promise to be good or to do something in exchange for another week or month or year of life. "What they promise is totally irrelevant, because they don't keep their promises anyway."
4. Depression	"Yes, me." First, the person mourns past losses, things not done, wrongs committed. Then he enters a state of "preparatory grief," getting ready for the arrival of death. The patient grows quiet, doesn't want visitors. "When a dying patient doesn't want to see you anymore, this is a sign he has finished his unfinished business with you, and it is a blessing. He can now let go peacefully."
5. Acceptance	"My time is very close now and it's all right." Doctor Ross describes this final stage as "not a happy stage, but neither is it unhappy. It's devoid of feelings, but it's not resignation, it's really a victory." (Kübler-Ross 1975)

Table 8-2. Subject Matter and Goals for Death Education for the Elderly.

SUBJECT MATTER	GOALS
Patients' rights	To provide the elderly patient complete and honest information about diagnosis, treatment, and prognosis.
The right to die	An informed patient in regard to legislation regarding the right to die — some states have passed such legislation.
A living will	A nonlegal document prepared well before the terminal illness stage, its purpose is to inform survivors of the wish to be allowed to die and not be kept alive by artificial means or heroic measures.
Legal matters	To provide assistance in taking care of legal affairs, and to encourage review of a will and insurance beneficiaries through the proper agency or organizations.
Emotional support systems (e.g., hospice)	No one should die alone. Many old people live alone, have no family, and need help in linking up with a significant other. Sometimes the health professional is the only significant other.
Postmortem care	Patients and families often live in fear and mystery about postmortem care. Families should be allowed to participate in closing the eyes and placing their loved one in a comfortable position immediately after death if they wish. They should be informed of physiological changes that will occur, such as rigor mortis, and of procedures that will take place in preparation for burial.
Autopsy	Decisions regarding authority for autopsy and release of remains should be a right of the dying; this also assists survivors.
Death certificate	The details of formal closure to a civil life require accurate information for governmental records and assure the dying person of his proper identity after death.
Funerals	To supply information about funeral costs and practices, and about the state's body disposal laws and public health requirements. To see that the older person's wishes regarding funeral, lying in state, cremation, or burial place are carried out.

NOTE: Adapted from Kalish (1981), Pennington (1978), Steffl (1976), and Wass (1980).

DEALING WITH LOSSES IN OLD AGE

For the older adult, physical losses are multitudinous. By the time individuals reach 60, they probably will have lost some physical abilities such as strength, vision, and hearing. They will also have experienced psychosocial losses such as a career, work, or family role and the death of a loved one. The list of losses is long and variable. Most aging adults have the potential for a large number of crucial losses (see Table 5-2).

The disequilibrium that occurs with a loss results in both mental and physical manifestations. An example of physical symptoms is seen in the spouse of the dying patient who, in the next year, has an increased incidence of illness. If chronic grief cannot be resolved, somatic symptoms evolve. When this grief-associated illness is extreme, the likelihood of terminal or debilitating disease is high (Burnside, 1969). The aged have fewer support systems and less physical strength for dealing with the changes occurring after a traumatic loss. Early assessment for problem areas and interventions is imperative for successful loss resolution.

A result of the study of grieving has been the recognition of ten stages of grief experienced by bereaved persons. The stages are shown in Table 8-3. For some, many of these stages may

be gone through in a few hours; others may require months. The whole process of successful grieving may require 1–2 years. Individual variations are common. When grief is not managed successfully, depression and/or physical illness will occur (Albert, 1979).

A natural support system is composed of family and close friends. When family is gone, the support system may expand to include health professionals and service personnel (barber, policeman, store clerk, etc.). This support seems to buffer the effect that stressors have to cause disease and enables the individual to protect self (Gelein, 1980). When a natural support system is lacking, a social system should be developed to meet these same needs. Individuals who do not have a support system network tend to have greater and more severe psychological symptoms than those who do have adequate support.

Situation

Mrs. W. H. was widowed by the unexpected cardiac death of her husband of 52 years. Her grieving was severe and was affected by the lack of natural support systems available in the new home they had moved to just six months earlier. She described herself as always having

Table 8-3. Stages of Grief.

STAGE IDENTIFIED	DESCRIPTION
1. Shock and surprise	Numbs comprehension; gives time for response.
2. Emotional release	How should my grief be expressed?
3. Loneliness	Acute awareness that person is gone.
4. Anxiety and physical distress	Concern over future and/or physical needs.
5. Panic	Thoughts are immobilized as grief occupies all.
6. Guilt	Questions about what else I could have done?
7. Hostility and projection	Accuses others of wrong judgment or mistreatment.
8. Lassitude	Suffering in silence with psychosomatic symptoms and suicide possible.
9. Resolution of grief	Working through grief and reestablishment of self.
10. Readjustment to reality	Adjustment to changed life status.
Time frame: May require 1–2 years of time to complete bereavement.	

NOTE: Adapted with permission from Albert, W.C. The management of grief. Unpublished paper (1979).

been "taken care of" by her husband who did all the planning and made all decisions. Suddenly she experienced the profound stage of wondering what she would do now? Had she let her husband do too much in his retirement and in the recent move? Did the stress kill him? She also blamed the new doctor they had called because he didn't demand hospitalization when her husband was short of breath. Mrs. W. H. was helped to ventilate her feelings of isolation, guilt, and anger by the visiting nurse. She was directed to a senior citizen's group and encouraged to make friends. During the first six months she wondered if she was mentally unbalanced because she felt like crying all the time. She was encouraged to think about her husband, and to remember both the good times and the bad, and then was always helped to come back to the present. This gave her permission to grieve and not be afraid of going insane. After 14 months, she was assessed as successfully finishing her grief work and accepting widowhood. She was driving her own car and was active in two social groups.

Another example of working through and acceptance was provided by an aging widow encountered at a conference:

When I asked the attractive white-haired lady across from me at a large breakfast meeting where she was from and how she happened to come to this part of the country, she said, "We came here to retire, we arrived on a Friday. On Tuesday, my husband died. It was our wedding anniversary. We had been married on a Tuesday. I didn't think I'd make it. I know every restaurant and coffee shop in town, even the clerks in all the shops in the shopping mall. I'll never forget the salesgirls at one of the stores — mainly because they listened and they were kind. Finally, I decided to try for a job. I didn't expect to get one. It has helped me so much in adjusting."

Widows and Widowers

The aging female who loses her husband faces not only a great personal loss but the added doom of widowhood. Widowhood presents special problems because of the dramatic change in the ratio of sex representation. The male population reduces significantly. The widow, who for years has been one-half of a mixed partnership, suddenly finds herself as one member of a female-dominated society (Schwartz and Peterson, 1979). The change requires adjustment in both social expectations and companionship roles. The widow who consequently develops a close, confident (nuturing) role with someone soon after the loss of a mate fares better than the individual who maintains an aloneness (Epstein, 1975; Gelein, 1980).

One man out of every six over age 65 is widowed. His opportunity for remarriage is high. He is more likely to remarry than a woman who loses a spouse. Up to half of the women in the same age group become widows and are less likely to remarry. Factors contributing to the lower incidence of older widows' remarrying are the decreasing number of available men, widowers' remarrying women much younger than themselves, and the unlikely marriage of older women to younger men (Kastenbaum, 1978).

Attitudes and Views of the Elderly toward Death and Dying

The consciousness of death changes from childhood through middle years and into old age. Kastenbaum (1978) identifies the loneliness characteristic of the old person who survives his peers. Death becomes a reality when one's spouse and friends are taken. Even though the surviving individual lives on, his losses are many. Separation after separation occurs as fewer and fewer friends or relatives remain. The surviving individual is more alone and constantly reminded that, ultimately, he too will die. This situation of being surrounded by losses provides a reality from which there is no escape. It is stated that the developmental task of preparing for death includes coming to some peace or satisfaction with what we have done with our lives (see Chapter 5).

Butler and Lewis (1982) describe the "life review" as sometimes being painful but also giving new significance and meaning to one's life: it helps in preparation for death by mitigating fear and anxiety, and it gives people an opportunity to decide what to do with the time left to them. A life review is a formal reminiscence of past accomplishments and crises. As the aged are helped through a life review, the "milestones" along the way provide reassurance that they lived and coped as best they could under the circumstances.

An "oral life history" is a talking reminiscence which assists the aged in coming to terms with their current situation and with the fact that they are aging. An oral life history consists of questions about two main themes: how one's life has been, and how it feels to be old. Culture and previous productivity seem to influence contentment with the aging process (Safier, 1976; Whalen, 1980).

The search for life's meaning may arouse tensions rather than, or as well as, equilibrium (Frankel, 1959). Even though some anxiety is useful, this can cause more problems. The implications, as seen by the authors are that the older person, especially the dying older person, may be so disappointed in himself that he sinks into a hopeless and fearful depression. In reminiscing and life review, the professional can assist the grieving, depressed, or dying person in sorting out his good works and strengths, and identifying the values he will leave behind.

Sooner or later each of us, if given time to review life, must sort out the meaning of life and face death (Steffl, 1976). When looking at overall family development, the developmental task of aging is adjustment to the loss of one's family, spouse, and significant others (Duvall, 1967). If previous developmental stages are unresolved or if the aged person becomes too uncomfortable from the stress of looking at his own life, he may use defenses of denial or anger to protect himself. We must respect his coping ability or lack thereof and not seek to expose him to stresses before the strength to face them is available. Time usually helps in the adjustment to a personal crisis.

Death is a realistic concern of the aged, and they will of necessity acknowledge death's possibility. Each individual may withdraw or actively prepare for death in much the same manner as he has approached living. Talking

about funeral arrangements or the disposition of earthly goods is not to be viewed as an abnormal obsession with death. Just as life review and reminiscing help one to accept oneself, allowing the individual to talk about plans regarding his death helps him to prepare for it with the assurance that his final wishes will be carried out (Neale, 1973).

HELPING THE AGED WITH GRIEF WORK

In the first stage of shock and disbelief, the survivor is stunned by the hurt and psychological stress of the loss. This stage can vary in time from minutes to days. In the second stage of developing awareness, the individual moves past shock to viewing the reality of loss. Spouses may cry, express anger toward the health care staff or others, or condemn themselves and feel unworthwhile or empty. During the third stage, working through grief begins, as the survivor makes funeral arrangements, settles the estate, and moves on to making decisions about life. Within 12 months successful grieving should be accomplished, leaving the individual ready to face new situations.

An assessment to measure the success of grieving of the survivor is based on how the deceased is remembered. The survivor should be able to recall and remember both good and bad about the deceased in a realistic manner (Engel, 1964). The initial visit to the griever should be prior to expected death when status and needs can be assessed. The first goal is to help the individual identify the relationship between the present crisis and stress (Fell, 1977). The health care personnel can support verbalization to relieve temporary tension and anxiety. If physical stress is very great, medication may be useful to insure proper rest. This is especially important at the time of death when the acute loss results in high anxiety, but it is important to allow measures to resolve the grief and not to overmedicate the aged so that grief work is retarded. Religious support should be considered. The appropriate clergy should be called according to individual desire. Clergy will assist in the expression of grief and foster the move toward preparing for service arrangements.

Involvement in funeral rituals has been criticized because of the expense incurred by those who are left with limited income. While the cost should not be excessive, the funeral service does serve to aid in the resolution of grief. A memorial service is a time to say the last goodbye. The surviving spouse and relatives are supported by the presence and the expressed concern of friends. The sympathy given at the funeral is usually therapeutic.

Sometimes the attention of others wanes too soon afterward and the griever is left alone (Fell, 1977). The nurse will have to seek resources and other contacts for the person. The survivor next needs to look at what or who is available as another avenue of gratification to fill the void left by the deceased. In reality, this substitution is neither easy nor complete, but as healing takes place, new interests are found which do fill the gap and living goes on. As resolution progresses the health care worker can appraise the present situation and plan for the future. The person should be encouraged about being able to successfully function at a new level with positive coping mechanisms. It should be suggested that periodically the individual will be confronted by a reminder of the bereaved and the bereavement, and that though this will be painful, his current strengths will foster continuing resolution (Fell, 1977). The process of remembering the deceased and then letting go is therapeutic. This intense "feeling" and then "releasing" assist the individual in moving on toward resolution of grief (Steffl, 1976).

On the anniversary of the death, wedding anniversaries, birthdays, or special holidays, the remembrances are especially painful. The nurse, care giver, or family can assist the survivor by contact and concern, and can help make specific plans for special days so that the griever will not be alone. Club and group activities can help a grieving person through the holidays more easily. Sometimes as the grieving person joins a group to gain help, he later becomes a helper. As one is successfully helped by socialization, the transition from the role of receiver to helper is common. The behavior of those in the supportive role has been observed during contact; later, as the grievers identify with the worker, they too begin to help others. This is especially true of widow-to-widow programs in which lay people help each other. Dependence on a professional is never reinforced in these groups; rather, they allow the individual to grow and utilize new strengths.

HELPING THE AGED AND THEIR FAMILIES THROUGH THE DYING PROCESS

The object of nursing care in situations where death is expected is to assist the dying and their loved ones. The dying person is the central theme of care for the loved ones, and activity is directed — for the first time — not to getting the person well but to caring until death occurs. This should not be viewed negatively, because *much* quality living can occur up to the point of death. The dying have many strengths in a time of crisis (see Table 8-1).

Open, honest communication is of utmost importance in caring for the aged dying. Communication with them demonstrates their importance and uniqueness. Communication allows them to be a part of the decision-making process concerning the time that is left and how to spend it (Putnam et al., 1980). Sometimes communication facilitates sharing the fears and unknowns of death, but death is not the only topic. Many day-to-day problems can only be solved by communicating. The nurse should not limit her concept of therapeutic communication to times when death is verbalized. The living-dying episode as described by Pattison (1978) shows that much of daily living is of prime importance. Assisting the individual in adjusting to current demands or solving everyday minor problems is therapeutic. The here and now of the problems of daily living causes us to be conscious of "living until death" and not "dying until death." When support systems are weak and life is fragile, the aged need honest expressions of care on a day in, day out basis.

Another aspect of care of the dying is the physical presence of being there. Topics of importance frequently surface when the care giver takes the time to be there or to have family and friends there and available. The care giver is exposed to a personal loss with close involvement. This is a time when the professional may share grief; it means getting involved. With the possible emotional risk also comes the possibility of great reward: first, the feeling of being truly helpful, and second, the personal growth which results from recognizing and resolving grief.

Honest communication means that the individual has a right to know the truth. Unless there has been a pattern of denial in previous life experiences, truth is desired. Sometimes this might include saying, "I don't know what will happen next in your case, but I'll be here to care for you," or "We can't really expect any more improvement."

The certainty of death is accepted; the time and place are not known. Most people contemplate a death which occurs late in life, after an illness with associated gradual deterioration. However, the events that lead up to an impending death are more apt to be unknown and cause personal anxiety. Identification of the usual changes and "caring" during the last hours will help acquaint nurses with their own feelings and with the opportunities for giving psychological, as well as physiological, support during death and bereavement periods.

Physical and Psychosocial Aspects of Nursing Intervention in Imminent Death

As expected death approaches, anticipatory grief is present. Both the dying person and the surrounding significant others should be encouraged to recognize and express the feelings of loss they are experiencing. Significant others who are removed by time or distance should be called so they may say goodbye for the last time. It is not possible to predict when death will happen so individuals who wish to be notified should be reminded to finish any necessary business while the dying person is still able to communicate.

The following needs have been identified by interviews and observations of mature adults facing imminent death: dignity, hope, pain-free comfort, freedom from suffocation, presence of others, place of choice, religious support, and a living will.

Dignity. Dignity is an attainable need in those facing death. We should admire their attitude and dignity in this last and most crucial loss (Saunders, 1978). In recent years, with the trend toward honesty in diagnosis, the individual has been more knowledgeable and involved in decisions about his care. Giving information early in treatment fosters both hope and realistic approaches to problems. The individual is approached with recognition and appreciation of his abilities. At this final phase, dignity is reinforced when the person is still talked to, listened to, and included in decisions about his care whenever possible.

Hope. Hope should be fostered at all times. Many patients have survived their doctors and nurses. We cannot predict the time of death — to do so is a fallacy. Patients who have been told they will die in six months have lived much longer and then have become angry because they had prepared for death sooner. The family and those in the support system have also responded negatively because everyone had been "over-ready" (Weisman, 1979).

Hope allows constructive living to continue. As the individual prays for a miracle, internal acceptance may be present and the prayer is really for eternal life or eternal peace.

The nursing intervention in hope is to allow expression of both the best and the worst that can happen. Hope includes both alternatives, with full recognition that the best is wanted although the worst may occur (Werner-Beland, 1980).

Pain-free Comfort. Many individuals identify the most common anticipated fear associated with death as being uncontrollable pain. The fears associated with cancer reinforce this. Much of society believes that cancer always causes severe pain. In reality, only about 40% of persons with cancer have severe pain, and current control measures reduce perceived pain to the point where this is a solvable problem. Based on the philosophy of St. Christopher's Hospice, pain medications should be given freely. The type and degree of pain are assessed at its onset, the appropriate medication and strength are given, and then these are increased as needed. Brompton's or hospice mix is given on a routine basis at designated intervals to keep the person free of severe pain (Stoddard, 1978). The emphasis is on control to prevent pain rather than on relieving pain when it occurs. It is important to again assess any new symptoms of pain, as the location and possible cause. It cannot be assumed that all pain is the same in quality or etiology. As imminent death approaches, pain needs may change. Medications may have to be given by injection or intravenously for better absorption. Family members may have to learn how to give injections — before the need becomes evident — if the person is cared for at home.

Morphine is currently being used both orally and intravenously for severe pain. Not long ago morphine administered orally was believed to be a poor drug for cancer pain, but recent studies have shown that when morphine is properly administered, it is equal in effectiveness to, or better than, Brompton's cocktail (Lipman, 1980). (Brompton's cocktail contains a variable amount of morphine, 10 mgm of cocaine, 2.5 ml. of ethyl alcohol (98%), 5 ml. of flavouring syrup and a varying amount of chloroform water for a total of 20 ml.)

Freedom from Suffocation. Another common fear that should be recognized and treated is fear of suffocating and being unable to breathe. Not all persons experience respiratory distress, but when it does occur it is frightening. Suffocation is associated with anxiety and helplessness. The nurse may request an order for oxygen by nasal prongs so that the flow of air is felt. Labored respirations are painful for the family to witness during this last stage, and oxygen administration satisfies this need.

Presence of Others. We say that one of the most important goals is not to let a person die alone, yet, many do — especially the elderly. Studies indicate that in the traditional hospital settings in previous years, terminally ill patients were placed in rooms far from the nurses' station and responses to the call lights were slow (Quint, 1967). During the 1960s and 1970s, nurses and society became more aware of death and associated fears. Some hospitals

have nurse specialists to work with terminal patients and their families. Few nursing homes have such specialists readily available.

The patient and family may request a private room, but the nurse should come frequently and assess their needs. By leaving the door open and communicating often and routinely, the nurse provides an important source of supportive care.

Frequently, as the person is dying, he becomes less interactive with others, mainly using one significant other. The nurse can take this cue and focus her care toward supporting this significant other because he has been selected as meaningful to the dying person. Asking about that individual's physical and mental well-being and the use of other support systems will facilitate the preservation of energy for dealing with the impending death.

Place of Choice. If given the opportunity, most people will choose to die in a familiar place with close friends. The hospice concept (discussed later in this chapter), borrowed from England and tempered the American way, gives evidence of the importance of this need. The hospice trend promotes a program of support for those who are terminally ill and want to die at home. Even when the patient remains in an institution, the philosophy of hospice care can be implemented with the same resolution benefits, that is allowing the patient as much family involvement as he desires and allowing him to be surrounded with the warmth of caring friends and perhaps even a pet.

Religious Support. There is a wide variation in the type of religious support needed by the dying aged and their family. This is best explained by differences in how individuals meet religious needs every day. In our society, the individual is allowed to worship in a personal fashion, and because of the cultural mix in this country, there are many different religious groups with unique traditions and mores regarding death and mourning (Watson and Maxwell, 1977). The health professional who avoids meeting religious needs frequently does so because of his own discomfort. When we face this task honestly and openly, we can meet the holistic needs of the aged.

First, determine what role religion has taken during previous situations and whether this has changed for the dying person. Most people will cope with or without structured religious support as they did in life (Weisman, 1979). For regular attenders church is often the place to seek solace with the Deity who transcends even this death struggle. For certain christian groups their belief is in a resurrected God who knows their innermost parts and thoughts, is with them, guides them even in the deepest trouble and is the eternal reassurance of ultimate power (Saunders, 1977). As health professionals, we can facilitate this continuing use of faith. Religious affiliation has also provided group cohesion. Fellow worshippers are a source of mutual consolation in times of grief.

The family's religious desires should also be determined. Even when the dying person has a separate or agnostic belief, the survivors may have distinct beliefs of their own. Providing access to a minister or priest will help when death is imminent. The presence of the clergy is desirable and important. Prayer is of great value. After the health professional's contact has ended, the religious community remains a continuing source of useful personal support.

A Living Will. Society has become more aware of death and terminal illness, and is establishing personal controls such as the living will. A living will can be drawn up by an individual whereby he communicates his desires about his eventual death situation. The person should be well and of an objective, clear mind when preparing the will. The will is appropriate for everybody, but it should definitely be prepared by individuals who do not want resuscitation or heroic measures undertaken in the event of impending death. By signing this form, they communicate a desire to allow the dignity and acceptance of inevitable death. They are relieving others of the burden of making a decision about survival with severe disability.

The Euthanasia Educational Council has produced a living will and suggested instructions see Figure 8-1 for a copy. The person should distribute copies of the signed document to his family, physician, and any other significant persons. Although many states have not recognized the legality of a "living will," it is usually honored because it promotes open discussion and acceptance of the dying individual's input into the decision. There should not be a focus on the fatal issue; rather, the emphasis is on quality of life up to death.

Physical Changes during Death and Nursing Intervention

When death is in progression, five changes are identified: loss of muscle tone, cessation of peristalsis, slowing of circulation, labored respirations, and loss of senses; lastly, there are the final signs of death. Each of the five changes requires specific nursing care (see Table 8-4).

THE HOSPICE MOVEMENT

Hospice is recognized as a way of dying, but actually it is a way of quality living.

Definition

Hospice is an ancient word which has a new meaning. Originally a medieval name for a way station for pilgrims and travelers where they could be replenished, refreshed, and cared for, hospice in the United States is described as an organized program of care for people going through life's last journey — dying and death. It is an interdisciplinary approach which provides palliative and supportive care for terminally ill patients and their families, either directly or on a consulting basis with the patient's physician or other community agencies such as a visiting nurse service.

The hospice movement evolved from a sense of responsibility to care for the dying. The first hospice in London, St. Christopher's Hospice, stimulated a philosophy of care which spread to the United States to involve both lay people and professionals. In 1974, Hospice, Inc., of New Haven, Connecticut, began and since then the movement has grown rapidly with formation of the National Hospice Organization to establish standards for local hospice programs. Programs vary; usually, the locally formed

To My Family, My Physician, My Lawyer and All Others Whom It May Concern

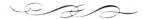

Death is as much a reality as birth, growth, maturity and old age—it is the one certainty of life. If the time comes when I can no longer take part in decisions for my own future, let this statement stand as an expression of my wishes and directions, while I am still of sound mind.

If at such a time the situation should arise in which there is no reasonable expectation of my recovery from extreme physical or mental disability, I direct that I be allowed to die and not be kept alive by medications, artificial means or "heroic measures". I do, however, ask that medication be mercifully administered to me to alleviate suffering even though this may shorten my remaining life.

This statement is made after careful consideration and is in accordance with my strong convictions and beliefs. I want the wishes and directions here expressed carried out to the extent permitted by law. Insofar as they are not legally enforceable, I hope that those to whom this Will is addressed will regard themselves as morally bound by these provisions.

Signed_____

Date _____

Witness_____

Witness_____

Copies of this request have been given to _____

_____

_____

_____

To secure extra copies for your own use and to give to friends, tear off this portion and mail to:

CONCERN FOR DYING
250 West 57th Street, New York, N.Y. 10019

Please send me _____ copies of a Living Will

Enclosed is my contribution of $_____ (tax deductible)

NAME _____
                        (please print)

ADDRESS _____

CITY _____ STATE_____ ZIP_____

See additional information on reverse side.

Figure 8-1. A living will.

To make best use of your LIVING WILL

1. Sign and date before two witnesses. (This is to insure that you signed of your own free will and not under any pressure.)

2. If you have a doctor, give him a copy for your medical file and discuss it with him to make sure he is in agreement.

   Give copies to those most likely to be concerned "if the time comes when you can no longer take part in decisions for your own future". Enter their names on bottom line of the Living Will. Keep the original nearby, easily and readily available.

3. Above all discuss your intentions with those closest to you, NOW.

4. It is a good idea to look over your Living Will once a year and redate it and initial the new date to make it clear that your wishes are unchanged.

35th printing
Revised May, 1978

IMPORTANT

Declarants may wish to add specific statements to the Living Will to be inserted in the space provided for that purpose above the signature. Possible additional provisions are suggested below:

1. a) I appoint _____
   to make binding decisions concerning my medical treatment.
   OR
   b) I have discussed my views as to life sustaining measures with the following who understand my wishes
   _____,
   _____,
   _____.

2. Measures of artificial life support in the face of impending death that are especially abhorrent to me are:
   a) Electrical or mechanical resuscitation of my heart when it has stopped beating.
   b) Nasogastric tube feedings when I am paralyzed and no longer able to swallow.

c) Mechanical respiration by machine when my brain can no longer sustain my own breathing.
d) _____

3. If it does not jeopardize the chance of my recovery to a meaningful and sentient life or impose an undue burden on my family, I would like to live out my last days at home rather than in a hospital.

4. If any of my tissues are sound and would be of value as transplants to help other people, I freely give my permission for such donation.

For additional copies of the Living Will, or the appropriate document in those states which have passed Living Will legislation, use coupon on reverse side.

Additonal materials available to contributors:

☐ Questions and Answers About the Living Will
☐ Selected articles and case histories
☐ A bibliography
☐ Information on films

The Concern for Dying newsletter is a quarterly publication reporting the most recent developments in the field of death and dying. It contains announcements of upcoming educational conferences, workshops and symposia, as well as reviews of current literature. The Newsletter is sent to anyone who contributes $5.00 or more annually to the CONCERN FOR DYING.

☐ I would like to receive the Newsletter.

A mini-will, a condensed version of the Living Will which can be carried in a wallet in case of accident or emergency, will be sent upon receipt of a contribution.

To obtain additional materials check above and fill in name and address on reverse side.

For information, call: (212) 246-6962

Figure 8-1. Reverse side of a living will.

Table 8-4. Physical Changes and Needs of the Terminally Ill.

PHYSICAL CHANGES	EXPECTATIONS AND NURSING CARE
1. Loss of muscle tone, manifests inability to control defecation and urination because sphincter muscles relax	May require urinary catheter. Clean perineum — use incontinent pads and deodorants, such as spray-on agents. Difficulty in maintaining position in bed. Fowler's position provides deeper ventilation of the lungs. If unconscious, position on side to promote mucus drainage; assess lungs; turn frequently. May have difficulty swallowing. Excess mucus causes gurgling sounds which family calls "death rattle" — oral suctioning may be done. Passive range of motion to allow muscle activity and decrease muscle aches. Lack of facial expression may be misinterpreted as not hearing or responding.
2. Diminished peristalsis, manifests lack of appetite, and abdominal distension	Frequent and thorough oral hygiene and sips of water are important; use of straw may be too difficult due to lack of muscle tone. Reduced peristalsis may cause flatus to accumulate in stomach and intestines resulting in distension and nausea; assess bowel sounds. Large amounts of H_2O cause vomiting — IV fluids are used to maintain hydration.
3. Slowed peripheral circulation so vital centers receive inadequate blood supply, manifested by reduced perfusion of blood	Irregular pulse. Variable blood pressure. Skin appears cyanosed or mottled — feels cold and clammy to nurse. Patient may feel warm. May require IV medication for pain. With circulation decreased, effectiveness of administered analgesics is decreased when given intramuscularly or subcutaneously. Give dose based on assessed need, not demand. As cardiac output falls to 1/2 normal, patient may have almost complete anuria; don't "fluid overload" with IVs.
4. Respiratory failure, manifested by slowed, irregular, or labored breathing	Difficult for family to witness. Oxygen by nasal cannula or mask may be helpful, humidified and used prn. As secretions collect, suction when needed to maintain airway. Cyanosis occurs and possible Cheyne-Stokes respiration.
5. Sensory alteration manifested by impaired visual, auditory, or oral response	Vision blurred: a well-lit room is preferred over a dark room; eyes may lack focus. Hearing — last sense to leave the body. Don't whisper — speak clearly and distinctly. Avoid impersonal talk. Assume patient hears. Touch when speaking to patient. Some may be conscious until moment of death; others are unconscious days or weeks; degree of consciousness alone is not indication of death.
Final Signs of Imminent Death:	Reflexes disappear; face assumes fixed position; pupils dilate; respirations are irregular with apnea; blood pressure drops; heart slows, with cessation of respiration and/or heartbeat with resulting death.

groups give home care to the terminally ill and support the families of those who are dying. There is a strong belief that even though nothing more can be done medically to prolong life, each individual has the right to quality life in the time that is left (Abbott, 1978; Carey, 1975; Kalish, 1981; Stoddard, 1978). Physical care and symptomatic relief of pain continue to be important, along with meeting the psychological, social, and spiritual needs of the patient and his family (Craven and Wald, 1975).

Characteristics of Hospice Programs in the United States

- Each hospice program is an autonomous, locally administered program of interdisciplinary care, including primary physician; nurse; social worker; physical, occupational, and speech therapists; spiritual support; trained volunteers; and other consultant services as needed.
- The unit of care includes the patient, the family, and significant others from the time of referral through death and a one-year period of bereavement.
- There is available 24-hour-a-day call for service without regard to ability to pay. Physical, emotional, and spiritual needs are assessed and cared for in the home, with emphasis on the quality of life.
- Pain and symptom control are evaluated and eased. The philosophy is to control pain not just to relieve it. Keeping the dying person free of pain allows him to live and interact with his family until death. It is not assumed that pain is to be suffered through as part of the dying process. (Adapted from Markel and Sinon, 1978)

Although the purpose of hospice is to allow the individual to die in his home with his own family, no one is expected to endure beyond physical and emotional capabilities in any setting. Most hospice programs coordinate efforts so that if family support is limited and institutional care is required, the patient is admitted to a hospital or nursing home and

visits by hospice personnel are continued. Some hospice programs are a coordinated effort between community and hospital, and some are located within hospital settings. The overall goal in the hospice concept is not only care of the dying, but care of the living, with emphasis on the fullness and quality of life until death occurs (Abbott, 1978).

SUMMARY

The vulnerability to loss and loneliness is increased in old age. Natural limitations are imposed when successive episodes of bereavement occur with fewer and fewer support systems. The numerous stresses and losses experienced by older persons, along with their diminishing resources and supports are reasons for nurses to assess, plan, and intervene by design in therapeutic grief work for the aged and their families.

Death becomes more imminent with advancing age; therefore, the gerontological nurse should be prepared to assist patients and their families in preparing for this developmental task. At this point in time, the recognition of feelings and behaviors, such as expected stages of grief work (e.g., Kübler-Ross' stages of dying), and death education for patients and their families constitute professional knowledge and skills for therapeutic care.

Finally, it must be understood that before they can help others nurses and other helping professionals have to first recognize and work through their feelings about aging, aged persons, dying, and death.

REFERENCES

Abbott, J.W. Hospice. *Aging* 38-40 (November-December 1978).

Albert, W.C. The management of grief. Unpublished lecture, College of Nursing, Arizona State University, Nov. 17, 1980.

Buckelew, B. Health care professionals versus the elderly. *Journal of Gerontological Nursing* 18(10): 560-564 (1982).

Burnside, I. Grief work in the aged patient. *Nursing Forum* 8(4): 416-427 (1969).

Butler, R.N. and Lewis, M.I. 3nd Ed. *Aging and Mental Health.* St. Louis: C.V. Mosby, p. 58-59 1982.

Carey, R.G. Living until death: a program of service and research for the terminally ill. In *Death, the Final Stage of Growth.* Englewood Cliffs, N.J.: Prentice-Hall, 1975.

Craven, J. and Wald, F.S. Hospice care for dying patients. *American Journal of Nursing* 75(10): 1816–1822 (1975).

Duvall, E. *Family Development.* Philadelphia: J.B. Lippincott, 1967.

Engel, G. Grief and grieving. *American Journal of Nursing* 9: 93–98 (1964).

Epstein, C. *Nursing the Dying Patient.* Reston, Va.: Reston Publishing, 1975.

Feifel, H.S. *The Meaning of Death.* New York: McGraw-Hill, 1959.

Fell, J. Grief reactions in the elderly following death of a spouse: the role of crisis intervention and nursing. *Journal of Gerontological Nursing* 3(6): 17–20 (1977).

Frankel, V.E. *Man's Search for Meaning.* Boston: Beacon Press, 1959.

Gelein, J.L. The aged American female: relationships between social support and health. *Journal of Gerontological Nursing* 6(2): 69–74 (1980).

Kalish, R.A. *Death, Grief and Caring Relationships.* Monterey, Calif.: Brooks Cole, 1981, pp. 174–190, 193–195.

Kastenbaum, R.J. *Facts about Older Americans* (DHEW Publication No. 79-20006). 1978.

Kübler-Ross, E. *On Death and Dying.* New York: Macmillan, 1969.

Kübler-Ross, E. *Death, the Final Stage of Growth.* Englewood Cliffs, N.J.: Prentice-Hall, 1975.

Lindemann, E. Symptomatology and management of acute grief. *American Journal of Psychiatry* 101: 141–148 (1944).

Lipman, A.G. Drug therapy in cancer pain. *Cancer Nursing* 3(1): (1980).

Markel, W.H. and Sinon, V.B. The hospice concept. *Ca–A Cancer Journal for Clinicians* 28(4): 225–237 (1978).

Neale, R.E. *The Art of Dying.* New York: Harper & Row, 1973.

Neugarten, B.L. and Maddox, G. *Our Future Selves: A Research Plan toward Understanding Aging.* A report of the Panel on Behavioral and Social Sciences Research of the National Advisory Council on Aging (DHEW Publication No. NIH 78-1444). Washington, D.C.: U.S. Government Printing Office, 1978.

Pattison, E.M. The living-dying process. In Garfield, C.A. (Ed.) *Psychosocial Care of the Dying Patient.* New York: McGraw-Hill, 1978.

Pennington, E.A. Post mortem care: more than ritual. *American Journal of Nursing* 78(5): 846–847 (1978).

Putnam, S. et al. Home as a place to die. *American Journal of Nursing* 80(8): 1451–1453 (1980).

Quint, J. *The Nurse and the Dying Patient.* New York: Macmillan, 1967.

Safier, G. Oral life history with the elderly. *Journal of Gerontological Nursing* 2(5): 17–23 (1976).

Saunders, C. Dying they live: St. Christopher's Hospice. In *New Meanings of Death.*

Saunders, C. Terminal care. In Garfield, C.A. (Ed.) *Psychosocial Care of the Dying Patient.* New York: McGraw-Hill, 1978.

Schwartz A.N. and Peterson J.A. Death, dying and grieving. *Introduction to Gerontology.* New York: Holt, Rinehart and Winston, 1979.

Steffl, B.M. Old age is not for sissies. In *Aging with Dignity: An Examination of Local, National, and International Concerns for the elderly.* Published proceedings of Hawaii Governor's Bicentennial Conference on Aging, Hawaii State Commission on Aging, 1976.

Stoddard, S. *The Hospice Movement.* New York: Random House, 1978.

Wass, H. Aging and death education for elderly persons. *Educational Gerontology, An International Quarterly* 5(1): 79–89 (1980).

Watson, W. and Maxwell, R. (Eds.). *Human Aging and Dying.* New York: St. Martin's Press, 1977.

Weisman, A.D. *Coping with Cancer.* New York: McGraw-Hill, 1979.

Werner-Beland, J.A. (Ed.). *Grief Responses to Long-term Illness and Disability.* Reston, Va.: Reston Publishing, 1980.

Whalen, P. Tu, solus, alienation and resocialization of the elderly. *Journal of Gerontological Nursing* 6(6): 348–353 (1980).

BIBLIOGRAPHY

Amster, L.E. and Krauss, H.H. The relationship between life crises and mental deterioration in old age. *International Journal of Aging and Human Development* 5(51): (1974).

Annas, G.J. Rights of the terminally ill patient. *Journal of Nursing Administration* 40–44 (March–April 1974).

Baird, S.B. Nursing roles in continuing care: home care and hospice. *Seminars in Oncology* 8(1): 28–37 (1980).

Brown, M. *Readings in Gerontology.* St. Louis: C.V. Mosby, 1978.

Dobihal, S.V. Hospice: enabling a patient to die at home. *American Journal of Nursing* 80(8): 1448–1450 (1980).

Gramlich, E.P. Recognition and management of grief in elderly patients. *Geriatrics* 87–92 (July 1968).

Grubruim, J.F. *Living and Dying at Murray Manor.* New York: St. Martin's Press, 1975.

Merriam, E. A conversation against death. *Ms* 80–83 (September 1972).

Wahl, P.R. Therapeutic relationships with the elderly. *Journal of Gerontological Nursing* 6(5): 260–267 (1980).

Walborn, K.A. A nursing model for the hospice – primary and self-care nursing. *Nursing Clinics of North America* 205–217 (March 1980).

Wald, F.S. Terminal care and nursing education. *American Journal of Nursing* 79(10): 1762–1765 (1979).

Wald, F.S., Foster, Z., and Wald, H.J. The hospice movement as health care reform. *American Journal of Nursing* 173–178 (March 1980).

Williams, F. To live until we say goodbye. *A Program Workbook on Death and Dying.* Tucson: University of Arizona, 1979.

Part III
Geropsychiatric Nursing

9
Mental Health and Mental Illness in Later Life

Irene Mortenson Burnside, R.N., M.S., F.A.A.N.

"I know you hurt, but there's nothing to bandage"

Donald D. Fisher, M.D. 1978

This chapter is an overview of mental health and illness in late life, and describes the state of the art in geropsychiatric nursing. The area is so broad and encompasses such a range of problems that only highlights can be given in a short chapter.

At this writing, there is no nursing textbook devoted exclusively to geropsychiatric nursing. The reader is referred to another handbook, an outstanding collection of papers by leaders in the field of mental health and aging, the *Handbook of Mental Health and Aging* (Birren and Sloan, 1980). Nursing does lag behind other disciplines in interest, concern, research, and literature about mental health in the elderly. However, with the influx and rapid production of books on aging written by nurses, it should not be long before there is an entire text on this subject edited by a nurse. At the present time, material can only be found in chapters of nursing texts (Burnside, 1978, 1980, 1981; Carnevali and Patrick, 1979; Good and Rodgers, 1980; Murray, Huelskoelter, and O'Driscoll, 1980; Weber, 1980; Werner-Beland, 1980; Yurick, Robb, Spier, and Ebert, 1980). Chapters also appear in textbooks which have been edited by nonnursing professionals (Birren and Sloan, 1980; Busse and Pfeiffer, 1977; Cowdry, in press; Eisdorfer and Friedel, 1977; Reichel, 1979; Rossman, 1979). The *Journal of Gerontological Nursing* and *Geriatric Nursing* both contain articles related to geropsychiatric nursing.

Geropsychiatric Nursing

Geropsychiatric nursing needs to be freed from traditional psychiatric nursing for three basic reasons: (1) many principles taught in psychiatric nursing do not apply to the older client and, therefore, are not effective; (2) adhering to tradition and to the original theoretical frameworks and/or rationales does not encourage creativity in developing new and more effective strategies; (3) a new body of knowledge is steadily accruing to be incorporated into the nurse's armamentarium.

While geropsychiatric nursing can use principles from psychiatry, they must be melded into the nursing process with the necessary adaptations. While we need not reinvent the wheel, we can surely change the spokes or rearrange them. Murray et al. (1980) have accomplished this well in chapters on geropsychiatric nursing in *The Nursing Process in Later Maturity.* Spier in *The Aged Person and the Nursing Process* (Yurick et al., 1980), organizes materials from other disciplines and applies the nursing process to cognitive aspects of aging.

One specific example in which nursing borrows principles spelled out by psychiatrists is in group work with the elderly. A group leader can use the principles of one of the pioneers in group therapy with the elderly (Linden, 1953) or of other psychotherapists (Beland and Poggi, 1981; Schutz, 1958; Yalom, 1970) and shape them into a particular kind of group modality for elderly patients (Burnside, 1978). Nurses are adroit at using eclectic approaches to group work (Burnside, 1984).

The Statistics

About one-third of the older population is very old, 75 years of age or over. This proportion will stay about the same for the foreseeable future if the mortality rate remains constant (U.S. Department of Health, Education and Welfare, 1979).

Surveys among noninstitutionalized elderly reveal a high number of mental disorders (Coe and Brehm, 1972). It has been estimated that approximately 15% of elderly who reside in the community are suffering from nervous disorders but are not hospitalized, while another 2-3% are in institutions because of their psychiatric problems (Busse and Pfeiffer, 1977).

Lowy (1980) reports, "The rate of people over 65 being treated in out-patient clinics did not increase between 1963 and 1971. It was 2.4 per 100,000 in 1971, compared to a 157 percent increase in services for all age groups in the same period." These statistics powerfully illustrate our continued lack of mental health care for the older person.

Burville (1971) states that in any group of medical and surgical patients, up to 50% of the group may have mental problems which are overlooked. In the geriatric patient, an underlying mental disorder can be masked by many somatic complaints (Mechanic, 1978); this is especially true in cases of depressed elderly, because depression is a frequent illness and it can be missed when the emphasis is on the presenting symptom, for example, lethargy or pain. Depressed elderly often quit eating, which frustrates families and care givers.

A study by Shuckit, Miller, and Hahlbohom (1979) in a Veterans' Hospital found that of 105 subjects, 38 were mentally ill and 12 of those cases had first been missed. The authors of the study suggest that some of the organicity could have been iatrogenic since the average subject received five different drugs and some were receiving as many as eleven (see Chapter 34 for a discussion of drug-related problems).

In summary, we must consider some findings which Harris (1978) extrapolated from a research study:

- Three million older persons, 13-15% of the older population, are in need of immediate mental health services.

- Seven million elderly live in conditions which are conducive to the development of mental illness.
- By 1980, 80% of those who need mental health services will not receive them, if present trends continue.
- The older population receives less than 2% of private psychiatric time and only 2.3% of total outpatient psychiatric services.
- The elderly suffer from poor diagnoses of mental illness and poor attitudes by professionals toward treatment of the elderly.
- Most elderly diagnosed as having functional disturbances can be helped; it is estimated that 15% of those with organic disorders can be treated.
- Under new Medicaid and Supplemental Security Income (SSI) reimbursement mechanisms, many elderly who need treatment are being transferred from hospital to community settings where treatment is not possible.
- Growing old is a difficult period of adjustment. Most of the difficulties that arise are treatable with minor counseling or interventions.

The need for nurses to become involved in improving the mental health of the aged is surely mandated by this information and by such staggering statistics.

Mental Illness in Later Life

Some of the facts about mental illness in later life which nurses must consider are:

1. Mental illness occurs more often in the older adult than in the younger person; 18-25% of older people have serious mental health symptoms.
2. The high rate of mental illness in nursing homes is well documented. Over 70% of nursing home residents have serious mental disturbances (Teeter, Garetz, Miller, and Heiland, 1976). Somewhere between one-quarter (250,000) and one-half (500,000

of nursing home residents have significant manifestations of senile dementia (Redick, Kramer, and Taube, 1973).

3. During the 1960s the deinstitutionalization phenomenon occurred as state mental hospitals all over the United States cleared their wards of elderly patients. By the 1970s many elderly patients had been reinstitutionalized in nursing homes. Cohen states that a new mental hospital has emerged in the communities of the United States and he calls it the nursing home (Cohen, 1979). The elderly constitute 40% of all these mental health referrals. This frail aged group receives care by persons who usually have little background in psychiatric principles and scant knowledge of gerontology/geriatrics.

4. Alzheimers Disease is the fourth or fifth leading cause of death in the United States (Katzman, 1976).

5. One out of four suicides in the United States is committed by persons 65 and over (Harris, 1978). Suicide occurs more often among white males in the 75 and over age group, while the white female suicide rate peaks in the 50–54 age group (Diggory, 1976); see Table 9-1.

6. Eighty-six percent of the elderly have chronic health problems of one kind or another (Butler and Lewis, 1978).

7. It has been estimated that between 2 and 10% of individuals over age 60 suffer from alcoholism (Shuckit and Pastor, in press). Most studies agree that alcoholism in the older age group increases with widowhood and for patients who come for medical or surgical treatment (Bailey, Haberman, and Alksne, 1965; Shuckit and Miller, 1976). Reviews of the residents of nursing homes indicate an alcoholism rate of nearly 20% (Graux, 1969), and surveys of general medical wards showed a rate of alcoholism which ranged from 15 to 20% (McCusker, Cherubin, and Zimberg, 1971; Shuckit and Miller, 1976).

Implications for Geropsychiatric Nursing

1. Nursing education must increase the geropsychiatric content of present nursing curricula; students need a better understanding of the mental health problems of

Table 9-1. Deaths and Death Rates for Suicide by Age and Sex: 1976.

AGE	NUMBER			RATE PER 100,000 POPULATION IN SPECIFIED GROUP		
	BOTH SEXES	MALE	FEMALE	BOTH SEXES	MALE	FEMALE
All ages	26,832	19,493	7,339	12.5	18.7	6.7
Under 1 year	–	–	–	–	–	–
1–4 years	–	–	–	–	–	–
5–14 years	163	126	37	0.4	0.7	0.2
15–24 years	4,747	3,786	961	11.7	18.5	4.8
25–34 years	5,064	3,716	1,348	15.9	23.6	8.4
35–44 years	3,759	2,557	1,202	16.3	22.8	10.2
45–54 years	4,541	2,990	1,551	19.2	26.2	12.7
55–64 years	4,005	2,826	1,179	20.0	29.8	11.1
65–74 years	2,772	2,094	678	19.5	34.0	8.4
75–84 years	1,406	1,096	310	20.8	42.7	7.4
85 years and over	371	299	72	18.9	47.5	5.4
Age not stated	4	3	1	–	–	–

SOURCE: *Facts of Life and Death*, U.S. Dept. of Health, Education and Welfare, 621-54-251, 1978, p. 46.

the aged and the management of those problems.

2. Scandals in nursing homes have been noted, but the nursing home population has been of little challenge to the nursing profession. Nurses from these agencies frequently tell of their isolation and professional loneliness (Chase, 1980). The need for educated, creative nurses in such facilities is critical. The nursing profession has given them little support. Geropsychiatric nursing consultants are rarely used in nursing homes in spite of the numerous mental health problems documented. Physical care continues to have priority over the management of mental health problems and/or psychosocial care in most long term care facilities.

3. There is a need for more articles in current nursing literature on care and management of persons which Alzheimer's disease (presenile and senile dementia). In fact, there is still little nursing research about senile dementia. Nursing lags behind geropsychiatry, neurology, and psychology in showing interest in the dementias and in contributions to the literature.

4. Nursing literature or research on suicide in the elderly is almost nonexistent.

5. The interrelationship of physical health and mental health is an important area for nurses to study and incorporate into geriatric protocols, nursing assessment, physical health assessments, and history taking.

6. The older person with a drinking problem has been ignored, and this is true in many settings. The problem of alcoholism in nursing homes is essentially a nurse-management problem. Often, nurses rely heavily on the assistance of police officers when alcoholic patients get out of hand. The fact that many of the organic brain syndromes may be attributed to alcoholism means that the prevention aspects are important. Nurses are referred to a nursing history adapted to the elderly by Heinemann and Smith-Di Julio (1979)

and to the case study, Case X, by Good and Rodgers (1980).

Overview of Nursing Literature

Four chapters in a book by Werner-Beland (1980) are helpful in understanding mental health problems of the elderly: "Effects of Grief Associated with Chronic Illness and Disability in Sexuality," "Grief and the Process of Aging," "Nursing and the Concept of Hope," and "The Burnout Syndrome of Nurses." Their changed body image may decrease self-esteem in the elderly; grief work is a common task of the aged; and burnout is one of the hazards of geropsychiatric nursing. For these reasons, the chapters mentioned are highly recommended to the reader.

A book by Good and Rodgers (1980) about clinical studies presents many of the problems "which beg for nursing solutions" and offers case studies for careful analytical reading and study. The book includes an excellent reference list on a variety of subjects including mental health, illness, and therapies. Another nursing text focuses on nursing management of the elderly client and is recommended for the management of individuals over 70 and their families (Carnevali and Patrick, 1979). This text is a comprehensive reference book and deals with common, but complex, problems which may occur in the aged client. The chapters on loneliness, pain, and powerlessness especially relate to mental health aspects of the aged.

Yurick et al. (1980) focus on the nursing process and the aged person, and offer an outline for gerontological education for nurses; one portion of their book is devoted to psychological factors which should be considered in curriculum planning (pp. 510-511). The book also contains a helpful table called "Guide for Assessing Developmental Tasks, Self-concept, and Coping Mechanism" (pp. 224-226). Because many elderly people have incorporated society's view into their own self-views, the assessment of self-concept is important. One particular strength of this table is the assessment of the relationship the aged person has with "significant others."

Murray et al. (1980) also focus on the nursing process in later maturity and devote one section of their book to emotional illness in later maturity and related nursing processes. The reader is referred to this for a chapter on "Withdrawal and the Schizophrenic Syndrome in Later Maturity," since that topic will not be covered here. The authors also include a fine chapter on group work with older persons and discuss the ways in which group work with the elderly differs from groups established for younger persons (pp. 113-114). The reader should also refer to Wells (1979) for data and information about commitment to gerontological nursing and existing educational programs.

While mental illness per se is not listed as the cause of death on death certificates, it is one of the most costly of illnesses in terms of money, care, and quality of life for the old person and the relatives. We are little prepared to deal with the problems of mental illness in later life. Katzman (1976) has reminded us that while Alzheimer's disease is not listed as a cause of death, it is indeed one of the major killers of the aged. The prevalence of depressed older individuals is well known to geropsychiatric nurses.

SUMMARY

The focus in this chapter has been on the high incidence of mental health problems and illness in the later years. The crisis areas in mental health of the elderly have been listed, along with a few directions which geropsychiatry might consider. The nursing literature is not a rich source of information for geropsychiatric nurses who will have to continue to borrow from the disciplines of geropsychiatry, neurology, psychology, and social work until nursing publishes textbooks in this specialized and sorely needed field.

REFERENCES

Bailey, M.D., Haberman, P.W., and Alksne, H. The epidemiology of alcoholism in an urban residential area. *Quarterly Journal of Studies on Alcohol* 26: 20-40 (1965).

Beland, D.I. and Poggi, R.L. Establishing newcomer's groups. In Burnside, I. M. (Ed.) *Nursing and the Aged* (2nd ed.). New York: McGraw-Hill, 1981.

Birren, J.E. and Sloan, R.B. *Handbook of Mental Health and Aging.* Englewood Cliffs, N.J.: Prentice-Hall, 1980.

Burnside, I.M. *Working with the Elderly: Group Process and Techniques.* 2nd Ed. Monterey, Ca.: Wadsworth, 1984.

Burnside, I.M. *Psychosocial Nursing Care of the Aged* (2nd ed.). New York: McGraw-Hill, 1980.

Burnside, I.M. *Nursing and the Aged* (2nd ed.). New York: McGraw-Hill, 1981.

Burnside, I.M., Waver-dyck, S., and Baumler, J. In *Working with the Elderly: Group Process and Techniques,* 2nd Ed. Monterey, Ca., Wadsworth, 1984.

Burville, P. Consecutive psychogeriatric admissions to psychiatric and geriatric hospitals. *Geriatrics* 26: 156-168 (1971).

Busse, E.W. and Pfeiffer, E. *Behavioral Adaptations in Later Life* (2nd ed.). Boston: Little, Brown, 1977.

Butler, R.N. and Lewis, M.I. *Aging and Mental Health.* St. Louis: C.V. Mosby, 1978.

Carnevali, D.L. and Patrick, M. *Nursing Management for the Elderly.* Philadelphia: J.B. Lippincott, 1979.

Chase, F. Personal communication (1980).

Coe, R.M. and Brehm, H.P. *Preventive Health Care for Adults.* New Haven, Conn.: College and University Press, 1972.

Cohen, E.S. Nursing homes – the new mental hospitals. *Generations* 1(4): 8 (1979).

Cowdry, E.V. *Care of the Geriatric Patient* (6th ed.). St. Louis: C.V. Mosby, in press.

Diggory, J.C. United States suicide rates 1933-1968: an analysis of some trends. In Shneidman, E.S. (Ed.) *Suicidology: Contemporary Developments.* New York: Grune and Stratton, 1976, pp. 25-69.

Eisdorfer, C. and Friedel, R.O. *Cognitive and Emotional Disturbance in the Elderly: Clinical Issues.* Chicago: Year Book Medical Publishers, 1977.

Fisher, D.D. *I Know It Hurts, but There's Nothing to Bandage.* Beaverton, Oregon, The Touchstone Press, 1978, p. 1.

Good, S.R. and Rodgers, S.S. *Analysis for Action: Nursing Care of the Elderly.* Englewood Cliffs, N.J.: Prentice-Hall, 1980.

Graux, P. Alcoholism of the elderly. *Review of Alcohol* 15: 61-63 (1969).

Harris, C.S. *Fact Book on Aging: A Profile of America's Older Population.* Washington, D.C.: National Council on Aging, 1978.

Heinemann, M.E. and Smith-Di Julio, K. Alcoholism. In Carnevali, D. and Patrick, M. (Eds) *Nursing Management for the Elderly.* Philadelphia: J.B. Lippincott, 1979, pp. 201-203.

Katzman, R. The prevalence and malignancy of Alzheimer's disease. *Archives of Neurolology* 33: 217-218 (1976).

Linden, M.E. Group psychotherapy with institutionalized senile women: study in gerontologic human relations. *International Journal of Group Psychotherapy* 3: 150-170 (1953).

Lowy, L. Mental health service in the community. In Birren, J.E. and Sloan, R.B. (Eds.) *Handbook on Mental Health and Aging*. Englewood Cliffs, N.J.: Prentice-Hall, 1980.

McCusker, J., Cherubin, C.F., and Zimberg, S. Prevalence of alcoholism in general municipal hospital population. *New York State Journal of Medicine* 71: 751-754 (1971).

Mechanic, D. *Medical Sociology* (2nd ed.). New York: Free Press, 1978.

Murray, R., Huelskoelter, M., and O'Driscoll, D. *The Nursing Process in Later Maturity*. Englewood Cliffs, N.J.: Prentice-Hall, 1980.

National Institute of Mental Health. *Referral of Discontinuation of Inpatient Services of State and County Mental Hospitals, U.S. 1969* (Biometry Branch, Statistical Note No. 57). Washington, D.C.: U.S. Government Printing Office, 1971.

Redick, R.W., Kramer, M., and Taube, C.A. Epidemiology of mental illness and utilization of psychiatric facilities among older persons. In Busse, E.W. and Pfeiffer, E. (Eds.) *Mental Illness in Later Life*. Washington, D.C.: American Psychiatric Association, 1973, p. 203.

Reichel, W. (Ed.). *Clinical Aspects of Aging*. Baltimore: Williams and Wilkins, 1979.

Rossman, I. (Ed.). *Clinical Geriatrics*. Philadelphia: J.B. Lippincott, 1979.

Schutz, W.C. *FIRO: a three-dimensional theory of interpersonal behavior*. New York: Holt, Rinehart and Winston, 1958.

Shuckit, M.A. and Miller, P.L. Alcoholism in elderly men: a survey of a general medical ward. *Annals of the New York Academy of Science* 273: 558-571 (1976).

Shuckit, M.A., Miller, P.L., and Hahlbohom, D. Unrecognized psychiatric illness in elderly medical-surgical patients. *Journal of Gerontology* 30: 655-660 (November-December 1979).

Shuckit, M.A. and Pastor, P.A., Jr. Alcohol-related psychopathology in the aged. In Kaplan, O.J. (Ed.) *Psychopathology in Aging*. New York: Academic Press, 1981.

Teeter, R.B., Garetz, F.K., Miller, W.B., and Heiland, W.F. Psychiatric disturbances in skilled nursing homes. *American Journal of Psychiatry* 133: 1430-1434 (1976).

U.S. Department of Health, Education and Welfare. *Facts about Aging*. Washington, D.C.: 1979, p. 542.

Weber, R. *Nursing the Elderly*. Reston, Va.: Reston Publishing, 1980.

Wells, T.J. Commitment to gerontological nursing. In Reinhardt, A. and Quinn, M. (Eds.) *Current Practice in Gerontological Nursing*. St. Louis: C.V. Mosby, 1979.

Werner-Beland, J.A. *Grief Responses to Long-term Illness and Disability*. Reston, Va.: Reston Publishing, 1980.

Yalom, I.D. *The Theory and Practice of Group Psychotherapy*, 2nd Ed. New York: Basic Books, 1975.

Yurick, A., Robb, S., Spier, B., and Ebert, N. *The Aged Person and the Nursing Process*. New York: Appleton-Century-Crofts, 1980.

10
Life Crisis Reactions, Depression, and Paranoia

Irene Mortenson Burnside

. . . the use of a classification of functional or organic, with or without demonstrable organic mental illness in the elderly, has always resulted in an impossible conceptual and clinical straightjacket.

Stanley Cath (1976)

In an effort to stay out of that impossible straitjacket, no attempt will be made in this chapter to delineate the nosology of the various types of depression or paranoid conditions in the elderly, because in a concise chapter such as this one, it would be impossible to do so [the reader should consult the *Diagnostic and Statistical Manual of Mental Disorders* (DSM III) list in the references]. Therefore, three specific areas in which nurses can demonstrate effectiveness have been chosen: life crisis reactions, depressive states, and paranoid conditions.

LIFE CRISIS REACTIONS

Blazer (1980) states, "The epidemiologist must organize the complex multifactoral processes that lead to the development of mental illness in later life." He suggests a turn of phrase "web of causation," which was originally coined by MacMahon and Pugh (1970). Such a concept of disease will take into account the predisposing factors and also the complex relationships between these factors and the outcome of the disease. Old age is a fertile ground for life crisis reactions to occur because of the many stresses and strains to be found in that particular stage of life. Some of the common stresses include: (1) the loss of a productive work role when retirement occurs, (2) reduced income, (3) the loss of spouse, (4) children leaving home (and even the immediate locale sometimes), and

(5) increased physical disabilities. These psychosocial losses and disappointments, "because of their implications for a life long pattern of behavior, are not easily set aside" (Renner and Birren, 1980). For an in-depth discussion of the mechanisms of stress, the reader should consult Renner and Birren (1980). For assistance in assessing functional symptomatology, see Table 10-1.

Loneliness

While there is controversy over whether old people are lonely or not, most nurses would attest to the fact that loneliness is a pervasive feeling expressed by their elderly clients. The experiences of loneliness, alienation, and loss of status were borne out in the survey sponsored by the National Council on Aging which found that 12% of those 65 and over felt that loneliness was a very serious problem for them (Harris, 1978). There are writings about nurses which hone in on loneliness in old age (Burnside, 1971; Carnevali, 1979; Clark, 1968; Harris, 1978). Widowhood represents an intense loneliness, a loss of emotional security, and an interruption of the fulfillment of basic needs (Payne, 1975).

Widowhood

Widowhood is one life crisis reaction nurses can expect to have to deal with constantly in their work with older persons. The reaction to the loss of a spouse will depend in part on the life-long character patterns of the survivor. Women seem to make a better adjustment than men do, perhaps because they are usually younger and because they often do some anticipatory

Table 10-1. Short Psychiatric Evaluation Schedule (Eric Pfeiffer, M.D.).

Please answer the following questions *Yes* or *No* as they apply to you now. Do not skip any questions. Occasionally a question may not seem to apply to you, but please *circle* either Yes or No, whichever is more nearly correct for you (NO = 0, Yes = 1).

1.	Do you wake up fresh and rested most mornings?	yes	NO
2.	Is your daily life full of things that keep you interested?	yes	NO
3.	Have you, at times, very much wanted to leave home?	YES	no
4.	Does it seem that no one understands you?	YES	no
5.	Have you had periods of days, weeks, or months when you couldn't take care of things because you couldn't "get going"?	YES	no
6.	Is your sleep fitful and disturbed?	YES	no
7.	Are you happy most of the time?	yes	NO
8.	Are you being plotted against?	YES	no
9.	Do you certainly feel useless at times?	YES	no
10.	During the past few years, have you been well most of the time?	yes	NO
11.	Do you feel weak all over much of the time?	YES	no
12.	Are you troubled by headaches?	YES	no
13.	Have you had difficulty in keeping your balance in walking?	YES	no
14.	Are you troubled by your heart pounding and by a shortness of breath?	YES	no
15.	Even when you are with people, do you feel lonely much of the time?	YES	no

Total Score:

To Be Completed by Interviewer

Patient's Name: Date

Sex: 1. Male   Race: 1. White
      2. Female   2. Black
                          3. Other

Years of Education: 1. Grade School
                             2. High School
                             3. Beyond High School

Interviewer's Name:

Scores from 0 to 3 imply an absence of significant functional psychiatric symptomatology. Scores from 4 to 5 constitute a borderland of uncertainty. One should be suspicious of possibly significant psychopathology, but other data from the history and from the remainder of the evaluation must be used to decide whether significant psychopathology exists. Scores greater than 5 are indicative of definite psychopathology, while scores of 10 or greater indicate extensive psychopathology.

SOURCE: E. Pfeiffer in E.W. Busse and D. Blazer (Eds.) *Handbook of Geriatric Psychiatry*, Van Nostrand Reinhold, 1980. Reprinted with permission of author.

rehearsals for the widow role (Verwoerdt, 1976). Nurses must be aware of the high risk of suicide after the loss of a spouse; it remains higher than average for five years following that loss (MacMahon and Pugh, 1970; Parkes, Benjamin, and Fitzgerald, 1969). For an in-depth discussion of widowhood and nursing interventions, the reader is referred to Burnside (1984).

Case History I

Mr. B. was a Caucasian male, aged 82, who had been hospitalized in nursing homes and acute care hospitals in two different cities for metastatic carcinoma, a prostatectomy (which he requested because he did not want to have a catheter), and bouts of extreme weakness and malaise.

The treatment focused on current medical problems, and Mr. B. had a kind and empathetic internist throughout the later months of his life. There was, however, little attention given to the depression he manifested, possibly because the physical symptoms of his depression also correlated so closely with the carcinoma condition (e.g., extreme weariness, sluggishness, slowed motions, disrupted sleep patterns, anorexia). His voice had been reduced to a whisper although the cause was never determined. The move from his home to a daughter's home 500 miles away resulted in an immediate confusional state, but the translocation trauma went unrecognized by the personnel caring for him. It was further compounded by the daughter's discarding all of his old and cherished belongings and replacing them with brand new ones (e.g., bathrobe, slippers, pajamas, radio, television set, etc.). Mr. B. confided to the student nurse that he had never gotten over the death of his wife who had died of cancer three years before. A favorite nephew had committed suicide recently. Mr. B. had "bereavement overload."

This case history of depression following a series of late life crises is not atypical. The staff responded almost entirely to the physical condition (see Table 10-1 for a short evaluation schedule).

DEPRESSIVE REACTIONS

Psychiatrists in their writings indicate that clinical depressive disorders increase in both prevalence and intensity with age (Butler and Lewis, 1981; Klerman and Barrett, 1973). Klerman suggests that it is possible that depression may increase enough in the future to become an age phenomenon, i.e., depression will become an even greater problem in mental health among the elderly population (Klerman, 1976). See Figure 10-1 for some components of the etiology of depression in late life.

Two excellent discussions of depression by Zung (1980) and by Stockwell (1968) are recommended. Zung (1980) states, "To understand depression of the elderly is to know the very fiber out of which the warp and woof of man's nature and destiny is woven." He

distinguishes between an endogenous depression and a reactive depression. Endogenous depressions occur in older persons when there is a family history of depression and there are no precipitating factors. These people respond to electro-convulsive therapy (ECT). In a reactive depression, the individual may be younger, there is no family history present, and there are precipitating factors. There is less self-pity and guilt in these individuals, and they do not respond to ECT. A bipolar depression, in which there are swings between mania and depression, is called a bipolar disorder, the average nurse will not have to care for persons with this disorder as they often end up in acute psychiatric units.

The symptoms of a depressive condition are most often confused with those symptoms found in dementia. This is an important area for the nurse practitioner. Depression is the most common psychiatric disorder that a physician is likely to encounter when he is treating an older patient, and it is the most likely condition to be overlooked or misdiagnosed (Epstein, 1976). The same may be said for nurses. It is true that even in day-to-day interactions, one will discover depressed individuals if one listens carefully. The following section discusses such a case. Two nurses were vacationing in a resort city, and they rented a condominium for the vacation. One of the permanent residents of the condominium, in an effort to be hospitable, dropped in for a social visit. Although a complete stranger, she quickly revealed the following history.

Case History II

Mrs. O., aged 61, was a Caucasian female who had been forced to retire much earlier than she had anticipated. She had received a head injury while on a cruise in the Caribbean, and the injury resulted in "multivessel aneurysms," as she described it, and incapacitating headaches. She also talked about her severe osteoporosis and about having received cracked ribs when someone came up behind her and lifted her off the ground rather suddenly with a strong squeeze. For one and a half hours the woman sipped a drink, smoked constantly, and talked

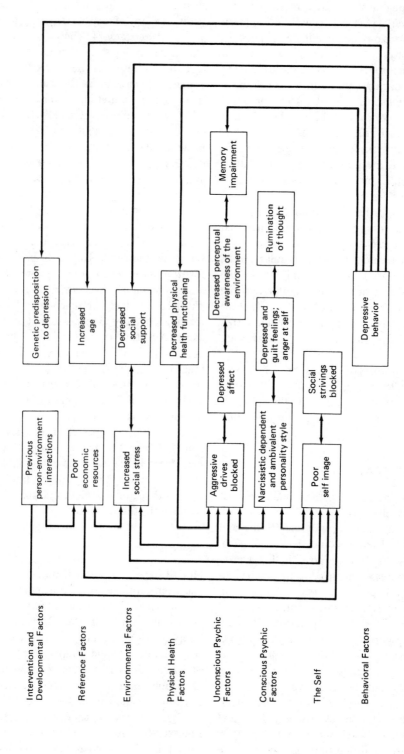

Figure 10-1. Some components in the etiology of depression in late life. Source: Dan Blazer in E.W. Busse and D. Blazer (Eds.) *Handbook of Geriatric Psychiatry*, Van Nostrand Reinhold, 1980, p. 262.

of her problems. Both nurses noted a slight slurring of speech as she spoke, and she stated that she enjoyed her Scotch very much. At one point, in describing her condominium, she stated she had put a low table on her lamp. In retrospect, the speech error seemed to fit her own life! Much of the focus of the theme of losses was on the stealing of a favorite cat which she had had for eight years. In her unhappiness, she had decided to move to another area of the city in hopes of finding more pleasant surroundings and a more competently run condominium.

The theme of losses, her unplanned early retirement, her preparation for her demise at the time of the head injury and subsequent surgery, the long discussion about her grief over her beloved cat, the preoccupation with her physical condition, her voice, and her lack of interests (some of which were undoubtedly due to her health and visual problems) indicated that Mrs. O. was struggling with her aloneness, with her inability to travel on long trips (which she had always enjoyed) because no one was willing to take the risk of traveling with someone in such precarious health, and with the loss of a work role. She had spent 18 years in a very responsible position, and as she herself described the abrupt termination of that job, "I was somebody, and then suddenly I was nobody" (said in a sad voice with bitterness). Each depressive reaction was related to definable life experiences which she related in great detail in her monologue conversation of one and a half hours. Two weeks later she was walking a frisky kitten on a leash! Then the woman was animated, and she spent that entire conversation telling how the kitten had really changed her life.

Vignette: Low Self-esteem

During a field trip to a private psychiatric hospital, a class studying the frail elderly received information about the importance of activities in the institutional setting. The recreation director had described the therapeutic results of bingo games and a way to use them as assessment tools (e.g., motor skills in placing the object on the square, reading and comprehending numbers, the ability to follow simple commands). Then she very poignantly described an older man who played bingo rather well but would not call out or acknowledge that he had the numbers for a bingo. His low self-esteem would not permit him to win or to accept a gift because he did not think he was worthy of winning. This occurrence was a pivotal point in his therapy and treatment plan because only then did the staff and personnel realize how very low his self-esteem truly was (Mesa Vista, 1980).

NURSING INTERVENTIONS

The following are some possible nursing interventions during depressive states in the aged:

- Promote a high level of self-esteem in these areas: self-identity, hopefulness, control, self-worth, and affiliations (Spier, 1980).
- Be alert for a client's feelings of depression which may occur in the early stages of the dementia process (Wells, 1977).
- If the state is a reactive depression, focus on mobilizing and helping the client to express emotions and to explore the role of ambivalence (Verwoerdt, 1976).
- In severely depressed, agitated, or even nihilistic cases, the psychotherapeutic stance may be "no more than the therapist's acceptance of disability. The patient is asked to give no more than his ability allows" (Langley, 1975).
- Avoid far-reaching decisions about the future (moving, selling one's home, etc.) if the depression is profound (Langley, 1975).
- Be alert for suicidal ideation (Murray, Huelskoetter, and O'Driscoll, 1980).
- Do not stifle the grieving process in the elderly (Agee, 1980).
- Recent losses to assess include: (1) relatives, (2) friends, (3) pets, (4) status, (5) funds, and (6) physiological changes (Libow, 1977).
- Be aware that the confused person may be suffering from depression (Cape, 1978).

- Decreasing the severity of physical illness will improve mental health and also decrease the high risk of suicide (Zung, 1980); therefore, complete physical assessments are necessary.
- Promote identification and resolutions of losses (Murray et al., 1980).
- Promote expressions of anger (Murray et al., 1980).
- Promote resolution of guilt feelings (Murray et al., 1980).
- Attend to physical symptoms (Murray et al., 1980).
- Encourage general hygiene (Murray et al., 1980).
- Encourage activities (Murray et al., 1980).
- Assist with electroshock treatment; give supportive care before and after the treatment (Murray et al., 1980).
- Work with the family and the health team (Murray et al., 1980).
- Improve the patient's general health (Stenback, 1980).
- Coordinate medical, psychopharmacological, sociotherapeutic, and psychotherapeutic measures (Stenback, 1980).
- Do not use drugs as substitutes for interpersonal and social modes of therapy (Crowley, 1979).
- Crisis interventions, if used, should be aimed at restoring the precrisis activity level (Stenback, 1980).
- Remember that pain may mask a severe depression; depression and chronic pain are often associated (Crowley, 1979).
- Compile a sexual history since depressed older males may have sexual difficulty and even be impotent (Finkle, 1976).
- Use a cautious attitude in therapy when the client is facing existential meaninglessness, suffering, and death (Stenback, 1980).
- Explore staff feelings regarding suicidal persons (Burnside, 1981).

PARANOID STATES

The classification of functional or organic source of mental disturbance is not easy as Cath (1976) has stated. One needs to remember that in organic states, there is an indication of some demonstrable pathology in the brain, while in a functional personality disorder or in functional disturbances, there seems to be nothing wrong organically. In fact, one is often amazed at the physical health of some of the aged persons who have mental illnesses. As a young student, I never ceased to be amazed at a paranoid old lady who was small and graceful, and always moved quickly. She would suddenly bolt across the long ward of the state hospital and leap onto the radiator to gallop on it, just as she had once ridden the white horses in the circus as a bareback rider. The frailty of her later years certainly had not affected her legs or balance — only her brain.

Although nurses often deal with paranoid behavior and must handle it in a variety of settings (Burnside, 1971, 1978), there really is not much in the way of statistics about its frequency or occurrence. Marjorie Fiske Lowenthal reported that 17% of individuals in her study exhibited symptoms of "suspiciousness" (Lowenthal, 1964). While there may be degrees of paranoid thinking, this chapter will focus on the management of suspiciousness.

Feelings of Persecution and Apprehension

Dr. Jack Weinberg (1975, p. 245) states that "primarily . . . paranoid states are the result of the resurgence of an individual's primitive hostile impulses toward the world and the people in it, both of which are beginning to fail him." The paranoid states are best characterized by the feelings the aged person has of being persecuted and of apprehension. Paranoia is a disturbing condition because of the suspiciousness and the ideation of persecution; it is disturbing not only to friends and relatives but also to the professionals who must care for that individual. Nurses are often disquieted by such behavior and may need to handle their own feelings about such clients. Weinberg (1975), who taught nurses about the projection defense whereby aged people project their losses onto others by stating that others are stealing objects, said very eloquently, "It is simpler to say that one is hated and not wanted because one is old, than to admit to oneself and others that one is incapable of coping with overwhelming odds." The case history of Mrs. E. describes some of the overwhelming odds against one woman.

Case History III

Mrs. E., an 82-year-old Caucasian woman, lives in the Island Home for Ladies with seven other frail, elderly women. Once a tall, large boned woman, she is now bent and moves about gingerly with a cane. Her increased hearing loss makes conversation or telephone calls impossible. She alienates most boarders and caretakers because she stubbornly and compulsively washes clothes and cleans her room. She is defensive and suspicious to overtures and/or suggestions for activity or medical attention.

Mrs. E. grew up in hillbilly country, where she was very poor; then she moved to the city and worked in a box factory until she married a widower with two children. She had a son in this marriage. She continued to work as a nurse's aide in a nursing home until age 75, her alcoholic husband having died 20 years earlier. Her life was a routine of work, washing, ironing, cleaning, and going to church. She looked forward to retirement and received the usual gold watch. She especially cherished the farewell letter about her years of service. One year after her retirement, she began complaining of noises in her head; she could not sleep, stayed up all night, and began wandering to find places "where everything wasn't shaking like an earthquake." She had lived in an apartment with her son for many years. Several years before her retirement, her fear of running out of clothes (because she had been deprived all of her life) and her aching feet prompted her to buy ten pairs of shoes — all nearly alike. During one visit, her stepdaughter counted twenty different coats in her closet — and she had always before been satisfied with one coat.*

Recently Mrs. E. during one of her walks ended up in the wrong house on the street and insisted she lived in that house; the police had

---

*Multiple purchases of the same item constitute a frequent complaint of the relatives of persons who have dementia.

to bodily remove her and return her to the Island Home for Ladies.

She was hospitalized several times for evaluation and has been managed fairly well with mild doeses of medication. Even during her moments of disorientation, she had been very resourceful (e.g., pinning her stockings to her slip when she lost her garters).

Mrs. E.'s early fire-and-brimstone Baptist and Methodist background ruled out any pleasurable interactions with men; yet she often remarked, "I don't think I'll ever remarry," or "Look at that old goat flirting with that young girl," which indicates a preoccupation with sexuality.

A thorough medical examination was sought because of severe halitosis; extraction of her remaining, terribly decayed remnants of teeth was recommended. She absolutely refused to have this done. Her son and daughter, who understood the problems and were willing to help her, were completely baffled because she refused to eat, stating that "there is not room anymore for food," and she refused her medications. She began to wander at night again.

Problems arise for the nurse when there is noncompliance regarding the medications prescribed for the aged paranoid individual. Sometimes medicines are not taken because of the fear of being poisoned (Burnside, 1980). The next case history describes an individual living independently who was not monitored regarding medications.

Case History IV: Paranoid Reaction and Somaticizing

Mrs. D. is a 69-year-old divorcee who came to the United States 34 years ago from Austria. She was diagnosed as paranoid schizophrenic ten months ago when she stopped taking the prescribed medications. She became decompensated, and her clinic physician sent her to an open psychiatric unit for stabilization and placement. Mrs. D. explained, "I lost my child and decided to let my husband go to marry his girlfriend and raise his child." Her suspicions included, "The boys are under my window at night and the paper boys sleep on my lawn. I also found my stove had been used during the day and that someone had been wearing my clothing and putting them back in my closet dirty — it must have been a woman because she wore my clothing, and my bed was messed up from sex — ugh." (She had shown flat affect in her life review until this point; then her face expressed extreme disgust.) She went on during the interview to describe a severe burn on her leg from knee to ankle; yet there was no trace of scar tissue on the leg. When her somatic concern increases, she requires a crutch to ambulate: this occurs when she is anxious or agitated. She ended the interview saying she was really a very happy person deep down inside. "I have to be silly so people can see that I am happy." She said she had survived three wars: World War I, World War II, and divorce. She equated the pain of that marriage and the loss of a child to having survived a war (Bryson, 1980).

Range of Symptoms

The symptoms to be found in a paranoid older individual may range from "mild querulousness to an unswerving conviction in the reality of a delusional system" (Burnside, 1981). Paranoia and depressive symptoms can be so intertwined with a dementia that the nurse may have a difficult time separating out all of the symptomatology for intervention strategies. One man in his 90s was depressed, delusional (people from the moon were after him), and also suffering from dementia. It was a real feat for the nurse to capitalize on his moments of lucidity and to support a very distraught family, who found it difficult to accept the bizarre behavior and thoughts of the once strong and powerful father figure. When he stated his wish to die, they no longer replaced the batteries for his pacemaker.

Verwoerdt (1976) reminds us that "at almost any point during the compensation of a grief reaction, paranoid elements may enter." He further explains the difference between the anger that may come out in a depression, which can be simply stated as "I am bad, you are good," but which the paranoid position changes to "I am good, you are bad" (Verwoerdt, 1976). As mentioned earlier, grief reactions are such common occurrences in late life that the nurse must be prepared to identify paranoid decompensation when she sees this during a grief reaction.

Management of Paranoia: Implications for Nursing

Management can be dealt with best if four different categories of intervention are considered: (1) situational and environmental manipulation, (2) identification and replacement of losses, (3) observation, and (4) psychopharmacologic strategies (Burnside, 1981). The clinical management of suspicious, paranoid individuals can be gleaned from the writings of psychiatrists, (Butler and Lewis 1981, Eisdorfer, 1980, Langley, 1975, Verwoerdt, 1976) and nurses (Bryson, 1980, Burnside, 1971, 1978, 1981.)

- Restore decision making and control to individuals whenever possible; especially try to allow greater decision making in institutions (Eisdorfer, 1980).
- Restore or prevent loss, especially hearing loss, but intervention in other losses is important also (Burnside, 1981). Seek the help of other professionals in this aspect of intervention.
- Special effort should be made with regard to loss of memory and memory retention, helping to organize belongings, and teaching the family about the problems. Use memory enhancement techniques (Eisdorfer, 1980).
- Observe for major environmental changes and trauma from relocation which may precipitate problems. Major environmental change can cause paranoid ideation (Eisdorfer, 1980). Be open about the manipulation of the environment (Butler and Lewis, 1981).
- Do not use drugs for the mildly suspicious; when drugs are used, they should be employed for a brief period and always with other psychosocial strategies (Eisdorfer, 1980).
- Since paranoia in old age is highly associated with sensory losses and may involve the sense of taste, there is absolutely no

point in giving these medications [phenothiazines] in pill form to paranoid patients. Such medication has to be given without the patient's awareness, and the nurse should know that all of the phenothiazines and Haldol do come in liquid form.

- Keep very close track of all the medications a patient is taking; do not treat patients in the outpatient clinic unless you are available for them for the following three weeks (Mannia, 1980).
- Watch for side effects from drugs. Two-thirds of the patients in one study developed parkinsonian side effects during drug therapy (Langley, 1975).
- The important aspect of management of paranoid individuals is "the maintenance of a personal relationship in a low emotional key" (Langley, 1975).
- Do not attempt to use logic regarding the folly of the delusional systems: it will fail and will produce emotional distress (Langley, 1975).
- Do not forget to be supportive of the relatives because having to live close to a paranoid individual can be a traumatic experience (Langley, 1975).
- Be absolutely honest with all paranoid patients (Butler and Lewis, 1977).
- The therapist stance is warmth with detachment, firmness, attentiveness, and being reasonable. Irony and humor are also valuable in working with paranoid individuals (Butler and Lewis, 1977).
- Develop a satisfying relationship with the individual: have a genuine caring attitude; increase the person's self-esteem; explore reality; reduce stress; intervene appropriately in the patient's behavior; and work with the family and other health team members (Murray et al., 1980).
- Paranoid persons, even those who live on their own, can be treated successfully in a day hospital setting (Mannia, 1980).
- The nurse must attend to sensory deficits (Burnside, 1981).

SUMMARY

This chapter has briefly described life crisis reactions and two common mental illnesses which occur in late life: depression and paranoia. Case studies which describe the conditions have been included, and literature sources have been cited to aid nurses in the care and management of such individuals.

REFERENCES

Agee, J.M. Grief and the process of aging. In Werner-Beland, J.A. (Ed.) *Grief Responses to Long-term Illness and Disability.* Reston, Va.: Reston Publishing, 1980.

Blazer, D. The epidemiology of mental illness in late life. Busse, E.W. and Blazer, D. (Eds.) *Handbook of Geriatric Psychiatry.* New York: Van Nostrand Reinhold, 1980, p. 261.

Bryson, J. Process recording, class: Working with the frail elderly. San Diego State University, July 18, 1980.

Burnside, I.M. Loneliness in old age. *Mental Hygiene* 55(3): 391–397 (1971).

Burnside, I.M. Gerontion: a case study. *Perspectives in Psychiatric Care* 9(3): 103–109 (1971).

Burnside, I.M. Eulogy for Ms. Hogue. *American Journal of Nursing* 78(4): 624–626 (1978).

Burnside, I.M. Adjustment to family losses: grief in frail elderly women. In Haug, M. and A.B. Ford. (Eds.) *The Physical and Mental Health of Aged Women,* New York: Springer, 1984.

Burnside, I.M. (Ed.). *Nursing and the Aged* (2nd ed.). New York: McGraw-Hill, 1981.

Burnside, I.M. Paranoid behavior in the elderly. In Burnside, I.M. (Ed.) *Nursing and the Aged* (2nd ed.). New York: McGraw-Hill, 1981.

Burnside, I.M. Suicide in the aged person. In Burnside, I.M. (Ed.) *Nursing and the Aged* (2nd ed.). New York: McGraw-Hill, 1981.

Butler, R.N. and Lewis, M.I. (Eds.). *Aging and Mental Health* (3nd ed.). St. Louis: C.V. Mosby, 1981.

Cape, R. (Ed.). *Aging: Its Complex Management.* Hagerstown, Md.: Harper & Row, 1978.

Carnevali, D. Loneliness. In Carnevali, D.L. and Patrick, M. (Eds.) *Nursing Management for the Elderly.* Philadelphia: J.B. Lippincott, 1979, pp. 501–513.

Cath, S. Functional disorders. An organismic view and attempt at reclassification. In Bellak, L. and Karasu, T.B. (Eds.) *Geriatric Psychiatry.* New York: Grune and Stratton, 1976, p. 141.

Clark, E. Aspects of loneliness: toward a framework of nursing intervention. In Zdaderad, L.T. and Belcher, H.C. (Eds.) *Developing Behavioral Concepts in Nursing.* Atlanta: Southern Regional Education Board, 1968.

Crowley, D. Pain. In Carnevali, D.L. and Patrick, M. (Eds.) *Nursing Management for the Elderly.* Philadelphia: J.B. Lippincott, 1979.

Diagnostic and Statistical Manual of Mental Disorders (DSM III). Washington, D.C.: American Psychiatric Association, 1977.

Eisdorfer, C. Paranoia in late life. In Busse, E.W. and Blazer, D. (Eds.) *Handbook of Geriatric Psychiatry*. New York: Van Nostrand Reinhold, 1980.

Epstein, L.J. Depression in the elderly. *Journal of Gerontology* 32: 278–282 (1976).

Finkle, A.L. Sexual aspects of aging. In Bellak, L. and Karasu, T.B. (Eds.) *Geriatric Psychiatry*. New York: Grune and Stratton, 1976.

Harris, C.S. *Fact Book on Aging: A Profile of America's Older Population*. Washington, D.C.: National Council on Aging, 1978.

Klerman, G.L. Age and clinical depressions: today's youth in the twenty-first century. *Journal of Gerontology* 31: 318–323 (1976).

Klerman, G.L. and Barrett, J.E. The affective disorders: clinical and epidemiological aspects. In Gershon, S. and Shopsin, B. (Eds) *Lithium: Its Role in Psychiatric Treatment and Research*. New York: Plenum, 1973, pp. 201–236.

Langley, G.E. Functional psychoses. In Howells, J.G. (Ed.) *Modern Perspectives in the Psychiatry of Old Age*. New York: Brunner/Mazel, 1975.

Libow, L.S. Senile dementia and "pseudosenility": clinical diagnosis. In Eisdorfer, C. and Friedel, R.O. (Eds.) *Cognitive and Emotional Disturbances in the Elderly: Clinical Issues*. Chicago: Year Book Medical Publishers, 1977.

Lowenthal, M. (Ed.). *Lives in Distress: The Paths of the Elderly to the Psychiatric Ward*. New York: Basic Books, 1964.

MacMahon, B. and Pugh, T.F. Suicide in widowhood. *American Journal of Epidemiology* 81(1): 23–31 (1965).

MacMahon, B. and Pugh, T.F. (Eds.). *Epidemiology: Principles and Methods*. Boston: Little, Brown, 1970.

Mannia, M. Personal communication (1980).

Mesa Vista Recreation Director. Personal communication (1980).

Murray, R.B., Huelskoetter, M., and O'Driscoll, D. (Eds.). *The Nursing Process in Later Maturity*. Englewood Cliffs, N.J.: Prentice-Hall, 1980.

Parkes, C.M., Benjamin, B., and Fitzgerald, R.G. Broken heart: a statistical study of increased mortality among widowers. *British Medical Journal* 1(5646): 740–743 (1969).

Payne, E.C. Depression and suicide. In Howells, J.G. (Ed.) *Modern Perspectives in the Psychiatry of Old Age*. New York: Brunner/Mazel, 1975, pp. 290–312.

Renner, J. and Birren, J.E. Stress: physiological and psychological mechanisms. In Birren, J.E. and Sloan, R.B. (Eds.) *Handbook on Mental Health and Aging*. Englewood Cliffs, N.J.: Prentice-Hall, 1980.

Spier, B.E. The nursing process as applied to the cognitive aspects of aging. In Yurick, A.G., Robb, S.S., Spier, B.E., and Ebert, N.J. (Eds.) *The Aged Person and the Nursing Process*. New York: Appleton-Century-Crofts, 1980.

Stenback, A. Depression and suicidal behavior in old age. In Birren, J.E. and Sloan, R.B. (Eds.) *Handbook on Mental Health and Aging*. Englewood Cliffs, N.J.: Prentice-Hall, 1980.

Stockwell, M.L. Depression: an operational definition with themes related to the nurse's role. In Zdaderad, L.T. and Belcher, H.C. (Eds.) *Developing Behavioral Concepts in Nursing*. Atlanta: South Regional Education Board, 1968.

Verwoerdt, A. (Ed.). *Clinical Geropsychiatry*. Baltimore: Williams and Wilkins, 1976.

Weinberg, J. Psychiatric aspects of aging. Lecture presented at the Andrus Gerontology Center, University of Southern California, Los Angeles, June 1970.

Weinberg, J. Psychopathology. In Howells, J.G. (Ed.) *Modern Perspectives in the Psychiatry of Old Age*. New York: Brunner/Mazel, 1975.

Wells, C.E. *Dementia* (2nd ed.). Philadelphia: F.A. Davis, 1977.

Zung, W. Depression. In Busse, E.W. and Blazer, D. (Eds.) *Handbook of Geriatric Psychiatry*. New York: Van Nostrand Reinhold, 1980.

11
Organic Mental Disorders

Irene Mortenson Burnside, R.N., M.S., F.A.A.N.

Working with people who have become cognitively impaired is difficult. But it is not impossible, and improvements in their ability to function can be achieved.

M. Hirschfeld (1977)

The variety of terms used to describe organic mental disorders (OMD) can confound the neophyte in geropsychiatric nursing. Just as we have become comfortable using the set of terms organic brain syndrome (OBS), a new set is introduced.

CLASSIFICATION OF ORGANIC MENTAL DISORDERS

The classification of the organic mental disorders was changed by the designers of the new *Diagnostic and Statistical Manual of Mental Disorders* (DSM III; 1977). The new manual's nosology deletes acute organic brain syndrome and chronic brain syndrome, although nurses will find these terms in common usage. Raskind and Storrie (1980) strive for a finer distinction in the terminology of the brain syndromes: dementia, in their usage, is roughly equivalent to the common term chronic brain syndrome, and delirium is roughly equivalent to acute brain syndrome.

The term "brain failure" is also currently used (Brocklehurst and Hanley, 1976; Caird and Judge, 1977; Cape, 1978; Judge, 1974). It is a term frequently used in the literature of the United Kingdom and Canada. Spier (1980) helps to simplify the use of terms regarding OMD, and she states that the utilization of the term "brain failure" falls into the realm of nursing diagnoses. The term "senile dementia" is still a currently recognized term and can be found in the *Glossary to the International Classification of Disease* (World Health Or-

ganization, 1946). The term "pseudodementia" is frequently used to describe the masked depression often seen in late life, "pseudosenility" is yet another term commonly found in the literature (Verwoerdt, 1976). This latter term is used to describe the reversible dementias (Libow, 1973). One cannot spend an entire chapter describing terms when space is so precious, but the multiple terms warrant explanation. Nurses may hear all of these terms, even "senility" which — perjorative as it is — is still frequently used by lay persons and may even occasionly be seen on a chart as a diagnosis.

This chapter will discuss diagnostic issues and common conditions found in persons with organic mental disorders. None of the problems can be discussed in depth because of the space problem; therefore, an extensive reference list is included to guide the reader to other writings gleaned from a variety of disciplines. Psychiatric nursing literature about care of the elderly with dementia continues to be scant; therefore, this chapter depends heavily on the geropsychiatric literature.* The reader is referred to Chapter 12 for a discussion of confusion in the elderly.

STATISTICS

Of all of the common chronic conditions which are becoming increasingly common, senile dementia affects the largest number of people. It is a progressive condition, and the peak age for the onset of senile dementia is 80-81; between one birthday and the next, about one of every twenty people will develop this condition (Gruenberg and Hagnell, 1976); see Figure 11-1. Note that in the years after 1947-1949,

---

*For an outstanding list of references about dementia, the reader should consult Edgar Miller's book *Abnormal Aging* (1977).

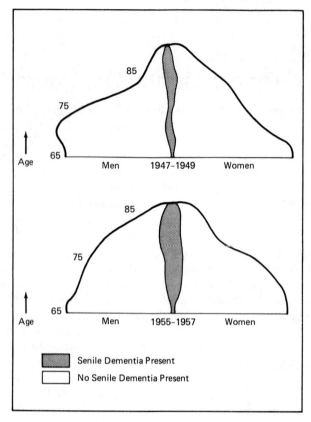

Figure 11-1. [Source: Ernest M. Gruenberg and Olie Hagnell. *Patterns of Disease among the Aged.* N.I.H. Publication No. 79-1407 (revised July 1978).

the number of persons with senile dementia in the population doubled for men and tripled for women. However, only one-third of all the people who die after age 80 have clinically recognizable signs of senile dementia when they die (Gruenberg, 1978).

It has been well documented also that the number of psychiatric problems in nursing homes is considerable (Eisdorfer and Cohen, (1982) Teeter, Garetz, Dailler, and Heiland, 1976). Over one million older Americans live in nursing homes, so the number of aged persons with mental problems, especially organic mental disorders, is high (Butler, 1982). The statistics in Table 11-1 indicate the number of referrals found by a geriatric crisis intervention screening team. The nonpsychotic organic brain syndromes comprised 59.5% of the problems, and the authors stated that these persons presented difficult nursing problems (Friedman and Bowes, 1971).

Katzman and Karasu (1975) indicated that 4.4% of the elderly population, or approximately one million people, have some degree of serious cognitive impairment. Among the aged with dementing illness, 60% have primary neuronal degeneration of Alzheimer's type; 15–40% have multi-infarct type (Eisdorfer and Cohen, in press). The two most common underlying brain disorders are (1) primary degenerative diseases of the brain (Alzheimer's type of presenile dementia and senile dementia) and (2) cerebrovascular disease, which is now called multi-infarct disease (Wang, 1977). All of the data clearly tell us that nursing has a great deal of work, thought, and research to do in these areas.

The severity of clinical findings and manifestations in the organic brain syndrome does not always correlate with the severity of the organic brain disorder (Wang, 1973; Wang, Obrist, and Busse, 1970). For example, a variety of psycho-

Table 11-1. Diagnosis of Geriatric Crisis Referrals.

DIAGNOSES	NUMBER
Manic-depressive illness, depressed type	1
Manic-depressive illness, manic type	1
Schizophrenia, chronic undifferentiated type	1
Schizophrenia, paranoid	1
Other paranoid state	3
Psychoneurosis, depressive neurosis	8
Psychoneurosis, anxiety neurosis	2
Senile dementia	1
Psychosis with cerebral arteriosclerosis	1
Cerebral arteriosclerosis	5
Cerebral thrombosis	1
Nonpsychotic organic brain syndrome with senile brain disease	36
Nonpsychotic organic brain syndrome with circulatory disturbance	18
Nonpsychotic organic brain syndrome with presenile brain disease	4
Nonpsychotic organic brain syndrome with brain trauma	1
Adjustment reaction of late life	7
Other social maladjustment	1
No mental disorder	6
Diagnosis deferred pending workup	1
Total	99

FOLLOW-UP RESULTS	NUMBER
Still in nursing home	29
Died in nursing home	3
Sent from nursing home to municipal hospital	2
Still in municipal hospital awaiting nursing home	2
Sent from municipal hospital to nursing home	2
Sent home from municipal hospital	2
Transferred from municipal hospital to state hospital	4
Still in voluntary hospital awaiting nursing home	1
Sent from voluntary hospital to nursing home	2
Sent home from voluntary hospital	1
Left voluntary hospital to live with neice in Florida	1
Still in proprietary hospital	2
Still in proprietary hospital, awaiting nursing home	1
Sent from proprietary hospital to nursing home	1
Still in government hospital (sigmoid neoplasm with mestastases found)	1
Sent from private psychiatric hospital to nursing home	1
Sent from private psychiatric hospital to old-age residence	1
Still in private mental hospital	1
Still in old-age residence	3
Still at home	16
Still at home with housekeeper	1
Still at home, awaiting nursing home	6
Still at home, attending mental hygiene clinic in another county	1
Still at home, attending mental hygiene clinic	3
Sent from home to nursing home	6
Sent from home to old-age residence	1
Sent from home to private mental hospital	1
Sent from home to state hospital	1
Sent from home to municipal hospital	1

SOURCE: Friedman, J.H. and Bowes, N. Experience of a geriatric crisis intervention screening team. *Journal of Psychiatric and Mental Health Nursing* 9(5):11–17 (1971).

NOTE: This study consisted of 99 patients seen over a 12-month period.

social factors, such as social isolation, depressions, and anxiety, can change the patient's behaviors and cognitive functions in ways similar to organic brain disorders (Wang, 1980); see Table 12-3.

DIAGNOSTIC ISSUES

The diagnostic issues and their importance in OMD are clearly stated throughout the geropsychiatric literature. The importance of the relationship between mental problems and physical problems means that a holistic approach is mandated for the professional nurse caring for these individuals (Cohen, 1980; Post, 1975; Roth, 1978; Sloan, 1980).

The following are symptoms commonly present in the mental decline of the elderly. Though they can be listed discretely, these symptoms overlap and a holistic approach is necessary for effective preventive as well as therapeutic intervention. For example, disorientation may be due to dizziness, a sensory impairment, or a nutrition deficiency.

Psychosocial	Cognitive	Physical
Anxiety	Confusion	Insomnia
Agitation	Forgetfulness	Anorexia
Hostility	Hallucinations	Dizziness
Irritability	Disorientation	Chest Pain
Depression	Poor Concentra-	Constipation
Loneliness	tion	Muscle
Unsociability	Thinking Dis-	Cramps
Bothersome-	turbances	Urinary Fre-
ness	Unusual Thought	quency
Uncooperative-	Content	Impaired
ness	Slowed Thought	Sensoria
Emotional	Processes	Diminished
Lability	Shortened Atten-	Locomo-
(Linden, 1976).	tion Span	tion
	Impaired Mental	Joint Pain or
	Alertness	Stiffness

Core symptoms to consider in screening and assessing for dementia are: (1) impairment of memory, (2) emotional stability, (3) impairment of judgment, (4) impairment of cognitive ability and (5) impairment of orientation (Glen and Cowley, 1974). A slightly different classification with an easy acronymn is JOMAC which stands for judgment, orientation, memory, affect, and cognition (Murray, Huelskoetter, and O'Driscoll, 1980). A nurse will need to understand how each of these symptoms is manifested so that she can intervene, as well as support and educate the family regarding dementia. Supporting the family may at times be the most realistic goal to strive for in persons with dementia (Harris, 1972). The symptoms are pervasive in any client who has diffuse impairment of brain tissue function. See Chapter 12 for assessment tools such as the Mental Status Questionnaire.

INTERRELATIONSHIP OF MENTAL AND PHYSICAL STATUS

The reader should consult Chapters 14 through 20 in this book for detailed explanations of physical changes occurring in the aged person. The interrelationship of mental and physical problems is important for the nurse doing assessments and also for the gerontological nurse practitioner. The direct relationship between organic brain disease and physical status has been pointed out by internists (Harris, 1972; Libow, 1973). Indeed, mental and emotional disorders are usually first manifested in physical complaints.

Nurses should become increasingly skilled in their ability to detect the potentially reversible mental changes in pseudosenility. Libow (1973) lists the common causes of pseudosenility. It is well to note that 30% of the individuals thought to have brain disorders may have reversible syndromes (Roth, 1978); see also Table 12-1). Besdine (1979) states that the 30% of the cognitive disorders which are medically reversible amount to about 300,000 persons. These are staggering figures, and nurses must begin to address the problems presented by these individuals.

DEPRESSION VERSUS DEMENTIA

"Depression as an affect or feeling tone, is a ubiquitous and universal condition which as a human experience extends on a continuum from normal mood swings to a pathological state" (Zung, 1980). Theoretically, dementia and depression are quite different, but in clinical practice, they may be quite difficult to separate (Eisdorfer and Cohen, 1978). While a depression may not be detected immediately, careful and persistent interviewing will clarify its presence (Post, 1975). The distinguishing features of dementia and depression have been succinctly tabulated by Zung (1980); see Table 11-2 for the differences between dementia and depression. Because senile dementia is a progressive illness, persons who show no change after six months would be suspected of having a depressive condition (Roth, 1978).

Suicide is particularly high in older people who have dementia. Evaluation of suicidal behavior is difficult in this group because many old people say that they would be better off dead, but they are not suicidal. The interview is not complete without an inquiry about self-destructive plans or suicidal ideation (MacKinnon and Michels, 1971). Depression may be observed in the early stages of Alzheimer's disease when the person is aware that something serious is happening.

Table 11-2. The Differential Diagnosis between Dementia and Depression.

DEMENTIA	DEPRESSION
1. *Affect:* Labile, fluctuating from tears to laughter, not consistent or sustained; may show apathy, depression, irritability, euphoria, or inappropriate affect. Normal control impaired; can be influenced by suggestions.	Depressed; feelings of despair which are pervasive, persistent; anxious, hypomanic. Affect not influenced by suggestion.
2. *Memory:* Decreased attention. Decreased memory for recent events. Confabulation. Perseveration.	Difficulty in concentration. Impaired learning of new knowledge. Decreased attention, with secondary decrease in recent memory.
3. *Intellect:* Impaired, decreased, as tested by serial 7s, similarities, recent events.	Impaired, but can perform serial 7s, remember recent events.
4. *Orientation:* Fluctuating with varying levels of awareness. May be disoriented for time, place.	May have some confusion, not as profound as in dementia.
5. *Judgment:* Poor judgment with inappropriate behavior and dress. Deterioration of personal habits and personal hygiene. Loss of bladder and bowel control.	May be poor.
6. *Somatic Complaints:* Fatigue. Failing health complaints with vague complaints of pain in head, neck, and back.	Typical complaints such as: • Decreased sleep • Decreased appetite • Decreased weight • Decreased libido • Decreased energy • Constipation
7. *Psychotic Behavior:* Mainly visual hallucinations; delusions.	May occur in psychotic depressions, with mainly auditory hallucinations; delusions.
8. *Neurological Symptoms:* Dysphasia, apraxia, agnosia.	Not present.

SOURCE: Zung, William K. Affective disorders. In E.W. Busse and D.G. Blazer *The Handbook of Geriatric Psychiatry* New York: Van Nostrand Reinhold, 1980.

ALZHEIMER'S DISEASE

Alzheimer's disease is used to describe senile dementia whether it occurs before or after the age of 65. If the disease occurs before the age of 65, it is called presenile dementia. After 65, it is known as senile dementia, Alzheimer's type (Cohen, 1980). It must be remembered that common names and common neuropathologic findings do not necessarily imply a common cause in the presenile and senile dementias. These two syndromes may have quite different causes (Butler, 1979, 1982).

There is some scattered evidence that genetic factors play a role in the Alzheimer's type of dementia (Katzman, Terry, and Bick, 1978; Larsson, Sjogren, and Jacobson, 1963). Some investigators in the field of dementia consider presenile and senile dementia as a continuum of Alzheimer's disease, which may be a genetic defect (Pearce and Miller, 1973; Terry, 1976). In a study in Sweden which is now classic, Larsson et al. (1963) found that relatives of patients with Alzheimer's disease have a higher frequency of Alzheimer's. Other researchers have reported this also (Heston and Mastri, 1977). Heston reports a higher frequency of Down's syndrome in these families (Heston, 1977). The neurofibrillary tangles, which are found in the brain and are diagnostic of Alzheimer's disease, are also found in persons who have Down's syndrome. Alzheimer's disease and its nursing care are discussed in depth by Bartol (1979) and Burnside (1979). See also the section "True Dementias" in Chapter 12.

The dementias associated with Parkinson's disease (one-third of the patients with Parkinson's disease develop dementia), multiple sclerosis, Huntington's chorea, Creutzfeldt-Jakob syndrome, and Pick's disease may have similar general presentations in the beginning, but they have different etiologies and different courses, and they respond differently to drug therapy (Eisdorfer and Cohen, in press). The brain changes found in autopsies of persons with Alzheimer's disease include: (1) neurofibrillary tangles, (2) atrophy of the brain, (3) loss of neurons, (4) granulovacuolar degeneration, and (5) plaque formation.

Gustafson and Hagberg (1975) have listed the various symptoms of dementia: (1) amnesia (reduced learning, retention, and recall of recent events and of the remote past) and confabulation; (2) disturbances of attention and concentration; (3) lack of initiative and spontaneity; (4) reduced stock of ideas (stereotypy and impoverishment of thoughts and associations); (5) increased reactivity, extreme selectiveness of stimuli (inability to survey, integrate, and analyze information; tendency toward catastrophic reactions); (6) disturbance of consciousness; (7) disorientation; (8) affective disturbances (e.g., emotional shallowness, reduced interests and awareness of own illness, affective bluntness, euphoria, affective lability, and increased irritability); (9) suspiciousness and paranoid tendencies; (10) aphasia (various disturbances of language); (11) agnosia (inability to understand nonverbal symbols); and (12) apraxia (incapacity for carrying out purposeful movements). The reader is referred to Burnside (1979) for a more detailed description of common terms used to describe behaviors, and also to Chapter 12 of this book.

Memory

Memory loss is usually the first symptom to appear in dementia. Recent memory should be studied, and patients should be aided in whatever way possible to remember the important things of daily living. Is it really important that the person learn the day, month, and year? Perhaps the emphasis on reality orientation classes is too enthusiastic for some individuals with low energy levels, and lower, more realistic goals that can be met should be set by the nurse. For example, it may be very important to help a person learn when it is morning or night or whether it is winter or summer (Besdine, 1979). The distinguished physician Richard Besdine also points out that sleep patterns change in old age and that the elderly tend to sleep for a shorter period of time and also less deeply. Yet what happens? We put them to bed earlier (Besdine, 1979)! (One might add that we expect them to sleep later in the morning too.)

COMMON PROBLEMS IN DEMENTIA

There are some very common nursing management problems in the care of individuals with organic mental disorders, and they constitute both the challenge and the frustration of nursing. Some of the problems which must be constantly monitored and managed include: (1) confusion and disorientation; (2) depressive states; (3) bizarre accusations or paranoid ideation; (4) nocturnal neurosis (Sundowner's syndrome); (5) incontinence; (6) wandering behavior; (7) drug reaction; (8) iatrogenic reactions, e.g., nosocomial infections, choking spells, bronchopneumonia; (9) aggressive behaviors; and (10) the alienation and loneliness experienced in dementia. In all of these, one should be alert to the consequences of such behaviors to the aged person, to family and friends, and to staff members. It goes without saying that the family will need support and education throughout the illness of the loved one because there will be a loss of social decorum, and when there is combativeness or sexual acting out, the families may need much support (see Chapter 12 for guidelines for care, as well as a discussion of wandering behavior).

Wandering

At this writing, there is little in the literature about wandering behavior; for nursing guidelines, refer to Burnside (1980); Cornbleth (1977); and Snyder, Kupprecht, Pyrek, Brekhus, and Moss (1978). Cape (1978) states that bemused wandering patients must have constant reassurance, comfort, and gentle encouragement; one should not confront them or argue with them: "They can only be led not driven." The following vignette beautifully describes problem solving in a small community (also see Chapter 12).

Vignette. "Willie Kunkle, 90 years old, was one of the sturdily independent men and women in a small village who were interviewed by Doris Schwartz. . . .He lived with his niece Elda, 80, and was as vigorous as a young man, but he was becoming forgetful. Willie could climb a towering oak and saw off a branch, but when he climbed down, he couldn't remember the way home. Aware of his wanderings and Elda's worry, the entire village held a meeting and made a plan. If Willie was missing, Elda was to phone the firehouse and the fire bell

would be rung twice to alert the town to start hunting. Whoever found Willie was to invite him home for a glass of wine, call Elda, and tell the firemen to sound the all clear. Their plan succeeded, and Willie Kunkle lived contentedly for another two years. . . .Could Willie Kunkle have survived those last two years, to age 92, if he'd been institutionalized as his memory faded? Probably he could have, but not in the contentment made possible by his neighbors' inter-dependent efforts" (Kelly, 1980).

Interviewing

Interviewing the elderly person with dementia is difficult, time consuming, and draining, even under the best of conditions. The exquisite pacing and sensitivity needed were well taught by Dr. Alvin Goldfarb; his skill in reducing anxiety and obtaining information resulted from his use of a conversational style.

During interviews with the chronically confused, "the trick is not to accept the local assessment" (Schmidt, 1975). The perception of the staff may be negative or based on a minimum of data. Their impressions can influence or even throw the new interviewer. In the assessment interview, the nurse must rely upon observations and listening skills. First interviews usually produce fear in the elderly person (Murray et al., 1980). The frail elderly require exquisite pacing by the interviewer, even to the point of having more than one interview to obtain the information. A geriatric nurse practitioner has sensitively described therapeutic approaches with the frail elderly during physical assessments (Robison, 1981). (See Chapters 14 through 20 in this book.)

The interviewer must work constantly to prevent a catastrophic reaction (Goldstein, 1942). A complaint of fatigue or exhaustion may occur because of the energy needed to preserve integrity and to cope with failing cognitive abilities (Murray et al., 1980; Sloan, 1980). The reader is referred to an excellent assessment of cognitive status by Spier (1980). She is one of the few writers to include color psychology in her writings about the environment for the cognitively impaired elderly. Arie (1973) says that the ability to ask the right questions is the basis for management of the person with dementia — it is also the crux of interviewing (see Chapter 7 on communication).

Sundowner's Syndrome

Cameron (1941), in a classic study, demonstrated that when demented patients were blindfolded, 13 out of 16 showed a severe distortion of their spatial image within an hour. This problem was called "nocturnal neurosis" by Cameron and has implications for nursing. Night nurses will have to be taught how to intervene effectively in this nocturnal sensory deprivation in the elderly. Cohen (1980) states that agencies fail to cope with the problem adequately.

Restraints

Ronald Cape, a geriatrician, feels that if nurses who are skilled in managing the confused elderly had rooms which were designed for this group of patients, the need for restraints would disappear (Cape, 1978). Bartol (1978) states that nurses can manage wards better by increasing interpersonal interactions and providing environments which are safe, comfortable, and structured; she has demonstrated ward management without the use of restraints. Space also appears to be an important variable in managing patients with dementia (Eisdorfer and Cohen, 1978).

Restraints may be used (1) to prevent wandering behavior, e.g., use of a "geri chair"; (2) to keep the patient from sliding out of a chair; and (3) to keep a patient quiet or prone in bed. (The reason for the restraint is usually to protect the patient, but that reason is not always sound or justified. The legal implications, of course, are great, which precludes taking risks that are sometimes necessary. Indiscriminate use of restraints encourages incontinence.)

Incontinence

Incontinence in geriatric psychiatry is almost wholly associated with dementia. Therefore, nursing must concern itself with the management of incontinence. The reader is referred to

Willington's fine book on incontinence (Willington, 1976), to a research study by Wells (1980), to a chapter by Wells and Brink (1981), and to comprehensive writings about the subject by Bartol (1980). Wells (1980, p. 27) wrote, "It would seem probable that the incidence of incontinence could have been reduced with enough staff who were knowledgeable in assessing and treating incontinence, with numerous suitable commodes and adjustable height beds, and with adequately designed toilets near to the patient areas." (See Chapter 29 on bladder and bowel rehabilitation.)

CAUTIONS

A patient who has an organic mental disorder may have difficulty in following directions and may therefore be unable to carry out the procedures in a therapy regime, e.g., a successful surgery for hip fractures. The reader is referred to Chapter 26 for further discussion of surgical problems in elderly clients. These individuals have a greater tendency to aspirate food so the chances for bronchopneumonia increase (Rossman, Rodstein, and Bornstein, 1974). Choking can occur from the rapid feeding that is often done by nurses aides who have too large a feeding assignment.

A person with organic mental disorder may also not have the ability to recognize or realize serious pathology in bodily changes and may therefore fail to report these changes (Rossman et al., 1974).

Reduced mobility and inability to handle the activities of daily living (ADL) can also be problems in working with these individuals. The sensory losses and their impact on behavior are well documented in the literature, and the nurse must pay close attention to the prostheses of these individuals and also to dentures which get lost or misplaced.

The inability to remember to drink or eat regularly is one of the areas which nurses should monitor carefully. Problems with medications are rampant, and this is another area in which these individuals need surveillance.

The elderly person who suffers from organic brain disease is especially susceptible to the side effects of the major tranquilizers, e.g., tardive dyskinesia (disfiguring, buccal, lingual masticatory movements) and akathisia (choreiform body movements).

TREATMENT MODALITIES

An excellent review of therapies by Folsom, Boies, and Pommerenck (1978) discusses the current modalities used (see Figure 11-2). These authors state, "Each person using these therapies must, however, inject a measure of his or her individuality into the process. That is a matter of style. It is part of being a person. It is also an important part of calling forth the individual who has withdrawn." Another excellent overview on therapies for older patients with cognitive impairment has been written by Eisdorfer, Cohen, and Preston (in press). The bibliography at the end of this chapter suggests added overviews for the reader.

Group Modalities

Voelkel (1978) compared a reality orientation (RO) and a resocialization (RS) group. The members of the RO group did not improve significantly, but the members of the RS group did. Voelkel stated, "It could be concluded that it is not the constant reminder of current information that improves mental status, but the coming together as a group in a social setting that makes the difference." She also felt that six weeks is too short a time for group life in working with moderate to severe mental impairment. See also Burnside (1978, 1980, 1981) for in-depth discussion of group work with the frail elderly impaired individual.

Nurses can improve environments and enrich them for the aged, even in custodial care settings. Mary Opal Wolanin's book on confusion is highly recommended for guidelines in assessment and care of the confused patient. (Wolanin 1981)

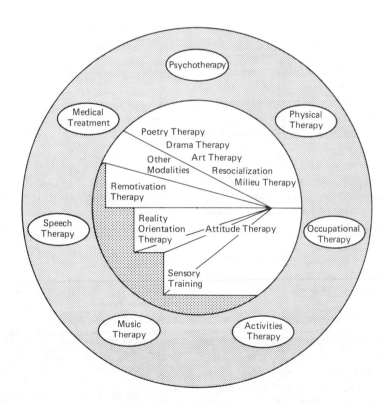

Figure 11-2. M. Weiner, A. Brok, and A. Sandowsky. *Working with the Aged: Practical Approaches in the Institution and Community*, p. 64. Copyright © 1978. Reprinted by permission of Prentice-Hall, Inc., Englewood Cliffs, N.J.]

Much has been written about the benefits of group therapy with the aged client suffering from organic mental disorders. There are conflicting reports on the benefits of reality orientation groups and remotivation groups. Whatever the results, one still has to commend group leaders who have the courage to begin groups and who try to maintain them when there is such a cloud of nihilism over many of the institutions in which old people are found.

Two nurses and a psychologist conducted an ego-enhancing group in a day care center, using an eclectic approach in an effort to extrapolate useful techniques from other forms of group modalities. A constant goal of the group was to improve the low self-esteem of cognitively impaired older individuals, and a model was designed for such groups. The leaders searched for the positive qualities of each member's strength, listened for individual group themes, and studied nonverbal behavior (Burnside, Baumler and Weaver-Dyck 1984).

MANAGEMENT

The implementation of psychosocial interventions falls under the aegis of nursing. To maintain a supportive caring environment and to constantly provide a therapeutic amount of sensory stimulation are obligatory for nursing if the alienation, loneliness, and fear in dementia are to be mitigated.

It is well for nurses to educate the general public, and especially older people, that dementia is not an inevitable consequence of longevity. It is a condition dreaded and feared by many. To assist nurses in interactions with clients and/or families, the following excellent pragmatic references are suggested: Burnside (1978, 1979, 1980, 1981) and Wolanin (1980). The baseline data needed for scientific study of senile dementia are simply not available (Butler, 1979). Epidemiological study is needed for these reasons: (1) to recognize the new patterns of the disease (for example, the increasing prevalence of chronic conditions brought on by the disease processes) and (2) to find preventable causes. We also need to know more about the incidence of new cases and the total number of both old and new cases. In additions, we need

to know familial patterns and environmental influences. Who escapes the disease? Nurses as observers, reporters, and caretakers could be instrumental in such investigations.

SUMMARY

This chapter has dealt with a tremendous problem in mental health in the aged and has highlighted some of the areas for nurses to consider. Nurses will need to be able to do comprehensive physical and psychiatric assessments. They will need to know both the theory and practice of gerontological and geriatric nursing. Nurses prepared at both the Masters and doctoral level in gerontology and geropsychiatry continue to be in great demand. The gerontological nurse will be an important part of the team in future geriatric assessment clinics (Busse and Blazer, 1980).

REFERENCES

Arie, T. Dementia in the elderly: diagnosis and assessment. *British Medical Journal* 4:540-543 (1973).

Bartol, M.A. Personal communication (1978).

Bartol, M.A. Nonverbal communication in patients with Alzheimer's disease. *Journal of Gerontological Nursing* 5:21-31 (July-August 1979).

Bartol, M.A. Psychosocial aspects of incontinence in the aged person. In Burnside, I.M. (Ed.) *Psychosocial Nursing Care of the Aged* (2nd ed.). New York: McGraw-Hill, 1980.

Besdine, R.W. *Medical aspects in the differential diagnosis of the cognitively impaired elderly.* Speech at the 4th Annual Psychiatry Symposium — Geropsychiatry, El Paso, Texas, January 18-20, 1979.

Brocklehurst, J.C. and Hanley, T. *Geriatric Medicine for Students.* Edinburgh: Churchill, Livingstone, 1976, pp. 59-62.

Burnside, I.M. *Working with the Elderly: Group Process and Techniques.* North Scituate, Mass.: Duxbury Press, 1978.

Burnside, I.M. Alzheimer's disease: an overview. *Journal of Gerontological Nursing* 5:14-20 (July-August 1979).

Burnside, I.M. *Psychosocial Nursing Care of the Aged* (2nd ed.). New York: McGraw-Hill, 1980.

Burnside, I.M., Ebersole, P., and Monea, H.E. (Eds.). *Psychosocial Caring throughout the Life Span.* New York: McGraw-Hill, 1979.

Burnside, I.M. Nursing and The Aged, 2nd Ed. New York: McGraw-Hill, 1981.

Burnside, I.M., Baumler, J., Weaver-Dyck, S. Group work in a Day Care Center: A Model in *Working with the Elderly, Group Processes and Techniques,* 2nd Ed. Burnside, I.M., Ed. Monterey, California: Wadsworth Publishing Co. 1984.

Busse, E. and Blazer, D.G. *Handbook of Geriatric Psychiatry.* New York: Van Nostrand Reinhold Co. 1980, pp. 249–272.

Butler, R.N., and Lewis, M.I. *Aging and Mental Health,* 3nd Ed. St. Louis: C.V. Mosby, 1982, pp. 283–219.

Butler, R.N. Research Leads and Needs. *Forum on Aging* Vol. 2, p. 116–251 (Nov. 1979).

Caird, F.I. Judge T.G. *Assessment of the Elderly Patient* Md. Ek. Philadelphia: J.B. Lippincott, 1979.

Cameron, D.E. Studies in Senile Nocturnal Delerium, *Psychiatric Quarterly* 15:47–53 (1941).

Cape, R. Aging, Its Complex Management, Hagerstown, Md: Harper and Row, 1978.

Cohen, G.D. *Fact Sheet: Senile Dementia.* Rockville, Md.: U.S. Department of Health and Human Services, 1980.

Cornbleth, T. Effect of a protected hospital ward area on wandering and non-wandering geriatric patients. *Journal of Gerontology* 35:573–577 (September 1977).

Diagnostic and Statistical Manual of Mental Disorders (DSM III). Washington, D.C.: American Psychiatric Association, 1977.

Eisdorfer, C. and Cohen, D. Cognitive impaired elderly differential diagnosis. In Storandt, M., Siegler, I.C., and Eliss, M.F. (Eds.) *The Clinical Psychology of Aging.* New York: Plenum, 1978.

Eisdorfer, C. and Cohen, D. Dementing illness in mid and late life. In Ebaugh, F.G. (Ed.) *Geriatrics for the Primary Care Physician.* Menlo Park, Calif.: Addison-Wesley, 1982.

Eisdorfer, C., Cohen, D., and Preston, C. Behavioral and psychological therapies for the older patient with cognitive impairment. *Behavioral Aspects of Senile Dementia.* Washington, D.C.: National Institutes of Health, in press.

Folsom, J.C., Boies, B.L., and Pommerenck, K. Life adjustment techniques for use with the dysfunctional elderly. *Aged Care and Services Review* 1:1–3 (1978).

Friedman, J.H. and Bowes, N. Experience of a geriatric crisis intervention screening team. *Journal of Psychiatric and Mental Health Nursing* 9(5): 11–17 (1971).

Glen, R.S. and Cowley, L.M. *Senile Psychoses – Aspects of Recognition and Management.* Sandoz Pharmaceuticals Publication for Scientific Exhibit, 26th Institute on Hospital and Community Psychiatry, Denver, Colorado, September 30–October 2, 1974.

Goldstein, K. *After Effects of Brain Injuries in War: Their Evaluation and Treatment.* New York: Grune and Stratton, 1942.

Gruenberg, E.M. *Patterns of Disease among the Aged* (DHEW Publication NIH 78-1410). Washington, D.C.: National Institute on Aging, 1978.

Gruenberg, E.M. and Hagnell, O. *The rising prevalence of chronic brain syndrome.* Paper presented at Symposium on Society, Stress and Diseases, Aging and Old Age, Stockholm, Sweden, June 14–19, 1976.

Gustafson, L. and Hagberg, B. Dementia with onset in the research period. *ACTA Psychiatrica Scandinavica* (Supplement 257): 1–71 (1975).

Harris, R. The relationship between organic brain disease and physical states. In Gaitz, C.M. (Ed.) *Aging and the Brain.* New York: Plenum, 1972, pp. 163–177.

Heston, C.C. Alzheimer's disease, trisomy 21, and myeloproliferation disorders: associations suggesting a genetic diathesis. *Science* 196:322-323 (1977).

Heston, C.C. and Mastri, A.R. The genetics of Alzheimer's disease: association with myeloproliferative disorders and Down's syndrome. *Archives of General Psychiatry* 34:976-981 (1977).

Hirschfeld, M. Nursing care of the cognitively impaired. In Eisdorfer, C. and Friedel, R.O. (Eds.) *Cognitive and Emotional Disturbances in the Elderly: Clinical Issues.* Chicago: Year Book Medical Publishers, 1977.

Judge, T.G. Drugs and memory. In Anderson, W.F. and Judge, T.C. (Eds.) *Geriatric Medicine.* London: Academic Press, 1974, p. 110.

Katzman, R. and Karasu, T.B. Differential diagnosis of dementia. In Field, W. (Ed.) *Neurological and Sensory Disorders in the Elderly.* New York: Stratton, 1975, pp. 103-134.

Katzman, R., Terry, R.D., and Bick, K.L. (Eds.). *Alzheimer's Disease: Senile Dementia and Related Disorders* (Aging: Vol. 7). New York: Raven Press, 1978.

Kelly, C. Quoting Doris Schwartz (editorial). *Geriatric Nursing* 1:2 (July–August 1980).

Larsson, T., Sjogren, T., and Jacobson, G. Senile dementia, a clinical sociomedical and genetic study. *Acta Psychiatrica Scandinavica* 39 (Supplement 167): (1963).

Libow, L.S. Pseudo-senility: acute and reversible organic brain syndromes. *Journal of the American Geriatrics Society* 21:112-120 (March 1973).

Linden, M.E. *Mental decline in elderly patients: treatment of selected symptoms.* Scientific exhibit presented at the National Association of Private Psychiatric Hospitals, Palm Springs, California, January 16-22, 1976.

MacKinnon, R.A. and Michels, R. The organic brain syndrome patient. *The Psychiatric Interview in Clinical Practice.* Philadelphia: W.B. Saunders, 1971.

Miller, E. Abnormal Aging: The Psychology of Senile and Presenile Dementia: London, Wiley, 1977.

Murray, R., Huelskoetter, M.M., and O'Driscoll, D. *The Nursing Process in Later Maturity.* Englewood

Cliffs, N.J.: Prentice-Hall, 1980, p. 528.

Pearce, K. and Miller, E. *Clinical Aspects of Dementia.* London: Tindall, 1973.

Post, F. Dementia, depression and pseudo-dementia. In Benson, D.F. and Blumer, D. (Eds.) *Psychiatric Aspects of Neurological Disease.* New York: Grune and Stratton, 1975.

Raskind, M. and Storrie, M.C. Organic mental disorders. In Busse, E.W. and Blazer, D. (Eds.) *Handbook of Geropsychiatry.* New York: Van Nostrand Reinhold, 1980.

Robison, B.J. Approaches to assessment of the frail elderly. In Burnside, I.M. (Ed.) *Nursing and the Aged* (2nd ed.). New York: McGraw-Hill, 1981.

Rossman, I., Rodstein, M., and Bornstein, A. Undiagnosed diseases in an aging population. *Archives of Internal Medicine* 133:366–369 (1974).

Roth, M. Diagnosis of senile and related forms of dementia. In Katzman, R., Terry, R.D., and Bick, K.L. (Eds.) *Alzheimer's Disease: Senile Dementia and Related Disorders* (Aging: Vol. 7). New York: Raven Press, 1978, pp. 71–85.

Schmidt, M.G. Interviewing the "old old." *The Gerontologist* 15:544–546 (December 1975).

Sloan, R.B. Organic brain syndrome. In Birren, J.E. and Sloan, R.B. (Eds.) *Handbook of Mental Health and Aging.* Englewood Cliffs, N.J.: Prentice-Hall, 1980, pp. 554–615.

Snyder, L.H., Kupprecht, P., Pyrek, J., Brekhus, S., and Moss, T. Wandering. *The Gerontologist* 18:272–280 (June 1978).

Spier, B.E. The nursing process as applied to the cognitive aspects of aging. In Yurick, A., Gera, S., Robb, S., Spier, B.E., and Ebert, N.J. (Eds.) *The Aged Person and the Nursing Process.* New York: Appleton-Century-Crofts, 1980, pp. 255–288.

Teeter, R.B., Garetz, F.K., Dailler, W.B., and Heiland, W.F. Psychiatric disturbances of aged patients in skilled nursing homes. *American Journal of Psychiatry* 133:1430–1434 (1976).

Terry, R.D. Dementia: a brief and selective review. *Archives of Neurology* 33:1–4 (1976).

Verwoerdt, A. *Clinical Geropsychiatry.* Baltimore: Williams and Wilkins, 1976.

Voelkel, D. A study of reality orientation and resocialization groups with confused elderly. *Journal of Gerontological Nursing* 4:13–18 (May–June 1978).

Wang, H.S. Cerebral correlates of intellectual function in senescence. In Jarvik, L.F., Eisdorfer, C., and Blum, J.E. (Eds.) *Intellectual Functioning in Adults, Psychological and Biological influences.* New York: Springer, 1973, pp. 95–106.

Wang, H.S. Organic brain syndromes. In Busse, E.W. and Pfeiffer, E. (Eds.) *Behavior and Adaptation in Late Life* (2nd ed.). Boston: Little, Brown, 1977.

Wang, H.S. Diagnostic procedures. In Busse, E.W. and Blazer, D.G. (Eds.) *Handbook of Geriatric Psychiatry.* New York: Van Nostrand Reinhold, 1980.

Wang, H.S., Obrist, W.D., and Busse, E.W. Neurophysiological correlates of the intellectual function of elderly persons living in the community. *American Journal of Psychiatry* 126:1205–1212 (1970).

Wells, T. *Problems in Geriatric Nursing Care.* Edinburgh: Livingstone, 1980, pp. 23–25.

Wells, T.J. and Brink, C. Continence. In Burnside, I.M. (Ed.) *Nursing and the Aged* (2nd ed.). New York: McGraw-Hill, 1981.

Willington, F.J. *Incontinence in the Elderly.* London: Academic Press, 1976.

Wolanin, M.O. *Confusion Prevention and Care.* St. Louis: C.V. Mosby, 1981, pp. 39–101.

World Health Organization. *Glossary to the International Classification of Disease.* Geneva, Switzerland: 1946.

Zung, W. Depression in later life. In Busse, E.W. and Blazer, D. (Eds.) *Handbook of Geriatric Psychiatry.* New York: Van Nostrand Reinhold, 1980.

BIBLIOGRAPHY

Burnside, I.M. You have been here before (editorial). *Journal of Gerontological Nursing* 6:377–379 (July 1980).

Farley, J.K. Responses to pathophysiologic disturbances in the aged. *Handbook of Clinical Nursing.* New York: McGraw-Hill, 1979.

Kayne, R.C. Drugs in the elderly. In Burnside, I.M. (Ed.) *Nursing and the Aged* (2nd ed.). New York: McGraw-Hill, 1981.

Lipowski, Z.J. A new look at organic brain syndromes. *American Journal of Psychiatry* 137:674–678 (June 1980).

Post, F. Dementia, depression and pseudodementia. In Benson, D.F. and Blumer, D. (Eds.) *Psychiatric Aspects of Neurologic Disease.* New York: Grune and Stratton, 1975.

Sideleau, B.F. Organic brain syndrome. In Haber, J., Leach, A., Schudy, S., and Sideleau, B.F. (Eds.) *Comprehensive Psychiatric Nursing.* New York: McGraw-Hill, 1978.

Wells, C.E. Chronic brain disease: an overview. *American Journal of Psychiatry* 135:1–12 (1978).

12
Confusion and Disorientation

Mary Opal Wolanin

O, let me not be mad, not mad, sweet heaven!
Keep me in temper; I would not be mad.

Shakespeare, King Lear
(act 2, scene 4, lines 287–289)

Confusion represents a constellation of behaviors that care givers recognize as a change from the usual and accepted. In classical cases there are easy distractibility, short attention span, loss of memory for recent events and later for remote events, and an inability to follow instructions. There is poor judgment in daily living tasks. All signs seem related to memory loss of previous events. There may be delirium with visual hallucinations in those persons who have acute brain syndrome. Confusion is a wastebasket, catchall term to describe any unusual behavior. It is an undesirable label.

The terms confusion and disorientation are often used interchangeably, but disorientation is a less abstract term for it describes a relation to time, place, and person which allows some precision in documenting behavior. It is more accurate to describe behavior by saying, "Mr. Smith is consistently disoriented to his surroundings," than "Mr. Smith is confused." Neither confusion nor disorientation describes total behavior, for few people are confused about everything or totally disoriented. There are degrees of confusion and disorientation. Both may be temporary or patchy in occurrence.

Confusion is found at all ages, but for the elderly it always is seen as a critical symptom. The assumption is made that it is a result of aging or senility and that there will be no improvement because aging is a permanent condition. Care givers may take away patient rights in the attempt to provide a safe environment. Mental status is used as an indicator for institutionalization.

INCIDENCE OF CONFUSION

There are three principal forms of confusional states which determine mental status: reversible, irreversible, and reversible superimposed on irreversible. Reversible confusional states are often referred to as acute brain syndrome or rapid onset type of confusional states. They are always secondary to some condition that can be improved, which will bring about elimination of the confusional state. Irreversible confusional states are found in about 50% of the institutionalized elderly and in a large number who are cared for by families. These are based on brain pathology and are progressive. Every person with irreversible confusional states is vulnerable to the same problems which cause reversible confusional states in all elderly, and the temporary nature is the same if recognized and treated. Irreversible confusional states are associated with multi-infarct brain disease, with about 20% of the incidence from that cause (Drachman, 1981). The incidence of confusional states due to Alzheimer's type of senile dementia is estimated at 10% in those over 65 years of age and 20% in those over 80 (Fox et al. 1975). Multi-infarct dementia and Alzheimer's disease account for 80% of the dementias of old age (Besdine, 1980). Reversible confusional states can be found at any age. Irreversible confusion and reversible superimposed on irreversible occur more in old age, that is, in the "old old."

REVERSIBLE CONFUSIONAL STATES

Signs and Symptoms

The rapid onset of a confusional state in connection with a change in an individual's physiological state, sensoriperceptual ability, emotional state, or environment is the first characteristic of reversible confusional states. There is a loss of memory for recent events such as surgery or an accident. There may be visual hallucinations and an inability to organize thinking or actions, yet the individual's orientation may be unimpaired. Memory loss prevents following directions or focusing on any subject for any meaningful time. Social graces may be unimpaired as the individual greets others and treats them in usual ways. Later the person can remember his own thoughts and actions as if he saw them on television.

Etiology

There are many causes of reversible confusional states which are secondary to some major change in the individual's physiology or emotional state. Table 12-1 lists conditions which cause brain failure (used in the same manner as cardiac or renal failure), while Table 12-2 lists factors such as sensoriperceptual change, emotional states, and change in physiological states which contribute to the rapid onset of confusional states.

Assessment for Reversible Condition

Reversible confusional states are secondary to etiological factors which are greater than the confusional state; however, the confused behavior may be the first sign of those factors. Assessment includes testing for mental impairment and comparing baseline information for recent changes in behavior. The testing can be done while the physical assessment is made. The patient's response to questions regarding history and life-style, as well as his ability to follow directions and maintain attention to the events around him, all indicate his mental status.

A complete physical examination, including vital signs, inspection, palpation, and auscultation, is necessary. A basic laboratory screening is recommended by Fox et al. (1975), which includes electrocardiogram, complete blood counts with red cell indices, thyroid studies, serum folic acid levels, fasting blood sugar, electrolyte studies, liver function tests, blood urea nitrogen, and if needed, computer assisted tomography and cerebrospinal fluid (CSF) protein. Less often considered are the functional vision and hearing abilities (Buseck, 1976; Wolanin and Phillips, 1980), but frequently they

are a key to the sudden onset when change has occurred. The nurse who is concerned with physiology may fail to consider recent events which have caused stress and which should be a part of the history.

Supportive treatment is needed to help the elderly person restore his contact with reality while physical and social problems are being assessed and treated. For example, Hilda Hammel, newly admitted to a six-bed ward in a nursing home, was frightened and apprehensive. She tried to cling to the nurse, saying, "Help me, help me," while admission procedures, examinations, and orders were in progress. She had been brought in because of wandering, incontinence, disorientation to time, and several underlying chronic conditions. The family could no longer manage her. A positive approach would be to have someone stay close to Hilda, touch her, and provide redundant cues of security such as, "Hilda, I am Mary Smith, your nurse. I'll be looking out for you; see my name tag. I will show you where I sit. This is your bed, and this is where we will put your things, etc." These kinds of statements help to orient the patient to his/her personal space. Space seems to play an important part in caring for confused individuals. Listening is also very supportive.

Treatment and Care

The treatment and care for problems of reversible and/or acute brain syndromes consist of treating the cause which differs in each case. The treatment for confusion secondary to dehydration is to relieve the dehydration while maintaining the safety of the person. The treatment for pernicious anemia, on the other hand, is to institute immediate and long term treatment with vitamin B_{12} replacement. For those problems listed in Table 12-2, the treatment is often interactional. The panic states which come with relocation, sensory overload, etc., yield only to reduction of the stress factors in the immediate situation.

The treatment for rapid onset and reversible confusional states must be instituted immediately. This means accurate assessment, screening diagnoses, close observation of the patient,

Table 12-1. Causes of Reversible Confusional States in the Elderly.

Drugs, therapeutic and nontherapeutic
    Anesthesia or surgery
    Therapeutic drug intoxication
    Other drug intoxication including alcohol
    Chemical intoxications; heavy metals such as arsenic, lead, or mercury; consciousness-
        altering agents; carbon monoxide

Metabolic conditions
    Azotemia, renal failure (diuretics, dehydration, hypokalemia)
    Hyponatremia (diuretics, salt wasting, intravenous fluids)
    Hypernatremia (dehydration, intravenous fluids)
    Volume depletion (bleeding, diuretics, inadequate fluids)
    Acid-base disturbance
    Hypoglycemia (insulin, oral hypoglycemics, starvation)
    Hyperglycemia (diabetic ketoacidosis, hyperosmolar coma)
    Hepatic failure
    Hypothyroidism
    Hyperthyroidism (especially apathetic)
    Hypercalcemia
    Cushing's syndrome
    Hypopituitarism

Hyperthermia
    Inability to lose heat in high ambient temperature
    Infection: pneumonia, pyelonephritis, cholecystitis, diverticulitis, tuberculosis,
        endocarditis

Hypothermia
    Unintentional or accidental, iatrogenic (in connection with surgery)

Hypoxia (decreased cerebral support)
    Ischemic hypoxia: acute myocardial infarction, congestive heart failure, arrhythmia,
        vascular occlusion, pulmonary embolism, hypotension, transient ischemia (TIA);
        ventilatory failure: chronic lung disease
    Anemic hypoxia: iron deficiency anemia, pernicious anemia; folic acid deficiency;
        gradual blood loss

Brain Disorders
    Trauma: subdural hematoma, concussion/contusion, epidural hematoma, intracerebral
        hemorrhage
    Infection: acute meningitis – pyogenic or viral; chronic meningitis – tuberculosis or
        fungal; neurosyphilis; subdural empyema; brain abscess
    Tumors: metastatic to brain, primary to brain
    Normal pressure hydrocephalus (NPH)

Pain
    Fracture; acute abdomen; fecal impaction or urinary retention

Stress
    Sudden changes in temperature, food habits, medication, or withdrawal of drugs

NOTE: Adapted from Besdine at al. (1980).

Table 12-2. Factors Which Contribute to Rapid Onset of Confusional States.

Sensoriperceptual

   Sensory deficits – diminished vision, diminished hearing, diminished sense of pain and touch, immobility

   Sensory overload or deprivation

   Lack of meaning in environmental patterns; panic, crisis (especially true in relocation)

Change in normal physiological functions

   Lack of sleep, fatigue, interrupted pattern of rest and activity

   Alteration in normal elimination patterns – impaction, colostomy; bladder problems such as retention, intubation, cystotomy

Loss of significant others, grief, depression

Stress, panic, crisis

---

and listening to what he has to say. Words interpreted as delirious ravings often hold the key to the cause when emotional problems are the cause. Calm, supportive, and gentle care is needed while the nurse explains and guides. Restraints cause panic states which increase the confusion.

Prevention

Prevention of reversible confusional states is now possible with the identification of the high risk elderly person. Predictors which are important and within the control of the nurse to recognize and decrease the threat can be found in Table 12-3.

IRREVERSIBLE CONFUSIONAL STATES

The true dementias of aging include Alzheimer's disease–(SDAT). The dementias have been called by various names throughout history. The most common of these are senility, senile dementia, organic brain disease, arteriosclerotic brain disease, and organic brain syndrome. The common element is progressive mental impairment and irreversibility even with expert diagnosis and treatment. The onset is usually slow and almost insidious. The person with a true dementia is noted by his family, employer, or friends to have failing attention span, memory deficits, and decline in mathematical ability, and he will make errors of judgment based on those symptoms. There will be irritability, poor orientation, and loss of one's sense of humor. Personality changes are noted. Usually the individual with increasing mental impairment is aware of his failing capacity and tries to compensate by various strategies such as confabulation which cover up the severity of the symptoms for a time. Progression often plateaus at a point and remains rather stable for a period, especially for the older person in a protected environment. Sudden change or physical illness can increase the rate of progress to a rapid and devastating confusional state which may require institutionalization unless the family can give almost constant supervision.

Incidence

The real incidence of disorientation or confusion must be extrapolated from small studies. No epidemiological survey has been conducted, but on the basis of studies with limited numbers of subjects, it is estimated that 10% of people over 65 have some degree of mental impairment. This rate grows higher with increasing age. After a leveling-off point in the 80s, those people who live to be 90 and over usually are the ones who do not show evidence of mental impairment. A

Table 12-3. Predictors of Confusional States in the Elderly (Reversible or Rapid Onset Forms).

Loss of sense of self (depersonalization)
Loss of continuity with life history

Distortion of time and light cues due to restricted environment, lack of familiar objects, disruption of sleep cycle (the hospital condition)

Loss of control because of:
  Sensory overload
  Sensory deficits (including kinesthetic deficits with immobility)
  Sensory deprivation
  Intubation (parenteral, nasogastric, catheter, suction, oxygen)
  Urinary problems: inability to empty or control bladder
  Fecal impaction
  Restraints

Disruption of pattern of daily living: food intake, mobility, sleep, orientation cues

Pain

Sexual expressions; rules of privacy and culture may not be observed (older men more prone to confusional states)

No contact with significant others

Drug and/or alcohol intake

Physiologic problems which interfere with cerebral support: hypoxia, dehydration, hypo- or hyperthermia, hypo- or hyperglycemia, hypotension, increased intracranial pressure

NOTE: Adapted from Wolanin and Holloway (1980).

survey of nursing homes (*Profile of Chronic Illness in Nursing Homes,* 1978) reported that 50-75% of the residents were mentally impaired. The *Long Term Care Facility Improvement Study* (1975) gave the incidence of confusion as 54%, with an additional 27% only occasionally confused. Forty-one percent displayed such typically inappropriate behavior as wandering or being disruptive. Also, of that group Marsden and Harrison (1972) estimated that 10-20% really had reversible conditions. Fox et al. (1975) found that 5 out of 40 patients referred from long term care facilities with dementia had reversible forms due to hypothyroidism, pernicious anemia, meningioma, and low pressure hydrocephalus. It is impossible to compile accurate figures since many confused people live at home with family support.

Etiology

At this time there is no known cause of SDAT although theories implicate genetics, neuro-

transmitters, aluminum, viruses, and various other factors. Multi-infarct disease is due to multiple occlusions of small cerebral arteries, often in association with hypertension or diabetes and atherosclerosis. Multi-infarct dementia is probably more common in men than women (Raskind and Storrie, 1980). The Alzheimer type of senile dementia or confusional states occurs in a more linear progression than multi-infarct assaults. Sudden change in the internal or external world of the patient can accelerate the progression. Three important pathological changes occur in the brain. They are neurofibrillary tangles, senile plaques, and granulovacuolar degeneration (Reisburg, 1981).

Prevention

The prevention of irreversible confusional states includes treatment for hypertension, diabetes, and atherosclerosis in order to prevent the multi-infarct assault. At this time, there is no certain prevention for the Alzheimer type of dementia. Avoidance of physiological changes, environmental changes such as relocation, or panic states can retard the rapid progress found with sudden change. Active people seem to have less of these confusional states, or perhaps people with less confusion are more active.

Research conducted in Sweden and in the United States as part of the Baltimore Longitudinal Study has shown that perhaps as much as 20% of the population now living will develop some severe dementia before death and that 50-65% of these people will have the neuropathological changes characteristic of Alzheimer's disease. Therefore, the 1% lifelong risk (and 4% risk for blood relatives) reported earlier may actually be as high as 10-13%, which makes this a fairly common disease, although not as common as other diseases of the elderly such as cancer and heart disease. It is estimated that Alzheimer's affects three to four million Americans at the present time. These data also conclude that close blood relatives run an increased genetic risk of developing Alzheimer's disease only when their relative developed the initial symptoms before age 65 (Mortimer and Schuman, 1981; National Institute on Aging, 1981).

Clinical Course of Alzheimer's Disease

Scientists are applying the newest knowledge and research techniques in histology, virology, immunology, toxicology, and biochemistry to study human brain tissue removed at autopsy in the search for the cause of Alzheimer's disease. Although there are promising clues such as the impact of slow viruses, the reduction of neurotransmitters, and the possible implication of aluminum, the cause of Alzheimer's disease is still unknown (NIH Publication No. 81-2252, 1981). Vasodilators and neuroleptic or antipsychotic drugs sometimes assist in management of the patient, but they do not alter the course of the disease. Cholinergic drugs are given to raise the level of acetylcholine, a neurotransmitter, and drugs to reduce the enzymes that break down acetylcholine are also being tried. Piracetam, a drug which improves memory and learning with animals, has not yet been approved for trial in the United States. Sodium fluoride is being administered in some tests to see whether it prevents the accumulation of aluminum in neuronal nuclei (Shore, 1981).

Though treatment has not been discovered which will cure Alzheimer's disease, supportive care can prolong the early stages before the more helpless and terminal stages begin. Supportive care can help the patient exist on a quite satisfying and productive level, and is often given within the family where love and understanding allow the older person to live life at his own pace, reduce his stress, and relinquish former functions when he is no longer able to handle them himself. The person who must be institutionalized is the one without family to take care of him, or one who presents a care burden to his family or a problem of safety to himself and others. Those who live alone require help — first in handling business affairs, then in handling the chores of daily living, and finally in maintaining existence itself. The progress of the disease has been divided into four stages: early, advanced, later, and terminal (Wolanin and Phillips, 1980).

Early Stage. The early stage of Alzheimer's disease is characterized by declining interest in the environment and in personal affairs; the inability to remember nouns (can recognize but not recall); difficulty in focusing on important events; a lack of social courtesies; and vagueness and uncertainty in initiating action. At this point the patient can live at home with supportive family care and a reduction in responsibilities. If he lives alone, he will need help from social agencies to keep his affairs in order. Attention to health care, with reduction of environmental change and stress, can prolong this stage. There will have to be assistance in paying bills and managing income. The individual may need a guardian and/or conservator to assist in protecting his interests. He should be encouraged to give up driving because it is common to forget the way home. Neighbors and friends can assist by being aware of any change in living habits which warrant increased vigilance. Relocation, change in residence, or illness will often be the point at which the patient slips into the advanced stage.

Advanced Stage. The advanced stage of SDAT is characterized by diminished ability to care for personal needs or affairs. There are obvious defects in memory, both in recall and in retention. Disorientation to time may be manifested between day and night. Appointments and usual days of celebration will be forgotten; personal possessions are misplaced and often hidden. There is an inability to remember simple directions. Health and hygiene are neglected.

The family can still care for the patient at this point if there is support for its members. The patient's role in the family is usually abandoned except for affectional ties. Institutionalization is required at this point if a supportive family structure does not exist. Business affairs must be turned over to a conservator or family member with power of attorney. This is a legal matter.

Later Stage. The patient in the later stage of Alzheimer's disease cannot find his way from one point to another, wanders aimlessly, is disoriented as to time and place, often mistakes the care giver for other persons, and deteriorates in ability to write and use fine motor skills. There will be problems in eating, dressing, and toileting. Communication becomes incoherent (Bartol, 1979), and nonverbal communication is used e.g., almost compulsive attempts to touch and examine objects with the hands and the mouth. Emotions also decrease.

At this point only a family with strong internal supports can maintain the 24-hour care which is required by the confused patient whose safety is in constant jeopardy. Institutionalization may become necessary. In the institution, the lack of familiar landmarks and faces usually results in a total loss of contact with the intact self. However, at this point the patient is still able to perform physical activities such as walking and some hand work, and enjoys music and some group activities. Care tends to be custodial, but reactions can surprise the care giver who continues to treat the patient as a human being with a life history and worth. The responsibility for personal hygiene is usually dependent on a care giver for every detail, and the care giver is responsible for planning care to maintain the physiology of the patient. Sleep will be impaired, and agitation and confusion are noted on awakening. The Klüver-Bucy-like syndrome is not uncommon in this stage of dementia (see Table 12-4).

Terminal Stage. The terminal stage of SDAT is the same as for any terminall ill patient who requires total nursing care. The patient is dependent on support for all physiologic processes. He is nonresponsive to communication, and does not recognize family or familiar objects. There is a gradual deterioration which is usually halted by death from an infection, renal failure, pneumonia, or decubitus. The family members undergo anticipatory grief at this point and require support from the staff and each other. Family members may not be able to tolerate seeing the mindless body which may give only wild shrieks and displays no natural signs. There is a tendency for them to abandon the patient.

Assisting Families

The family of the older patient with SDAT may consist only of an aging spouse who attempts to care for the patient up to the advanced or later stages of confusion and disorientation. If there are supporting family members, this is possible; if not, the nurse should anticipate the struggle that will occur in the remaining spouse's heart and mind when care can no longer be safely given. Supporting the family member is important to prevent abandonment with institutionalization. Social agencies which can assist should

---

Table 12-4. Klüver-Bucy-Like Syndrome in Final Stage of Alzheimer's Disease.

1. Hyperorality — extremely strong tendency to touch and examine all objects with the mouth

2. Loss or decrease of emotion

3. Bulimia — a morbid hunger which leads to drastic changes in dietary habits

4. Visual agnosia (may already be present)

5. Hypermetamorphosis — an attempt to touch every object in sight in a compulsive manner

SOURCE: Klüver, H. and Bucy, P. *American Journal of Physiology* 119:352–353 (1937).

be invited in to help during the period when institutionalization takes place and during the period of anticipatory grief. A few minutes of support to the family may save its members from complete disruption. The situation must be discussed with complete honesty so that necessary preparations can be made. A lifetime is drawing to a close, if not physically at least from a relational standpoint when human interaction becomes a problem.

General Guidelines for the Care of the Patient with Alzheimer's Disease

The following guidelines apply to professional care givers and to families; they are relevant to all the dementias (adapted from Burnside, 1979; Wolanin and Phillips, 1980):

- The patient should be prepared carefully for any change. No change in geography, residence, life-style, food, medication, or social situations should be made without taking into consideration the principle of *no abrupt change.*
- Physical health should be maintained with adequate diet, exercise, and sunlight. Exercise should be regular and should follow a pattern.
- A routine should be maintained; the patient's world must be dependable to avoid surprises.
- Social stimulation and change should be introduced in small increments to avoid overload. Avoid placing the patient in crowds.
- Communication and affectional ties with others should be maintained. Every channel of communication, including touch, sensory stimulation without overload, eye contact, and frequent identification by name, should be used (Bartol, 1979; Kazmierczak, 1975).
- Health measures to be monitored are nutrition, dental care, foot care, and the use of properly fitted shoes.
- The use of drugs should be avoided.
- Positive reinforcement should be used to maintain social and physical skills. Praise when praiseworthy.

- Time cues such as calendars, clocks, newspapers, magazines, reality boards, and trips outdoors to maintain orientation should be provided. Celebrate special events such as anniversaries and birthdays.
- Simple organization should be maintained without adding complex ideas, activities, or conversations.
- The client should be assisted to organize affairs such as getting legal assistance, storing valuables and important papers, and delegating power of attorney or a conservator.
- Humor and laughter should be used frequently with the client.
- When deterioration in toileting occurs, bowel and bladder programs should be consistent and routine.
- Garments which are familiar should be utilized until dressing becomes a problem; then substitute shirts, pants, and skirts with few buttons, velcro fasteners, and elastic waistbands. Use parkas with gloves attached for outdoors in winter.
- The family will need support and, in turn, will support the patient.
- Sudden changes should be avoided.

SPECIAL PROBLEMS OF THE CONFUSED PATIENT

Agitation

All personnel dread the agitated patient. Agitation is a sign of helplessness and loss of control at any age. With memory loss and disorientation, there are more instances of loss of control for the confused person. He reacts in a panic state, which is frightening in an adult and bewildering in an elderly person. Agitation often breeds return panic by those who are onlookers. The first reactions are to contain, restrain, and silence. This is dangerous. The less force used, the better, for force frightens still more. Quiet reaction by one member of the staff who accepts the agitation calmly can take a great deal of the panic out of the situation. Reasoning is often impossible and should not be attempted until the patient is calm. Listen to what the patient is saying. He is usually trying to communicate the reason for his agitation. He is lost, has lost something, feels that his dependable world is slipping away, or frequently has a physiologic need such as emptying his bladder, relieving his thirst, or finding comfort from pain. Offering a glass of water for a drink and taking one oneself can lead to quieter actions (at times, they can lead to the throwing of a tumbler, which should be plastic or paper). Being led gently to a more brightly lit area and sitting in a rocker can relieve some of the tension. Exercise should be obtained if possible. Listen. What is the patient saying? Respond to his feeling which is often fear about what is happening to him. Staff who can do this well should be the ones who handle such situations and teach other personnel.

Kales (1975) found that normal aging was associated with decreased sleep. For patients with chronic brain syndrome (SDAT), total sleep time was highly correlated with intellectual function. Patients with Alzheimer's disease awakened from REM sleep in a state of delirium or agitation lasting 5-10 minutes which Kales felt might reflect their inability to tell the difference between dreaming and reality.

Screaming and Moaning

Repetitive screaming, moaning, babbling, or sing-song calling for someone or something such as baby, baby, baby is not an uncommon sound in the corridors of long term care facilities. Such behavior is upsetting and aggravating to families and staff, and unfortunately they often respond by retaliating behavior such as shushing the person by threats and physical abuse. This, of course, makes the situation worse and adds to the problem.

This perseveration (constant repetition of a word or a phrase) has no simple definitive cause or simple solution. Some possible causes are the fear and uncertainty that accompany cognitive loss, pain which cannot be communicated, relocation, the fear of being alone, the belief that one is dying, anger, profound loneliness, and profound disorientation. The best approach is to look for causes and for patterns of the behavior (time of day, etc.), document them, and then in staff conference with a team

approach try various strategies which include a calm environment, adequate personal space, listening for lucid comments, and sitting with, holding, and/or touching the patient. Music therapy and behavior modification techniques may be helpful. Most important is a warm, gentle, caring staff. Staff will need to share their feelings and pool their creative abilities to reach the patient and give support to families and to each other (Burnside, 1981; Wolanin and Phillips, 1981).

Wandering

Wandering is behavior which seems to have no aim — it is purposeless activity. It should be seen as a need of the body for exercise and of the person to know his environment, a chance to explore. Usually, personnel and family are very uncomfortable with allowing freedom; often the need for physical activity is misinterpreted and the patient is restrained. One alternative is to offer physical activity which includes some group exercises and walking as far as the patient can tolerate. Rocking chairs also offer physical activity with kinesthetic value for the person who cannot walk but needs activity. Confusion makes the patient quite anxious. Activity reduces anxiety.

If a patient leaves the grounds or institutional perimeters, his safety becomes a community affair. Most patients have a reason for leaving — a need for exercise, for exploration, or to do some personal errand — and some simply do not realize that the boundaries have been crossed. One caretaker should "catch up" with the wanderer and approach by keeping in step with him. A confederate can be in the background, but two people are threatening to the patient and will often agitate him. After falling in step and walking a short distance, the staff member or family member can turn and retrace steps gradually; usually the patient will accompany without any further question. The use of force is poor judgment and will result in agitation. For institutions that do not have fences or walls, special training in working with wanderers will enable staff to be comfortable with this approach.

REVERSIBLE CONFUSION SUPERIMPOSED ON IRREVERSIBLE CONFUSION

Reversible confusion superimposed on irreversible confusion will not be discussed here in detail for obvious reasons. Knowledge and skill for assessment of this condition require application of a combination of the principles and guidelines already discussed. The nurse should be alert to, and aware of, the additional reversible stress and confusion which may occur when an 85 year old with advanced senile dementia is suddenly moved. For example, Mrs. Mayme Hicks, age 88, was institutionalized with advanced senile dementia. In a protective environment with definite routines and supportive staff, she managed very well and improved to the point that staff, in their desire to help, moved her to a floor with increased demands in the activities of daily living and decision making. The relocation was devastating, and Mrs. Hicks became very confused about time and place, apathetic, and fearful of the people around her including staff. Until an assessment conference was held to analyze what had happened in relocation, some staff simply believed that Mrs. Hicks' dementia was "getting worse."

Nurses should also be alert to superimposed reversible confusion when persons with any degree of dementia are suddenly ill with high fever, dehydrated, or having a problem with medications.

SPECIAL NEEDS OF THE CONFUSED PATIENT

A Structured Environment

In the guidelines, the need for maintaining a routine in the patient's daily pattern of life was stressed. There must be *no sudden changes.* This is as important in the surroundings. The world must have an element of dependability about it. The same thing should be done each day at the same time in the same place with the same people. Change should be introduced with only one element varying at a time. Big changes, such as relocation, can be neutralized

by careful planning and preliminary discussion, asking the family to accompany the patient, letting him carry his own personal belongings, and helping to place them in as nearly the same place as they were in the previous site. Personal clothing should be used until new garments must be introduced. Personnel should be introduced one at a time starting with one person and adding the second and third only as the patient adapts. Every element of the old situation and environment which can be brought with the patient to the new should be prominently displayed during the adjustment period. All moves should be made in daytime and at a time of day when the patient is usually most alert (never during nap time or just before a meal). No one should have to face a new dining room and a new home at the same time.

Space and Privacy

The more the patient is disoriented, the greater is the need for keeping visible boundaries around space. There is less chance for the feeling of panic which comes from not knowing where one is. The space must have limits, but it should be large enough to allow for exercise, preferably walking in well-fitted shoes and in open air and sunshine. There should be a chance for exploration of the environment. Constant attendance is inhibitive and seen as restraint. The patient should be able to sit alone if he desires and to have the feeling that there are no prying eyes. The need for safety precautions often prevents such privacy. Families should be allowed to visit in a private place.

Reducing Disorientation

The use of reality therapy on a 24-hour-a-day basis (Hahn, 1980) can reduce the amount of disorientation. We all need constant reminders of where we are and what day it is. The young active person has many reinforcing cues which are lacking in institutional life. A deliberate effort to provide cues should be part of the social and physical environment of the frail elderly. Reality orientation techniques are helpful if carried out carefully and consistently.

Reality orientation is a basic technique in the rehabilitation of persons having a moderate to severe degree of memory loss, confusion, and time-place-person disorientation. Therefore, it is a beginning phase of rehabilitation for those who are confused and disoriented. The philosophy is that each individual patient should make the maximum use of his assets. The best use of a person's abilities is made when rehabilitation is begun as soon as possible. Reality orientation has two phases: 24-hour reality orientation for any confused person and classroom reality orientation for any who need intensive sessions for gross confusion.

The orientation process is in effect 24 hours a day while one is performing activities of daily living. Concrete, basic, current, and personal information is presented to the patient, beginning with his name, where he is, and time references. Each contact the staff has with a patient will be utilized to improve his awareness of person, time, and place. Each confused patient should be told where he is going, the occasion, and what is expected of him in the same manner that one would respond to any patient (see Table 12-5 for guidelines).

Nowakowski (1980) has theorized that the disorientation of the patient, who was clear mentally before hospitalization, is due to nursing response to the behavior of the patient. If the disorientation is simply noted and no attempt is made to reach the "solid self" behind the behavior, the patient will continue to be disoriented. Nowakowski introduced working with the patient to reach the "solid self," the decision-making self responsible for issues in his own life. Her intervention was to restore the patient's right and ability to make some important decisions, and the results were to relieve the disorientation. Certain predictable persons would be disoriented, such as those who were dependent, persons with intense fusion with their spouses, those who had had no significant information about their own health care from providers and family, persons who did not ask questions about themselves, those for whom families and care givers gave too much assistance and communication was directed "at" the patient instead of "to" him, cases where the focus was on what was wrong with the patient, and those instances in which there were important decisions to be made. Nowakowski (1980) placed these predictable situations into three categories: (1) persons who have abdicated decision making to others on important issues, (2) persons who have experienced disruption of meaningful relationships, and (3) persons with intense marital fusion.

Table 12-5. Guidelines for 24-hour Reality Orientation.

1. A calm environment is needed.
2. There should be a set routine.
3. Give clear, simple responses to residents' questions. Questions asked of residents should be clear and simple also.
4. Talk clearly to residents, not necessarily loud and not as to a child.
5. Direct residents around by clear directions. If need be, guide them to and from their destinations.
6. Remind them of the date, time, etc.
7. Do not let residents stay confused by allowing them to ramble in their speech and actions.
8. Be as firm as necessary.
9. Be sincere.
10. Be consistent.

SOURCE: Shannon, Margaret. Return to reality. *Atlanta Journal and Constitution Magazine* (January 9, 1972).

Socialization and Resocialization

Maintaining human contact with significant others is extremely important for every person with changes in mental status that are termed confusion. Families should be encouraged to maintain this contact, and in their absence, surrogates should take over the task of keeping the elderly person in touch with his life history. One staff member acting in a primary relationship should develop an interaction which allows the patient to identify that person as one who will be his advocate and who will be a harbor in an uncertain sea. If there is a change of staff, the new surrogate should be introduced by the old one, and a transition period to establish an acquaintance should be allowed before the old surrogate leaves. There should be closure. In one nursing home, each staff member from administrator through the housekeeping and cooking staff leaves his/her job for 15 minutes at a scheduled time every day to interact on a one-to-one basis with a patient. The change in both the patients and the staff has been dramatic. The actual transformation has not required more staff, but those who are in the agency have a different relationship and the patients have improved markedly in social interaction. Some staff members simply sit and hold a hand or share a cup of coffee.

Most institutions have group activities. The confused patient may not be able to handle group activities at first and may require one-to-one interaction (Ebersole, 1976). Later, joining in resocialization groups, remotivation groups, exercise classes, and music classes enables the confused patient to extend his range of contacts. Music classes or sessions (Kartman, 1977) offer a means of reestablishing contact with one's life history and kinesthetic communication with one's own body. The SAGE program has succeeded in this aim (Dychtwald, n.d.) as rhythms start feet stamping and hands clapping, revive memories of happier active times, and lead to group exercise.

The principle behind all resocialization is that the patient has lost his self-initiating abilities and must be helped to regain them. It is satisfying to know at least one other person and to laugh and touch in a group. Group activities have been explored in depth by Burnside (1978).

Physiological Needs

The confused elderly person forgets or he would not be termed confused. He has lost contact with his previous experience and cannot bring it to consciousness to assist with making decisions and judgments. The physiology of daily existence may be entirely neglected, with the need for food and fluids unnoticed. Notes are written to remind oneself, but the notes are forgotten. Someone must take responsibility for nutrition and elimination. Incontinence usually results from forgetting to go to the toilet and even forgetting where it is. Between the time the patient starts to the toilet or drinking fountain and his arrival, he can forget his mission. Sleep and rest are often taken in short naps, rather than a single eight-hour bedtime period, or in the daytime with nighttime wandering. Adequate daily exercise and activity can change part of this pattern, but poor sleep is a common pattern for the confused elderly. Hypnotics given at night are rarely the answer because they cause daytime "hangovers" (Jenkins, 1976) rather than nighttime sleep, and often lead to nighttime agitation. Nurses know the demands of the biological organism. Planning will insure that those needs are met even when the patient's own ability to meet them is diminished (Eliopoulos, 1979).

Mental Status Evaluations

The busy practitioner seeks shortcuts for evaluating mental status by using some simple, standard questionnaire types of tests. Simple tests should be seen as just that — some tests do not allow for variables (which prevents people from giving correct answers in any situation) such as anxiety in the testing situation, anxiety in the presence of a physician, lack of energy due to illness, inability to hear the question, and lack of access to the information sought. For someone who does not celebrate birthdays, checking age by subtracting the birth date from the present date requires manipulating four figures which necessitates a pencil and paper for many people and a hand-held calculator for others. The person with diminished vision does not have access to news of the political scene. The care giver who uses these simple tests is warned to be sure he is not testing anxiety levels, lack of sensory input, sensory deprivation, or lack of access to information when he arrives at a simple numerical answer that is used to indicate the extent of organic brain damage.

Mental status evaluations are designed to test remote memory, recent memory, orientation, and logical memory. There may be an effort made to use calculations such as subtraction. Logical thinking may be tested by asking the meaning of proverbs which are common to our culture. The nurse is encouraged to test these components of the mental status evaluation in a natural manner in connection with everyday care, in a nonthreatening situation, and with appropriate consideration to ethnicity. Perlin and Butler (1963) test mental status and retention with a simple mental status evaluation which is based on giving the patient something to remember and later asking for its recall. This is followed with questions about birthplace, schooling, and age at certain turning points in life. There should be a question about mother's maiden name and who the president was at the time of the first job. Orientation is tested for time, date, place, and person (person of the interviewer). Recent memory is tested with questions regarding present home and recent

events such as, Where were you a week ago? How many meals have you had today? Logical memory is tested by reading a story and asking the patient to repeat it.

The MSQ (Mental Status Questionnaire; Kahn, Goldfarb, Pollack, and Peck, 1960) is a ten-item test of orientation to place, time, recent memory, and calculation questions such as age, birth date, and what year it is (see Figure 12-1). The questions require access to rather precise information, especially in relation to time orientation, and to general information in relation to the names of presidents.   In Canada, the name of the prime minister is substituted. Substitutions which can be made for the institutionalized patient who does not have access to such information include asking him to show you the way to a landmark in the building such as a nurses' station, the bathroom, or the dining room.

Pfeiffer (1981) offers a newer version called the short portable mental status questionnaire for the assessment of organic brain deficit in elderly patients (see Figure 12-2). The Pfeiffer test has been tested for validity and reliability with correlations of 0.82 and 0.83, and with 92% agreement between the test and clinical diagnosis when the test indicated impairment

MENTAL STATUS QUESTIONNAIRE

1. Where are we now?	Place
2. Where is this place (located)?	Place
3. What is today's date — day of month?	Time
4. What month is it?	Time
5. What year is it?	Time
6. How old are you?	Memory — recent or remote
7. What is your birthday?	Memory — recent or remote
8. What year were you born?	Memory — remote
9. Who is the president of the United States?	Memory — general information
10. Who was president before him?	Memory — general information

If the person makes 0-2 errors, we say that organic mental syndrome or brain syndrome is absent or mild; 3-8 errors, brain syndrome is moderate; 9-10 errors, brain syndrome is severe.

Note: Modified from Kahn, R.L., Goldfarb, A.I., Pollack, M., and Peck, A. Brief objective measures for the determination of the mental status of the aged. *American Journal of Psychology* 117:326-328 (1960).

Figure 12-1. Mental status questionnaire. [Note: Modified from Kahn, R.L., Goldfarb, A.I., Pollack, M., and Peck, A. Brief objective measures for the determination of the mental status of the aged. *American Journal of Psychology* 117:326-328 (1960).]

PFEIFFER'S PORTABLE SHORT MENTAL STATUS QUESTIONNAIRE

What is the date today? _____
　　　　　　　　　　　　 month　　　　　　day　　　　　　year

What day of the week is it?

What is the name of this place?

What is your telephone number?

What is your street address (if the patient does not have a telephone)?

How old are you?

When were you born?

Who is the president of the United States now?

Who was president before him?

What was your mother's maiden name?

Subtract 3 from 20 and keep subtracting from each new number all the way down.

Scoring requires that information be verifiable. The special scoring takes into account the amount of schooling the patient has had; for instance, an extra error is allowed if there was only a grade school education and one less error if the patient had more than a high school education. Blacks are allowed an additional error.

The following criteria were established if the patient was white and had some high school education:

0-2 errors	Intact intellectual functioning
3-4 errors	Mild intellectual functioning
5-7 errors	Moderate intellectual impairment
8-10 errors	Severe intellectual impairment

(Pfeiffer, 1975).

Figure 12-2. Portable mental status questionnaire (Pfeiffer, 1975).

and 82% for no mental impairment. This test measures mental impairment rather than organic brain damage.

Another approach to the detection of brain syndrome is through a series of double simultaneous stimulations of the face and hand, the Face-Hand Test (FHT). Its value to the practitioner is in screening for brain syndrome and evaluating its severity (see Figure 12-3). Failure to report the touch on the back of the hand is presumptive of cortical neuronal loss.

When one test suggests a more severe chronic brain syndrome than the other, it is possible that cognitive functioning can be improved to the level of the better performance. At times an improvement in a coexisting affective disorder will reveal that the patient has more resources than suggested by either the FHT or the MSQ (Goldfarb, 1974).

The caution is repeated that these tests do not replace observations under normal situations for the patient and they do not take into consideration the sensory deficits of the aged, his culture, life-style, and other variables. These can be tested in the real-life setting where the patient is observed by family and nurse for the same memory defects, recent and remote memory, orientation and recall, and retention. The nurse has the advantage of seeing patients' reactions in their own environment which shows their continued adaptability. All of these tests may be used to assess both reversible and irreversible confusion and disorientation according to the preference of the practitioner.

FACE-HAND TEST

1. Right cheek——————— left hand		
2. Left cheek——————— right hand		Initial trials. Response evaluated in context of further trials.
3. Right cheek——————— right hand		
4. Left cheek——————— left hand		
5. Right cheek——————— left cheek		Teaching trials. Almost always correctly reported. Examiner informs or reinforces response that there were two touches.
6. Right hand——————— left hand		
7. Right cheek——————— left hand		Incorrect response and stimulation not reported; felt but displaced, projected, or located in space – is presumptive of brain damage.
8. Left cheek——————— right hand		
9. Right cheek——————— right hand		
10. Left cheek——————— left hand		

The Face-Hand Test includes two series of ten trials each, one with eyes closed and one with eyes open.

The subject sits facing the examiner with his hands on his knees, and is given the following instructions: "I am going to touch you. Point to where I touch you." It is necessary that the instructions be specific on how to respond as verbal response leads to fewer errors than pointing. The subject is then touched with one or two brisk strokes on the cheek and dorsum of the hand.

The most common error is extinction, in which one of the stimuli is not perceived, almost always the hand. If this type of response is made on any of the first four trials, the subject is asked, "Anywhere else?" This compels the subject to consider the possibility of more than one stimulus. The concept of twoness is also reinforced by the symmetric stimuli trials, which should be perceived correctly to indicate a valid procedure. If errors are made on trials 5 and 6, it indicates that the subject has a sensory impairment or is unable to follow instructions. The second most common error, and indicative of more severe pathology, is displacement, in which one stimulus is displaced to another part of the body, most often the hand stimulus being displaced to the opposite cheek. The most severe, and relatively rare, form of error has been termed "exsomesthesia," in which a stimulus is displaced outside the subject's body.

Figure 12-3. Face-Hand Test. [Note: From Goldfarb, A.I. The evaluation of geriatric patients following treatment. In Hoch, P.H. and Zubin, J. (Eds.) *Evaluation of Psychiatric Treatment.* New York: Grune and Stratton, 1964, p. 291.]

REFERENCES

Bartol, M.A. Non-verbal communication in patients with Alzheimer's disease. *Journal of Gerontological Nursing* 5(4):21-31 (July-August 1979).

Bayne, J.R.D. Assessing confusion in the elderly. *Psychosomatics* 20(1):43-53 (January 1979).

Besdine, R. et al. Senility reconsidered, treatment possibilities for mental impairment of the elderly. Report of task force sponsored by NIA. *Journal of American Medical Association* 244(3):259-263 (1980).

Burnside, I.M. *Working with the Elderly: Group Process and Techniques,* 2nd Ed., Monterey, Ca.: Wadsworth, 1984.

Burnside, I.M. Alzheimer's disease – an overview. *Journal of Gerontological Nursing* 5(4):14-20 (1979).

Burnside, I.M. Organic brain syndrome. In Burnside, I.M. (Ed.) *Nursing and the Aged.* New York: McGraw-Hill, 1981, pp. 172-200.

Buseck, S. Visual status of the elderly. *Journal of Gerontological Nursing* 2(5):34-39 (1976).

Drachman, D. Summary of mini White House proceedings. *ADRDA Newsletter* 1(1):4 (1981).

Dychtwald, K. *Exercises for Lifelong Health and Well Being.* Berkeley, Calif.: Senior Actualization and Growth Exploration Project (SAGE), n.d.

Ebersole, P. Problems of group reminiscing with the institutionalized aged. *Journal of Gerontological Nursing* 2(6):23-27 (1976).

Eliopoulos, C. *Gerontological Nursing.* New York: Harper & Row, 1979.

Fox, J. et al. Dementia in the elderly – a search for treatable illnesses. *Journal of Gerontology* **30**(5): 557-564 (1975).

Goldfarb, A.I. *Aging and Organic Brain Syndrome.* Fort Washington, Pa.: McNeil Laboratories, 1974.

Hahn, K. Using 24 hour reality orientation. *Journal of Gerontological Nursing* **6**(3):130-135 (1980).

Information on Aging No. 25 (April 1982).

Jenkins, B.L. A case against "sleepers." *Journal of Gerontological Nursing* **2**(2):10-13 (1976).

Kahn, R.L., Goldfarb, A.I., Pollack, M., and Peck, A. Brief objective measures for the determination of the mental status of the aged. *American Journal of Psychiatry* **117**:326-328 (1960).

Kales, J.D. Aging and sleep. In Goldman, R. and Rockstein, M. (Eds.) *The Physiology and Pathology of Human Aging.* New York: Academic Press, 1975, pp. 187-202.

Kartman, L.L. The use of music as a program tool with regressed geriatric patients. *Journal of Gerontological Nursing* **3**(4):38-42 (1977).

Kazmierczak, F.G. et al. Communication problems encountered when caring for the elderly individual. *Journal of Gerontological Nursing* **1**(1):21-27 (1975).

Klüver, H. and Bucy, P. *American Journal of Physiology* **119**:352-353 (1937).

Long Term Care Facility Improvement Study: Introductory Report, Office of Nursing Home Affairs. Washington, D.C.: U.S. Department of Health, Education and Welfare, 1975.

Marsden, C.D. and Harrison, M.J.G. Outcome of investigation in patients with presenile dementia. *British Medical Journal* **2**:249-252 (1972).

Mortimer, J.A. and Schuman, L.M. (Eds.). *The Epidemiology of Dementia.* N.Y. Oxford University Press 1981.

National Institute on Aging. *Special Report on Aging, 1981.* Bethesda, Md.: 1981.

National Institute of Health. *The Dementias.* Publication #81-2252 For Sale by Supt. of Documents U.S. Gov. Printing Office, Wash. D.C. 20402, 1981.

Nowakowski, L. Disorientation – signal or distress. *Journal of Gerontological Nursing* **6**(4):197-202 (1980).

Perlin, S. and Butler, R.N. Psychiatric aspects of adaptation to the aging process. In Birren, J.E. et al. (Eds.) *Human Aging, a Biological and Behavioral Study.* Washington, D.C.: U.S. Government Printing Office, 1963.

Pfeiffer, E. A short portable mental status questionnaire for the assessment of organic brain deficit in elderly patients. *Journal of the American Geriatrics Society* **23**(10):433-439 (1975).

Pfeiffer, E. The psychosocial evaluation of the elderly patient. In Busse, E.W. and Blazer, D.G. (Eds.) *Handbook of Geriatric Psychiatry.* New York: Van Nostrand Reinhold, 1980, pp. 278-279.

Profile of Chronic Illness in Nursing Homes, 1973-75 (DHEW Publication No. PHS 78-1780). National Center for Health Statistics Series 12, No. 23, 1978.

Raskind, M.A. and Storrie, M.C. The organic mental disorders. In Busse, E.W. and Blazer, D.G. (Eds.) *Handbook of Geriatric Psychiatry.* New York: Van Nostrand Reinhold, 1980, pp. 309-310.

Reisberg, B. *Brain failure: An Intro to Current Concepts of Senility.* New York: The Free Press, 1981, p. 17.

Shannon, M. Return to reality. *Atlanta Journal and Constitution Magazine* (January 9, 1972).

Shore, D. Search for new treatment methods. *The Advocate* **2**(2):1-2 (1981).

Wolanin, M.O. and Holloway, J. Relocation trauma. In Burnside, I.M. (Ed.) *Psychosocial Nursing of the Aged* (2nd ed.). New York: McGraw-Hill, 1980.

Wolanin, M.O. and Phillips, L. *Confusion: Prevention and Care.* St. Louis: C.V. Mosby, 1981.

13
Prevention of Mental Illness in Later Life

Irene Mortenson Burnside
Bernita M. Steffl

Proving that mental illness can be prevented, especially in aged persons, is extremely difficult — evidence for it has rarely been sought.

Charles M. Gaitz and Roy V. Varner (1980)

Prevention is an important role for all nurses who care for the elderly, wherever they are employed. It is imperative to designate specific areas for more effective intervention in the prevention of mental illness is later years. This chapter is about prevention and health care. Our present health care and services were criticized with acumen by a nurse in Aldous Huxley's book *Island* (Huxley, 1962):

So you think our medicine's pretty primitive? That's the wrong word. It isn't primitive. It's fifty percent terrific and fifty percent non-existent. Marvelous antibiotics — but absolutely no methods for increasing resistance, so that antibiotics won't be necessary. Fantastic operations — but when it comes to teaching people the way of going through life without having to be chopped up, absolutely nothing. And it's the same all along the line. Alpha Plus for patching you up when you're starting to fall apart, but Delta Minus for keeping you healthy. Apart from sewage systems and synthetic vitamins, you don't seem to do anything at all about prevention. And yet you've got a proverb: prevention is better than cure.

At an international symposium it was emphatically stated that the age of retirement is not too late for prevention. One physician said, "Old age is not given to us like youth; we must conquer it" (Richard, 1980).

The concepts of levels of prevention, holistic health, and high level wellness are workable

(Steffl, 1981) but have been laid aside when it comes to preventive mental health for the aged, perhaps because in our production-oriented society, the industrial athlete is the center of attention. The lack of interest in mental illness is described by Talbott (1979): "Every other disease — cancer, kidney disease, hypertension — has a constituency. But the chronically mentally ill have no constituency. Everybody would just like them to disappear, their families, the press, even the medical profession." All of this is perhaps even more true if the chronically mentally ill person is also old.

The general principles for a preventive approach, according to Gaitz and Warner (1980, p. 969), include the following:

- Early diagnosis of, and therapeutic intervention in, both physical and mental disorders are necessary at all stages of life.
- Early in the life cycle, improve mental health education and counselling; make medical and psychiatric care more easily available.
- Promote attractive functional medical and psychiatric facilities for the elderly.
- Reduce physical and mental chronicity through improved discharge planning and continuity of care.
- There should be greater utilization and coordination of multidisciplinary professionals.

Primary prevention (i.e., complete prevention of the occurrence of disease) is not often realistic in old age, nor is it likely that the state of health after age 50 will be that described in the widely accepted World Health Organization

(1947) definition: "Health is a state of complete physical, mental, and social well-being and not merely the absence of disease." Leavell and Clark (1965) Other levels of prevention, however, are necessary, feasible, and effective.

Experts in the field of geropsychiatry point out that depression and similar states are possible sources of all pathology and important elements in aging (Fessard, 1980); see Chapter 9 for a discussion of depression. It is important to prevent stress and to regulate tension at all ages, but preventive aspects of care is frequently lacking in old age. Specialists are trained in preventive aspects, but we still are not seeing enough "Individualized collective prevention" for older individuals in medicine or nursing. (*CASE Center*, 1980).

There are indeed some very specific measures to maximize mental health in old age, even for the frail elderly. Prevention is necessary and possible at every stage of life. Nurses can assume three roles: advocate, assessor, and intervenor. The nurse is a key professional who can promote good nutrition, physical exercise, cessation of smoking, and reduction of stress. Poor physical health, with its many vicissitudes, leads to loss of a sense of well-being and depletes the emotional bank. Hypertension leads to serious and sometimes deadly results. Untreated, it may cause cognitive decline (Wilkie, 1971). A procedure as simple as monitoring blood pressure is an important strategy of prevention of cognitive decline.

ROLE OF THE NURSE

Advocate

Nurses need to be advocates for the mental health needs of the aged client or patient. However, older people and all of us should act as advocates for legislation and should exercise our votes. We can have a say in our destinies. Health insurance, transportation, housing, and legal and protective services are all current national concerns indirectly related to mental health. Whether we are thinking about ourselves or others, we owe it to ourselves to know about a patient's rights in institutional settings for the aged (see Appendix A for patient's rights and Chapter 1 for the nurse's role of advocate, assessor, and intervenor).

Assessor

The nurse must be able to assess constantly the health status of the aged client. It is well known that falls and relocations have long term and serious consequences for elderly persons; confusional states can occur concomitantly with either a fall or a sudden move (Wolanin and Holloway, 1980). Nurses do not generally perceive themselves as responsible for preventive environmental controls, and often neglect to use the authority and autonomy that they do have to manipulate the environment and personal space for the elderly. An example of such neglect on the part of nursing personnel can be found in Case History I in Chapter 10. The nurses in the acute hospitals and the nursing home failed to manipulate the environment: they did not educate the daughter about the importance of old, cherished objects, nor did they intervene in the confusional states. There were no strategies to prevent the translocation shock (also see Chapter 10 regarding manipulation of the environment for aged persons with paranoid problems).

Intervenor

Studies indicate a consistent high rate of misuse of medications by the elderly. See Chapter 34, p. 925. A nurse who is knowledgeable about the use and abuse of drugs (both those prescribed and those sold over the counter) and alcohol can be a powerful change agent. Iatrogenic disease and nosocomial infections not only compound physical problems for the elderly but are frightening to them and mentally devastating (an infection acquired in the hospital, e.g., staphylococcus infection following surgery or bladder infection resulting from use of a catheter, is usually referred to as a nosocomial infection). Nurses can be effective in preventing such infections and consequences of institutionalization.

SPECIFIC PROGRAMS

Outreach

Assisting the elderly, especially the frail elderly with mental health problems, to maintain ties with a confidant or significant other can be an important role for the nurse. Sometimes the nurse is the only link to a significant "lifeline" for the lonely, old, sick, and poor person. We hear much about outreach these days, but professionals themselves are not always sure what outreach entails. In this chapter, the authors use outreach to mean all of the following: case finding, assessment, evaluation, crisis intervention, creating linkages, and maintaining follow-up services to promote and maximize the highest possible level of wellness and well-being. Outreach is especially important in suicide prevention among the elderly because the increasing suicide rate (National Council on Aging, 1978) among elderly men is another problem with clear implications for nurses (see Table 9-1 for an indication of the seriousness of this problem).

The Vial-of-Life program has become a state-wide effort to save lives and enhance relationships between the elderly and the law in Michigan. A plastic vial containing vital medical information about the individual is placed in the refrigerator, where in case of need for emergency medical treatment, emergency personnel can check before proceeding with treatment. This voluntary program was developed by a sheriff in Monroe County, Michigan in 1975. Information about the program is available from any Michigan State Police Post (Wayne State University and University of Michigan Institute of Gerontology Newsletter, June 1980).

Some outreach methods are not expensive or complicated. Such a simple addition as a telephone may be a tremendous asset to promote and maintain human contact; it can alleviate much of the isolation and loneliness that elders may experience.

Retirement, Re-careering, and Recreating

Retirement is a crucial crossroad: it is a warning that old age is fast approaching. In our society,

nobody wants to get old; they just want to live a long time (see Case History II in Chapter 10 which describes the devastating effects of forced early retirement upon a career woman). We all need to take more responsibility in preparing for retirement and possible re-careering.

There are vast, untapped, life-enriching resources in the humanities, literature, music, and applied arts. These must be more accessible to the aged, especially the present cohort groups who did not have the opportunity for education that many of us take for granted. Schools are noting increased enrollment in classes which provide short and long term opportunities for retirees. Elderhostel is a new concept of a short term live-in education at colleges and universities which focus on history and a wide variety of topics. This concept needs expansion.

A discussion program for older members of a community was assembled by the National Council on Aging and supported by the National Endowment for the Humanities. It is called *Senior Center Humanities* and can be used by voluntary discussion leaders with groups of 20 persons or less for weekly meetings over a period of eight weeks. The thesis behind the program is that the humanities have a special ability to stimulate in the aged person a quest for self-discovery (National Council on Aging, 1980).

In many instances, the elderly need assistance in learning how to "recreate" (Atchley, 1980). The roots of the present cohort groups are in the work ethic, and it is difficult for them to allow themselves playtime even when they are retired and have opportunities in recreational or occupational therapy classes.

Legal and Protective Services

In planning for legal and protective services, it is important, for example, to know the difference between a guardian and a conservator. It is also important to plan for a second backup when making a will — a responsible person, guardian, or executor — because frequently the significant other may have problems or die, which leaves many costly legal entanglements for the family.

Nurses should also work closely with the police department. This is especially true in the case of wanderers who may live in the precinct or the aged with marginal adaptations to community living. Police are often the first ones on the scene, so such individuals should have an identification bracelet showing at least a name and address. Firemen can also be very useful in helping with fire safety, education, and first aid demonstrations for older persons in the community.

EDUCATION NEEDS

Some of the training needs in the area of prevention of mental illness include: (1) models for in-service education, (2) professional staff orientation in the field of mental health and aging, (3) continuing education, and (4) better teaching materials, especially videotapes, cassettes, films, etc. Many instructors still must spend much of their time designing videotapes, writing teaching modules, and searching for hard-to-find materials.

Glaring needs that still remain in psychosocial caring and mental health include: the poor quality of dying of many institutionalized aged persons; the high frequency of incontinence, decubitus, and use of restraints; the poor grooming of many elderly; poor dental care; and inadequate or poorly functioning prostheses (Burnside, 1972).

Regarding the staffing problem, the shortage of qualified registered nurses in nursing homes continues, and data show that mental health problems are rampant there. The continued use of foreign nurses with language difficulties is another problem, especially on the night shift. Many incompetent nurses are able to find work with the elderly because no one else chooses to hire them.

Education for Nurses

As stated earlier, firemen and policemen can provide some training needs when called upon. Nursing still has a major job to do in motivating nursing students to work in the field of gerontological nursing. Schools are turning out only a handful of nurses educated at a master's level, with skills as clinical specialists or gerontological nurse practitioners (Kane et al., 1980; Wells, 1979). State board examinations as yet do not mandate content on aging (Gunter and Miller, 1979).

We will have to bring nursing knowledge to bear on many of the mental health problems associated with the aged population. We still do not have an organized areas of scientific and professional activity in nursing which focuses on the mental health of the aged person. True, research on mental health and aging is divided among a variety of scattered fields, but nursing could "borrow" and lean on some of the work of other professions more heavily than it currently does until a body of knowledge by nurses is established. There is also room for much more creativity in teaching nurses about aging (see Figure 13-1).

Should nurses be educated in geropsychiatry? Yes, but they also need a sound foundation in the physical health problems of the older adult and skills in assessment, so that they can detect when mental health problems have an organic origin. The ideal educational pattern would be for nurses to have a background in the developmental life cycle, normal aging process, pathophysiology of aged persons, physical assessment and history-taking skills, and then intense clinical experience working with the mentally ill older client and with tools and techniques in rehabilitative nursing. For a comprehensive overview of rehabilitation knowledge and skills applicable to gerontological nursing, see Chapters 28 through 32.

Burnout syndrome is common among nurses working with long-term illnesses and in long-term care facilities. It is often ignored but needs more attention because the mental and physical energy level of the nurse has a direct relationship to the level of care and well being of the patient (Beland, 1980).

SUMMARY

The report of the President's Commission on Mental Health — Task Panel on the Elderly (DHEW Publication No. HDS 80-20960, 1980) which was chaired by Dr. Eric Pfeiffer, describes

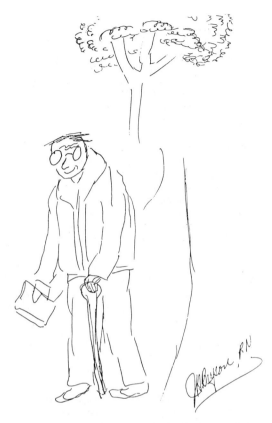

Figure 13-1. Drawing of centenarian by Jim Bryson, R.N. One of the authors (IMB) has consistently used drawings of the aged self for a teaching experience for students. In this particular class, the students were asked to draw themselves as centenarians. Despite the cane and the slightly stooped posture, there is an upbeat quality to this student's drawing. It rather reminds one of the upbeat ending of the excellent film *Peege,* when the trace of a smile crosses Peege's face in the last part of the film. (Courtesy of Jim Bryson, R.N.)

(3) more emphasis on effective preretirement and postretirement education programs, (4) a major program of public education to work on ageism, (5) the prevention of unnecessary institutionalization, (6) crisis intervention programs available at a community level for high risk elderly who may develop mental illnesses, (7) a comprehensive, long term social service system to be developed in communities, and (8) special assistance for frail elderly with severely reduced physical and emotional capacities due to extreme old age, and regularly monitoring of these high risk elderly.

This chapter, while not covering all areas of prevention in depth, has offered some specific areas in which nursing could excel. Two areas in which nurses can demonstrate their expertise include: caring for the institutionalized, chronically mentally ill and being advocates, assessors, and intervenors for the frail elderly in the community — those persons of extreme old age who have lost much physical and/or mental capacity and are in very dependent positions. These people need the personalized attention, advocacy, and long term care that nurses can offer them. This is a formidable goal for the profession to work toward.

Finally, it seems appropriate to remember that "the aged are us" (Eisdorfer, 1979) — that is, if we are lucky. We all need to begin to prepare for mental health in old age. Sister Constance, S.S. J.D. who writes for the *Canadian Institute of Religion and Gerontology Newsletter,* describes preparation for fulfilling retirement as a trilogy of trilogies. It says nine things. The first of the trilogies is to think in terms of three careers. Launch out into the first and keep two ideas stored away for future use. The second of the trilogies is to have three hobbies, a long term one, and engrossing shorter term one, and a pickup hobby. These can lead to lasting friendships and faraway places, and can tide you over rough spots. The third of the trilogies is to have an interest in elderly people in three types of circumstances: have concern and become known in a large institution; have a part in some organization concerned with the elderly; and have a friend who is old (*Canadian Institute of Religion and Gerontology Newsletter,* 1978).

six major areas of concern: (1) prevention, (2) services, (3) training, (4) research, (5) minorities, and (6) mechanisms for implementation. The committee focused on three objectives for prevention: (1) preserving the physical and mental health of the elderly, (2) keeping the mildly ill from becoming more seriously ill, and (3) keeping the severely ill from having prolonged illness. The eight recommendations made for preventive programs were as follows: (1) teaching the elderly effective ways to cope with the aging process, (2) training the elderly for new or continuing roles in the community,

Alex Comfort (1976) says it this way:

As an "old" person, you will need four things: dignity, money, proper medical services, and useful work. They are exactly the things you always needed. As things are today, you won't get them, but there is no divinely ordered reason why you should not. So, either set out now to see that you do get them or work to force society to change its posture — or do both.

REFERENCES

Atchley, R. (Ed.). *Social Forces in Later Life* (3rd ed.). Belmont, Calif.: Wadsworth, 1980.

Beland, I.L. Burn-out syndrome in nurses. In Werner-Beland, J. (Ed.) *Grief Processes in Long-term Illnesses.* Reston, Va.: Reston Publishers, 1980.

Burnside, I.M. Accoutrements of aging. *Nursing Clinics of North America* 7(2):291–301 (1972).

Canadian Institute of Religion and Gerontology Newsletter 5(2):1 (1978).

CASE Center for Gerontological Studies Newsletter 4:5–6 (March–April 1980).

Comfort, A. *The Good Age.* New York: Crown Publishers, 1976.

DHEW Publication No. (HDS) 80-20960. *Mental Health and the Elderly: Recommendations for Action.* Report of the President's Commission on Mental Health: Task Panel on the Elderly and the Secretary's Commission on Mental Health and Illness of the Elderly. Washington, D.C.: U.S. Government Printing Office, 1979.

Eisdorfer, C. Cognitive loss and the aging process. Lecture at The Symposium on Geropsychiatry, El Paso, Texas, January 18, 1979.

Fessard, M. *CASE Center for Gerontological Studies Newsletter.* 4:5–6 (March–April 1980).

Gaitz, C.M. and Varner, R.V. Preventive aspects of mental illness in later life. In Birren, J.E. and Sloan, R.B. (Eds.) *Handbook of Mental Health and Aging.* New York: Van Nostrand Reinhold, 1980.

Gunter, L. and Miller, J. Gerontic nursing education. In *Power in Action.* Kansas City, Missouri: American Nurses Association, 1979.

Huxley, A. *Island.* New York: Harper & Row, 1962, p. 75.

Kane, R.L., Solomon, D.H., Beck, J.C., Kelly, E. and Kane, R.A. *Geriatrics in the United States: Manpower Projections and Training Considerations.* Santa Monica, Calif.: Rand Corporation, 1980.

Leavell, H.R. and Clark, E.G. Preventive Medicine for the Doctor in the Community. New York, McGraw-Hill, 1965, p. 14.

National Council on Aging. *Fact Book on Aging: A Profile of America's Older Population.* Washington, D.C.,: 1978, pp. 159–161.

National Council on Aging. *Senior Center Humanities* (a program of the NIA). Washington, D.C.: 1980.

Richard, J. *CASE Center for Gerontological Studies Newsletter.* 4:5–6 (March–April 1980).

Steffl, B.M. Prevention measures and safety factors for the aged. In Burnside, I.M. (Ed.) *Nursing and the Aged* (2nd ed.). New York: McGraw-Hill, 1981.

Talbott, J. Quoted in Psychiatry on the couch. *Time* 100:81 (April 2, 1979).

Wayne State University and University of Michigan, Institute of Gerontology Newsletter, 205 Liberty Court, Detroit, Mich. Number 18, June 1980, p. 10.

Wells, T.J. Nursing committed to the elderly. In Reinhardt, A.M. and Quinn, M.D. (Eds.) *Current Practice in Gerontological Nursing.* St. Louis: C.V. Mosby, 1979.

Wilkie, F.L. and Eisdorfer, C. Intelligence and blood pressure in the aged. *Science* 172:959–962 (1971).

Wolanin, M.O. and Holloway, J. Relocation confusion: Intervention for prevention. In Burnside, I.M. (Ed.) *Psychosocial Nursing Care of the Aged* (2nd ed.). New York: McGraw-Hill, 1980.

Part IV
Physical Changes and Physical Assessment of Older Individuals

14
The Initial Health Assessment: An Overview

Linda Ellison Jessup

"Clinical protocols for older age groups are needed ... they act as both an educational tool and a method for audit and peer review"

Pearson and Kotthoff (1979).

During the last three decades, with the expansion of nurses' academic preparation to include an understanding of the scientific "whys" of care, the modern nurse's theoretical grasp of anatomy, physiology, and pharmacology has generally far exceeded her ability to apply this information clinically. Unequipped with the tools needed to collect coherent physical data with precision, the nurse has consequently been crippled in her ability to sift and order information, to discuss findings authoritatively, and to determine sound courses of action. Nursing education is belatedly moving to correct this deficit and to emphasize the need for examination and assessment skills which augment the communication and decision-making capabilities of nurses. Nowhere is this advance more urgently needed than in working with the elderly patient.

In old age there are multiple disorders, and the various protective mechanisms of the body are compromised and begin to give way. Symptoms present differently in the old, and unprepared clinicians often miss diagnoses. In older persons, serious diseases and conditions such as tuberculosis, appendicitis, or heart attack may proceed in silence (Butler, 1979). In addition, the older person is usually not all sick or all well at any one time; therefore, the ability to assess these changing states of health is essential to gerontological nursing.

The prospect of performing a succinct, yet accurate and comprehensive, evaluation of an elderly person can seem overwhelming initially. After all, 60 or more years of living encompass a wealth of experiences which have tempered these hardy survivors, just as heat tempers fine steel, making it more resilient, durable, and able to withstand time. Additionally, every individual is a complex and intriguing unknown at first, a puzzle to be investigated. Imagine yourself to be a skilled detective, with the task of reconstructing events in the complicated mystery of identifying this person, discovering why he is the way he is, and deciding how things can be better for him (see Figure 14-1).

The "investigation" or initial health assessment involves the use of three different approaches: (1) the patient history, (2) the physical examination, and (3) the necessary laboratory work and diagnostic procedures. As the investigator you are looking for facts, a chronology of developments, and clues suggesting obvious or hidden hazards, such as illnesses, allergic or severe emotional reactions, and other potential problems. You are also searching for

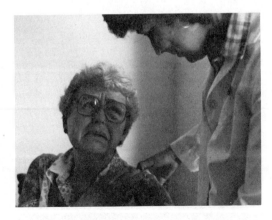

Figure 14-1. The nurse is a detective of sorts, attempting to discover who the patient is, why he is the way he is, and how his health and living situation might be improved.

obscure treasure, such as unrecognized strengths, sound self-care practices, buried interests, and untapped potentials.

The patient history yields primarily subjective information about the person's past, his present circumstances, and his prospects and hopes for the future. Both the physical examination and the laboratory and diagnostic procedures provide objective information about the individual's condition at a specific point in time. When the pertinent data are gathered in a systematic fashion and organized into a useful outline for easy retrieval, this collection constitutes the data base.

The data base is, then, the material from which a working hypothesis is constructed. If this material is of poor quality, then the case built with it will be shaky, inadequate, and perhaps inappropriate. If, on the other hand, the data are complete and of high quality, they become a solid foundation for building a sensitive, sensible care plan, which effectively addresses the concerns of the patient, the nurse, and the physician, while utilizing the patient's resources and those of his support system as efficiently as possible.

Compiling an adequate data base on an elderly person requires patience, a willingness to verify facts by means of old records or "witnesses," such as family members or close friends, and an ability to integrate information. Such a process generally requires several interactions with this mysterious stranger.

THE OBJECTIVES OF ASSESSMENT

There are three central reasons for assessing an elderly person, all of which must be treated as inseparable elements of comprehensive care and none of which can be claimed as the exclusive domain of any single health profession. These are:

- to discover what is wrong with an individual's state of health;
- to discover what is right, functional, and promising about an individual's state of health;
- to determine what system of care will be the most suitable for the individual, immediately and on a continuing basis.

Differentiating normal from pathological processes facilitates intelligent initiation of action for dangerous, distressing, or correctable problems. Clearly, while much disability in the elderly is very real and must be addressed forthrightly, much disability is self-imposed due to fears of falling, having a heart attack, looking silly, or "losing one's mind." Other disability may be imposed by the people around the elderly adult, by preconceived notions of the proper behavior "at his age," and by either neglect or overprotection. Finally, some disability is imposed by environmental barriers, such as an absence of handrails, ramps, or adequate transportation. Without a thorough process of data collection and organization of the physical, psychological, and socioeconomic aspects of an individual, it would be difficult indeed to distinguish many truly pathological problems from the multitude of external factors which isolate older people and which may limit an otherwise very functional person's sense of "being able" to get around and to cope with the routine demands of daily living.

Equally as important as the process of discovering pathology and problems is the simultaneous identification of what resources each elderly person brings to this period of his life. Unfortunately, assessment still remains largely unexploited by nurses and physicians alike as a powerful tool for maximizing an individual's sense of self-worth, for building on his strengths, and for engaging his interest and, as much possible, his responsible participation in his own care. For nurses especially, with their unique orientation toward health in its broadest sense, the assessment process offers the opportunity to learn more about each elderly person as a special individual within an intricate life context.

Of the genuine physical and mental disabilities with which many aging adults are faced, it is important to keep in mind that some of these problems can be corrected completely, some can be adjusted to with adequate support, and the rest can be put into perspective. The challenge of the assessment process itself is to differentiate the real limitation from the illusory and to determine, with the patient himself, the most acceptable route to take in coping with the problems.

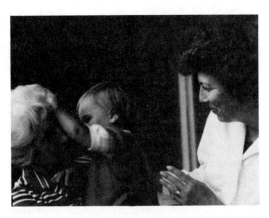

Figure 14-2. Every interaction, however casual, offers the nurse new opportunities to "fine tune" her assessment of the aging person's physical, mental, social, and emotional functioning.

Ongoing Assessment

For the skillful professional, assessment becomes internalized, a way of approaching problems and interacting with others at all times, rather than a technique which is turned on only for special occasions. An apparently casual conversation can be, in fact, highly purposeful communication. Every bath, every walk down the hall, every home visit offers the opportunity to refine and modify one's perception of the individual and his ever-changing status (see Figure 14-2).

The nurse elicits information about the person's functioning, his feelings about himself, his interactions with others, and his life, encouraging expression of his thoughts and concerns, paying attention to her own hunches, and pursuing those worries, signs, or symptoms which seem to merit a closer look. The three elements that are present in the initial assessment — history taking, examination, and further diagnostic measures — are recognizable in a sometimes modified form in the continuing process of assessment and are equally applicable to physical, social, and psychological phenomena.

PHYSICAL EXAMINATION

Many examiners deliberately choose to begin the "hands on" portion of the physical examination at the onset of the contact by measuring the vital signs — the respiratory rate, pulse rate, arterial blood pressure, and temperature — in spite of the fact that patient apprehension may cause the initial measurements to be abnormally elevated. This approach may be both strategic and utilitarian in design if the nurse utilizes the opportunity to build on the familiar, the expected, and the peripheral, demonstrating with gentle deftness what the subject can expect in terms of touch, explanations, and support during the examination proper.

This initial period of purposeful handling serves as an introduction to the examiner's style and as an "icebreaker," decreasing the initial tension and desensitizing the patient to being systematically touched. It also provides a measure of the degree of stress the patient is experiencing, as well as an opportunity to gauge how he tolerates that pressure and how rapidly and to what levels these indices will drop as he relaxes. Explaining to him that a single measurement of his vital signs is informative only when compared with previous or subsequent readings helps to prepare him for the fact that the examiner will be repeating the pulse and blood pressure determinations later in the examination, as well as during successive visits.

As a general rule, it is important to remember that the vital signs of older people display a wider range of variation from the accepted physiological norms than they do in any other age group of younger adults. As a result, it is of great relevance to establish readings which are "normal" for each person as a basis for accurate assessment in times of ill health.

Temperature. The route for measuring body temperature is determined by the needs of the situation and by the ability of the person to cooperate with and tolerate the procedure. The recording variations of normal in the aged are as follows:

Oral readings	34–37.4°C (93.2-99.3°F)
Rectal readings	Approximately one degree higher than the oral measurement on the same person
Axillary readings	Approximately one degree lower than the oral measurement would be, with a difference of up to 1.6°C between the right and left side in many subjects

Obviously, in order to make the data on a person's temperature comparable, the route used to measure the temperature should be noted; comparisons of repeated readings must be corrected for variations related to the route used (where this changes); diurnal variations must be taken into account; and if axillary temperatures are recorded, the same axilla should be used each time.

In addition to the wider range of baseline temperatures encountered in the elderly, there are two other extremely important differences in the evaluation of temperature readings for this age group.

1. While fever in old people nearly always indicates an infectious or inflammatory condition, the absence of fever in an old person in no way eliminates the possibility of an infection. The elderly simply do not always respond (especially to a pernicious, low grade pneumonia) with fever. Other signs and symptoms, such as unusual fatigue, sudden confusion, or weakness (perhaps manifested by a fall), must also be considered in this respect as possible indicators of infection.
2. Hypothermia occurs fairly frequently in old age. It may be accidental, the result of a severe illness such as a stroke or virulent infection, or due to neurological disease. In hypothermia, all parts of the body feel cold to the touch, including those portions which have been covered by clothing. If a temperature is recorded as 35°C (95°F), which is the lowest reading on most clinical thermometers, the temperature should be repeated immediately, rectally, with a special, low reading thermometer. Mild hypothermia = 32-35°C (90-95°F) and indicates the need to prevent further heat loss. Serious hypothermia = less than 32°C (90°F) and requires immediate medical evaluation (Rango, 1980).

Fever has the same significance in the elderly that it has in the young, although its presence may not be detected in an old person whose normal reading falls well below the standard norm.

For instance, a gentleman whose temperature in good health ordinarily hovers between 34.2°C (approximately 94°F) and 35.4°C (95.8°F) would manifest a rather high fever if he ran a temperature of 38°C (100.4°F); see discussion of hypothermia in Chapter 38.

Pulse Rate. Because of the frequency of irregular rhythms in the elderly, an old person's radial pulse should be palpated for a full 60 seconds for accuracy. Howell reports that pulse rates may be as low as 44 beats per minute or as high as 104 beats per minute in active, seemingly healthy old men, with a tendency for the rate to slow with age, beginning in the early 60s (Howell, 1975). Like temperature readings, documentation of the normal pulse rate during a period of good health is valuable information to have on record for later comparison. In one individual, a pulse rate of 80 beats per minute could actually be a tachycardia, while in another it might indicate a mild bradycardia. In any event, rates as low as 30 beats per minute in any individual are definitely pathological.

The force of the pulse should be noted in addition to the rate and the rhythm. Radial arteries in elderly people often feel unusually hard, indicating the Mönckeberg type of arteriosclerosis which is generally thought to be unrelated to occlusive vascular disease elsewhere (Caird and Judge, 1979).

Respiration. The normal respiratory rate in the elderly approximates the adult norm of 16-20 breaths per minute. Similarly, the depth and the regularity of respirations are noted discretely, along with the presence of adventitious sounds (i.e., wheezing, sighing, grunting, or audible rales) and the use of accessory muscles. Respiratory movement of the chest wall is less pronounced in older people (see Chapter 23), which may make counting the respiratory rate visually less reliable.

Blood Pressure. Arguments have raged for years over what the limits of "normal" arterial pressures should be in the aged (see Chapter 21 for discussion and specific limits). Because of the lack of research dealing specifically with arterial hypertension in this age group, treatment continues to be initiated at a wide variety of levels, depending upon the beliefs of the physician, the condition of the patient, and the causes of the hypertension.

For the initial blood pressure determination, it is necessary to take readings in both arms. Normally little difference will be noted when the pressures obtained are compared. If, however, a significant discrepancy is discovered, an obstruction of the innominate artery or an abnormality such as an aortic aneurysm may be suggested.

All elderly people, but especially those taking antihypertensive medications or those with complaints of syncope or light-headedness when getting up from a sitting or lying position, should have their pressure measured first in a supine position and then again immediately after standing (or, if falling is a possibility, sitting up). Ordinarily the cardiac output decreases upon standing, which results in a slight drop in the systolic pressure. In a person experiencing orthostatic hypotension, however, there will be a dramatic drop of 30 mm Hg or more when he stands, with a somewhat smaller drop when he sits up. A standing systolic level of 100–110 mm Hg frequently gives rise to symptoms of cerebral insufficiency. Any febrile illness can cause such unexpected episodes of hypotension.

Every nurse must be aware that no blood pressure reading in the elderly should be accepted as reliable unless a compatible palpatory blood pressure reading is obtained first. Especially when dealing with older people, in whom extremely high systolic pressures are frequently encountered, a phenomenon known as the "auscultatory gap" can easily deceive unwary examiners. For example, if the blood pressure reading is determined by auscultation alone, the nurse may first detect the sounds at a high level, perhaps 210 mm Hg, only to have them suddenly disappear at 180 mm Hg and ultimately reappear at 130 mm Hg. If the nurse has inflated the cuff only to 170 mm Hg, she will assume that 130 mm Hg is the systolic pressure rather than the true reading of 210 mm Hg.

To determine the palpatory systolic pressure, the radial pulse is palpated and the pressure in the cuff is increased quickly to a level of about 30 mm Hg above the point at which the radial pulse disappears. As the cuff is slowly deflated, the palpatory systolic reading is taken at the point at which the pulse reappears. The cuff is then deflated completely and remeasured by the usual method of auscultation. Generally, the systolic pressure determined by auscultation is slightly higher than the point at which the radial pulsations are first palpable. If the palpatory reading is consistently somewhat higher, however, it should be accepted as the prime reading for the systolic pressure.

LABORATORY WORK AND DIAGNOSTIC PROCEDURES

The final step in the initial health assessment is the use of carefully selected studies to detect some common, perhaps asymptomatic, conditions (such as anemia, a low grade urinary tract infection, diabetes, gastrointestinal bleeding, or pulmonary tuberculosis). Other procedures may be helpful in confirming or ruling out specific problems which the examiner has reason to suspect may exist on the basis of the history or the physical findings. The nurse has an obligation to weigh the need for each test in terms of the urgency of the problem, the clinical condition of the elderly subject, the risk of the procedure itself, the cost of performing the test, and its potential for providing the information which is desired.

Organizing these investigations around the suspected problems to maximize their appropriateness, and grouping the procedures to minimize repetition, number of trips to the laboratory, cost, and discomfort to the subject, the examiner should deliberate the nature and limitations of each procedure. The least complex, most comprehensive studies are usually done first, followed by more detailed tests if their use is warranted.

Finally, laboratory tests, x-rays, microbiologic and immunologic studies, and endoscopic and electrographic procedures must all be kept in perspective. These analyses, however sophisticated, are simply additional ways of extending the senses of the examiner and providing her with more sources of information against which to consider the clinical findings and the elderly individual's account of his symptoms. Laboratory errors are not uncommon, however, and no conclusions should ever be drawn on the basis of a single laboratory result.

In general, all investigations which are considered to be appropriate should be performed. Except in situations in which the dangers or demands of the procedures are contraindicated because of the precarious mental or physical condition of the subject, or situations in which the outcome will not change the management of the problem, age alone is not usually an acceptable reason for denying an individual the benefits of a full investigation of his problem(s). Aging is a continuous fact of life, not a pathological process, and the skilled nurse will use every means at her disposal to enhance the quality of all the lives she touches.

SUMMARY

The initial health assessment provides a wealth of information with which the nurse can evaluate the physiological, functional, and developmental well-being of the elderly patient. Collection of these data allows the nurse to establish contact with the individual on a physical, emotional, and verbal level. It offers her the opportunity to hear both what is said and what is not said, to understand what used to be, and to help the elderly person himself better appreciate "what is left, not what is gone" (Steffl, 1979). She can interpret the manifestations of aging for him in light of his body's continuing ability to adapt, to utilize its resources in new ways, and to compensate for losses. In addition, the nurse can educate the aging individual in terms of the active measures he can take to make himself more secure and to protect himself from identifiable hazards that menace certain aspects of his life.

The material in these chapters on physical assessment can serve as a foundation for the chapters on medical-surgical and other aspects of gerontological nursing in this book. The bibliography at the end of this chapter applies to all of Part IV and is offered as a general knowledge base and as a supplement to specific documentation.

REFERENCES

Butler, R.N. *Medicine and Aging* (NIH Publication No. 79-1699). Washington, D.C.: 1979.

Caird, F.I. and Judge, T.G. *Assessment of the Elderly Patient* (2nd ed.). Los Altos, Calif.: J.B. Lippincott, 1979, p. 32.

Howell, T.H. *Old Age: Some Practical Points in Geriatrics*. London: H.K. Lewis, 1975, p. 26.

Pearson, L.J. and Kotthoff, M. *Geriatric Clinical Protocols*. 1979, pp. 11-18.

Rango, N. Old and cold: hypothermia in the elderly. *Geriatrics* 93-96 (November 1980).

Steffl, B.M. *Nursing care of the elderly*. Paper presented at the 4th Annual Psychiatry Symposium — Geropsychiatry, El Paso, Texas, January 18-20, 1979.

BIBLIOGRAPHY

Adams, G. *Essentials of Geriatric Medicine*. New York: Oxford University Press, 1977.

Agate, J. *Geriatrics for Nurses and Social Workers* (2nd ed.). London: William Heinmann Medical Books, 1979.

Bates, B. *A Guide to Physical Examination*. Philadelphia: J.B. Lippincott, 1974.

Brocklehurst, J.C. *Textbook of Geriatric Medicine and Gerontology* (2nd ed.). New York: Churchill Livingstone, 1978.

Caird, F.I. and Judge, T.G. *Assessment of the Elderly Patient* (2nd ed.). Calif.: Pitman, 1979.

Cape, R. *Aging: Its Complex Management*. Hagerstown, Md.: Harper & Row, 1978.

Carnevali, D.L. and Patrick, M. (Eds.). *Nursing Management for the Elderly*. Philadelphia: F.A. Davis, 1980.

DeGowin, E. and DeGowin, R.L. *Bedside Diagnostic Examination* (3rd ed.). New York: Macmillan, 1976.

Fowkes, W.C. and Hunn, V.K. *Clinical Assessment for Nurse Practitioners*. St. Louis: C.V. Mosby, 1973.

Futrell, M., Brouender, S., McKinnon-Mullett, E., and Brower, H.T. *Primary Health Care of the Older Adult*. North Scituate, Mass.: Duxbury Press, 1980.

Hoffman, A.M. *The Daily Needs and Interests of Older People*. Springfield, Ill.: Charles C. Thomas, 1970.

Howell, T.H. *Old Age: Some Practical Points in Geriatrics* (2nd ed.). London: H.K. Lewis, 1975.

Kart, C.S., Metress, E.S., and Metress, J.F. *Aging and Health*. Toledo, Ohio: Addison-Wesley, 1978.

Krupp, M.A. and Chatton, M.J. *Current Diagnosis and Treatment*. Los Altos, Calif.: Lange, 1974.

Morgan, W.L. and Engel, G.L. *The Clinical Approach to the Patient*. Philadelphia: W.B. Saunders, 1969.

Pearson, L.J., and Kotthoff, M., Geriatric clinical protocols, Philadelphia, J.B. Lippincott Company, 1979, p. 11.

Prior, J.A. and Silberstein, J.S. *Physical Diagnosis: The History and Examination of the Patient* (5th ed.). St. Louis: C.V. Mosby, 1977.

Reichel, W. (Ed.). *Clinical Aspects of Aging.* Baltimore: Williams and Wilkins, 1978.

Rossman, I. *Clinical Geriatrics* (2nd ed.). Philadelphia: J.B. Lippincott, 1979.

Steinberg, F.U. *Cowdry's The Care of the Geriatric Patient* (5th ed.). St. Louis: C.V. Mosby, 1976.

Yurick, A.G., Robb, S.S., Spier, B.E., and Ebert, N.J. *The Aged Person and the Nursing Process.* New York: Appleton-Century-Crofts, 1980.

15
The Health History

Linda Ellison Jessup

You don't get old all at once. You notice
the first wrinkle, the first gray hair . . . but
you are too busy living to really think of
"when you'll be old."

Rose Rudin, 1974

The first and possibly the single most important element of the initial health assessment is the patient's history. The complete patient history details the development of an individual's state of health, from birth to the present, according to his ability to recall facts and according to his perception of events. Consequently, it is primarily a subjective account, which is made as accurate as possible by a process of systematic questioning and careful clarification of information by a skilled and sensitive interviewer. The history is a brief biopsychosocial biography in outline form, with several important purposes.

The first, and most obvious, purpose of a patient history is to determine what is healthy about a person and what has the potential to improve his health status, as well as to identify what is unhealthy and what has the potential to erode his level of wellness.

Second, a comprehensive understanding of an individual facilitates a kind of "bonding," which stimulates the care provider to become professionally invested in the patient. This investment forms the basis for a therapeutic relationship as well as for a truly personalized approach to care (see Figure 15-1).

Third, a thorough history makes the physical examination much more meaningful and challenging, by suggesting problems and possibilities to investigate further and with extra care. A good history prevents the examination from becoming a dry, mechanical procedure and permits the examiner to correlate the physical

findings with information gathered earlier. Ultimately, these combined data will also serve as a guide for additional laboratory and diagnostic work and for the development of an effective plan of care.

Fourth, asking questions in an ordered fashion insures against overlooking major information and helps the examiner to organize findings for coherent written and verbal presentation.

Finally, obtaining as complete a history as possible has a benefit to the older adult which can be consciously used to maximize and extend the value of the interaction beyond its traditional usages: that is, the process of remembering, of recounting earlier life experiences, of reaching back into the past, and of struggling to arrange events in a chronological sequence can be an excellent vehicle for memory stimulation and the process of "life review," as Butler calls it (Butler, 1974). History taking is a purposeful, systematic approach to reminiscing. It often has a priming effect, setting into motion the recall of significant events which have lain buried for many years. "Why, I haven't thought of that for ages!" is a frequent exclamation of older individuals during history taking.

Life would be much easier for everyone if every patient were able to provide an accurate, complete, and comprehensive health history. Unfortunately, reality is usually far from this ideal. Often older persons are first seen by health care providers only when they develop an acute problem. The history may have to be gathered in several stages or obtained entirely from a family member of friend who is familiar with the patient and his problems. Old charts supply data which augment the information from the patient and the family. Past records are especially helpful in documenting the duration of symptoms which have persisted for long periods of time (Burnside, 1980). In any event, an initial

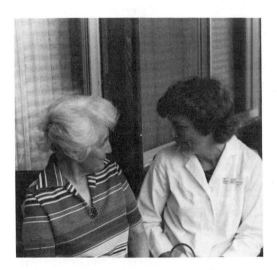

Figure 15-1. A comprehensive understanding of the older person catalyzes a kind of bonding. This emotional investment not only forms the basis for the therapeutic relationship but also results in a personalized approach to care.

patient history follows a logical, preset order; the elements of this history will be discussed in the following sections.

THE PATIENT PROFILE

A patient-centered approach to care, logically enough, should begin with the patient profile, a brief, personal description of the individual whose history follows. In spite of the fact that this section precedes the rest of the data, it is only when the data-collecting process is complete that the interviewer, equipped with these facts along with his personal observations of the patient, can distill this knowledge into a very succinct, pertinent, introductory profile paragraph.

Appropriately enough, the term "profile" is used in an artistic sense, outlining a person quickly from an angle that shows his prominent, distinguishing features. Thus, this crucial paragraph serves to sketch the subject briefly by using visual and informational cues, first to identify and then to introduce the individual to all who have reason to read the record and work with him. It should be kept in mind that the way in which this profile is written may

well help to shape the attitudes of those who care for the individual. The description can be dull and mechanical, brusque, judgmental, or even antagonistic in tone. It can diminish concern, obscure understanding, and even provoke prejudice against the elderly person (perhaps treatment of this kind should be renamed the "impatient profile").

The profile also offers the interviewer a prime opportunity to put into practice the "art" of nursing. This approach entails describing the new patient in terms that emphasize his individual uniqueness as an interesting and valuable human being, and sets a sympathetic tone for the care he will receive. Making the effort to discover and record a few special qualities, interests, and problems which characterize this person clearly communicates to subsequent readers that this elderly person is deserving of their time and effort.

The patient profile, while always important, becomes absolutely essential when a patient is unable to communicate effectively for himself. For the elderly person who is aphasic, disoriented, severely depressed, or even unconscious, knowing something about his life assists care providers to relate to him more appropriately and to look beyond the limits of his impairment and see the outline of an individual human being. Since a variety of personnel may be involved in the care of a single elderly person, a brief, readable, and accurate profile reduces the need for repetitive questions, engages the care provider's interest in the patient, and guards against errors of mistaken identity.

The first sentence of the profile identifies the person by name, age on admission, birth date, sex, ethnic or racial background, marital status, and distinguishing reasons for needing care. This single sentence helps to establish a mental picture of the patient which clearly differentiates him from others on the basis of age, physical characteristics, and any other unique characteristics of this patient. It also tells us how he should be addressed or what he wishes to be called.

The remaining information in this sentence and in the rest of the paragraph begins to color and add depth to our perception of the individual. His environment, life-style, habits, temperament, present family structure, and support systems are included.

The Source

A succinct description of the source of the interviewer's information — be it the patient, a friend, a family member, or an old record — should be given. A judgment about the reliability of the informant is also important. Knowing that the subject was "alert, cooperative, and had excellent recall for past events" or that he was from the outset "confused, suspicious, and reluctant to divulge information" helps the reader to better evaluate the history that follows.

PRESENT HEALTH STATUS

The Chief Complaint and the Present Problem(s)

The segment of the history dealing with the chief complaint and present problem(s) is collected in precisely the same form and for the same purposes for the older person as it is for any other age group. The primary objectives are twofold: first, to establish the chief complaint, a brief statement or two about what the patient perceives as being the major reasons for needing care and the duration of this problem to date; second, to elaborate and describe in meticulous detail the present problem from the time of onset to the time of the interview.

When caring for the elderly, who are characterized clinically by the occurrence of multiple and chronic health problems, it is useful to be aware that the chief complaints are generally of two types. The first type involves those "complaints" in which a symptom or a series of symptoms is as yet undiagnosed. This is often a new or acute problem. For example,

Chief Complaint: "I've been getting dizzy for about the last month, especially when I reach high for something."

Chief Complaint: "My heart just starts pounding in the middle of the night and wakes me up. It happened last Saturday night, the night before last, and last night.

The second type of chief complaint concerns symptoms which result from changes in already well-established disorders, such as

Chief Complaint: Diabetes — I'm urinating large amounts of water again. It began yesterday morning.

Chief Complaint: Hypertension with congestive heart failure — "Just walking across the room makes me terribly out of breath. X 6 days.

Chief Complaint: Eczema — "My arms broke out and have been itching since my son called about his divorce, about three days ago."

Present Problem. Many symptoms in the elderly are extremely nonspecific in nature and should be investigated with that fact in mind. A patient who becomes bedridden because he "can't walk" may be suffering from conditions as diverse as arthritis, a cerebrovascular accident, coronary disease, an acute respiratory or urinary tract infection, an emotional disorder, or a drug toxicity. In order to disentangle the actual problem from the other possibilities, the interviewer's questions should be clear, simple, and to the point, and should follow a systematic order in delineating the present problem and characterizing the precise nature of the symptoms.

At times, when documenting an older person's present health, it may be possible to determine the exact nature of a symptom from which the person is suffering, but one may discover that the elderly person is unable to remember how long the symptom has been present. Conversely, sometimes the interviewer can establish that something has been wrong for a specific period of time, but may find that the patient just can't seem to pin down precisely what the problem is. Not only can the patient be quite vague about such details, but on occasion, the perceptions of patients and their family members may even be in conflict on these points.

Being able to resolve these inconsistencies requires tact, patience, and persistence on the part of everyone involved, and an awareness by the nurse of such psychological mechanisms as denial, displacement, or projection. A person's perceptions in defining disability should also be taken into consideration. For example, what one person or family considers to be "moderate hearing loss," others may consider being "deaf as a doornail," even though the clinical impairment is the same.

Sometimes, determination of the subject's condition before the onset of the problem can be helpful in getting a feel for the nature of the illness and the degree of disability it has caused, while revealing a rough estimate of the time which has passed since it began. "Why, he was out most every day this spring, turning over his garden." "She never did have a strong back. May sons have carried in her groceries for years, but at least she was able to go to the store until a few weeks ago." "I haven't been able to crochet baby clothes for my last grandchild like I did for all the others because of my hands."

Old records, of course, are another invaluable resource since they often help to document or to rule out the previous existence of important symptoms such as a cough, weight gain or loss, headaches, or mental deterioration.

The rapidity with which a person becomes ill or disabled is one more valuable indicator of the nature of the present problem. Symptoms which appear suddenly suggest an infectious process or an obstructive problem (vascular, renal, or gastrointestinal), while symptoms which have developed over months or even over years are more likely the result of some gradually progressive condition.

The diffuse nature of many of the symptoms manifested by the elderly and the difficulty the interviewer may have in determining the duration of certain problems create some special challenges. In spite of these obstacles, utilizing additional sources of information, relating the change in the individual's condition to his previous state, and determining the speed with which the problem has occurred will often allow the interviewer to define the presenting problem with surprising accuracy.

THE PAST HEALTH HISTORY

Obtaining and recording a past health history of an elderly individual is structurally the same as for any other person, in that the information collected deals with the person's

General health
Childhood and adult health and illness
Immunizations and tests
Allergies
Medications
Accidents, hospitalizations, and surgical procedures
Habits and risk factors

Still, this portion of the history is substantially different for the older subject because there are simply more data to draw upon and more ways in which this information can be utilized to enhance the care of the elderly person.

General Health

The topic of the past history is usually introduced by the examiner's inquiring, "In general, how would you say your health has been in the past?" Here one is interested in learning the person's overall assessment of his total health experience, emotional as well as physical, and good health as well as ill health. For example,

General Health: Mrs. G. characterizes her health as, "Pretty good. I've never been terribly ill."

General Health: Mr. T. describes his overall health as, "Excellent! I'm as strong as a mule."

Although only the patient response is recorded, the examiner encourages clarification, seeking to understand the elderly subject's perception of himself in relation to his health experience.

Obviously, an individual's self-image, developed over a lifetime, as primarily a robust or a fragile person, as a helpless victim or as a strong, capable man or woman, has an impact on how he reacts to any current or future threat to his integrity. Kahn, Zeman, and Goldfarb (1958) report that persons who are resourceful and who show an assertive approach to specific problems tend to have fewer somatic complaints regardless of their true medical status; persons who appear to be more passive in their orientation seem to have more complaints and anxiety about their status.

The nurse has ample opportunity through this and subsequent portions of the interview to develop a sense of whether a patient tends to maximize, minimize, or respond fairly realistically to symptoms. This assessment will help her to navigate astutely through the rest of the patient's account of both the present and the past, as well as to anticipate the individual's emotional responses to immediate and future problems.

Childhood and Adult Health

Establishing the occurrence or avoidance of a whole array of childhood illnesses has a dual purpose. Fifty years ago, diseases such as smallpox, diphtheria, pertussis, tuberculosis, and other highly contagious infections were commonplace. Polio (all three antigenically distinct types), rubella, rubeola, and mumps are other communicable diseases against which many elderly people may have acquired immunity over the years. Yet it cannot be assumed that all people 65 years and older are automatically protected against all of these illnesses. Thus, the first reason for determining which "childhood illnesses" the individual has actually manifested is to get an idea of the subject's immunity to specific communicable diseases.

The second reason concerns the nature of some of these illnesses. Many early problems are characterized by an acute phase that subsides, only to resurface or to be followed by serious sequelae in later years. Tuberculosis is one such disease which may reactivate at any time and progress to chronic destructive tuberculosis without further exposure to infection (Balchum, 1971). Since it can also remain asymptomatic or manifest itself in an atypical manner, an accurate history may be the first clue that the

disease exists. Syphilis acquired in adolescence or during adulthood is still another highly destructive disease which, if not adequately treated, can affect almost any organ system after years of latency.

Immunizations and Tests

An important area of preventive care often overlooked in the elderly is that of current immunization status. Determining the degree of protection an older person has acquired by means of active infection or immunization requires skillful questioning and perhaps delving into old records.

Because the development of vaccines is relatively recent, few of the elderly have ever received the initial series of vaccinations on which to base later boosters. As a result, a vaccination program of selected, important immunizations may be necessary in later life. For an older person who lives with, or is in frequent contact with, young children (especially if their immunization status is not complete), antibody titers can be run to insure that his immunity against measles and mumps is adequate.

The danger that these childhood diseases pose to a vulnerable elderly person should not be underestimated. One of the most seriously ill patients this author has ever seen was a 72-year-old gentleman with mumps. He had participated in a recreation program for a group of retarded children. Rubeola (measles) also is not infrequent in adults and can be quite severe. If diphtheria and polio reappear as significant menaces because of the decreasing pool of adequately vaccinated children, large numbers of old people will be at serious risk.

Tetanus, while not contagious, is a threat throughout one's lifetime since the *Clostridium tetani* bacillus is universal in distribution. The bacillus is found mainly in soil and in animal and in human feces, so complete protection is recommended for all who are not allergic to the vaccine and is vital for the elderly who live in rural areas, who garden, or who are active outdoors. After the initial series, boosters at intervals of 10–12 years have been shown to give a high level of immunity against this often fatal infection (Tindall, 1971).

Influenza, with its ever-changing varieties, is one of the few communicable diseases for which vaccination of the elderly has been given high priority and a great deal of publicity. In an effort to lower the high mortality rate, due in large part to respiratory and cardiac complications, it is common practice to vaccinate this high risk population before the flu season.

Tuberculosis, on the other hand, continues to be a little recognized but insidious threat to the health of the elderly. Statistics show that over the last 30 years, the peak prevalence of tuberculosis has shifted from young adulthood to old age, and that for people 65 and over, the new active case rate is actually double that of the total population (Balchum, 1971). In older people, chronic tuberculosis has been demonstrated to arise most commonly from a reactivation of an initial primary infection implanted years before, although a primary infection can be contracted at any age.

The date of the most recent film and tuberculin test and the results should be noted in this portion of the past history (or in the section on risk factors, if a risk appraisal is done) along with any other tests for regionally endemic diseases. The dates of each of the previous vaccinations and boosters are also listed in this section.

Allergies

Unfortunately, allergic reactions are no respecters of age. In fact, because older people tend to use more of a drug or a greater number of drugs than younger people, they run an increased risk of allergic responses. As a general working rule, it may be said that any drug can cause trouble at any time in a person's life and that even a long history of usage without incident does not preclude a drug from suspicion as the cause of an allergic reaction.

Cross-sensitization also poses a very real problem for the elderly, if only because they have had so many opportunities to be exposed to a multitude of antigens. For example, many people are allergic to a para-amine group found in sulfonamides and in many local anesthetics. The same para-amine group is a common ingredient in hair dyes. Thus, a negative history of drug exposure to sulfa drugs or to local anesthetics does not necessarily mean that a drug reaction will not result from the elderly person's first contact with one of these medications.

Therefore, when compiling the history of previous allergic reactions, care should be taken to include both systemic and localized responses to:

- Medications (injected, oral, or topical)
- Food and drink
- Natural agents (plants, insects, animals, etc.)
- Cosmetics (creams, lotions, hair dyes, permanent waves, perfumes)
- Household or work-related substances (detergents, fumes, chemicals, etc.)

Asking about asthma, hay fever, and skin rashes may seem redundant, but it is frequently productive, since these manifestations might not have been perceived as being allergic in nature or identified as a link between a reaction and the causative allergen.

Allergic reactions to foods, natural agents, and occupational allergens appear to be much less common in the elderly. Either there is less opportunity for exposure to these substances, or the person, through experience, has simply learned to avoid them.

When a previous or possible allergy does come to light, it is vital to note the offending substance, a description of the reaction, and any treatment the person received for it. A detailed description of the reaction is critical in determining if a true allergic reaction occurred.

Medication

As a crucial part of the initial data base, every patient should be asked about the medication he takes on a regular and occasional basis. In fact, having him actually bring the medications with him is a great aid to the interviewer and a help in determining what education is needed to improve compliance with the therapeutic regime. Compiling a flow sheet of all the drugs an older person takes may astound and horrify nurses and physicians since it is not unusual for them to number from 20 to 30 different substances! It stands to reason that toxic reactions and other medication-related complications are frequent causes of hospitalization in this population. With a large number of overmedicated, undermedicated, and irregularly medicated older people mixing over-the-counter drugs with prescription drugs (often prescribed by several different physicians, each unaware of the other medications the patient is taking) a veritable pharmacological mine field is created. Obviously, the longer an elderly person is left to wander blindly over this hazardous terrain, the more numerous are the potential dangers, and the greater is his chance of detonating a serious reaction.

These medical mine fields also exist in institutions under the eyes and noses of the physicians who prescribe them and the nurses who administer them. It goes without saying that there is no excuse for irresponsible drub administration under these controlled and, supposedly, protective conditions. Conducting a regular review of all of a patient's medications, be he an inpatient or an outpatient, questioning the necessity for each, and eliminating all but those which are essential, would prevent a great deal of unnecessary suffering. It would also reduce the tremendous cost of unnecessary drugs, not to mention the enormous sums of money which are expended in trying to repair the damage of medication-related reactions (Kayne, 1978).

Whether an older person is self-sufficient or institutionalized, new symptoms, a deterioration in his condition, or changes in his behavior may well be drug induced. The medications the individual is taking should come under sharp scrutiny at such times, in addition to regular interviews. In the elderly, chronic laxative use and routine analgesic abuse are frequently discovered and may help to explain a serious potassium depletion or even chronic renal failure (Caird and Judge, 1979).

Conversely, drugs that are prescribed but not taken, or not taken correctly, may explain a recurrence of congestive heart failure, atrial fibrillation, an anemia, or an exacerbation of arthritis. Cutting the number of medications to the bare essentials and simplifying the regimen as much as possible tend to increase compliance,

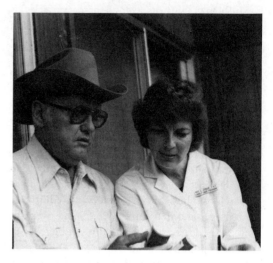

Figure 15-2. Drugs, whether obtained by prescription or over the counter, often constitute a chemical mine field for the elderly person.

and thus the therapeutic effect, while reducing the risk of dangerous reactions.

Accidents, Hospitalizations, and Surgical Procedures

Accidents and surgical procedures can occur at any age, and they too are important indicators which may shed light on a person's current symptomatology. For example, surgery for a "growth" 15 years ago might well increase one's index of suspicion regarding the findings of an enlarged liver and anemia at present. "Arthritis" in a wrist, the site of a fracture years ago, may well be degenerative rather than rheumatoid in nature. By the same token, an episode of confusion which occurred around an accident, an operation, or an acute illness several years earlier may suggest that the same patient's present disorientation is also stress induced and temporary, or it may have represented the first signs of chronic brain syndrome, which is now much more apparent (Caird and Judge, 1979).

A caveat is in order here about a patient's account of any episode of illness or previous medical procedure. As a rule of thumb, no diagnostic term used by an informant to specify a health problem is ever accepted at face value by the cautious interviewer. It is always more valuable to have at least a minimal description of the problem, in terms of the date of its occurrence, the symptoms, the course, the treatment, and any sequelae, than it is to have a diagnostic label.

Thus, any diagnosis used by the informant is identified clearly as being a direct quotation, and if the interviewer has any question about the validity of the label, it is followed by a brief description of the problem. Even with major health problems, as Caird and Judge (1979) note, "It is not unusual for patients to be largely or completely unaware of what illness has taken them to hospital in the past or what operation has been performed. This is only rarely due to impaired memory on the part of the patient, and much more often to impaired communication on the part of the doctors."

Regardless of origin, misconceptions about the true identity of earlier episodes of illness or about the nature of injuries suffered in an accident are common. As a result, the experienced interviewer is cautious in accepting a previous diagnostic conclusion without corroborating evidence.

The date, location, and cause of all hospitalizations are recorded. In addition, a careful obstetrical history is included when working with the aged female adult.

Habits and Risk Factors

Ordinarily, "social habits" such as smoking, drinking, and the habitual use of chemicals are noted in the section of the history dealing with habits and risk factors. Unless a major problem is evident, this information is usually passed over rather swiftly. For the health practitioner who believes that care can and should be a search for the elements which constitute the healthiest, most satisfying life-style possible for an individual, this portion of the interview can be made infinitely more serviceable.

This author believes that it is the proper role of health care personnel to be involved in helping people to change their life patterns which appear to be directly related to chronic illness and traumatic death. Too often dismissed

as "over the hill" or "too set in their ways to change," older people tend to be overlooked as candidates for even the most rudimentary evaluation of risk factors. This attitude smacks of ignorance and prejudice, since research has documented that a willingness or an ability to modify old behavior patterns and even learn new ones is far more directly linked to an individual's basic personality structure, his motivation, and an understanding of the pitfalls of his current life-style than it is to his chronological age. In any event, unless we — together with the older person — can define what habits increase his risk of illness, death, or disability, the chance of his making the choice to alter these habits is remote.

An evaluation of risk factors can be very complex or very simple, depending on the individual, his circumstances, and the environment in which he lives. Some basic indices which are particularly valuable for identifying problem areas are given in Table 15-1.

Some Special Considerations of Risk Factors.
Diet. Poor nutrition in the elderly is an all too common occurrence in the United States today. The absence of an adequate diet seriously jeopardizes the precarious balance between health and illness in the frail older person, yet nutritional deficiencies are very difficult to detect clinically unless they are extreme. As with other high risk age groups in which dietary factors assume critical importance, senescence is again a time for careful reevaluation by the health care provider, in conjunction with the older person, of food buying, preparation, storage, and intake patterns.

In examining this aspect of the person's life, the nurse should be very conscious of the many factors which affect the nutritional practices of older people. Meals may come to be the highlight of an old person's day, or they may be perfunctory and often forgotten. Many elderly people eat mechanically and only because they know they "should" or to "break up the day" which stretches long and bleakly before them.

Food preferences are generally pronounced in this population, although poverty or physical

Table 15-1.

EXERCISE

1. What do you do for exercise?
2. How often do you exercise?
3. How long do you exercise at a time?
4. Why do you stop this activity at that time?
5. Would you say that you are inactive, somewhat active?
6. Is this degree of activity a change for you?
7. Are you satisfied with this level of activity? (i.e., Are you able to do what you need to do, what you like to do?)

WEIGHT

1. How long have you weighed _____ ?
2. Have you been gaining, weight, losing weight, or staying the same over the last 12 months? (If gaining or losing, discover if this is intentional and how much weight has been gained or lost in a year's time.)

DIET

1. How many hot meals do you eat per week?
2. What are your sources of meals?
   a) What is the number per week prepared by yourself?
   b) What is the number per week prepared by family members, friends, or neighbors?
   c) What is the number per week prepared by an organization (Meals on Wheels, local senior center, Salvation Army, church, club, etc.)?
3. How much do you spend on food for yourself each week?
4. How much do you spend on pet food each week (if applicable)?
5. What do you eat for breakfast, lunch, dinner, snacks (based on a recent, normal day)?
6. What are your favorite foods? Do you eat them often?
7. What foods do you like least?
8. Do you ordinarily eat alone or with someone else (number of times per week)?

SMOKING*

1. At what age did you begin to smoke?
2. What do you smoke (cigar, pipe, or cigarettes)?
3. What was the most you ever smoked? For how long?
4. How old were you when you stopped smoking (if applicable)?
5. How long have you smoked in all?
6. Have your smoking habits changed recently?

ALCOHOL CONSUMPTION

1. What alcoholic beverages do you drink?
2. How much do you drink in a day? In a week?
3. Do you ever drive when you've been drinking?
4. Have you ever blacked out while drinking?

DRUG USE*

1. What drugs or medicines (both prescribed and over the counter) do you take regularly? Occasionally?
2. What medicines are there that have been prescribed but that you don't take?
3. How do you take _____ ? (Go through each medication.)
4. What is this medication for? (Go through each medication.)
5. Do you know any precautions regarding this medicine?

MOTOR VEHICLES

1. Do you drive?
2. How long have you been driving?
3. How much do you drive, or travel by car or truck each week?
4. What percent of the time do you wear seat belts when you are in a motor vehicle?

SUICIDE

1. Would you describe yourself as always, often, seldom, or never depressed?
2. Has anyone in your family ever committed suicide?

PROSPECTIVE TESTS

Have you ever had a:

		Date	Results
1.	proctosigmoidoscopy?		
2.	blood test for diabetes?		
3.	EKG?		
4.	chest x-ray?		
5.	TB skin test?		
6.	breast examination (men and women)?		
7.	urinalysis?		
8.	vaginal examination and Pap smear?		
9.	eye exam?		
10.	dental check?		
11.	hearing test?		

*See the section entitled "Some Special Considerations of Risk Factors" for further elaboration.

problems may limit the consumption of foods that are the most satisfying to the person. Sweet foods may predominate in the diet, possibly as the result of atrophy of the taste buds for sour, salty, and bitter flavors. There is some evidence that the taste buds for sweetness deteriorate last, so that highly sugared foods may ultimately become the one flavor that is still appreciated. When the senses of smell and taste are dimmed, the nurse must remember that the person's ability to detect food spoilage is also diminished.

Evidence of defective nutrition demands a search for the cause. Alcoholism is synonymous with dietary deficiency. Economic hardship is shamefully widespread among the elderly in our society, as is the lack of transportation and "task services" to ease the chores of shopping and even of food preparation, if such aid is needed.

Some lifetime dietary habits are truly bizarre and difficult to change, although nutritional supplements to balance intake may be accepted by the eccentric eater. When a person is still faithfully following a high potassium or low calorie diet or therapeutic regimen prescribed decades ago, which is no longer appropriate, a more adequate diet must be prescribed and will probably be followed with equal dedication. Malnutrition which is secondary to mental deterioration, alcoholism, and severe neurosis or psychosis will require continuous close dietary supervision and support.

Making a home visit for a firsthand assessment of the food situation of an elderly person in whom poor nutrition is suspected may provide a wealth of information about his present life and diet. A kitchen with few supplies and little recent evidence of eating suggests a serious degree of nutritional deprivation, while the number of stairs to be climbed, the gas or electrical services which have been discontinued, the distance from public transportation, and other situational clues may point to obvious causes and suggest some rather straightforward remedies.

Many older patients are almost pathetically grateful that a nurse will take the time and show the interest to visit them at home as part of the assessment process. Being on their "own turf," in combination with this demonstration of the nurse's concern, frequently engenders the courage necessary for an elderly person to reveal a problem which has seemed shameful or unacceptable previously. The relief of having the nurse recognize a distressing situation, which the individual has been hesitant to admit, is sometimes profound.

Smoking. Because respiratory problems are frequent, often disabling, and not uncommonly life threatening in the elderly, a major causative culprit like smoking is always considered seriously. In fact, of all the factors influencing lung disease in the aged, smoking is by far the most significant (Balchum, 1971).

A long term smoking habit is more common in the males of this earlier era, often dating back to the days of World War I or even to their preteen years. Whether male or female, however, the duration of the habit and the largest quantity of tobacco smoked for an extended period of time are vital information.

Pipes and cigars are less often implicated than cigarettes in respiratory disorders, since they are less often inhaled, but the regular use of any kind of tobacco (or alcohol) definitely increases the risk of oral cancer. In fact, oral cancer is considered a disease of older people because 90% of it occurs in persons over 45 years of age, and the average age of occurrence is about 60. With their longer exposure to smoking, men in this age group are twice as likely to develop oral cancer as women. Unfortunately, this ratio will probably change with the increase in tobacco consumption among women of all ages (Carbone et al. 1974).

The reason for change in a smoking habit is of interest because it may signal a deeper change in underlying factors or a swing in the fortunes of the individual. A decrease in the number of cigarettes or cigars smoked in recent years or months may be due more to the economics of living on a limited income or to poor health, for example, than to a desire to reduce the habit.

An increase in smoking, on the other hand, may be in response to increased stress, as other aspects of the person's life undergo changes which are disturbing or which represent a decrease in the satisfaction that he receives from other sources. In any event, these underlying factors should be taken into account when suggesting that the individual modify his smoking pattern (Burnside, 1976).

A final consideration for the nurse is the smoker whose eyesight is failing, whose mental condition is deteriorating, or whose use of consciousness-altering chemicals (such as alcohol, analgesics, hypnotics, or sedatives) multiplies the risk of smoking by adding fire hazard to the other dangers of this habit.

Alcohol Abuse. Alcoholism among the elderly, both men and women, constitutes an ever-growing menace to the health of this population. It is an addiction with many faces in older people, and its effects undercut the already reduced physical, psychological, and social resources on which the elderly person must depend to survive.

Aneurin (vitamin B_1) deficiency, which produces sensorimotor neuropathies, myelopathy, and encephalopathy, is commonly caused by chronic alcoholism in the older person. The clinical picture may contain one or several of the associated symptoms. Pain in the legs, burning or tingling in the hands, and peripheral weakness and wasting are due to the neuropathy, while the myelopathy can produce disorders of the cardiac muscle and eventual heart failure. Chronic alcoholism has also been implicated in the demineralization of bone and increased bone fragility, which frequently result in the fractures of a variety of bones. Since intoxicated people also tend to fall more than sober ones, many fractures are due to trauma, although some are due to the osteoporosis alone (Spencer and Lender, 1979).

In the presence of brain damage, alcohol may produce severe disorientation. If a patient is taking tranquilizers, alcohol will potentiate the effects of the drug, with potentially tragic results. Any person who is known to drink frequently or in large amounts should thus use such medications only under careful supervision and should be fully aware of the dangers of mixing these chemicals.

Alcohol abuse may be a new or a long term problem. Its presence may be obvious, suspected, or very difficult to detect. Drinking may be acknowledged as a problem by the patient and his family, or it may be totally denied by either or both parties. The nurse is well advised to be direct and nonjudgmental in questioning the subject about the quantity and frequency of alcohol consumption, and to keep in mind that a relative's account, especially that of a spouse, is not necessarily more reliable than the patient's (Wattis, 1981).

Note: A distinction should be made here between the alcohol abuser and the elderly person who uses alcohol with discretion and in small amounts. There are many older people for whom a small amount of alcohol provides a great deal of pleasure. A small glass of sherry or a cocktail before dinner may stimulate a poor appetite, promote relaxation, and be an important time for socialization, either in an institutional setting or at home. For the older person who has difficulty falling asleep, a small glass of port or a light white wine may be enjoyed after a warm bath or before a back rub to help promote drowsiness.

Despite the great span of time covered in the past health history of an older person, generally speaking the elderly are uniquely suited to retrace the events of a lifetime. Just as the body automatically seems to adjust to conserve energy and just as the gaze becomes directed downward, thereby reducing the less agile old person's risk of falling, so too does the mind's eye seem involuntarily to become directed backward, at times viewing the past with more ease, objectivity, and clarity than it sees the present.

Obtaining the past health history, as well as the three segments which follow it and which also deal with the past — the family history, the personal and social history, and the review of systems — is frequently facilitated by this apparently adaptive orientation of looking more to the past than to the future.

THE FAMILY HEALTH HISTORY

The attention of the interviewer now shifts to the fertile topic of the aging individual's family constellation. By this time in the interview, many of the subject's family members will already have been mentioned, and a fair amount of information will be known about the relationships between the elderly patient and certain family members. Using this knowledge as a takeoff point, the interviewer now proceeds to ask systematically about the age, health, and whereabouts of each member, and each person's role — past and present — in the life of the subject.

Next, the family tree or "pedigree" is drawn, which illustrates relationships graphically (see Figure 15-3). Whenever feasible, drawing the family diagram with the older subject's active help and involvement produces a more accurate diagram and is an enterprise which many elderly people thoroughly enjoy. Being able to actually see one's pedigree frequently stimulates the individual to reconstruct the genealogical history scrupulously, accounting for siblings and children who died early in life, common-law partners, separations, illnesses, and deaths of more peripheral relatives. Valuable insights into family patterns of illness or behavior may be experienced by the patient as he traces his lineage and views graphically his place in the constellation.

From the standpoint of the history taker, the objectives of the family health history are ordinarily fourfold:

1. to discover the existence of familially transmitted disorders (either genetic or situational) which might have significance for the patient's present or future health;
2. to determine the past or present existence of contagious diseases in the family, such as tuberculosis, rheumatic fever, etc.;
3. to learn about the other family members and their relationship to the patient;
4. to learn about the experience the patient has had, through his family, with marriages and separations, births and deaths, and illness and care.

With the elderly, the first goal decreases in importance for predictive medical purposes since nearly all of the diseases which are known to be genetic will have appeared by this time if they are going to manifest themselves at all. Exceptions to this rule are Huntington's chorea and familial polyposis of the colon (McKusick, 1978).

The occurrence of common disorders in later life in which genetic factors are suspected to play a part, including certain forms of hypertensive disease, coronary artery disease, a variety of cancers, gout, mental illness, allergic disorders, and even obesity, should be investigated with special care for two reasons. First, a family tendency toward stomach cancer or hypertension secondary to pheochromocytoma, for example, may have some bearing on the elderly patient's "heartburn" or his high blood pressure readings. Second, and perhaps even more important, the experience of the patient with one or more relative's illnesses may affect the older patient's perceptions of his own symptoms.

One might expect, for instance, that a patient with bronchitis, whose grandfather and brother both died of lung cancer, will be likely to react with more anxiety to his own cough than will a person without this grim family experience. Asking the question, "Has anyone in your family ever had an illness like yours?" may uncover a familial connection that would not have been found in any other way.

The interpersonal relationships within the family assume great significance in the care and sustaining of an elderly person, and thus must also be carefully evaluated. Learning who the family members are and which ones are, or have been, especially important to the aging person becomes crucial in understanding who actually constitutes this person's physical and emotional support system. One needs to determine how willing and able those family members are to assist the elderly individual, and what kind of guidance they will need to do this job well.

PERSONAL AND SOCIAL HISTORY

The personal and social history constitutes the adhesive that binds the personal elements of the individual's account into a more cohesive narrative, and fills in, or delineates, any important biographical gaps which remain. Many of the items of health and illness which have been touched upon now slip into place and move

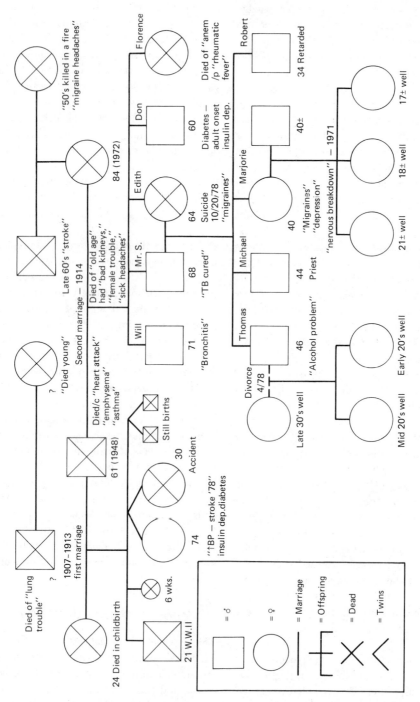

Figure 15-3. An example of a family tree.

into perspective in relation to the subject's over-all life experience and his present circumstances.

The personal and social history is constructed to provide the interviewer with an opportunity to explore and clarify her/his understanding of the evolution of this novel individual and of the critical influences which have helped to shape his development through time. The ways in which this person has functioned, made his way through successive stages of life, and adapted to crises which have arisen come into focus in this section. His reactions to, and ways of dealing with, major challenges (such as leaving home, marriage, getting or losing a job, becoming a parent, the death of a crucial family member, retirement, and gaining or losing significant material goods) command the interviewer's attention as she follows the patient's lead through these private milestones.

During this part of the interview, the nurse simultaneously corrects any previous misconceptions, reviews the chronology of events, and inserts, eliminates, or expands information to present as pertinent and recognizable a description of the person as possible. If care has been taken throughout the interview to foster a relationship of sincere interest and trust, the elderly patient is often willing to be very candid about sensitive topics at this point and may reveal concerns which he would have refused to discuss earlier. For purposes of clarity and access to data, the personal and social history is organized into two parts: the current life situation and the past development.

The Current Life Situation

In dealing with an old person, obtaining a complete description of his present living situation assumes primary importance. Circumstances which relate directly or indirectly to the individual's present health may well surface at this time. For example, it would be helpful to know of a recent move to an apartment from the family home, which coincides with a depressive episode and the development of an iron deficiency anemia, or to know that a pneumonia developed after the gas and electricity had been turned off in an elderly person's home for nonpayment of bills. Clearly the individual's physical and social environment must be well understood in order to treat a problem and to work out a reasonable plan of care and health maintenance measures with which the person and family are willing, and able, to comply.

An adequate description of the current life situation will include information about the following aspects of the person's life:

- *Home and family.* What is the physical living situation in the community for this person? Who is at home, and how are his relationships with those at home?
- *Present occupation and economic status.* Many elderly people work long after they reach retirement age. Some are compelled to work by necessity, while others work to stay active or because they enjoy it. Hobbies and "sidelines" may become major occupations as time becomes available and may even become unexpectedly lucrative. In any event, assessing the person's financial resources, his health insurance provisions, and his sources of income is of great importance.
- *Social and community activities.* Important friends, colleagues, clubs, religious activities, and organizational involvements provide a reading of the degree to which a person is isolated or is a participant in social relationships. If no such links exist, it is useful to discover if the isolation is preferred or disliked, self-inflicted or imposed by other factors. Where ties exist, they can often be tapped as support sources.
- *Sexual patterns.* Sexual attitudes, felt needs, and inhibitions are extremely variable in the elderly, changing with fluctuations in the subject's well-being, the availability of a desirable partner, and the opportunity to gratify one's sexual urges in a satisfying and personally acceptable manner. Some older people are reluctant to talk about sex; others seem genuinely amused or flattered by the raising of a topic which may simply no longer interest them much. Still others welcome the chance to express their concerns and explore the normalcy

of very vigorous sexual feelings. The interviewer's job here, as at other points in the interview, is to open the topic for consideration in an inviting and accepting way, often beginning with a broad and more impersonal statement. For example, the interviewer might say, "Many times, as people age, they notice changes in their need for closeness, for touching, for affection, and for sex. Some people experience increases in these needs, while others discover that some of these desires are diminished. Have you felt that your needs have undergone a change within, say, the last five years, Mrs. Miller?" A sensitive interviewer also comments on any strong feeling she encounters in dealing with this topic, rather than simply dropping the subject. Embarrassment, guilt, enthusiasm, enjoyment, disgust, and loneliness can all be acknowledged and explored with the patient, as can unsatisfied areas of need. Often, older people may lack the vocabulary to discuss sexual subjects fluently, and some will reflect the strong prejudices and even fears toward masturbation, sexual fantasies, and intercourse that characterized the era in which many of their attitudes were formed. The nurse identifies areas of patient interest where further education and interpretation are indicated, makes arrangements to return to the topic again, and includes this need in the plan of care.

- *Leisure activities.* Discovering how an individual enjoys himself — how he plans and uses his spare time — offers a special view of a person's world. Travel, vacations, special interests, and developing creative abilities may make this part of the person's life more exciting and gratifying than ever before. Decreased responsibilities and too much empty time, on the other hand, may weigh oppressively on a person's spirit and decrease his sense of self-worth.
- *The activities of daily living.* The interviewer and older person verbally "walk through" the routine of an average day, recording what happens from the time the individual awakens in the morning until he falls asleep at night. Included in this sequence are items such as eating patterns, rest times, socializing, working, and being active.

Worthy of special note in the overall current life situation segment is the identification of unresolved problems, significant interpersonal conflicts (especially involving a spouse, family member, or close friend), and additional circumstances in the person's life which cause him real concern. Recent changes, especially losses, may figure prominently in an older person's health and illness status. Therefore, any current dislocations in the life of the individual should be recorded, the date of the change given, and the person's reaction to the event noted.

Past Development

Childhood. The past development of the elderly patient begins with his birth and the setting into which he was born. The date and place of his birth, as well as subsequent major moves of the family, are noted. His parents' occupations and their relationships with each other, with the patient, and with others in the family receive attention, as do the relationships between the subject and his siblings.

Since adolescence in our society frequently is a turbulent time, involving breaking away from the family, forming initial relationships with the opposite sex, and making decisions about one's future, this period is analyzed with special care given to how the individual handled these complicated developmental tasks associated with this level of maturity.

Some helpful questions may touch upon the kinds of expectations the family held of the subject and the kinds of responsibility he was expected to assume at home. Asking about how affection was shown and how limits were enforced often triggers insights into the emotional tone of the person's home life, and sometimes helps to explain long established behavior patterns.

Educational and Occupational History. The educational and vocational preparation of the individual is detailed in this section, including the dates specific programs were completed, the credentials earned, and the age of the subject at the time of each major achievement. The interviewer also describes the person's military service (i.e., age, rank, conditions of discharge, etc.) and his regular work experience, including the jobs he has held, his successes and failures with the work itself, and his relationships with his fellow workers, superiors, and subordinates. If the individual has retired, his age and the circumstances at the time of retirement, as well as his reactions to retiring, are often highly significant and should be recorded.

Marital and Family History. Since the names, ages, and health of the patient's immediate family members have already been recorded under family health, the intent of this portion of the past development is to explore the most significant relationships this person has experienced from the time of early adulthood to the present. This exploration involves attention both to the details of these bonds as they developed over time and to the impact that they have had on the elderly person and his life. The way in which he has reacted to the birth of a grandchild, the death of a spouse, or the departure of a dear friend or family member to a distant location is always at least as important as the event itself.

Included in this aspect of the older person's development is a description of present and past marriages, with separations, divorces, and the death of spouses noted. The ties that grew as children were born, as they matured and expanded their horizons, and as they left home and married are elicited by careful questioning as well. If the patient has never married and if he has lived with a companion for an extended period of time, then the living arrangements and the nature of this relationship are also considered here.

The interviewer specifies the individual's age at the time an important bond was established, the age of the significant individual, the history and general character of the relationship, and the dates or ages at which major events occurred.

Changes in a relationship brought about by illness, conflict, separations, death, or simply by the normal process of maturation are often especially revealing. Finally, of course, when dealing with an emotion-laden topic such as important relationships, the alert interviewer learns a great deal simply from paying attention to what the subject chooses to discuss.

MAXIMIZING THE USES OF THE COMPREHENSIVE HEALTH HISTORY

Traditionally the process of history taking has focused on the meticulous collection of information about past illnesses, accident, and medical interventions, and it has traditionally ended with the pinpointing of immediate and potential medical problems for further investigation. For the nurse who tends to have prolonged, intimate contact with the older patient, however another equally vital dimension of information is also needed to flush out this data. If the nurse is to fully support the elderly patient's adaptation to the demands of the present and if she is to facilitate his continuing growth, then information regarding the emotional experiences of this individual must also be collected and analyzed.

As the history unfolds, the nurse searches the patient's account, his facial expressions, and his physical responses for evidence of his feelings about these past events. She notes apparently unresolved fears and conflicts, as well as examples of successful adaptation and coping behaviors.

Identifying and Utilizing Coping Patterns

Ordinarily, by the time an individual reaches 65 years of age or more, his patterns of coping with stress (while by no means cast in cement) are identifiable. Thus, when a symptom or an illness presents itself, each elderly person will attempt to handle the threat in his own way, based on his own highly personalized frame of reference.

For example, some people react by worrying about the problem. They are anxious during the day and unable to rest at night. Others deny that a problem exists and go blithely about their business, disregarding appointments, dietary and activity limits, and treatment measures. Some people attack adversity with relish, insisting upon obtaining all the information they can get, following the regimen with ferocious loyalty, and generally mobilizing their internal and external resources to conquer the threat. Still others become angry and resentful or retreat into depression.

Whether an older person employs a variety of responses to stress or whether one response predominates, the nurse who looks for this information in the history can anticipate the patient's reaction to present or future health problems, illness, or disability. She can also evaluate current behaviors and expressions of feeling against the background of the person's past reaction patterns. The insights gained from this process will enable the nurse to treat these responses consciously and thus with the considerate, sympathetic attention each elderly person needs and deserves.

Building on Past Experiences

Utilizing her knowledge of an elderly person's history, the nurse can approach almost any new situation by way of the patient's past experiences. To explain a new procedure, such as establishing an intravenous line in a patient who has never experienced this before, a comparison can be drawn to a similar procedure. "Mrs. Hollings, I am going to start an intravenous feeding in your arm, which will supply the fluids you need until you can take them by mouth again. Starting this feeding is very much like having a blood sample taken from your arm, except that the needle will be secured in the vein and you'll be getting something instead of giving something for a change."

It is not generally reassuring for elderly people to be faced with an innovative approach to some aspect of their lives. A new drug, new experts, or new procedures evoke a burst of apprehension and anxiety at the prospect of having to master new tasks, adjust to unfamiliar patterns, and relate to strangers. Stressing the familiar aspects of any new person, place, or technique or emphasizing continuity establishes a bridge which helps the older person cross

from the known to the unknown more safely and securely. In this way, the patient can bypass many of the ominous chasms of fear and uncertainty that lie in his path when he sets foot in unfamiliar territory.

When introducing oneself to an older person, a nurse might say, "Good morning, Mr. Davis. I'm Mrs. Donahue. I will be continuing the care you've been receiving from Mrs. Smith. I, too, am a registered nurse." Another helpful approach is to ask the patient to make the connection with the familiar. Asking, "Do I remind you of anyone you've known before?" or "Have you ever shared a room before?" helps to tie the past to the present, making it seem more familiar and thus more manageable. Obviously, anticipating a change and taking the time to prepare the individual for it by introductions, a visit to look at a new room, or even rehearsing for a procedure or a situation, are also ways to establish continuity.

In the same way, emphasizing the patient's past experience, and especially his successes, gives the nurse the opportunity to point out the elderly person's competence and durability. For example, if a new drug is to be introduced into a patient's life, the nurse might say, "I see from your record that you're an old hand at taking medications, Mr. Davis. That experience will come in handy because when you go home on Friday, you will be taking this small, but important white tablet, called 'digitalis,' with you. We will be talking about how Dr. K. wants you to take it and what the medicine does so that you'll really understand it before you leave."

Asking an older person to use his previous experience to search for solutions or ways of looking at things which worked for him earlier in his life increases his sense of control and eases his adjustment to a new situation. For example, "Mr. Lee, you mentioned to me once that after your wife's death, you handled the pain of that first year by living 'one day at a time' and by getting very involved in the church choir. Do you think that a similar approach to the next few months, while your hip heals, might be helpful? We even have a singing group here that could surely use a good baritone voice."

Building on the patient's past experiences, the known and the successful from other eras, the nurse can assist the elderly person to allocate and channel his vital energy resources where they are needed the most. He can thus be helped to avoid some of the tremendous energy drain due to the anxiety which tends to surface in unfamiliar situations. His physical and mental efforts are then free to focus more productively on the business of getting better, on continuing adaptation and personal development, and on maintaining contact with his environment and the people in it who matter to him.

STIMULATING THE PROCESS OF LIFE REVIEW

One final, nontraditional use to which the health history can be put involves the need of the aging adult to continue to grow, to adjust to changes and losses, and to find meaning in having lived. Old age is a time when there is still vital developmental work to be done — the work of reviewing one's life, "searching for purpose, reconciliation of relationships and resolution of conflicts and regrets" (Butler, 1974). This process of coming to terms with one's life has been called by Erik Erikson (1950) the stage of "ego identify vs. despair," and the successful resolution of this work prepares the individual to experience "a personal sense of the entire life cycle" and, ultimately, to accept death without fear (Butler, 1974).

Life review is, of course, an ongoing process which extends far beyond the limits and the immediate purposes of the comprehensive health history. Yet history taking constitutes a potent vehicle for beginning and encouraging this vital process. As the older individual works at recounting the milestones in his life, the interviewer's job becomes to elicit important information, to clarify the sequence of events, and to knit the pertinent elements into a coherent, chronological outline.

Simultaneously, the interviewer can seek out submerged, emotional content in these significant events by such comments as, "Let's see then, you must have been 25 when you returned from the war. Was it difficult to step back into

your family life again?" or "Am I correct in thinking that your fifth child was born in 1945, while you were still receiving treatment for tuberculosis? Do you think that that early separation from her for the next two years affected your relationship?" This process is helpful in establishing the accuracy and order of the historical data, as well as in unlocking the memories and feelings which have been tucked away for years but which are too important to have been lost.

Long after the formal history-taking process is over, the nurse can continue to support the aged person as he feels his way back through these memories. She can sustain him through the grief and depression, the resentment, and even the suspicion that these recollections may generate, and she can reflect his gratification and perhaps exhilaration over his contributions and accomplishments.

The nurse can also reassure the older person and his family too that he is not "going crazy" or "becoming senile," and she can dignify the process of reviewing his life by interpreting it as genuine work, as well as an important sign of growth. By legitimizing the elderly person's need to reminisce, it is often possible to actively involve important family members in the remembering process. Visiting meaningful places with his family, and reviewing old photographs and other memorabilia, may help the patient to set and attain some specific, desired goals as he wraps us the "loose ends" of a lifetime. Expanding the review in this way, far beyond the patient's health history, may create an opportunity for self-fulfillment, revived intimacy, and the transmission of an emotional and genealogical legacy of inestimable value to the older person and to those who care about him.

REFERENCES

Balchum, O.J. The aging respiratory system. In Chinn, A.B. (Ed.) Working with Older People, a Guide to Practice. *Clinical Aspects of Aging*, Vol, 4 (Government Publication No. 1459). Rockville, Md.: U.S. Department of Health, Education and Welfare, 1971, pp. 23, 119, 120.

Burnside, I.M. Mental health and the aged. *Nursing and the aged*. New York: McGraw-Hill, 1976, p. 139.

Burnside, I.M. Interviewing the aged. *Psychosocial Nursing Care of the Aged* (2nd ed.). New York: McGraw-Hill, 1980, pp. 5-33.

Butler, R.N. Successful aging and the role of life review. *Journal of the American Geriatrics Society* 22(12):531-534 (1974).

Caird, F.I. and Judge, T.G. *Assessment of the Elderly Patient* (2nd ed.). London: Pittman Medical Publishing Company, 1979, pp. 23-26.

Carbone, V.J. et al. Gastrointestinal tract and liver. In *Current Diagnosis and Treatment*. Los Altos, Calif.: Lange Medical Publications, 1974, pp. 316-390.

Ebersole, P.P. Reminiscing and group psychotherapy with the aged. In Burnside, I.M. (Ed.) *Nursing and the Aged*. New York: McGraw-Hill, 1976, pp. 214-230.

Erikson, E.H. *Childhood and Society.* New York: W.W. Norton, 1950, pp. 228-229, 231.

Kahn, R.L., Zeman, F.D., and Goldfarb, A.I. Attitudes toward illness in the aged. *Geriatrics* 13:246-250 (1958).

Kayne, R.C. (Ed.). *Drugs and the Elderly*. Los Angeles: University of Southern California Press, 1978, pp. 1-7.

McKusick, V.A. *Mendelian Inheritance in Man* (5th ed.). Baltimore: John Hopkins Press, 1978, pp. 206, 323.

Mezey, M. et al. The health history of the aged person. *Journal of Gerontological Nursing* 3(3):47-51 (1977).

Reichel, W. (Ed.). *Clinical Aspects of Aging.* Baltimore: Williams and Wilkins, 1978, pp. 129-132.

Rudin, Rose. Old People Write of Aging. In *Aging: An Album of People Growing Old.* by Shura Saul, New York: John Wiley and Sons, 1974, p. 128.

Spencer, H. and Lender, M. The skeletal system. In Rossman, I. (Ed.) *Clinical Geriatrics* (2nd ed.). Philadelphia: J.B. Lippincott, 1979, pp. 467-468.

Steel, K. Evaluation of the geriatric patient. In Reichel, W. (Ed.) *Clinical Aspects of Aging.* Baltimore: Williams and Wilkins, 1978, pp. 3-12.

Tindall, J.P. Geriatric dermatology. In Chinn, A.B. (Ed.) Working with Older People, a Guide to Practice. *Clinical Aspects of Aging*, Vol. 4 (Government Publication No. 1459). Rockville, Md.: U.S. Department of Health, Education and Welfare, 1971, p. 23.

Wattis, J.P. Alcohol problems in the elderly. *Journal of the American Geriatrics Society* 29(3):131-134 (1981).

16
The General Appearance of the Aging Person

Linda Ellison Jessup

The most chilling cold is not measured on a thermometer but in the human soul.

M.O. Wolanin (1981)

Many external clues — some subtle others striking — signal the gradual move from adulthood to senescence and call forth the awareness that marked changes are similarly occurring beneath the surface of the aging person's skin. Less often perceived or appreciated either by the older individual or by the observer, however, is the remarkable way in which the aging organism spontaneously adapts itself to, and compensates for, a great many of these alterations.

Perhaps the first signs that the observer notices are the obvious changes in hair and skin, although the age of onset of these ectodermal signs varies considerably from person to person. Gray or white hair may, banner-like, herald the first real recognition that a parent, friend, or offspring is "moving on in years." Thinning hair, a receding hairline, or baldness broadcast this same message. Similarly, wrinkling of the skin, although due to a complex mix of physiological and environmental events (such as sun exposure, smoking, or dieting), acts as an intricate road map of sorts. The convoluted topography of the epidermis traces the long distance traveled by the individual, from the smooth horizons of childhood to the weathered path of senescence, scarred and rutted by the trek through life.

In terms of supporting the aging process, these external alterations are extremely useful in that they constitute "psychic stimuli," documenting the physical reality that death, the ultimate destination, lies unavoidably ahead. Thus, by their very presence, graying hair and wrinkles set in motion a great variety of anticipatory responses in the aging person and in those around him, which are means of preparing to deal with the inescapable conclusion of man's finiteness. Anguish, rejection, depression, and despair may constitute a painful part of the individual's reaction to his obvious mortality. However, once the nearness of his own death has been accepted, a compelling urgency to live the remainder of his life with exquisite awareness, to tie up loose ends, and to savor the totality of his personal experience, including death, may also give this bittersweet period tremendous significance.

For the evolving adult himself, the first portent of involution may precede the external signs of aging by many years and be received with vague dismay. This sign, beginning as early as the third decade, is the decline of one's formerly boundless energy resources, which diminish almost imperceptibly at first as the years pass by. Only when the discrepancy between what a person can do and what he used to do becomes marked, does the full impact of this change make itself felt. For individuals who have relished activity for its own sake or who feel seriously limited by their new fatigability, the evaporation of energy is a troubling, frustrating loss indeed.

Gait

The body's unconscious response to the older person's decreasing energy reserves can actually be observed in several aspects of an individual's general appearance. Energy conservation, in fact, constitutes one of the primary characteristics of the aging organism, and its influence is especially notable in the altered motor activity of the elderly person. Gone is the bounding heel-toe gait of youth, the sinuous spring and rollicking bravado of unchecked vitality. Gone are the extravagantly swinging arms, working pendulum-like to propel the exuberant youngster along his endless trajectory.

Instead, as energy wanes, the gait smooths out to a shorter, flatter, more measured step. The older person's arms swing less freely, and are kept slightly flexed and closer to his body. He moves more slowly in general, often starting off initially with a few stiff, jerky steps, which become smoother as the joints limber up and as he reaches his habitual pace and rhythm. In addition, the gait widens laterally, becoming broader based and, thus, more stable.

This steadying aspect of the altered gait again commands the observer's attention since it points to still another primary characteristic of the aging body responding to the many retrogressive changes it is undergoing — that of the development of new ways of protecting itself. Just as the organism adapts to conserve energy, so too it automatically adjusts to protect the elderly person from falling, a hazard which becomes magnified in terms of being more feared, more likely, and more treacherous as the years go by.

Reflexes

Unfortunately, many of the protective features acquired in childhood and middle age disappear at senescence, leaving the aged person increasingly susceptible to trauma. The brisk, sure reflexes of youth slow markedly, muscles waste, and joints stiffen, making it more difficult to regain one's balance quickly or to catch oneself if a misstep occurs. Proprioception and sensorimotor receptors function with less sensitivity, while the maladaptive return of the "parachute reaction" (straightening of the spine and simultaneous extension of the arms to reestablish one's balance), a reflex action often seen in toddlers, also serves to increase the possibility of falling.

At the same time, the elderly person's vision or hearing may decrease, which dims his ability to perceive potential hazards in his path or around him. The generous layer of subcutaneous tissue which padded his frame earlier in life, and protected his strong and resilient long bones from bumps and blows, is thinner now and covered by the easily torn parchment of aging skin. Even the bones themselves are more brittle, especially in inactive older people, predisposing the aging skeleton to fractures.

Posture

The remarkable response to the changes which result in the increasing vulnerability of old age takes several forms. The center of gravity is lowered by means of the wider gait, by a slight degree of flexion of the knees, and by an actual decrease in height, giving the old person added stability and a broader base to compensate for his loss of agility and protective reflexes.

Osteoporotic changes of the vertebral column result in a loss of height by shortening the spine and lead to a gradual ventral curving of the thoracic segment. This kyphosis forces the head to move from its former upright position, from which the gaze in youth was carelessly, optimistically directed up and out, to a more jutting, bowed position, in which the eyes are involuntarily guided downward and outward, toward the ground directly ahead of the individual. Irregularities in the path, which can be disregarded by the high stepping, fast moving younger person who can rely on his fine reflex response to a stumble, are thus more likely to be seen and avoided by the slower moving, broader-based older person whose vision is providentially directed downward.

If, in spite of these adjustments, the aged individual should fall, his posture of flexion — flexed neck, body, arms, and knees — often serves to have him already halfway positioned into a protective ball, like a fighter or an acrobat. His brittle extremities are then splinted against his own bulk, and some of the shock can be absorbed by the more abundant padding of the trunk and hips. On the other hand, if the old person, having lost his balance, has time to initiate the "parachute response," much of the protective advantage of the flexed stance is lost in the straightening of the trunk and the outthrust arms.

The overall appearance of the aging person clearly identifies him as being "old" in the eyes of those around him, people who constitute a potential support system. Interestingly, the combination of certain attributes — smallness, frailness, and hesitance — serves to elicit attention, concern, and often, assistance, regardless of the age of the person manifesting these characteristics. A younger person of either sex may spontaneously yield his seat to an older person. A stranger may take the arm of an elderly individual trying to make his way off a curb and across a street. Thus, these protective social responses, triggered by visible features in the person's general appearance, may also be said to support the aging process. Perhaps instinctively, other people recognize the aging person's rapid fatigability and physical vulnerability; thus, on occasion, these can serve to reduce the risk of certain environmental hazards.

The General Inspection

The physical examination begins the moment the examiner first glimpses the patient, and it continues during the introductions and throughout the taking of the complete health history. The signs of aging and the compensatory responses are noted, including the person's posture, his motor activity (both voluntary and involuntary), and the nature and stability of his gait. His appearance, be it kempt or disheveled, and his facial and physical responses to the examiner are also revealing. Does he seem nervous, in pain, seductive, or fearful? Does he speak clearly in a modulated tone of voice, or does he talk loudly, listen with his head consistently inclined to one side, or become unintelligible? Does he walk gingerly, as if his feet hurt him; does he hide his mouth behind his hand when he speaks or smiles? Does he smell of urine? Can he move with ease — stop, sit, stand, bend over to untie his shoe, and undress himself without difficulty? Does he appear to be well nourished, underweight, or obese? Is he pale, perspiring, or tearful? Is he breathing hard, wheezing, or coughing when he enters the room?

Just as the individual's demeanor and behavior are vital indicators of his status, so too are his surroundings a clue to his social and emotional reality. Are there plants, pictures, cards, or memorabilia present in his room, or is it barren of human caring touches and suggestive of emotional isolation? Does he read mysteries, the Bible, or Thoreau? Does he whittle, solve crossword puzzles, visit with passers-by, write poetry, watch television? Is the bottle of pills on his bedside table medication that he's taking in addition to the drugs that are ordered? Are there boxes of peanut brittle, chocolates or salted nuts on the table of the patient who is obese or in heart failure?

The general inspection is a period of making purposeful, alert observations discreetly, observations which are often especially keen since this elderly individual is as yet an unknown to the examiner. The senses of the examiner are highly receptive and "fresh" at this point in the encounter, thus making possible a sensitivity which can be consciously utilized and developed to capture elusive clues.

Jotting down these initial impressions unobtrusively but immediately is (in the author's experience) an invaluable aid, since these first signs may subside as the patient relaxes and be forgotten, or they may be obscured by more compelling, dramatic findings and the total mass of information gathered. Such impressions must not be lost because they suggest leads to pursue more thoroughly as the examination proceeds; and, not infrequently, these fleeting perceptions prove to be crucial messages, suggesting, augmenting, or clarifying other findings.

Later, in the process of implementing the plan of care, the older person may be encouraged to wear properly fitting, rubber-soled footwear, instead of floppy slippers, and may be taught to use walking aids if these are indicated. Regular exercise, which will decrease the reabsorption of calcium from the bone, and an adequate diet, which will supply all the essential nutrients (including calcium and vitamin D) for both sound bone structure and good health in general, might be discussed as well. "Accident-proofing" his surroundings, in terms of securing torn rug edges, throw rugs, and loose stairboards, as well as improving the lighting in a person's living quarters, for example, may add significantly both to his real security and to his sense of safety.

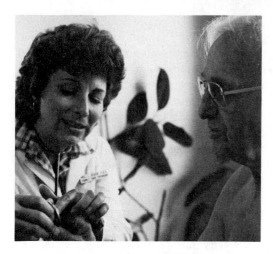

Figure 16-1. The concern and competence displayed by the nurse facilitate the rapid development of a trust relationship. This climate of confidence provides the perfect opportunity for the nurse to educate the individual about himself, emphasizing the ways in which his body continues to adapt and stressing his functional abilities.

Appreciating the marvelous mechanism of his own body, in spite of its shortcomings and retrogressive changes, and being helped to use his ingenuity to compensate even more effectively for the changes he is undergoing helps to nurture confidence in the older adult. His body has not deserted him! He is not falling apart! Such an approach, accompanied by a constant attitude of respect for every aspect of his person, facilitates a feeling of wholeness, preparedness, and even self-admiration, and frees the older person from the tyranny of self-loathing and personal alienation.

REFERENCES

Freehafer, A.A. Injuries to the skeletal system of older persons. In Chinn, A.B. (Ed.) Working with Older People: A Guide to Practice. *Clinical Aspects of Aging.* Rockville, Md.: U.S. Department of Health, Education and Welfare, 1971, pp. 180–193.

Howell, T.H. *Old Age, Some Practical Points in Geriatrics* (3rd ed.). London: H.K. Lewis, 1975.

Morgan, W.L. and Engle, G.L. *The Clinical Approach to the Patient.* Philadelphia: W.B. Saunders, 1969, pp. 80–81.

Rossman, I. Human aging changes. In Burnside, I.M. (Ed.) *Nursing and the Aged.* New York: McGraw-Hill, 1976, pp. 81–91.

Witte, N.S. Why the elderly fall. *American Journal of Nursing* 1950–1952 (November 1979).

Wolanin, M.O. The older adult and drug therapy. Part I. *Geriatric Nursing* **2:**410 (November–December 1981).

17
The Integument

Linda Ellison Jessup

No longer the good fit it once was, the wrinkled skin is public evidence of aging.

Ashley Montagu (1971)

The integument refers to the nails, hair, and skin. Observation of the nails tells us a great deal about the physical and psychosocial status of older patients, their daily living competence, and the kind of nursing care they receive.

NAILS

Normal Changes

The finger- and toenails of aging people often have well-marked, longitudinal striations. The significance of this is not known. The toenails especially tend to thicken (possibly in part due to old fungal infections) and to appear increasingly yellowish in color. Although the fingernails may become markedly curved downward in normal individuals and give the illusion of clubbing, observing the angle of the nail bed carefully corrects mistaken impressions.

Physical Examination

In the inspection and palpation of the nails, the angle of the nail bed must always be noted. An angle of 160°, which when viewed from the side looks like this ⌒, is normal in any adult, while a straightened angle ── of 180° or more ⌐ indicates true clubbing. In early clubbing, the nail base loses its characteristic firmness and feels spongy or fluctuant. Later it becomes visibly swollen.

Clinical Considerations

The color of nails is helpful in detecting the dusky blue tinge of cyanosis, but pallor of the nail bed is an extremely imprecise indicator of anemia.

Clubbing indicates a prolonged lack of systemic oxygen brought about by cardiopulmonary disorders or sudden development of bronchocarcinoma. Its presence is always abnormal, and an explanation of the cause should be sought.

Fungi are often present in the toenails of asymptomatic older people. These conditions rarely cause concern when proper foot care and well-fitting shoes are the rule, unless the elderly person is diabetic. If a fungal infection becomes active, secondary bacterial invasion is an ever-present danger.

HAIR

Normal Changes

As individuals age, changes in the color and the distribution of hair are early and prominent indicators of advancing years. Major notable normal changes are:

- Graying or whitening as pigment cells become less efficient
- Generalized thinning of the hair (including the pubic and axillary areas) progressing to partial or total baldness in some men
- An increase in facial hair in women around the nose and chin, and in the "moustache" area, with a change in the hair from soft to bristly
- A decrease in facial hair in men

Physical Examination

The hair and scalp should be examined with great care; the patient's comb or an applicator should be used to part the hair systematically at

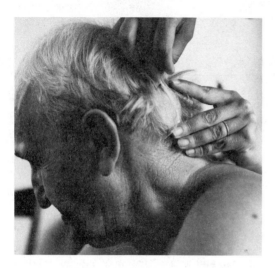

Figure 17-1. The "hands-on" portion of the examination begins with the meticulous exploration of the hair and scalp. This often neglected activity serves to relax and reassure an anxious subject, while uncovering problems from lice to malignant melanomas which might otherwise remain undiscovered.

one-eighth inch intervals so that both can be observed clearly over every aspect of the head. This careful, methodical approach is warranted because important, clearly visible lesions may otherwise remain hidden from view. People often find this portion of the examination to be soothing. It generally reassures and relaxes, and provides an opportunity to discuss the patient's feelings about his appearance. Evaluation of the rest of the body hair comes with examination of the torso, abdomen, and extremities.

Clinical Considerations

The character and color of the hair are noted as the hair is manipulated. In fairly severe cases of hypothyroidism (myxedema) the hair is coarse, dry, and brittle. Fine, soft hair, on the other hand, is typically found in hyperthyroidism, and very oily hair is characteristic of parkinsonism.

Hair loss due to hereditary alopecia is found in about 40% of all men and is characterized by generalized thinning, symmetry, and a posterior march of the anterior hairline. Neurotic hair pulling may result in asymmetrical bald spots. A fungal infection of the scalp or secondary

syphilis produces an irregular, patchy hair loss, resulting in a "moth-eaten" look. A sudden, total loss of hair, termed "toxic" or "symptomatic alopecia," sometimes follows a severe illness or major emotional trauma.

The presence of hair on the feet and legs constitutes a reassuring sign since its existence is good evidence that no significant peripheral vascular disease or ischemic condition is present. The increased production of adrenaline in Cushing's syndrome, however, may result in an excessive growth of hair on the upper lip, chin, and sideburn areas of the face.

The scalp and other hair-covered areas may manifest the loose scaling of seborrhea in people with abnormally oily skin (or with Parkinson's disease), and these same areas may play host to such friendly visitors as lice. More often observable than the shy adult insect are the eggs, or "nits," which tend to be distributed like tiny, tenacious pussy willows on the hair stems, especially in the areas behind the ears, on the crown of the head, and along the occiput.

Localized areas of redness and tenderness, both above and below the hairline, together with thickness and pulsations of the superficial temporal arteries suggest the underdiagnosed, painful, but treatable condition of giant cell arteritis. Randomly scattered sores and scratches on the scalp are sometimes self-inflicted and may have psychological significance.

Sebaceous cysts resulting from the blockage of a sebaceous gland are frequently found on the scalp as smooth, round nodules attached to the skin. Other skin lesions such as ulcerations, raised growths, and pigmented lesions must be carefully examined, meticulously described, and evaluated since skin cancers are common among the elderly; melanomas and basal cell carcinomas, especially, may otherwise go unnoticed until they are quite advanced.

SKIN

Far from being a simple bag-like covering which contains all the paraphernalia that constitutes the human organism, the skin is a remarkably sensitive indicator of emotional and physical conditions. In fact, it has been said that "the skin is the mirror of the mind," a reminder that the complex interrelationship of these two vital components of every human being is reflected externally for the astute to observe.

Decades of interaction between an old person's genetic make up, biochemistry, diet, and emotions on the one hand, and his environment and life experiences on the other, produce a composite of alterations in his integument, making it impossible to single out only those changes due to aging per se. The recognition of the "normal" changes seen in older skin and their differentiation from the abnormal require more vigilance in the older age group than in any other. Because of color changes and the proliferation of benign growths common to aging skin, abnormalities which are readily apparent in the young may not be so obvious in the elderly.

A healthy skin is the single most extensive protection people of any age possess. Under ordinary circumstances, the skin renews and heals itself, serves to regulate body temperature, assists in the process of excretion of body wastes, and acts as an extensive sensory receptor. Clearly, meticulous attention to this marvelous outermost layer commands high priority in care of the aged.

Normal Changes

- The overall picture of the aging integument is one of generalized thinning, but with marked thickening occurring in localized areas.
- Aging skin seems drier up to age 60, then the water content increases somewhat.
- The wrinkled, dry appearance of the skin is not due solely to dehydration, but also to loss of cells, loss of subcutaneous fat which reduces the stability of body temperature regulation, decreased sweat and protective sebum on the skin surface, and a thickening and fragmentation of the elastic fibers in the light-exposed areas ("senile elastosis") resulting in the parchment-like, yellowed appearance of fair-skinned people's facial skin.
- The skin atrophies, leaving little support for the blood vessels, which may result in easy bruising and spontaneous develop-ment of "senile purpura" which are often restricted to the arms and neck.
- Circulation to the skin itself is reduced. Thus, when bruising has occurred, rapid phagocytic activity does not take place, free red cells persist for some time, and the usual progression of color changes in a healing ecchymosis is retarded. Skin breakdown occurs more easily and is restored more slowly.
- Variations in pigmentation are noted with age in light-skinned races. They become paler overall and develop lentigo senilis (so-called liver spots) on the dorsal aspects of the hand and wrist areas, and less often on the face and ankles. These spots have nothing to do with the liver.
- There is a marked increase in the size and number of growths on the skin, most of which are benign such as skin tags and seborrheic keratoses, xanthelasmas, and syringomas, but the potential for malignant growths is, obviously, also greater (Tindall, 1978; Wells, 1978).

Physical Examination

The skin is examined under a strong light by observation and palpation. Daylight or non-fluorescent light is preferable, since fluorescent light tends to mask the red tones of a rash or the rosy undertone of healthy dark skin and to impart a yellowish cast to the skin. All of the body skin should ultimately be surveyed as the examination progresses, i.e., behind the ears, the entire neck, the lips and inside of the mouth, the palms of the hands and the soles of the feet, between the digits, the axillae, and the anal and genital regions. Obviously, examination of the skin must be frequent and ongoing, during bathing, back rubs, foot care, and dressing or undressing of the elderly patient.

Places where sagging and skin folds cause deep creases to form, such as under breasts, pendulous abdomens, or in the groin, constitute areas of special concern. These are warm, dark, moist hideaways — perfect incubators for skin breakdown and for bacterial and fungal growth unless they are inspected frequently, and kept clean and dry.

In aged persons who spend more than a day or two in bed at a time, or who stay in one position much of the time, the pressure areas of the buttocks, sacrum, elbows, knees, and heels should be examined for reddening on a daily basis.

Any lesion should be measured precisely, described in detail, and sketched on the examination record for later comparisons. The nurse must determine and document the following characteristics for a complete description of the lesion. Where is it located? What kind of a lesion is it, in dermatologic terms? What color is it? Is there evidence of increasing size, a change in color, or the development of satellite lesions? What is its shape? Is the border discrete or diffuse, and is it raised? Is there a discharge? Is it attached to the top layer of skin or does it penetrate to deeper layers? Is it painful, erythematous, warmer than the surrounding tissue? Does it have a tendency to bleed easily? If there is a rash, is it generalized or localized? Does it clearly demarcate a clothing, cast, tape, or bandage line?

Clinical Considerations

Itching (pruritus) is perhaps the most common, distressing condition of elderly skin. Most pruritus is a common, poorly understood condition, sometimes called "winter itch," which may be very difficult to relieve. It is aggravated by cold, dry, wintry weather, by exposure to sun and wind, by frequent bathing, and by rough fabrics or wool. Pruritus is a vague symptom, and often the only signs are scratch marks on the skin surface. Dryness and scaliness, which appear as an ashy gray color in dark skin, may also be obvious.

Sometimes generalized itching seems to have psychogenic origins. Certainly any pruritus is aggravated by emotional upset and tension. The examiner should pursue the most visible possible causes and attempt to rule out:

- scabies — a history of intense itching at night, along with telltale vesicles and pustules in irregular "runs" or burrows, 2-3 mm long, along the sides of fingers, on the heels of the hands, on the wrists, and around the midriff;

- pediculosis — infestation of any hair-covered area of the body, including eyebrows and lashes, best identified by a distribution of white "nits" which adhere tightly to the hair stem and look like minature pussy willows;
- intertrigo — confined to the body folds, especially of obese people; the area is erythematous, superficially denuded, soggy, and often fissured; there may be a history of seborrheic dermatitis, and an underlying diabetic condition should be ruled out.

Other general medical conditions which may be the cause of persistent itching are arteriosclerosis, diabetes mellitus, uremia, internal neoplasms, polycythemia, hepatic and biliary cirrhosis, and even thyrotoxicosis. Examination for these should be pursued when pruritus stubbornly persists in spite of improved atmospheric and systemic hydration, lubricating ointments, reduced bathing with soap and hot water, and other nursing measures.

Common dermatoses are another frequent cause of pruritus. Whether or not an allergic reaction is a new development, older people characteristically respond differently from younger patients. For example, discoid or nummular eczema is more common in the elderly than is flexural eczema, and sometimes small patches of eczema suddenly seem to explode, becoming generalized to the whole face, an extremity, or the torso. The cause of this eruption may be emotional stress or a topical medication for the condition to which the patient has suddenly become allergic. In fact, contact dermatitis is more often caused by topical medicines in older people than by occupational or natural agents. For some allergens, such as poison ivy, sensitivity actually appears to decrease with age.

When there is itching and swelling around the thin, delicate tissue of the eye orbits, the nurse should immediately consider the possibility of a contact dermatitis. This sensitive tissue often serves as an early indicator of an impending contact reaction.

Systemic drug reactions occur in people of any age, and although such authorities as

Leopold (1965) maintain that injections and orally administered medications are less often dermatitis producing than are epidural applications, he also warns that any drug can cause a rash even after years of trouble-free use. The large number of medications used by the elderly and the danger of cross-sensitization with chemicals in medicines and other substances result in frequent systemic drug reactions in older people (Brady, 1978; Leopold, 1965; Lofholm, 1978). Rashes on dark skin may be very difficult to see, so the examiner must sometimes rely more on the sense of touch to detect hidden skin changes (Rubin, 1979).

Neoplasms

Neoplasms, literally "new growths," seem to proliferate on the skin of the aging individual. There is a highly significant correlation between aging and long years of exposure to radiation in the development of both benign and malignant lesions. Caucasians have the highest incidence of skin changes. Persistent exposure to sunlight increases the incidence of new growth formations.

Seborrheic keratoses are the most common tumors which worry the elderly, although they are completely harmless and are easily removed for cosmetic reasons. These lesions occur primarily on the trunk and less often on the face or scalp. They are greasy, wart-like or flat growths which range in color from a very dark brown to a murky yellow. Little blackheads may be observed within the lesions. They tend to grow in areas irritated by belts or bras and are sometimes mistaken for malignant melanomas.

Skin tags, or papillomas, are little outpatchings of skin which typically occur on the sides of the neck, the cheeks, and under the arms. They seem to develop more commonly in women and sometimes appear in crops. While removal is a minor undertaking, they are best left alone unless they are disfiguring.

Sebaceous hyperplasia is an acne found in elderly males, predominating around the orbits and developing into giant sized, shiny, waxy yellow tumors. These lesions result from a sudden increase in the activity of the cutaneous glands and often measure 10–12 mm in diameter.

Unlike the acne of puberty, the comedones (blackheads) are not inflammatory. Ironically, it is a good sign if many of these lesions develop at once, since the skin cancers which they may resemble (basal cell carcinomas) do not appear in groups. They can be surgically removed if they become unsightly.

Basal cell carcinoma is the most common and least malignant form of skin cancer. These lesions occur on the light-exposed skin of fair-skinned people. They rarely metastasize but should be completely removed. Follow-up is necessary because of the likelihood of recurrence. These tumors are nodular, or nodular-ulcerative, glossy lesions with raised, pearly borders across which blood vessels can be seen to extend. They are painless, bleed easily, and are usually skin colored, but there are brown- or black-pigmented varieties which may be confused with seborrheic keratoses or melanomas.

Actinic (solar) keratoses are premalignant lesions which may develop into squamous cell carcinomas unless they are removed. Actinic keratoses often come in groups, masquerading as reddish patches of dry or rough skin with a silver-white adherent scale. They may also appear light gray or brown, and are generally less than a centimeter in diameter. Three clues which should alert the nurse examiner as to their true nature are: (1) the age and skin color of the patient, (2) their propensity for sun-exposed areas, and (3) their persistence over a long period of time.

Squamous cell carcinoma occurs less frequently but is a more menacing lesion because it has the potential to metastasize. It is a flesh-colored lesion, nodular and wart-like in appearance, which may ulcerate painlessly. As it increases in size, the border becomes elevated, with a rolled appearance, and the center becomes depressed. If an imaginary line were drawn from the patient's ear lobe to the corner of his mouth, it would be found that about two-thirds of all skin cancers occurring above that line would be of the basal cell type, whereas about two-thirds of the skin cancers developing below that line would be of the squamous cell type. The lower lip is a particularly troublesome spot for squamous cell carcinoma because of the excellent blood supply (Tindall, 1978).

Malignant melanoma is the most dreaded of the skin cancers because of its tendency to metastasize rapidly. The majority of melanomas arise from preexisting lesions on the feet, legs, hands, back, and trunk. They are flat or slightly raised, brown, blue, or black in color, and may be intermingled with other colors (red, brown, or white). The margin is irregular with a notched border. Fortunately, melanomas occur less often in older people than squamous or basal cell carcinomas, but because they are so dangerous, they must be sought with vigilance and treated immediately.

Decubitus Ulcers

Decubiti are a special type of ulcer caused by impairment of the blood supply and by inadequate tissue nutrition due to prolonged pressure over prominent bony areas. Pressure sores are much more easily prevented than cured, and their prevention constitutes a never-ending challenge to nursing care. The skin overlying the sacrum and hips is most often involved, but decubiti also occur on the occiput, ears, elbows, heels, and ankles. Debilitated, paralyzed, bedfast, or listless older patients are at great risk. Any reddening or abrasion of the skin over a bony prominence must be noted and considered an immediate problem. Prevention of skin breakdown requires good nutrition and hydration, relief of pressure, frequent changes of position, stimulation of circulation by increased activity and massage, and well-lubricated, clean, dry skin (see Chapters 33 and 37).

Herpes Zoster ("Shingles")

A reactivation of an old varicella (chickenpox) virus infection is the cause of this cruel affliction of the elderly. It typically involves one or more sensory nerve pathways. Intensely painful vesicles on erythematous bases occur unilaterally along the path of the nerve. The most common distributions occur on the trunk and the face, although the most dreaded site involves the ophthalmic branch of the trigeminal nerve, with almost certain involvement of the cornea. Local lymph glands may be tender and swollen.

Following the acute phase of the infection, postherpetic pain may persist as an agonizing kind of "phantom" pain for months or years, long after the lesions have disappeared. Elderly persons over age 70 and those with underlying leukemia, lymphoma, or myeloma are most vulnerable.

REFERENCES

Brady, E.S. Drugs and the elderly. In Kayne, R.C. (Ed.) *Drugs and the Elderly.* Los Angeles: University of Southern California Press, 1978, pp. 1-7.

Leopold. Allergy. In Freeman, J.T. (Ed.) *Clinical Features of the Older Patient.* Springfield, Ill.: Charles C. Thomas, 1965, pp. 414-419.

Lofholm, P. Self-medication by the elderly. In Kayne, R.C. (Ed.) *Drugs and the Elderly.* Los Angeles: University of Southern California Press, 1978, pp. 8-28.

Montagu, A. *Touching: The Human Significance of the Skin.* New York: Columbia University Press, 1971, pp. 5-7, 102-103.

Rubin, B.A. Black skin. *RN* 42(3):31-35 (1979).

Russell, D. Skin diseases. In Pearson, L.J. and Kotthoff, M.E. (Eds.) *Geriatric Clinical Protocols.* Philadelphia: J.B. Lippincott, 1979, pp. 325-378.

Tindall, J.P. Geriatric dermatology. In Reichel, W. (Ed.) *Clinical Aspects of Aging.* Baltimore: Williams and Wilkins, 1978, pp. 331-356.

Wells, T.J. In geriatric patients that "minor" skin problem could be trouble. *RN* 41(7):41-46 (1978).

18
The Head and Neck

Linda Ellison Jessup

May you demonstrate old age is not a defeat but a victory.

Ethel Percy Andrus

The face of a healthy, elderly person is generally bright, expressive, and alert, with moderately symmetrical features. The eyes and head tend to turn spontaneously, albeit perhaps somewhat slowly, toward activity, light, and sound. Facial expression is a sensitive reflection of mood and feelings in any person. Interest and friendliness as well as pain and withdrawal may be written in the lines of the face and the lift of the head. In an older person, the somewhat forward thrust position of the cranium angling slightly downward is due to the bowing of the thoracic vertebral column that occurs with aging.

Abnormal facies which characterize important disorders in older people, are the "moon" face and excessive facial hair of Cushing's syndrome, the enlarged and coarsened features of acromegaly, or the flat, seemingly emotionless expression of parkinsonism. The periorbital edema of allergy, the nonpitting edema of myxedema, and the pitting edema of nephrotic syndrome are critical observations, as are any asymmetries of a single feature and the paralysis or drooping of one side of the face.

The examination of the head and face of the older patient does not differ from that of any mature individual. (*Note:* Only when the examination process, technique, or observation merits special attention in its application specifically to the elderly person, will it be discussed under "Examination" in this chapter. The reader is encouraged to consult a general guide for the details and sequence of the complete physical examination for "normal" adults.)

While carefully inspecting the head and gently palpating the entire skull, the nurse should keep in mind that old injuries to the cranium resulting in unconsciousness or an amnesic episode may have been forgotten by, or unknown to, the patient. Questioning the origins of scars or lumps and noting these important evidences of damage may be the only way significant past or recent trauma will come to light.

A fine, side-to-side or up-and-down resting tremor of the head and arrhythmic deviation laterally of the fingers may indicate a condition known variously as "essential," "familial," or "senile" tremor. The tremor intensifies with deliberate movement such as using a spoon or cup, and although it is a benign and very slowly progressive disorder, the social embarrassment an individual suffers because of spills and poor fine motor control may indeed be crippling (Locke, 1971).

THE EYES

The eye is so well constructed that it can be expected to function efficiently throughout and even beyond the lifetime of its owner (which is why eye banks are possible). It is a cheering fact that many older individuals have fair to excellent vision, and in studies which have been conducted, over half the eyes examined at autopsy in elderly people revealed normal findings (Kornzweig, 1979).

Still, a variety of changes in the eyes occur regularly with the advance of years, although the age at which alterations appear varies widely from person to person. The ability to see is so important for the pursuit of well-being and pleasure throughout life that regular examination is mandatory.

Normal Changes

Normal changes in the eye involve increasing sclerosis of the ciliary muscles, making them less able to expand or contract as vigorously as before, decreasing the size of the pupillary aperture, increasing the amount of lens opacity, and decreasing the elasticity of the lens making it less able to become convex enough to clearly focus the image of near objects on the retina (presbyopia). Gradual corneal degeneration, gradual retinal sclerosis, and retinal atrophy, probably brought about by vascular changes, particularly arteriosclerosis, are common. Other frequent findings are a thin grayish or white ring encircling the inner edge of the corneal border (the arcus senilis), increased droopiness of the eyelids due to the loss of elasticity of the skin plus the pull of gravity, and decreased tear production by the lacrimal gland which contributes to drier and less lustrous eyes (Kasper, 1978). Many of these modifications tend to decrease the amount of light that the pupil admits at the very time when more light is required to compensate for the clouding of the lens, and this may seriously reduce night vision.

Physical Examination

Visual acuity tests the person's ability to perceive detail. Though the Snellen test is helpful, in old age determining whether the individual can see what he wishes to see and needs to see is of utmost concern. Can he perceive the examiner's facial expression (happy, sad, angry, tongue out) from 10 feet or 2 feet away? Can he read newsprint or headlines? Is he able to pursue pleasurable and necessary activities, such as sewing, tying a fishing fly, driving a car, using a stove, or regulating a thermostat? What about his color vision? Can he correctly perceive street light signals, identify his belongings, or enjoy the kind of art he prefers?

Peripheral vision deficits such as a residual hemianopia must be taken into consideration, especially if the person drives or lives alone. The selection of visual tests depends upon the individual's life-style. The results should be discussed, with advice about how to avoid accidents and suggestions for fully using the vision that is retained.

The extraocular muscles of most elderly people display normal parallel eye movements to all six cardinal fields of gaze. However, many individuals with Parkinson's disease or severe brain dysfunction, as well as a few normal individuals, may be unable to show an upward conjugate motion. Patients who do not comprehend the examiner's instructions will frequently follow the glow of a penlight or the position of the examiner herself, thus inadvertently demonstrating the state of the extraocular muscles. When the subject is encouraged to gaze downward, "lid lag" (a rim of sclera glimpsed between the upper lid and the iris), a sign of hyperthyroidism, and the coordination of the inferior muscles are noted.

The eyelids in older people often manifest the irritating condition of ectropion (outward rotation of the lower lid margin) and entropion (turning inward of the lower lid). Both problems produce considerable tearing and discomfort, although the mechanism for each differs. In the former, the punctum is turned outward, and the eye no longer drains properly; in the latter, the movement of the lashes against the sensitive cornea and bulbar conjunctiva abrades them. Both conditions are surgically correctable.

Since the conjunctiva becomes thinner and more fragile in old age, the nurse examiner will notice that subconjunctival hemorrhages occur rather frequently. The cause is often unknown but may be the result of a sneeze, cough, or other unexceptional event. Conjunctivitis may develop "silently" in elderly individuals and continue unnoticed because of diminished pain sensation. Because of less efficient tear production, the increasingly delicate conjunctiva is more vulnerable to cold, wind, and dust. This susceptibility is heightened by conditions which result in incomplete lid closure. The development of a pterygium, a wedge-shaped thickening of the bulbar conjunctiva, which usually grows from the nasal side of the eye toward the cornea, is of no concern unless it actually encroaches upon the pupil and thus obstructs vision.

The cornea may appear somewhat less translucent, even smoky, in the older patient. Oblique illumination or fluorescein stain assists the examiner in identifying corneal abrasions or ulcers. These lesions are not uncommon in this population and are usually due to trichiasis.

Corneal scars, seen as superficial grayish-white opacities, result from old injuries and should not be confused with the deeper opacity of a cataract which is visible only through the pupil.

Oblique illumination of the anterior chamber casts a characteristic, crescent-shaped shadow on the opposite side of the iris if this space is abnormally shallow. A shallow anterior chamber predisposes the eye to glaucoma. This finding and any previous history of glaucoma or episodes of hazy vision contraindicate the use of mydriatics and necessitate an ophthalmological consultation. The pigmentation of the iris often becomes markedly irregular. Areas of normal coloration are replaced by pale brownish patches.

The elderly routinely manifest smaller pupils. Often the margins are slightly irregular. The pupils should be equal in size and should constrict visibly (if not quite as quickly or vigorously as in younger adults) to direct and consensual stimulation as well as to accommodation.

Ophthalmoscopic Examination

The clarity of the lens determines to a large degree whether or not the internal portion of the eye can be visualized by the examiner. Any opacity situated near the center of the lens will impair the patient's vision, and obviously if the individual has difficulty seeing out, the examiner may have trouble seeing in. The red reflex will be interrupted by even a tiny cataract, corneal scar, or vitreous opacity casting a dark shadow on the corresponding portion of the reflection, while a dense cataract or vitreous hemorrhage will eliminate the red reflex completely.

If the examiner experiences difficulty in visualizing the inner eye, asking the subject to look through a pinhole punched through a piece of cardboard can be useful. If the elderly person's vision is improved to near normal by this technique, then the visual pathway all the way to the retina is intact and the examiner can rest assured that there are no significant obstructions in the media (Caird and Judge, 1979).

The normal appearance of the optic disk does not change significantly in the elderly. Marked whiteness of the whole disk, with an absence of the tiny disk vessels from at least a segment, suggests optic atrophy — especially if comparison with the other disk shows that they differ in appearance. Pallor with cupping of the temporal side of the disk is characteristic of glaucoma. The pallor appears as the condition increases in severity.

Papilledema is a phenomenon which is rarely observed in the aged, probably because of the reduction in mass of brain tissue. Space-occupying lesions thus have more room to expand before intercranial pressure increases significantly to produce the hyperemic disk with blurry margins and numerous tortuous capillaries typical of papilledema. Thus, the absence of these signs does not eliminate the possibility of serious hypertension or an expanding lesion.

"Copper" and "silver" wiring and increased tortuosity of the retinal vessels occur so commonly in the elderly that they are considered unremarkable. Nicking of the veins at arteriovenous crossings, retinal hemorrhages, and "cotton-wool" exudates, however, may all indicate a harmful degree of hypertensive disease.

The area of the macula is always carefully scanned for the exudates, microaneurysms, and occasional small hemorrhages of diabetes. Deposits of black pigment, whether few or many, are worthy of note since their presence may signify macular degeneration with resulting loss of vision.

Clinical Considerations

Presbyopia, farsightedness caused by a loss of elasticity of the lens, is frequently noted first in middle age, with the disconcerting discovery that the print in the telephone book is too fine to see and the "arms aren't long enough" anymore to allow one's eyes to focus clearly on certain reading materials. This condition is usually refrangible.

A cataract (of which there are many classifications) involves a partial or total loss of transparency in any part of the crystalline lens. It is the leading cause of blindness in the United States and affects, to some degree, 90% of the people over 70 years of age (Hirschman, 1977). Cataracts develop gradually, obstructing vision only when they develop in the center of the lens. The most promising treatment is the surgical implantation of an artificial lens to replace the natural one. Traditional correction with glasses, following surgical removal of one or both lenses, and the use of contact lenses have many adaptational disadvantages not shared by the quick, permanent procedure of lens implantation. It must be pointed out that this surgery is still being investigated in terms of duration of success.

Senile macular degeneration is usually bilateral and probably results from vascular changes in the retina. The macula constitutes the center of retinal vision for the perception of fine detail. Central blindness is a relatively benign condition which can be compensated for by the use of magnifying spectacles or a magnifying glass for reading and close work.

Degeneration of the mid- and far periphery of the macula is a more serious loss, resulting in tunnel vision. This condition produces a dangerous loss of side vision and may be so severe as to make it impossible for the subject to see the eyes or ears of the examiner while gazing at the nose. Such restricted vision is irritating and creates a dangerous hazard especially in traffic.

Glaucoma takes many forms, all of which involve a pathological elevation of the intraocular pressure due to some obstruction of the anterior chamber angle. If the disease is not treated early and adequately, damage to the retina or optic nerve will result in irreversible blindness. Acute glaucoma is caused by a sudden blockage of the anterior angle, creating excruciating pain, a perception of halos or rainbows around lights, and vomiting which may mislead staff into focusing on the gastrointestinal symptoms. The pupil is dilated and forced open by the pressure. The globe is hard, the eye is reddened by ciliary injection, and the cornea appears steamy. This condition constitutes an ocular emergency.

Chronic glaucoma, of both the open- and the closed-angle types, is more insidious and thus more likely to be overlooked. Open-angle glaucoma results from a defect in the outflow of aqueous humor, progressing gradually without dramatically high intraocular pressures.

The patient may suffer from vague headaches and continually wipe his glasses in an effort to clarify his "smeared" vision. He may seek frequent refractions or suffer from tearing of the involved eye(s).

Closed-angle glaucoma is characterized by intermittent attacks of high pressure, lasting a short time and resolving spontaneously. Unless the condition is identified and treated, adhesions develop with each episode, gradually obliterating the angle. Since the intraocular pressure fluctuates with this type of chronic glaucoma and the pressure builds gradually with open-angle glaucoma, repeated routine tonometry readings are the best method for identifying victims before irreversible damage results.

Additional Considerations

The important facts to ascertain about any symptom involving the eye are the duration of the problem, whether it developed suddenly or gradually, and whether it affects one or both eyes. Any rapid partial or complete loss of sight is considered an emergency. Occlusion of the major retinal vessels most often produces sudden blindness.

In the elderly, eyes should be examined and tonometry performed at yearly intervals. A change of lenses may be required as often as every 3-5 years. Visual changes which occur more rapidly than this require evaluation by specialists. Very heavy pipe or cigarette smokers sometimes experience failing vision which clears up when smoking is reduced. This condition is referred to as "tobacco amblyopia."

Since sight may diminish so gradually that its loss is hardly noticed, and since the activities of the elderly may become so narrow and routine that they come to rely on their eyes less and less, an accident or withdrawal from the world beyond structured and familiar living quarters may be the first clue of serious visual deterioration.

THE EARS

Hearing and equilibrium are both considered in the evaluation of the ears. The external and middle portions of the ear function strictly to conduct vibrations to the inner ear; the inner ear contains some structures which serve to transmit these impulses to the acoustic nerve and other structures which help to maintain balance, coordinate body movements, and provide awareness of the position of the body in space.

Happily, most people retain auditory function adequate for hearing and good communication purposes throughout their lives. Yet most, if not all, elderly people experience some diminution in hearing. The loss may be slight and at times even unnoticed by the person himself. Because hearing loss occurs so commonly in the later years, difficulty in hearing or deafness is often accepted by professionals and by older people as an inevitable part of the aging process. This attitude frequently prevents the discovery of remediable problems, and contributes to the tragic sensory and social isolation of elderly individuals. The ears of an older person should be examined and hearing evaluated at regular 1-3 year intervals, unless there are complaints and problems.

Normal Changes

- Atrophic or sclerotic changes in the tympanic membrane are common in the elderly, resulting in a somewhat dull, retracted, whitish or gray appearance. These changes do not seem to cause any appreciable loss of hearing.
- A variety of degenerative changes in the cochlea and neurons of the higher auditory pathways constitute the primary cause of hearing loss due to the aging process. The most important condition resulting from deterioration of these structures is presbycusis, a bilateral, progressive, sensorineural loss which begins in middle age. Typically, the ability to hear high frequency sounds is affected first, so that whispers, certain consonants, and the sibilants become unintelligible. Middle range frequency reception, containing most of the sounds of speech, may go next, and eventually low frequencies may be lost.

Physical Examination

The pinna of the elderly adult plays host to some lesions which are not encountered in a young person. Basal cell and squamous cell carcinomas may be encountered on the pinna, although the more dangerous squamous cell type is most commonly found in this location. Any small, crusted, ulcerated, or indurated lesion which does not heal promptly should be biopsied. The small, chronic, and painful nodule of chondrodermatitis helicis, found primarily in men and located most often in the helix of the right ear, should also be biopsied to distinguish it from cancerous lesions. Tophi (deposits of uric acid) present as hard nodules on the rim of the helix or antihelix of a person with gout (Bates, 1974).

When cerumen obscures the view of the posterior portion of the external canal and the tympanic membrane, it must, of course, be removed to permit visualization. Impacted cerumen in an elderly patient usually contains a large amount of keratin and is difficult to soften adequately. Evacuating cerumen with a curette and then irrigating the canal with a lukewarm hypertonic solution of saline are usually effective (as long as the tympanic membrane is intact). The external canal should always be dried well after irrigation. The manipulation of the ear during the cleansing process generally causes the walls of the canal and the membrane to appear reddened temporarily.

Any accumulation of cerumen which completely occludes the ear canal will produce a significant conductive hearing loss, so that accurate hearing evaluation is impossible until the cerumen has been removed. This simple procedure sometimes instantaneously restores a gratifying degree of hearing to a patient who may have considered himself "deaf" or "hard-of-hearing" for years.

Testing for auditory acuity must be performed in a quiet setting and involves the use of the examiner's voice and three frequencies of tuning forks, 512, 1024, and 2048 Hz. To test for spoken voice perception, the examiner stands slightly behind the patient and speaks in a normal voice while occluding the opposite ear canal, asking the patient to respond to questions or to repeat a series of words. If the subject experiences difficulty with either or both ears, the test should be repeated facing him and within visual distance, to determine his spontaneous willingness and ability to "lip-read."

The Weber test is used to indicate whether the hearing sensitivity is the same or different in both ears. When a conductive loss exists, but sensorineural function remains, the patient perceives the tone in his "bad" ear. Older people may become bewildered and give a false response unless they understand that such a result is possible. If sensorineural function is lacking in one ear, the tone can only be perceived in the "good" ear. The Weber test alone does not indicate whether a hearing deficit is conductive or sensorineural, it only indicates whether a discrepancy exists between the two ears.

The Rinne test, given in conjunction with the Weber test, helps to clarify the clinical picture by demonstrating the ratio between a bone-conducted tone and an air-conducted tone for each ear. In a normal ear, the ratio of air conduction to bone conduction is 2:1 (a "positive" Rinne). A "negative" Rinne results when bone conduction is greater than air conduction.

An audiological workup is indicated whenever a hearing loss, tinnitus, or pain of unknown etiology exists. The correction provided by a hearing aid and the functioning of the instrument itself must be checked periodically and reevaluated if the patient is to obtain maximum benefit from his prosthesis.

Clinical Considerations

Many conductive hearing losses are correctable since they may involve such conditions as the occlusion of the ear canal by cerumen, edema, or growths; perforations of the tympanic membrane; serum or pus in the middle ear; or fixation of the middle ear bones. A purely conductive loss is always only a partial loss since the auditory nerve is undamaged; thus the individual can still hear if sound reaches the inner ear.

Sensorineural losses are nearly always irreversible. Partial sensorineural losses tend to affect certain frequencies, leaving transmission of some frequencies intact. This kind of a deficit, found in occupational deafness or presbycusis, distorts sounds because only parts of a whole complex are transmitted. Nevertheless, if enough midfrequency reception remains, amplification may assist in comprehending speech even where sensorineural loss is involved.

Most hearing losses are "mixed losses," especially in older adults who have histories of infection with residual scarring, ototoxic medications, occupational noise, and degenerative changes due to aging. Otosclerosis, which causes fixation of the stapes in the oval window, is generally a disease of youth and results in a conductive disorder. If untreated, it may progress later to involve the cochlea, thus adding a sensorineural component which may result in total deafness.

Systemic problems also affect an older person's hearing. Diabetes mellitus often produces a gradual sensorineural loss similar to that of presbycusis. High blood pressure may induce or increase tinnitus. Ototoxic drugs, such as large amounts of aspirin or aspirin compounds, quinine, some diuretics, and aminoglycosides, have the potential to damage the auditory nerve or the vestibular system. The symptoms and prognosis of ototoxicity vary considerably, depending upon the specific drug, the quantity taken, and the duration of consumption. An older person's hearing may also deteriorate if there is frequent exposure to a great deal of noise, emotional upset, or smoking, or if he develops a cardiovascular disorder.

Vestibular involvement, such as Meniere's disease, is manifested by nystagmus, nausea, and vomiting. These occur in response to intermittent attacks of severe vertigo which may cause falling. Initially there is a unilateral fluctuating hearing loss for low frequency sounds. It is gradually progressive and often accompanied by a low pitched tinnitus.

The elderly often complain of "itchy ears" and may traumatize the epithelium of the external canal and tympanic membrane by attempting to scratch with hair pins or other objects. The itching is often due to the reduced lubrication of the epithelium by the sebaceous and cerumen-producing glands, resulting in a white, flaky wax. If no perforations are present, it may be relieved by the application of a little lubricating oil. Chronic external otitis, due to a bacterial or fungal infection or to a chronic dermatitis, may also cause pruritus. These conditions may be differentiated by noting the reddening and thickening of the epithelium and sometimes by the presence of an aural discharge.

Upper respiratory infections and allergies can produce acute or chronic otitis media in the elderly, with or without eustachian tube dysfunction and a temporary hearing loss. Any sudden loss of hearing is considered an auditory emergency, and any aural discharge or increase in granulation tissue in the external auditory canal requires immediate medical attention.

Additional Considerations

Frequently, hearing loss encountered in testing older persons appears to be quite disabling, but it may not always be accompanied by complaints of deafness or perceived as a limitation to communication. Conversely, other individuals may complain bitterly of being "deaf" and, by their behavior, demonstrate a retreat from the attempts of others to communicate with them, when audiological profiles indicate only a mild to moderate loss.

The nurse must assess the elderly individual's hearing in a context of psychosocial abilities and motivation, determining whether voices are heard but word discrimination is difficult (a sensorineural component), whether hearing improves in a noisy environment (conductive component), or whether it becomes worse in the presence of background noise (sensorineural component). It is also helpful to determine whether the person has difficulty talking to individuals (moderate to severe loss or decreased speech discrimination) or whether the difficulty occurs primarily in a group situation (a sensorineural loss or asymmetrical impairment). Is hearing on the telephone difficult because of reduced speech discrimination (sensorineural) or is it improved, especially with amplification? How much volume is needed to listen to a radio or TV (conductive)?

These details provide the basis for seeking further consultation and for maximizing the potential hearing of older individuals (Farrell, 1979).

THE NOSE

Normal Changes

- The sense of smell may diminish with age, a subtle change with some important implications (see Chapter 6 for further discussion).
- As the subcutaneous tissue, which tends to round and soften the facial features, begins to thin and sag, the features of the aging face appear more prominent and produce the angular, craggy look that photographers and artists seek to capture. The nose, which seems to protrude more sharply, may manifest bumps and deviations hitherto unnoticed. Some degree of septal deviation is common in adults, but most septal displacements do not completely obstruct either nasal passage.

Physical Examination

The patency of each naris is checked by closing the opposite side with a fingertip while the patient inhales with his mouth closed. Perforations of the septum, lesions, masses, and polyps are best detected by gently pushing up the tip of the nose with one thumb while occluding one naris with a penlight. When looking through the open naris, lesions on the septum will be transilluminated and light will shine through any perforations.

The olfactory nerve (cranial nerve I) is tested by obscuring the vision or utilizing the test substances in a manner so that the contents cannot be visualized. Test first with subtle, natural aromas such as flowers, orange peel, banana, fish, coffee, or onion, and then with the more pungent odors of perfume, alcohol, or ammonia.

Clinical Considerations

Nosebleeds may be spontaneous, minor events in the elderly, but they may also be insidious sources of blood loss and a life threatening condition. Hypertension, a dry mucosa, hot weather, or capillary fragility due to a vitamin C deficiency may serve as predisposing factors for nosebleeds. Nosebleeds usually originate in Kiesselbach's plexus, a vascular network in the anterior septum, and are usually precipitated by minor trauma such as picking at the nose or a blow. Those originating in this area are usually easy to stop with pressure to the area and the application of cold compresses. However, if this small amount of blood loss is a frequent occurrence, such as in the neurotic individual who persistently picks at his nose, the total blood loss may be significant enough to result in anemia.

More threatening is the sudden, profuse hemorrhage from the posterior portion of the nose. Vessels in this region are large and belong to the external carotid artery system. In the older individual with rigid, arteriosclerotic vessels (especially the hypertensive patient), a vessel occasionally ruptures, inundating the nose and throat with blood. The patient should be positioned upright if possible, leaning slightly forward, and encouraged to avoid swallowing blood, which will irritate the stomach and cause vomiting. This is a terrifying situation and a true emergency. The patient must be taken to a location where the posterior portion of the nose can be packed properly, suction and oxygen are available, and replacement blood can be given if necessary.

Excessive dryness of the nasal mucosa is a frequent complaint of the elderly. Since much of the ability to warm and moisturize inspired air has been lost, irritating crusts form on the dry mucosa; breathing through the nose becomes uncomfortable, and mouth breathing (with all its detrimental effects) may result. The older person may pick his nose to get relief, thus traumatizing the tissue further. Increasing the environmental humidity and keeping the nasal mucosa lubricated often provide considerable relief from this condition.

THE MOUTH AND THROAT

The mouth serves varied and vital functions throughout life, most of which are taken for granted until a problem draws attention to this complex structure. Respiration, nutrition, hydration, the senses of taste and texture, and effective communication all depend to a large degree upon the health and proper operation of the mouth and throat. The mouth usually remains structurally and functionally sound for a lifetime, but few individuals reach their seventh decade with all 32 teeth intact.

Much of the knowledge we now possess about mouth care and prevention of oral problems, along with advances in modern dentistry, has come too late to benefit our current elderly population. Still, yearly examination, meticulous oral hygiene, dental care, proper fluid intake, and a well-balanced diet are essential measures to preserve the remaining structural integrity and useful function of the teeth and mouth, and ultimately, of the entire body.

Normal Changes

The mouth is one of the most sensitive areas of the body and is almost constantly in use. Many age-related changes are visible in this "gateway to the body." These changes are strongly influenced by chronic illness, past dental health, and familial factors. In general, the following changes occur (Elfenbaum, 1971):

- Some vertical wrinkling of the perioral skin, due to a loss of elasticity, resulting in the "purse string" appearance of the mouth
- Wearing down of the tooth surfaces due to long use
- Hardening of the teeth due to increased calcification and a loss of moisture, and at times the breaking off of cusps
- Yellowing from absorption of fluorides in food and stained cracks in the enamel of old teeth
- The reabsorption of gum tissue around the base of the teeth, due to a loss of moisture, fat, and elasticity in this soft tissue
- A thinning and decreased vascularization of the buccal mucosa, imparting a "varnished" sheen to the surface of this tissue

- A progressive decrease in the number of taste buds, particularly on the sides of the tongue
- The appearance of varicosities on the ventral surface of the tongue
- A decrease in the secretion of saliva, as the epithelial lining of the mucous glands degenerates, and secretion of a more mucoid, thicker consistency of saliva
- A deficiency of ptyalin, the enzyme in the saliva that begins the digestion of starch in the mouth and converts it to dextrose and maltose (thus increasing the work of the gastrointestinal digestive process)

Physical Examination

The examination of the mouth and throat begins with an evaluation of the function of speech, the ability to chew efficiently, and to swallow. Tone of voice, ability to articulate words, hoarseness, unusual voice quality, or any speech defect should be noted during the examination.

To facilitate examination for occlusion of the teeth, the examiner demonstrates closing the teeth and sliding the mandible forward and from side to side to detect restricted movement of the jaw. The temporomandibular joint is palpated as the patient makes exaggerated chewing motions, and the clicking or crepitus which is often associated with generalized arthritis or severe overclosure of the jaws is noted. Firm pressure and percussion of the joint with the examiner's middle finger should elicit localized tenderness suggestive of temporomandibular joint syndrome.

Evaluation of the ability to swallow is vitally important because difficulty leads to rapid and severe dehydration. Drooling of saliva, dribbling of liquid intake, coughing, or having to swallow several times to pass a small amount of liquid requires immediate attention. The dangers of aspiration make it necessary that suction be available for this test, especially in stroke patients or where a problem is suspected.

The mouth and throat are inspected with a tongue depressor and a good light. The examination should first be carried out with all prostheses in place, and these should be checked for articulation and fit; then, when they have been removed, the dentures and surfaces covered by them should be meticulously examined.

The gingivae should be pink and firm, without redness, swelling, or breaks in their surface. The gum margins should be sharp around the teeth and should not bleed easily. In dark-skinned people primarily, but also occasionally in individuals with fair complexions, a brownish line along the gum margins and brownish dappling of the buccal mucosa are normal findings. However, this configuration should be investigated further, since a similar color pattern may also be found in Addison's disease. A bluish or black line along the gum margin is never normal and may be an indicator of lead, bismuth, mercury, or arsenic poisoning.

Dryness of the lips and mouth and a dry tongue with longitudinal furrows are excellent indicators of systemic dehydration. The multiple deep fissures of the so-called scrotal tongue are normal but pose a problem of hygiene, since food particles tend to get trapped in them. A coated tongue, contrary to some belief, is not an unhealthy sign in the elderly, neither is the atrophy of the papillae around the sides of the tongue abnormal. A bright red shiny tongue (without papillae) may indicate a deficiency of vitamin B_{12}, niacin, or iron and is distinctly abnormal, as opposed to "geographic tongue" in which scattered patches of smooth red tissue contrast with areas with regular papillate surfaces. This benign condition may change its map-like pattern over time for reasons that are not yet understood.

Next, the examiner puts on gloves to carefully palpate the tongue, the gingivae, and lesions, and the U-shaped area under the tongue in the floor of the mouth where cysts, salivary gland calculi, and malignant neoplasms are most likely to occur. Any area of induration should arouse suspicion, as should any ulcer or nodule which has a cracked crust and which fails to heal within two or three weeks. The teeth are percussed with a gloved finger for tenderness, and the consistency of the saliva is noted.

Testing for the twelfth cranial nerve (hypoglossal) function requires that the patient be able to protrude and extend his tongue in the midline and move it from side to side. True fasciculations are rare but can be seen when the tongue is in the mouth and at rest. The ninth (glossopharyngeal) and tenth (vagus) cranial nerves should be tested at the conclusion of the examination of this area because the test involves triggering the gag reflex. Vagus nerve paralysis is noted when the subject says "ah" and the soft palate on the paralyzed side fails to rise while the uvula deviates to the uninvolved side. With an intact vagus nerve, both sides of the soft palate elevate equally and the uvula stays midline.

Testing for taste provides information about the elderly person's present level of interest in food and his dietary pattern. Substances must be in solution to be tasted, and the four easily identified sensations are sweet (sugar), sour (lemon), salty (sodium chloride), and bitter (quinine). The examiner dips an applicator in a vial of the test solution, places a drop or two of the liquid on the subject's tongue, and asks, "What does this taste like to you?" Sweet flavors are registered mainly at the tip, sour at the sides, salt at the tip and sides, and bitter at the back. The patient should rinse his mouth out with clear water between tastes.

While surveying the hard palate, a lobulated, bony outgrowth in the midline may be observed. This is probably a torus palatinus, a benign growth which develops during adulthood in some people. A hard nodule which is not situated in the midline suggests a tumor.

The soft palate, uvula, anterior and posterior pillars, tonsils, and posterior pharynx are inspected last. The mucosa of these structures should be light red in color; free of inflammation, swelling, lesions, or exudates; and symmetrical. The tonsils in an older person, if they have not been removed, are often atrophied and may not be visible unless they are enlarged in response to an infectious process.

Clinical Considerations

Unusual voice tones need special attention. Hoarseness may be idiosyncratic in a few cases due to an upper respiratory infection; it may indicate dysfunction of the vagus nerve; it may result from the chronic irritation of smoking or alcohol ingestion (the "smoker's" or "whiskey" voice); or it may suggest cancer of the larynx. Hoarseness which persists after two weeks of voice rest must be thoroughly investigated by a physician. A monotonous, soft voice with rapid, somewhat slurred speech is characteristic of parkinsonism. Pseudobulbar palsy produces a monotonous, nasal speech which has a very harsh quality.

Speech and the enunciation of words may be distorted by missing teeth, poorly fitting dentures, a painful tongue, a mouth lesion, paralysis, temporomandibular joint ankylosis, or a lifelong speech impediment. These causes must be differentiated from those originating in the central nervous system, such as the various aphasic states in which there is impaired ability to understand, sequence, or use language properly.

Temporomandibular joint syndrome is an underdiagnosed condition producing a wide variety of head, neck, and shoulder pains. It has been dubbed "The Great Imposter." This syndrome mimics such diverse problems as migraine headaches, vertigo, tinnitus and other ear problems, tic douloureux, and neck or shoulder spasms. Some people have difficulty opening their mouths, while in others the mouth springs open and is difficult to close. Patients with this condition often have a history of wandering from physician to physician seeking relief from their misery.

The lips, as the most exposed portion of the mouth and as a transitional tissue, are vulnerable to solar and chemical influences as well as to systemic conditions. Carcinoma of this area usually involves the lower lip and should be suspected with any sore or crusting lesion which does not heal. Angular stomatitis (cheilosis) results from the maceration of the skin at the corners of the mouth, followed by fissuring and cracking. Although sometimes due to vitamin deficiencies (the B complex) or to a secondary infection of Candida or bacteria, cheilosis is most often caused by the overclosure of the mouth in edentulous patients or in those whose dentures are improperly fitted, which results in an overlapping skin surface where saliva collects. This perpetual dampness and the rubbing together of the skin surfaces cause the tissue to break down.

The lips and buccal mucosa may suggest anoxia if they are dusky blue and anemia if they are very pale. Patchy brown pigmentation of the buccal mucosa in fair-skinned people may be indicative of Addison's disease. The appearance of bright red petechial spots in this area is always a potential danger signal, signifying an abnormality of the hemopoietic system, capillary fragility, or an abnormality of the blood elements (Elfenbaum, 1971).

Painful little aphthous ulcers (canker sores) often appear singly or in groups on the oral mucosa, showing up as small round or oval white ulcers surrounded by a reddened ring. These lesions are easily distinguished from the painless white or gray patch of leukoplakia, a keratosis of the epithelium which must be carefully described and monitored because it can become malignant. Moniliasis, too, can involve the oral mucosa. Typically the white curd-like patches can be scraped off, leaving a raw and even bleeding surface. Infrequently moniliasis presents as an irregular erythematous area which is shiny without the distinctive curdy appearance, in which case culturing out the yeast establishes its identity.

Oral cancer constitutes a special concern in this population. About 90% occurs in persons over age 45, with 60 as the average age of incidence. Malignancies can develop anywhere on the oral mucosa. The lips and tongue (especially the less obvious base and sides of the dorsal aspect of the tongue) are the most frequent sites. Since squamous cell carcinoma is the most common type of cancer of the oral cavity (90%), early detection is essential. A history of chronic smoking or alcohol use increases the risk of oral cancer substantially, and a history of syphilis seems to increase the risk of cancer of the tongue (Carbone et al., 1974).

Saving as many teeth as possible and even preserving roots help to distribute the functional load and reduce the loss of as much as 1 mm of bone per year in the critical lower jaw (Wasser, 1980). Partial dentures and overdentures (dentures made over nerveless roots) are preferable to full plates, especially in the lower jaw, because

dentures destroy bone. The expanse of the maxilla is great enough so that upper dentures are usually tolerated fairly well because the pressure is distributed over a relatively large area, thus decreasing bone loss. In the mandible, the area covered is small and the bone is easily overloaded by the function of the prosthesis. Dentures must be relined and refitted at frequent intervals to minimize avoidable stress on the jaw structure and to prevent the "collapsed denture" appearance which is stereotypical of the aged face.

Much tooth loss in the elderly is due to the insidious process of periodontal disease, which attacks both the soft tissues of the gingivae and the bone. Hyposalivation, poor oral hygiene, and a diet high in carbohydrates also contribute to the ever-present problem of tooth decay. Destruction spreads along the surface of the tooth in older people, rather than boring into the body of the tooth as it does in young people, and thus becomes almost impossible to repair (Elfenbaum, 1971).

Systemic dehydration contributes to the reduction in salivary flow and to the production of a gummier saliva which reduces the irrigation of food particles from the teeth, does not buffer as effectively against dental caries, encourages the formation of plaque, and results in shrunken, dehydrated oral tissues which cannot hold even the most well-made dentures in place. Food must be masticated longer to become moist, and swallowing is more difficult because the bolus of food is less well lubricated. Mouth breathing, some antihypertensive medications, and a variety of physical and emotional conditions (diabetes, postclimacteric syndrome, and poor nutrition, for example) also serve to reduce saliva production.

The bright red spots surrounded by gray, hyperkeratotic epithelium on the mucosa of the hard palate of heavy smokers are inflamed mucous glands. This condition is called "nicotine stomatitis."

THE NECK

The neck is an important crossroad of the body. It is a small, but very complex area encompassing vital circulatory and respiratory

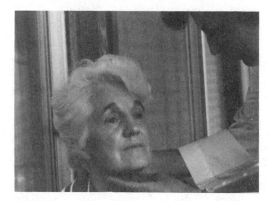

Figure 18-1. The neck is a small, but very complex crossroad of the body, which contains the major transport systems of blood, lymph, nerve, and respiratory passages. This remarkable structure also houses a physiological "highway patrol" which sets up roadblocks to infection, permits the important surveillance activities of the head, and regulates the metabolic rate of the body.

channels, major endocrine glands, the nerve trunk which connects the brain to the rest of the body, and a chain of lymph nodes which act both as indicators of local and generalized infection and as roadblocks to the passage of infection from one area to another. The rotation of the head on the neck constitutes a useful safety device permitting a scanning action which enlarges the field of vision. Examination is facilitated by the generalized loss of subcutaneous tissue which appears in most elderly people, causing the neck to appear thinner and bringing the underlying structures more clearly into view (see Figure 18-1).

Normal Changes

The cervical range of motion and ability to flex the head anteriorly to rest the chin on the sternum are often reduced in the elderly. Osteoporotic changes of the cervical vertebrae, and shrinkage and sclerosis of the tendons and muscles combine to produce a more limited range of motion and increased resistance to passive neck movements.

The vessels in the neck and the pulsations of the jugular veins and carotid arteries are usually more easily observable in older people. Because of the dilatation and elongation of arterial walls

and the generalized sclerosis of vascular interna, some increased tortuosity of the vessels in the neck and slightly more forceful cervical pulses may be considered normal.

The lymphatic response to infection is reduced in older adults. Prolonged and repeated traumas and infections over the years cause the tonsillar lymph nodes in the neck (often calcified by old tuberculous disease), as well as some axillary and femoral nodes, to become permanently firm and palpable. In older people these nodes are characterized by being small (less than 1 cm in diameter), smooth, and nontender. Other palpable nodes should be regarded with suspicion, and a search should be made for the cause.

After age 25, there is a gradual decrease in thyroid function. Whether this diminution is due primarily to the effect of aging on the thyroid or occurs secondarily as a result of the aging process on the pituitary, is still unclear. In any event, some atrophy of the thyroid gland occurs, along with a lowered basal metabolism rate, a decreased breakdown of circulating thyroid hormone, and a decrease in the total amount and configuration of urinary neutral 17-ketosteroid excretion.

Physical Examination

Examination of the neck proceeds as it would for any adult. Manipulation of the carotid arteries must be gentle to prevent an undesirable slowing of the cardiac rhythm and a sudden decrease in the blood pressure.

The jugular veins are not normally distended when the patient sits upright. In the elderly individual reclining at a 45° angle, it is not uncommon to note the left jugular vein and pulse elevated several centimeters above the level of the right jugular. This unilateral elevation normally results from an elongated aortic arch which exerts pressure on the left innominate vein. With a deep inspiration, the two pulse pressures should be seen to equalize. Thus, in order to obtain a reliable measurement of venous pressure, the level of jugular vein filling should always be taken on the right side during inspiration. The venous pulse is observed closely for the double beats of a normal sinus rhythm. Variation from this rhythm must be carefully described and monitored.

The arterial pulses are helpful for timing the cardiac cycle, for noting the unusually forceful pulsations of thyrotoxicosis, hypertension, and aortic regurgitation, and for detecting the expansile pulsation of a carotid aneurysm. In the older person, occasionally a pulsation suggesting an aneurysm may be felt above the right clavicle. This condition may be the result of the elongation of the aorta with the resultant buckling of the carotid, especially if the person is hypertensive and arteriosclerotic.

The movement of the head is normally less than that in younger people. Existing movement should be evaluated for symmetry, freedom from discomfort, and safety. Even when a significant degree of cervical spondylosis prevents flexion of the neck, lateral movement should be relatively free if nuchal rigidity is not present.

The muscles should be palpated for spasm, since posterior cervical muscle tension may frequently produce occipital headaches, especially in women. Weakness of the lower face muscles is tested by watching for symmetrical contraction of the fibers of the platysma as the patient is asked to lift his head from the pillow against resistance from the examiner's hand. Similarly, sternocleidomastoid strength is noted by asking the patient to turn his head against the examiner's resisting hand. This maneuver is part of the test of the accessory nerve (the eleventh cranial nerve).

Although the thyroid is usually not visible or palpable in older individuals, asking the subject to tilt his head straight back and swallow may bring an enlarged thyroid into view. Since the thyroid ascends during swallowing, any nodule or enlargement that moves upward is probably related to this structure.

After the salivary glands, lymph nodes, thyroid, cervical pulsations, and trachea have been palpated, the carotid arteries and the thyroid gland are auscultated for bruits.

Clinical Considerations

As the head moves through positions of flexion and extension, and through lateral and rotary movement during the process of the examination, the nurse should be alert for signs or complaints of dizziness or pain in the neck and shoulder region. Dizziness may result from an inner ear disturbance, or it may be due to stenosis of the carotid arteries, caused by arteriosclerosis, which deprives the brain of vital blood.

Often elderly persons notice an attack of dizziness or momentary unconsciousness when the head is tipped back, as if to look for something on a high shelf, causing a temporary cutoff of blood to the brain as the vessels "kink." If present, high pitched bruit over the bifurcation of the carotid artery should be discernible unilaterally or bilaterally. This condition is usually operable if the blood flow is compromised significantly.

Aching, tingling, or a sharp, shooting pain in the posterior neck is often due to cervical spondylosis, and results in voluntary and involuntary limitation of cervical movement. If the pain radiates to the shoulder, arm, or hand, hyperextension of the neck and flexion of the head to the involved side often intensify this discomfort. Compression of the nerve roots or the spinal cord by degenerating cervical disks may give rise to corresponding neurological signs, depending upon the structures involved.

Thyroid malfunction is less clearly defined and thus more deceptive in the elderly because many suggestive symptoms may be attributed to common manifestations of aging. For example, hypothyroidism often presents in the older person as weakness, dryness of the skin, cold skin and an intolerance to cold, impaired memory, constipation, coarse hair, and the loss of the normal arrangement of the eyebrows. Because one or any combination of these signs and symptoms may be due to other factors, special attention should be paid to the key indicators of slow cerebration, a husky voice, and slowly relaxing reflexes.

Hyperthyroidism also appears in a different form in old people. The ocular symptoms which are prominent indicators in middle-aged patients are rarely present. The key evidence is concentrated in the nervous and cardiovascular systems of the elderly. Thus, agitation, restlessness, weight loss, a fine tremor, continuously warm moist skin, a tachycardia which does not disappear during sleep or after rest, and rapid reflex relaxation all assume primary importance in detection. An enlarged or nodular thyroid, a systolic bruit heard directly over the gland itself, or a continuous venous hum heard in the supraclavicular areas, are highly suggestive of an overactive thyroid.

A neoplasm must be considered with any thyroid nodule(s) or a gland which does not move upward freely with swallowing. A careful search for associated lymphadenopathy must be made, including palpation of the midline Delphian nodes which enlarge with thyroid cancer or subacute thyroiditis.

An elevated venous pressure, manifested by abnormally distended jugular veins bilaterally (i.e., the venous level is over 4 cm above the sternal angle with the subject reclining at a 45° angle), may be due to right-sided heart failure, constrictive pericarditis, tricuspid stenosis, or an obstruction of the superior vena cava.

REFERENCES

Bates, B. *A Guide to Physical Examination.* Philadelphia: J.B. Lippincott, 1974, p. 62.

Burnside, I.M. The special senses and sensory deprivation. In *Nursing and the Aged.* New York: McGraw-Hill, 1976, pp. 380–395.

Caird, F.I. and Judge, T.G. *Assessment of the Elderly Patient* (2nd ed.). Philadelphia: J.B. Lippincott, 1979, pp. 57, 59, 67, 69.

Carbone, J.V. et al. Gastrointestinal tract and liver. In Krupp, M.A. and Chatton, M.J. (Eds.) *Current Diagnosis and Treatment.* Los Altos, Calif.: Lange Medical Publications, 1974, pp. 316–390.

Elfenbaum, A. Dentistry for the elderly in health and illness. In Chinn, A.B. (Ed.) Working with Older People, a Guide to Practice. *Clinical Aspects of Aging,* Vol. 4 (Government Publication No. 1459). Rockville, Md.: U.S. Department of Health, Education and Welfare, 1971, pp. 337–353.

Farrell, D.E. Hearing deficit. In Pearson, L.J. and Kotthoff, M.E. (Eds.) *Geriatric Clinical Protocols.* Philadelphia: J.B. Lippincott, 1979, pp. 120–124.

Hirschman, H. Intraocular lens implantation: faster, more complete rehabilitation of the cataract patient. *Journal of the American Geriatrics Society* 25(1):35–38 (1977).

Kasper, R. Eye problems in the aged. In Reichel, W. (Ed.) *Clinical Aspects of Aging.* Baltimore: Williams and Wilkins, 1978, pp. 391–402.

Kornzweig, A.L. The eye in old age. In Rossman, I. (Ed.) *Clinical Geriatrics.* Philadelphia: J.B. Lippincott, 1979, pp. 369–390.

Locke, S. Neurological disorders of the elderly. In Chinn, A.B. (Ed.) Working with Older People, a Guide to Practice. *Clinical Aspects of Aging,* Vol. 4 (Government Publication No. 1459). Rockville, Md.: U.S. Department of Health, Education and Welfare, 1971, pp. 45–49.

Wasser, V.E. Personal communication (1980).

19
The Chest, Abdomen, and Genitourinary System

Linda Ellison Jessup

A sound heart is the life of flesh.

Old Testament, Proverbs 14:30
King James Version

CHEST

The Breasts

Regardless of age, sexuality is an important and ongoing aspect of physical, social, and psychological existence. Sexual identity develops from infancy on. It is less dependent upon anatomical structure than cultural expectations. Therefore, by the time one reaches senescence, the reality of one's womanliness or manliness is so deeply embedded in self-concept as to be central to the rest of the personality.

It is devastating when medical and nursing personnel treat individuals as asexual beings. The best way to acknowledge and to reinforce the existence of the older person's sexuality is to treat the breasts with the scrupulous concern that they merit at any age. The breast of the older female generally continues to be an important erogenous zone throughout the later years, especially in women who have the opportunity to continue to be sexually active.

History taking and the examiner's matter-of-fact observations open the way for the embarrassed, worried, or reluctant patient to voice questions and concerns about sexuality. Examining the reproductive parts of the anatomy conveys more clearly than words that these continue to be integral and functional parts of each person's being.

In women, breast cancer is found most frequently in menopausal and postmenopausal women. Still, 1–2% of all carcinomas of the breast occur in men. Because of the ease with which breast tissue in both men and women can be examined, bypassing this procedure is rarely justifiable.

Normal Changes. The major change of aging involves atrophy of normal breast tissue, which results in sagging and some regression in the structure and size of these appendages.

Physical Examination. A thorough examination of the breast includes visual inspection followed by bimanual palpation, with the subject in both the upright and the supine positions. Minor variations in the size or height of the breasts or a slight deviation of a nipple is normal. Any major discrepancy should be noted and investigated. Having the patient lean forward to let the breasts fall freely may expose an area of retraction. Having her sit erect with hands pushing in at the waist as firmly as possible will contract the pectoral muscles and reveal dimpling which might otherwise go unnoticed.

When pressure is applied to the breast toward the nipple, any fluid secreted should be noted and perhaps collected for cytology studies, especially if the discharge is bloody. The point at which pressure applied produces the secretion should also be described with care, since a dilated duct or small tumor may be palpable at the site. Finally, the nipple is closely inspected for very small erosions which may be the only sign of a Paget's carcinoma. This cancer is a rare one, which is often mistakenly treated as a dermatitis or as an infection.

Inspection continues while the subject raises her arms over her head, followed by palpation of the axilla as the examiner lowers the subject's arm to its dependent position. Any axillary mass should prompt a search of the hand, arm, front, and back chest wall to determine if an infection or other trauma might account for enlarged nodes (Bates, 1979).

Bimanual palpation of the breast tissue by quadrants is followed by palpating the tissue against the rib cage, once again moving systematically from quadrant to quadrant. Because pre- or postmenstrual hypertrophy is no longer a problem and cystic mastitis is rare in old age, any palpable lump should be treated with great suspicion. To guide the examiner's efforts, the relative incidence of carcinoma, according to location in the breast, is shown in Figure 19-1 (Wilson, 1974, p. 367).

Clinical Considerations. Acute mastitis, manifested by a painful, erythematous and edematous breast, is uncommon in the elderly. These symptoms in the older age group suggest a highly malignant inflammatory carcinoma, especially if the axilla is involved and there is lymphadenopathy. A notable exception to this involves older men who wear suspenders. The chronic irritation produced by the rubbing or snapping of these elastic bands can precipitate episodes of acute mastitis which is extremely uncomfortable but easily remedied.

Gynecomastia, the noninflammatory enlargement of one or both breasts which is often seen in adolescent boys, also occurs in elderly men. Although the development of this condition often causes psychological distress, it is usually transient and of little significance. In occasional cases, gynecomastia may also be a

sign of serious testicular tumors or a bronchogenic carcinoma. It may result from hormonal stimulation, the administration of certain drugs (such as digitalis, isoniazid, and phenothiazines), or the incomplete destruction of estrogen due to liver dysfunction. Thus, the appearance of gynecomastia, while generally benign, must be monitored carefully while it persists.

Fibroadenosis, either unilateral or bilateral, is sometimes seen in men over 50 years of age. The typical fibroadenoma is a small, disk-shaped mass appearing under the areola, which is movable, firm, and often somewhat tender. In spite of the fact that this neoplasm is completely benign, it must of course be distinguished from carcinoma of the breast.

Carcinoma of the breast occurs in both elderly men and women and usually presents as a "lump." Although the signs may vary and occur in different constellations from person to person, the following criteria are helpful for evaluating and describing any mass:

Highly Suspicious Signs	*Generally Benign Signs*
Hard to stony hard	Soft to firm
Nontender	Tender to painful
Fixed	Movable
Poorly delimited margins	Discrete margins
Unilateral	Bilateral
Rapid Growth	Slow growth
Dimpling, retraction, or peau d'orange skin	Normal overlying skin

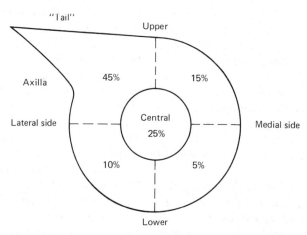

Figure 19-1. Incidence of breast cancer according to location.

The involvement of the lymph nodes in the area is an important factor in the determination of a diagnosis. At times, an unexplained, enlarged node may be the first clue that a tumor exists. All findings, including precise measurements of any mass, must be recorded and mapped on a drawing of the breast for purposes of referral, consultation, and future reference.

The Respiratory System

The respiratory system controls the ability to be physically active. In old age, respiratory disease and respiratory signs and symptoms are more frequent and of increasing importance because they manifest the cumulative effect of air pollution, smoking, occupational inhalations, and lung disease. Respiratory disease is a major cause of acute illness and chronic disability in the elderly, often limiting vital oxygen to the organism, stressing the heart, and threatening life itself (see Figure 19-2).

Though the respiratory system is often impaired in later life, it is actually well constructed, and should function and last throughout a long lifetime. It is important for nurses to realize that chronic respiratory symptoms

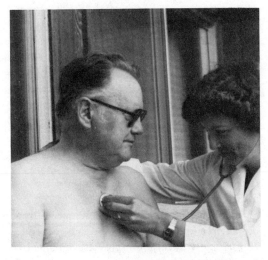

Figure 19-2. The respiratory system largely determines an individual's ability to be active, mentally and physically, throughout a long lifetime. Normal elderly people are free from any chronic respiratory symptoms and they do not become short of breath with moderate exercise.

such as a cough, sputum production, and shortness of breath are not normal in aging, nor is shortness of breath with moderate exercise.

Normal Changes. The lungs of the elderly are larger because of decreasing elasticity and force of recoil. Their vital capacity is decreased, and their residual volume after complete expiration is greater. The aged lung has larger alveoli and often shows thickening of the alveolar membrane. There is a relative loss of capillaries, producing a slight decrease in diffusing capacity.

The mobility of the chest wall decreases due to reduced muscle strength, alterations in the nature and distribution of elastin, and reduced lung elasticity. As a result, the older person has to expend more energy (about 10% more than a younger person) to stretch the chest wall and lungs during inspiration. In spite of these common changes, ventilation generally remains adequate to meet the demands of ordinary activity in the normal elderly person (Balchum, 1971).

Physical Examination. The entire thorax should be inspected, with the patient bare to the waist, for overall observation of conformation and respiratory movements of the chest and back. The general nutrition, musculature, and skin condition of the older person are also easily evaluated at this time. As in younger adults, the muscular development on the side of handedness is frequently more pronounced in those who have been very active physically. Moles and skin lesions on the chest and shoulders should be noted.

An increased anterior-posterior diameter may be found in older people with a marked degree of kyphosis, especially if the chest is rather short. This can usually be distinguished from the "barrel chest" of emphysema by a careful history and by signs of obstructive respiratory disease. Excursion of the chest is usually minimal, but localized restrictions of movement which suggest a large lesion in the underlying lung are noticeable with very precise observation, especially during deep inspiration. The respiratory movements, however slight, should be symmetrical and regular 16-20 breaths per minute without the use of accessory muscles. Intercostal bulging or retractions are always abnormal.

Palpation of the chest begins with the trachea. Deviations from the midline are usually due to the same conditions which displace the trachea at any age, with the exception of benign deviation due to upper dorsal scoliosis, which is generally associated with old age. The muscles of the thorax are systematically palpated for soreness, crepitus, and masses. The costochondral junctions are tapped for the tenderness of costochondritis, and the xiphoid process is pressed to elicit the distinctive arthritic pain which is sometimes mistaken for angina by elderly patients. The ribs are palpated and compressed for point tenderness and for the remote pain caused by a fracture. Friction rubs may be less noticeable to the touch because of decreased lung expansibility, while fremitus may be more marked.

Percussion often reveals generalized hyperresonance in the thorax of the kyphotic or emphysematous individual. Flatness or dullness elicited in areas which are normally resonant, however, continues to be a reliable indicator of pleural fluid, fibrotic thickening, or pulmonary consolidation in the underlying area.

Auscultatory findings may be more difficult to determine in the elderly because the intensity of breath sounds (and thus their quality) may be subdued and because the patient may be unable to take the necessary number of deep breaths requested by the examiner. Meticulous attention to the *length* of the inspiratory and expiratory phases is necessary to distinguish the longer inspiratory phase of vesicular breath sounds from the longer expiratory phase of bronchial breathing or the more equal phases of bronchovesicular breathing. Wheezes, rubs (best heard laterally), rales, and rhonchi are often heard; voice sounds, especially whispers, are helpful in detecting areas of pulmonary consolidation, infarction, effusion, and atelectasis.

Clinical Considerations. Sometimes older people are surprisingly unaware of respiratory symptoms such as a cough of long duration, chronic breathlessness, or pleuritic pain. Determining whether or not sputum is produced is sometimes the best indicator that a productive cough indeed exists, because while coughing and breathlessness may be obvious to the examiner, the patient may deny their existence. Perception of pleuritic pain also seems to be diminished in the elderly, so that its absence can never eliminate the suspicion of pneumonia in this population (Caird and Judge, 1979). The following nursing observations and assessments are needed in caring for the older patient with respiratory problems.

First, the presence or absence of a cough requires careful evaluation because coughing serves a critical protective function. Therefore, the strength of the cough must be consciously noted. No cough or a weak cough in the patient with respiratory problems increases the risk of respiratory infection and respiratory embarrassment because of inability to clear secretions from the bronchi. Patients with frequent single or paroxysmal coughing spells may become exhausted rather quickly, especially when coughing interferes with sleeping. Nutrition and hydration are affected rapidly if intake is constantly interrupted and/or severe coughing triggers the gag reflex resulting in vomiting. The nature of the cough — dry, brassy, productive — and whether it is produced voluntarily or involuntarily are also crucial considerations.

Second, the sputum is the single best indicator of the cause, status, and course of the respiratory problem. Clear, mucoid sputum suggests that no severe infection exists, while purulent sputum signals an infectious process. Bloodstained, purulent sputum may be caused either by bronchitis or by a bronchial carcinoma, while bloodstained mucoid sputum is more likely due to a pulmonary infarction. In hemoptysis, the sputum is bright red and frothy, indicating damage to the alveoli or a bronchial ulceration such as that caused by tuberculosis, bronchiectasis, a lung abscess, or a malignancy.

Third, the pattern of respiration needs to be observed and documented. Periods of apnea alternating with respiratory cycles building to a maximum, then decreasing again to apnea (Cheyne-Stokes respirations), are more characteristic of dyspnea of cardiac rather than respiratory origin. This kind of breathing is found occasionally during the normal sleep of aged individuals. Prolonged expiration and rapid inspiration are typical of chronic obstructive pulmonary disease. Normal respirations may also be interrupted by the pain of thoracic movement from pleurisy, bruised or inflamed muscles, fractured ribs, or acute abdominal problems.

Fourth, the type of breathing should be noted. Stertorous breathing (snoring) may result from vibrations of the secretions in the upper respiratory tract during a severe illness. This sound has been called the "death rattle" and may be a grave prognostic sign. Stridulous breathing is the high pitched whistling or crowing sound caused by the passage of air through a partially closed glottis. Kussmaul breathing — deep, regular, sighing respirations — signifies air hunger. It should not be confused with the sighing respirations of psychoneurotic origin, in which respirations are normal but frequently interrupted by long, deep sighs. Dyspnea may be a sign rather than a symptom. The patient may not be aware of it, and the examiner's first clue may be the subject's pausing for a breath in the middle of a sentence. Other unmistakable signs of difficult breathing are anxiety and an expression of distress. Breathing may become more rapid (tachypnea) and may include the involvement of accessory muscles such as the scaleni and sternocleidomastoids. It may also be accompanied by flaring of the nostrils, movements of the lips and chin, and a hunching of the shoulders with the hands or forearms braced on the thighs. (See Chapter 23 for common respiratory conditions in old age.)

The Cardiovascular System

Throughout the ages, the human heart has been imbued with spiritual and emotional considerations far beyond its physiological reality. In most cultures, this pulsating muscle symbolizes the nucleus of one's being and one's integrity as a person. Thus, the health or impairment of this organ carries overtones of human soundness beyond physical changes. Although the lungs, the kidneys, and the liver are as essential for survival as the heart, none are vested with an equal romantic aura nor do they receive as

much concern as people grow older (see Figure 19-3). Unfortunately, concern for cardiovascular health develops too late in life. Nurses are prime witnesses to the impact of years of cardiac abuse: the ravages of high cholesterol and triglyceride diets, smoking, obesity, and stressful living patterns.

Normal Changes. In spite of ominous official statistics on heart disease, the heart remains a powerful, resilient pump which functions admirably throughout a long lifetime for most people, sometimes against overwhelming odds. Because of the incredible amount of work that the heart does nonstop from before birth until death, the wear and tear on it are registered in certain distinct anatomical changes.

The heart size of normal old people (i.e., without hypertension or clinical disease) is the same or smaller than it was in middle age. As energy declines and demand is decreased, the heart muscle actually atrophies. Even a hypertrophied heart may shrink with prolonged bed rest, illness, or malnutrition.

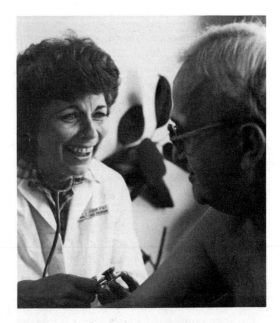

Figure 19-3. The human heart is imbued with spiritual and emotional connotations which go far beyond its anatomical importance. The quality of life for an older person may have as much to do with being "warmhearted," "stouthearted," "bighearted," or "lighthearted" as it does with actual cardiovascular functioning.

Sclerosis and thickening of the endocardium and valve leaflets occur where constant hemodynamic stress is greatest (i.e., more in the left ventricle). The resulting poor closure ("incompetence") of the leaflets of the mitral, tricuspid, and pulmonic valves may produce a murmur simulating acquired heart disease. This malocclusion is usually not important unless there is also preexisting valvular disease, in which case it can produce congestive heart failure.

Calcification and the proliferation of elastin produce a narrowing of the small arteries; however, with the decreased demand, this development is usually not a problem. Dilatation and lengthening of the aorta and the great muscular arteries occur, with a decrease in their tone and elasticity making them more prominent and tortuous.

The following physiological adjustments made by the heart are mentioned to explain functional features we notice in older adults.

- There is generally a decreased cardiac reserve which means that the aged heart reacts poorly to either sudden or prolonged stress.
- A generally decreased cardiac output results in a slower heart rate, which is highly variable (between 44 and 108 beats per minute).
- The blood flow through the coronary vessels decreases by one-third by age 60, thus delivering less oxygen to the cardiac muscle. Additionally, the ability of the myocardium to utilize oxygen is decreased.
- The myocardium is slower to recover its contractility and irritability. This delay poses no problem if there is adequate recovery time between beats, allowed for by frequent pauses while climbing stairs, for example, and a generally slower pace for all activities. The myocardium reacts poorly to a tachycardia, whatever the cause, and an older patient can quickly slide into heart failure without even a rise in his blood pressure if the rapid beat is sustained.
- The myocardium is less sensitive to atropine and more sensitive to carotid sinus stimulation. Interestingly, elderly persons undergoing an episode of tachycardia are often observed instinctively massaging their necks, thereby slowing the heart action by activation of the carotid sinuses.
- There is an increase in the pulse wave velocity in the normotensive aged, reflecting the increased rigidity of the medium and larger arteries.
- The pulse rate tends to slow with age, beginning in the early sixties (although this is extremely variable; see "Vital Signs" in Chapter 14).
- The loss of elasticity in the arterial vessel walls increases the systolic pressure and decreases the diastolic pressure, while the lability of vasopressor action increases both in systolic and diastolic pressures. Thus the usual picture for the elderly individual without a history of cardiovascular disease is a rise in systolic pressure and either a rise or a fall in the diastolic pressure.

Physical Examination. The first step in the examination of the cardiovascular system is simply the evaluation of general health and vitality. Noting the vascular pulsations and the degree of tortuosity of the vessels in the head, neck, and extremities is generally facilitated by the decrease of subcutaneous tissue. At the same time, the hands and feet are examined for cyanosis confined to the digits, indicating a reduced peripheral blood flow which is often due to decreased cardiac output. Where cyanosis is suspected, the color of the tongue and the inner surface of the lips should also be checked. They are sensitive indicators of arterial hypoxemia.

Palpation is used to confirm the physical findings suggested by the observations. The hands of older people are usually dry and cool to the touch. Cold hands indicate reduced blood to the periphery. The presence or absence and symmetry of the carotid, radial, femoral, dorsalis pedis, and posterior tibial pulses are determined. The carotids, the aorta (as the abdomen is palpated), and the popliteal arteries are palpated for the expansile pulsation of an aneurysm. The absence of a pulsation suggests an arterial obstruction in or near a pulse point; however, the foot pulses in the elderly are often not detectable. When a pulse is hard to find, skin changes, cold reddish-blue feet, loss of hair on the toes and lower legs, and experiences of intermittent claudication are sought as evidence to confirm or rule out the suspicion of obstruction.

The pulse rate, character, and rhythm are again noted for a full minute; the examiner generally compares the radial and apical pulses, noting any marked difference between these findings and the initial reading taken at the beginning of the encounter. The presence of edema in the extremities and the sacral area (if the person is not ambulatory) is appropriately included at this time, and the blood pressure is again measured, with the patient's position indicated by diagrams on the record (e.g., ⚓︎ , ⚓︎ , ⚓︎) and the right or left arm Ⓡ or Ⓛ specified.

The point of maximal impulse (the PMI) is palpated next, and the entire precordial area is felt with the finger pads in order to detect any other precordial pulsations, lifts, or heaves. The palmar surface of the hand (at the base of the fingers) is then used to search for thrills, although both thrills and precordial pulsations are less obvious in older adults. It must be kept in mind that the PMI may be displaced by a marked kyphoscoliosis of the spine, so that left ventricular hypertrophy is often more reliably indicated by an apical beat that is powerful and sustained than solely by the location of the apex. Percussion is sometimes useful in detecting gross cardiac enlargement in this age group, but more often it simply provides a useful orientation regarding the position of the heart.

Normal heart sounds in the elderly are identical to those of younger people, and they are auscultated through all seven auscultatory areas, with the examiner listening first to the first sound, then to the second, and noting changes which occur with the respiratory cycle. Since these cardiac sounds may be fairly loud or remote because of emphysema or some skeletal malformation, the examiner must decide if faint heart sounds are due to poor heart function or to some structural cause.

Any murmurs, extra heart sounds, reversed or fixed splitting, clicks, or snaps should be meticulously described as to location, character, and radiation, and diagrammed to indicate the shape or point of occurrence in the cardiac cycle. Although approximately 60% of the elderly have systolic murmurs, most of which are probably functional, some are not. All diastolic murmurs are assumed to be abnormal. Consultation must always be sought by nurse examiners to help validate the nature of any heart sounds which are not clearly within normal limits.

Clinical Considerations. The identification of the prime warning symptoms of cardiac disease in older patients is often misleading for the examiner who lacks special knowledge of geriatrics. For example, sudden severe dyspnea rather than chest pain may be the presenting symptom of an acute myocardial infarction in the elderly, while any chest pain in the elderly, however mild, needs attention because cardiac pain, whether from angina or a myocardial infarction, may be considerably less severe even with serious damage in this age group. Therefore, more emphasis is placed upon the location of the pressure or pain, its relation to exercise, and the radiation of the pain since these characteristics do remain the same. Other indicators such as dyspnea, diaphoresis, heart rate, and blood pressure are also significant in corroborating cardiac involvement.

The appearance of edema in one or both legs is a far more frequent occurrence in older people than in the young. It may be due to incompetent venous valves, blockage in the return of venous and lymphatic fluids, chronic nephritis, or cirrhosis. The cause of dependent edema must be carefully ascertained to avoid the inappropriate use of powerful cardiotonic or antihypertensive medications when the problem is not due to ineffective cardiac function. Edema due to cardiac factors is bilateral (although it may be asymmetrical on occasion because of a secondary obstructive process) and usually of fairly recent onset.

Shortness of breath due to heart disease may manifest itself primarily as extreme fatigue, rather than as an obvious breathing problem. Orthopnea, especially paroxysmal nocturnal episodes, tends to occur with the classic experience of being awakened to breathe and needing to sit upright to obtain relief. These events are terrifying and well remembered by the patient.

Two other common symptoms which suggest cardiac problems are the recent development of a cough and fainting (i.e., syncope). The wheezing and/or cough of early left-sided failure is nearly always a recent occurrence, while a bronchitic cough has a history of many years. Syncope, a brief loss of consciousness which occurs with walking or simply at rest, may be due to sudden cessation of cardiac output resulting from a Stokes-Adams attack or (rarely) from severe aortic stenosis. Medications such as phenothiazines and guanethidine may also be causative factors (Caird and Judge, 1979).

As mentioned previously, the controversy over what constitute the upper limits of normal blood pressure in the elderly well person showing no signs of cardiovascular damage from hypertension has yet to be resolved. American cardiologists tend to believe that high blood pressure exists when a persistent reading of 170/95 or higher is found (Harris, 1971). British experts tend to accept a higher upper limit of blood pressure in otherwise healthy, elderly people, ranging from 195/100 in men over 60 to 200/110 in women. Caird and Judge (1976) caution that "neglect of the normal range of blood pressure in the elderly leads to many old people being unnecessarily treated with drugs of high potency to relieve symptoms attributed to high blood pressure, while neglect of the second problem (postural hypotension) leads to many incorrect diagnoses of cerebral vascular insufficiency." Overall, a consistent rise in blood pressure, a persistent elevation to an unacceptable level, a blood pressure accompanied by AV nicking and tortuosity, or other cardiovascular stigmata of hypertension, should have immediate attention (see Chapter 21 for common cardiovascular conditions).

THE ABDOMEN

The Gastrointestinal Tract

Of all the body's systems, the gastrointestinal tract is the most common source of chronic distress in the elderly. As Sklar (1971) and other researchers have shown, probably more than half of all these complaints are without a detectable, organic cause and are due more to poor life-style patterns of nutrition, hydration, and exercise, and to psychological patterns of depression and preoccupation with fears of illness, aging, bodily functioning, and death, than to actual disease processes. Still, the determination of the cause of a gastrointestinal complaint requires careful, patient, and sometimes repeated investigation since in this age group the symptoms of both benign and dangerous diseases are often atypical, seemingly trivial, and frequently difficult to distinguish from each other.

It is important for nurses working with the elderly to know the following:

- The types of gastrointestinal problems older people manifest do not differ greatly from those of younger people.

- The death of an aged person is almost never due to the "wearing out" of the gastrointestinal tract (which, even when diseased, could generally continue to sustain life).

- The mortality rate from gastrointestinal disease, due primarily to malignancies, biliary tract disease, intestinal obstruction, and finally peptic ulcer, is not as great in the elderly as popularly thought (about one-third that from cardiovascular causes).

- Changing established life-style patterns must be done gradually and cautiously, since the frail, elderly person may be unable to tolerate too sudden a change to optimal hydration, vigorous laxation, a diet high in fiber, or a significant increase in exercise.

Normal Changes. Separating the external factors which affect gastrointestinal function from the intrinsic factors of aging per se is an almost impossible task. Tooth loss, deterioration of the senses of smell, taste, and sight, an increase or decrease in appetite due to social and psychological factors, and changes in the pattern of activity may or may not be age related. Yet each of these elements has an impact on this sensitive and complex system.

While research on the structural and physiological changes of aging has resulted in few, and even then sometimes contradictory, findings, there is a fair amount of agreement about the following observations:

- The esophagus presents decreased motility with aging (which can lead to dilatation and delay in emptying and can result in spasm, esophagitis, and gastric esophageal reflux).
- Within the stomach, there is a decrease in mucosal thickening, a decrease in total acid secretion, and a decrease in motor activity. The latter causes reduced hunger contractions and delayed emptying (seven hours versus three hours for younger adults). The output of digestive enzymes is decreased as well, but ample quantities remain available for digestive processes. *Note:* The pernicious anemia sometimes found in the elderly is probably caused by the atrophy of the gastric mucosa, which secretes the hydrochloric acid and "intrinsic factor" necessary for vitamin B_{12} absorption.
- There is muscular and mucosal atrophy throughout the large and small intestines.

Despite the prevalence of constipation in this age group, there is no good evidence of major changes in the motor or secretory activity of the colon or rectum. Similarly, where liver disease is not present, liver function does not change significantly, nor does there seem to be a relationship between biliary calculi and aging in the absence of gall bladder disease. Finally, although many old people prove on investigation to be nitrogen deficient, this deficit is probably the result of a diet low in protein rather than a problem with absorption (Sklar, 1971).

Physical Examination. Although the abdominal wall of an older person tends to be less taut than that of a younger one, the same techniques are used to reduce voluntary or involuntary tensing, thus permitting optimal examination. To this end, the room should be warm, and the patient should be supine, draped, and comfortable. The head and popliteal space should be supported on small pillows so that the spine is flexed slightly, and the examiner should take care to warm his hands and stethoscope before touching the abdomen.

Other steps which facilitate examination are to reverse the order in which palpation and auscultation are usually performed, with auscultation being carried out first (before the abdomen is manipulated); to begin with light palpation before proceeding to deeper pressure; and to examine any portion known or suspected to be tender, last. Inspection of the abdomen will be easier with the examiner on the patient's right side and the light source either opposite or at the patient's feet.

Auscultation should never be hurried through since vital information may be overlooked unless time is taken to listen with care. An abdominal murmur may be heard if an aortic aneurysm is present, and bruits and rubs are occasionally heard in the splenic or hepatic regions or elsewhere over the abdominal area. A hepatic rub suggests a neoplasm of that organ, and a peritoneal friction rub, which is often palpable as well, indicates inflammation of the underlying serous membrane. If good peristaltic sounds are not immediately audible below and to the right of the umbilicus, the examiner must sit down and listen for at least five minutes, stimulating peristaltic action by flicking the abdominal wall if necessary. Weak tinkles are not evidence of good peristalsis, while increased peristaltic sounds may indicate either the increased bowel activity of diarrhea or an early obstruction.

Light abdominal palpation requires scouting the entire abdominal wall, beginning at the pubes and working upward to the costal margin in order that a grossly enlarged liver or spleen not be overlooked. Determining the presence of direct or rebound tenderness, muscle rigidity, and masses is done first with light pressure; then, deeper palpation is employed. The femoral pulses are palpated for synchronous beats (to rule out the presence of a coarctation of the aorta, and aortic aneurysm, or a thrombosis of the aorta or of the common iliac artery). Any femoral lymphadenopathy is also noted at this time.

The kidneys are felt for but should not be palpable unless they are enlarged or the older person is very thin. The aorta may be palpable in an elderly person as a soft pulsatile area in the midepigastrium no more than 4 cm wide and extending down to the pelvic brim. Pressure on this great vessel normally produces some tenderness. An aortic aneurysm is substantially wider and usually reveals a bruit on auscultation, which can be followed down the common iliac arteries to the groin. Aneurysms may be single or multiple, so if a large pulsation with lateral expansion is felt, the examiner should estimate its width and palpate carefully down the length of the aorta to the pelvic brim in a search for additional areas of dilatation (Caird and Judge, 1976).

Finally, percussion is used to demarcate the area of hepatic dullness and any other sites of dullness which have been located.

Clinical Considerations. As the gastrointestinal tract becomes an increasing target of major concern, the complaints encountered by the nurse examiner most commonly involve bowel function, problems with eating and appetite, and abdominal pain. Each symptom must be investigated thoroughly and, if the problem persists, repeatedly.

A great many people become preoccupied with their bowel habits as they grow older. The reasons for this intense focus may stem from a variety of subconscious motivations — from sexual sublimation and a need to control at least one's own body processes, to boredom, depression, or more severe psychiatric distur-bances — or may result from actual changes in bowel function. The elderly person's definition of what constitutes "constipation" or "diarrhea" is essential information for the nurse to determine, as is a good look at the feces itself.

While there is no good evidence that constipation is a function of aging, physical inactivity, decreased dietary bulk and fluid intake, certain medications, systemic diseases (such as hypothyroidism), and any central nervous system damage are among the most common causes of hard, dry stool formation in this age group. Sudden, unexplained changes in bowel habits should provoke suspicion of an organic problem (i.e., a tumor, neurogenic problem, or painful anorectal disease), while a long term history of chronic constipation is more likely to be amenable to life-style changes and the establishment of a reasonable evacuation routine.

Diarrhea in the elderly is always of significance, and its appearance requires immediate attention. Not only is fecal incontinence extremely distressing to any lucid adult, but also the rapid loss of fluid and electrolytes poses a real threat to the frail individual's precarious well-being. Diarrhea may be due to an intestinal infection, the side affects of iron or antibiotic ingestion, the misuse of cathartics, metabolic or neurologic disease, carcinoma, or colitis. This sign may also be associated with fecal impaction, which is not infrequently coupled with the concomitant retention and overflow of urine as well. Determining the underlying cause of this development and protecting against dehydration and skin breakdown are obviously very high priorities.

Problems with the ingestion of food and fluid may result either from a loss of appetite or from actual difficulty with the mechanics of chewing and swallowing. Having a baseline weight for any person complaining of eating difficulties is vital, both for an initial assessment and for monitoring the severity of the problem objectively. The onset of the symptoms, whether they developed recently in someone who ate well previously or whether they developed gradually over weeks or months, is often indicative of the cause. Broken or abscessed teeth, poorly fitted dentures, a sore throat or tongue, or temporomandibular joint pain should be clearly differentiated from the sudden development of choking, slowness in eating, and impaired speech due to a neurological insult. Increasing trouble swallowing first solid foods and then even liquids over time, on the other hand, should raise suspicions of some kind of neoplasm.

The sudden development of anorexia similarly suggests an acute infectious process, gastrointestinal disorder, or perhaps the shock of an important loss. A gradual loss of appetite, however, generally indicates the development of a lesion such as an ulcer or a malignancy, or the onset of a depressive illness. Sometimes a person has an established pattern of depression which has accompanied other illnesses or incidents occurring earlier in his life, and which may be reactivated by a similar event occurring in senescence. Any such previous anorexic episode may help to interpret the current problem.

Additional Considerations. Assessing a complaint of abdominal pain in the elderly often poses special problems for two reasons. The first involves the difficulty frequently encountered in obtaining an accurate history of the pain, in terms of both detailing the chronology of the symptoms and tracing the original location and subsequent radiation of the pain to other sites. The second reason involves the interesting phenomenon once again of a markedly diminished perception of abdominal pain in many elderly people, which may cause this symptom to be minimized or overlooked entirely. Complicating matters further, because the abdominal muscles are frequently weak and flabby, the abdomen may be incapable of displaying true rigidity in response to peritoneal irritation. This important sign may, instead, be replaced by distension as the underlying bowel becomes inflated, although supersensitivity of the overlying skin, localized tenderness, rebound tenderness, and absent bowel sounds all retain their usual significance.

Trying to establish a general sense of the onset and duration of the pain in gross terms (i.e., hours, days, months, or years) is sometimes successful, while linking an increase or decrease in the intensity of discomfort to other symptoms and identifying the areas of tenderness may help considerably in pinpointing the site of the problem. For example, pain related to the ingestion of food or to vomiting is likely to be located in the stomach or small intestine, while pain which is relieved or intensified by defecation or associated with a change in bowel habits is probably located in the large bowel.

The prudent nurse keeps in mind the major causes of gastrointestinal disease while collecting historical and physical data and while helping to improve the health practices of the individual to eliminate many of the problems which can be remedied by life-style alterations. In a series of major studies (Leeming, Webster, and Dymock, 1978; Strauss, 1979) of elderly patients with gastrointestinal complaints, there has been a high degree of concurrence with the classic Sklar (1971) study in which 56% of the distressing symptoms were found to be "functional" (i.e., without any identifiable physical basis), 11% were malignancies, 10% were due to peptic ulcer disease (the same incidence as found in younger people), and 7.7% resulted from gall bladder disease.

Three other potentially problematic conditions were discovered in the course of these studies but the symptoms these patients were experiencing were felt to be attributable to the following circumstances in only a few cases. Diverticulosis was found in 20% of the population, there was a high incidence of hiatal hernia (unspecified), and rectal polyps were identified in 5% of these elderly people. *Note:* The larger polyps, 1 cm in size or larger, were removed since they can become a source of occult blood loss and since rapid growth suggests a malignancy potential (Sklar, 1971).

THE GENITOURINARY SYSTEM

There are probably no greater forms of personal human tragedy and humiliation than the disorders of urinary control and sexual performance. Too often these losses are accepted, equated with "old age," and denied the careful inspection and investigation they deserve. Urinary tract infections are secondary only to pulmonary disease as a cause of infection in the elderly. They often act as an insidious drain on the older person's pride, energy, and physical reserve when they are overlooked, as they frequently are. Additionally, nocturnal frequency and incontinence of urine are extremely important as causes of disability, fatigue, and sexual isolation.

Normal Changes

The Kidneys. Because these delicate filtration-concentration units are subjected over a lifetime to constant hemodynamic stresses and often to episodes of infection and trauma, it is no wonder that the kidneys definitely show evidence of change directly attributable to wear and tear as early as the fourth decade. As an individual continues to age, progressive degeneration and atrophy of renal tissues, unrelated to disease, make these organs less able to respond quickly or as effectively to sudden changes in the acid-base balance or to alterations in the volume of renal blood flow. Thus, the following changes occur (Kahn and Snapper, 1971):

- The glomeruli undergo differing degrees of hyalinization, which decreases their ability to filter as efficiently as before and reduces the renal plasma flow, by age 90, to about half that of a healthy 20 year old.
- The blood urea nitrogen, resulting from the catabolism of amino acids, rises at age 70 to approximately 21.2 mg% (from 12.9 mg% at age 30 or 40) because of less effective filtration.
- The tubules seem to be even more compromised by involutionary changes than the glomeruli and are thus less able to concentrate the filtrate.
- The renal response to acidosis caused by excess ammonium chloride is much slower in the elderly.
- The normal diurnal excretory pattern may be lost, resulting in the development of nocturia (this change may be compounded by a variety of factors, including disrupted sleep patterns, systemic conditions such as diabetes and cardiac failure, ingestion of liquids late in the day, long acting diuretics, or lower tract obstructions and infection).

Lower Urinary Tract. Because of the tendency of the prostate to gradually enlarge in about three-quarters of all aging men (65 and over), the dangers of infection and obstruction are increased. Hormonal changes and the decreased resistance of the epithelium of the urethra and bladder in aging women also increase their vulnerability to infection over the years. (Regular, thorough cleansing of the genitalia may also decline with the development of weakness, tremulousness, a loss of vision or the sense of smell, obesity, social isolation, or the lack of bathing facilities, thereby increasing the exposure to concentrations of pathogens in the genital area.)

The Genitalia. With old age there is a loss of hair and subcutaneous fat in the pubic region in both sexes. The external genitalia sag more in the male. The testes become smaller and less firm. Sperm production and the volume and viscosity of seminal fluid all decrease gradually. The labia of the female flatten, and the skin becomes thin, shiny, and avascular. The vaginal introitus often shrinks (especially in a woman who has become sexually inactive), the vaginal epithelium thins and appears pale, the rugae disappear, and lubrication diminishes. The uterus atrophies and may become so small that it is difficult to palpate bimanually. The endometrium atrophies but always retains its ability to respond to hormonal stimulation (Birnbaum, 1971).

Physical Examination

Palpation for the kidneys and bladder are included as part of the examination of the abdomen. As noted earlier, the lower poles of the kidneys are felt only rarely on deep palpation in very thin persons or when an abnormal kidney is enlarged by hydronephrosis, polycystic disease, or a neoplasm. The kidneys will descend during deep inspiration, and the examiner, supporting the subject's loin posteriorly (i.e., between the rib cage and iliac crest) and pressing deeper than when searching for the liver, may feel the kidney as it slips back up into place on expiration.

A grossly distended bladder may be visible on inspection, or it may be palpated in the suprapubic region, unless the subject is obese. More often, however, a tense bladder or a bladder enlarged by chronic retention is best detected by percussion in the midline. In acute retention, pressure over the bladder produces suprapubic tenderness and the urgent sensation of needing to void, while in elderly women, retention with overflow may be detected by incontinence occurring when the person stands. The disappearance of a midline mass after voiding or catheterization obviously confirms the identification of the mass as a full bladder. A uterine mass, too, is generally midline, but it is usually harder and often nodular. An enlarged ovary rises laterally to the midline and tends to be asymmetrical. Any lateral pelvic mass or any abdominal mass which becomes painful or increases in size must be precisely described as to size, location, consistency, mobility, and tenderness, and should be referred for further medical evaluation.

Examination of the genitalia involves visualization and palpation of the accessible structures and should never be omitted for reasons of modesty or expedience. In the elderly male, a carcinoma may be hidden beneath a tight prepuce, on a testis, or in the prostate. Phimosis, testicular swelling, hydrocele, and herniations are important to identify, as is any evidence of acute or chronic infection. The size, shape, consistency, mobility, and tenderness of the prostate should be meticulously determined on rectal examination, of course.

In the elderly female, since the clitoris and Bartholin's glands are favorite sites for malignancies to occur, these areas should be inspected and palpated with special care. Any patches of leukoplakia on the membranous surface of the vulva must also be noted and reported as a malignant precursor. The vulvar area is often found to be erythematous, edematous, and sometimes ulcerated in older women displaying "senile" or atrophic vulvitis secondary to estrogen depletion. Scratching in response to the irritation produces trauma and may cause secondary bacterial infections as well. This condition may also be an indicator of unregulated diabetes mellitus, a fungal infection, an allergic reaction, pernicious anemia, leukemia, hepatitis. Obviously, such underlying causes should be ruled out if possible before beginning symptomatic treatment; any lesions and urethral or vaginal discharges should be cultured and/or examined microscopically.

A bright red urethral caruncle protruding from the urethral meatus is a frequent finding in postmenopausal women, and prolapse of the bladder, the uterus, or the rectum is usually obvious when inspecting the vaginal introitus or when asking the subject to "bear down." This relaxation of the pelvic muscles and ligaments can usually be attributed originally to childbearing. Sagging of these structures increases with aging because of the loss of tonus and hormonal stimulation, resulting in complaints of low back pain, heaviness in the pelvic area, and problems with proper bowel and bladder function. Prolapse of some degree constitutes the single most common complaint in the older female and may be the cause of cystitis, constipation, stress incontinence, or urinary retention.

A rectal examination, identical to that done at any age, is an important final step of the physical examination of this area. Although the pelvic examination is beyond the scope of this chapter, at least a single finger bimanual exam and Pap smear should be performed routinely at five-year intervals or so. Usually, in asymptomatic elderly females, the vagina is atrophic; the cervix, uterus, and adnexa are rarely palpable; and it is unusual to gain significant information from such an examination. Still, in any woman with urinary retention or incontinence, a vaginal discharge, or vaginal bleeding, medical attention must be sought. In fact, in this age group, vaginal bleeding constitutes a quasi-emergency and can never be ignored (Birnbaum, 1971).

Clinical Considerations

Nurses dealing with elderly individuals who display symptoms of a urinary disorder need to make some careful distinctions in assessing the problem. Dysuria, when it occurs, for example, is usually a good indicator of an acute infection in either sex. However, since pain is either not present or poorly perceived in many cases, a urinary tract infection should always be considered whenever an unexplained fever, incontinence, or an increase in urinary frequency develops.

When urinary frequency is the main symptom, paying close attention to the quantity of urine voided as well as to the pattern of time intervals may provide valuable clues as to the underlying problem. For example, repeated small amounts of urine may signal a urinary tract infection or an irritative lesion of some kind, while numerous, large amounts of urine probably signify uncontrolled diabetes or chronic renal failure.

Requiring more than two trips to the bathroom per night is often accepted without question as being normal for an older person, yet the use of prescribed diuretics or tea, coffee, and other fluids ingested in the evening often are the cause of this exhausting disruption of sleep. Giving short acting diuretics in the morning and limiting liquids — especially those with a marked diuretic action — in the evening may reduce nocturia significantly. Nocturia in elderly men, associated with hesitancy and the diminution in force of the stream of urine, post-micturition dribbling, poor control, or overflow incontinence, on the other hand, points to prostatism as the probable source of difficulty. Conversely, a decrease in urinary frequency associated with a decreased volume of urine may be due either to developing cardiac failure, kidney failure, or the retention of urine because of obstruction.

Incontinence constitutes one of the most important causes of disability in this age group and may be the sole reason for a family to institutionalize an elderly relative. Investigating the circumstances under which wetting occurs may help to separate tremulousness in handling a bedpan or urinal from the overflow of prostatism or retention, and from incontinence due to infection or to a neurological cause. If constipation is also a problem, fecal impaction may be producing the urinary dysfunction. If the bathroom is too far for the subject or if he has trouble ambulating or very little warning of the need to urinate, a bedside commode may prevent accidents (Caird and Judge, 1974).

REFERENCES

Balchum, O.J. The aging respiratory system. In Chinn, A.B. (Ed.) Working with Older People, a Guide to Practice. *Clinical Aspects of Aging*, Vol. 4 (Government Publication No. 1459). Rockville, Md.: U.S. Department of Health, Education and Welfare, 1971, pp. 113–123.

Bates, B. The breasts and axilla. In *A Guide to Physical Examination* (2nd ed.). Philadelphia: J.B. Lippincott, 1979, pp. 186–199.

Birnbaum, S.J. Geriatric gynecology. In Chinn, A.B. (Ed.) Working with Older People, a Guide to Practice. *Clinical Aspects of Aging*, Vol. 4 (Government Publication No. 1459). Rockville, Md.: U.S. Department of Health, Education and Welfare, 1971, pp. 149–155.

Caird, F.I. and Judge T.G. *Assessment of the Elderly Patient* (2nd ed.). Philadelphia: J.B. Lippincott, 1979, pp. 40–47.

Harris, R. Special features of heart disease in the elderly patient. In Chinn, A.B. (Ed.) Working with Older People, a Guide to Practice. *Clinical Aspects of Aging*, Vol. 4 (Government Publication No. 1459). Rockville, Md.: U.S. Department of Health, Education and Welfare, 1971, pp. 81–98.

Kahn, A.I. and Snapper, I. Medical renal diseases in the aged. In Chinn, A.B. (Ed.) Working with Older People, a Guide to Practice. *Clinical Aspects of Aging*, Vol. 4 (Government Publication No. 1459). Rockville, Md.: U.S. Department of Health, Education and Welfare, 1971, pp. 131–140.

Leeming, J.T., Webster, S.P.G., and Dymock, I.W. The upper gastro-intestinal tract, small bowel and exocrine pancreas. In Brocklehurst, J.C. (Ed.) *Geriatric Medicine* (2nd ed.). New York: Churchill Livingstone, 1978, pp. 344–357.

Sklar, M. Gastrointestinal diseases in the aged. In Chinn, A.B. (Ed.) Working with Older People, a Guide to Practice. *Clinical Aspects of Aging*, Vol. 4 (Government Publication No. 1459). Rockville, Md.: U.S. Department of Health, Education and Welfare, 1971, pp. 24–130.

Strauss, B. Disorders of the digestive system. In Rossman, I. (Ed.) *Clinical Geriatrics* (2nd ed.). Philadelphia: J.B. Lippincott, 1979, pp. 266–289.

Wilson, J.L. Diseases of the breast. In Krupp, M.A. and Chatton, M.J. (Eds.) *Current Diagnosis and Treatment*. Los Altos, Calif.: Lange Medical Publishers, 1981, pp. 406–409.

20
The Musculoskeletal and Nervous Systems

Linda Ellison Jessup

"What the eyes see, the ears hear, and the fingers touch, gives our minds the shape of the ordinary or macroscopic world of the senses. Every person, due to his structure and experience, sees it a little differently."

Stuart Chase, (1954)

THE MUSCULOSKELETAL SYSTEM

Building and maintaining the body's musculoskeletal integrity are not subjects that usually receive much conscious thought until that system either sustains an injury or begins to falter. Often such an awakening occurs later in life, at which point most people tend to view "fractures" as being synonymous with "falling," and both occurrences are seen as major disasters, if not a death sentence. The dread that these specters inspire may be sufficient to cause an individual to severely curtail his activities and interests, and may throw him into despair if he does, in fact, sustain such an injury. Curiously, on the other hand, joint or muscle pain, bunions, and structural deformities of the digits are too often considered the price of longevity and accepted, without professional evaluation, as inevitable. Nurses have the opportunity to play a major part in separating real information from misinformation and in making people aware that the development and promotion of optimal structural integrity should begin ideally with good prenatal care and continue throughout life.

Most adults, for example, might be dismayed to realize that breaking the neck of a brittle femur by a sudden twist may actually precede a fall or other accident, while becoming overly cautious, venturing out less, and becoming increasingly sedentary in an effort to reduce the risk of accident may hasten bone resorption and actually leave bones more vulnerable to fractures. They might also be surprised to know that most falls do not result in fractures; that preventative measures — such as a diet which supplies adequate protein, calcium, and vitamins A, D, and C, and fairly vigorous exercise patterns — are effective in maintaining strong skeletons and connective tissues throughout life; and that when older people do suffer fractures, they usually still possess a tremendous potential to heal, often with an abundance of callus formation (Aloia, 1981).

Normal Changes

Muscles.

- As aging progresses, muscle fibers decrease both in number and in mass. The more prominent muscles of the arms and legs may appear to be thin and flabby, while the corresponding loss of bulk in the small muscles is especially noticeable in the hand which becomes thin and bony, with deep interosseous spaces.
- While muscular strength decreases overall, along with endurance and agility, it does not diminish to the degree one might expect in proportion to the loss of muscle bulk. The muscles are not normally sore, their strength should be symmetrical, and the occasional muscle twitching (fasciculation) which can sometimes be seen when a muscle is at rest is not accompanied by severe weakness or wasting.
- The older person's movements generally decrease in number and slow down with age, due to involuntarily changes of the extrapyramidal system. A resting tremor may be present.

- There is an increase in muscle rigidity, especially in the extremities and the neck, which reduces the range of motion slightly. The legs are more resistant to passive movement than the arms, and the proximal aspects of the limbs are more rigid than the distal aspects.
- Defects in conjugate upward gaze and convergence of the eyes occur normally in some older people. The pupils accommodate more slowly and respond more sluggishly to light.
- There is some shrinkage and sclerosis of tendons and muscles which decrease the briskness of the tendon reflexes. Ankylosis of the ligaments and joints also combines with these changes to draw the older frame into the slightly flexed posture characteristic of later life.

Joints.

- There is some noninflammatory deterioration and abrasion of the articular cartilage of weight-bearing joints (osteoarthritis), giving rise to new bone at the joint surface, which is universally present and demonstrable histologically in people over 20 years of age.
- The degree of articular tissue change increases with age, although only a small proportion of people with radiologic changes actually experience local symptoms.

Bones.

- There is a progressive reduction in total bone mass throughout later life, probably a result of bone resorption. The vertebral column and intervertebral disks actually shrink and become bowed forward, producing a loss of height and contributing to the posture of general flexion (see description of general appearance in Chapter 16).
- Collagen fibers, which are necessary as a matrix upon which minerals are deposited to give bones their hardness, as well as for the healing of the soft tissue which

surrounds bones and joints, are less elastic, thicker, and thus less mobile (Grob, 1971).

Physical Examination

The examination of the back ordinarily begins with the subject supine. The examiner watches the individual respond to the request to turn to each side and then to sit up. The spine can then be inspected, with the normal cervical, thoracic, and lumbar curves noted. If there is a marked degree of kyphosis or scoliosis, the possibility of it displacing the heart should be kept in mind during the evaluation of the cardiovascular system. Lordosis may also make the aorta easier to feel and must thus be taken into account in assessing a possible aortic aneurysm. Each of the vertebral spines should be pressed or percussed for tenderness affecting on the spines themselves and not the spinal muscles. Such localized tenderness is the sign of an acute process of the involved vertebrae, such as a recent fracture or vertebral collapse due to inflammatory or metastatic disease (Caird and Judge, 1979).

The upper dorsal muscles, i.e., the trapezius and scapular muscles, are inspected and palpated for tenderness and wasting, and the sacrum is examined for edema and pressure lesions. Reddening of the skin is also looked for over the greater trochanters and buttocks, over projecting vertebral spines, between the knees, and on the malleoli and heels.

Finally, the range of motion of the back is noted, along with muscle spasm and pain with motion. The subject is then asked to sit, thereby testing the power of the spinal musculature and the hip flexors, as well as their ability to coordinate in arriving at and maintaining a sitting position. Patients with parkinsonism, for example, will have great difficulty maintaining a sitting posture when they are displaced sideways or backwards, and they have more trouble moving from a lying to a sitting position than they do walking.

The upper extremities are inspected and palpated for their temperature (may be cool but should not be cold) and evidence of cyanosis, indicating the status of the peripheral circulation. The fingertips are also observed for nail pulsations, a sign rare in this age group but one which can indicate a pulmonary heart disease, and clubbing, a sinister sign when it develops in an older person, suggesting bronchial carcinoma. The position of the hands is noted at rest, along with any tremor at rest or when in motion. Heberden's nodes on the dorsolateral aspects of the distal interphalangeal joints are usually hard and painless, and may or may not be associated with osteoarthritis in other joints (see Figure 20-1).

The skin is observed for the presence of "senile purpura," bruising which is often seen on the dorsum of the hand and forearm of institutionalized elderly people, but rarely on those living at home. These lesions are characterized by their purple color and by having at least one straight edge. "Senile scars" are white areas in the dermis which have spider-like strands branching out where old tears of the dermis have been repaired.

The palms are also examined for wasting or thickening of the palmar fascia and Dupuytren's contracture, by having the subject first extend and spread the fingers of both hands, then make a fist with the thumbs across the knuckle.

All the joints of the upper extremities are examined in turn; each joint is inspected while it is supported and at rest, with the least possible degree of pain and muscle spasm. Symmetrical joints should be compared with each other for deformities (i.e., swelling, contractures, or ankylosis), the size and contour of the joint, and the color and temperature of the overlying skin. Areas of tenderness, thickening of the synovium, fluctuating areas of effusions, and crepitus are located by palpation. The range of motion with both active and passive movement is also checked.

The muscles are gently squeezed between the examiner's thumb and index finger to elicit tenderness or to detect the unusual hardness of a tonic contraction. Muscle strength is finally tested by having the subject push and pull against the resisting hand of the nurse, then grasp and squeeze her hands, and by comparing one hand or arm with the other.

The examination of the lower extremities begins with the observation of the subject's gait and assessment of his footwear (stockings, slippers, and/or shoes). It is important to check these articles of clothing both for fit and for stability, to determine if garters are worn, and

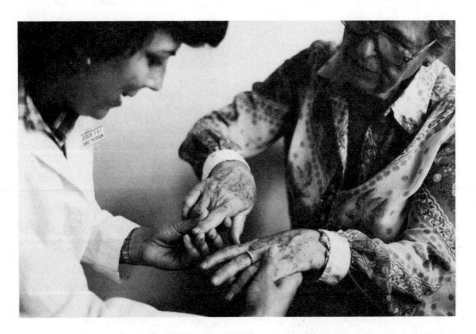

Figure 20-1. Pain in the joints or muscles and structural deformities of the digits are often accepted by the elderly, without professional evaluation, as inevitable.

to note if there is evidence that circulatory return is reduced by them. If walking aids are used, their use must also be evaluated. Floppy slippers, poorly fitting shoes, and the misuse of crutches, canes, and walkers can all put an older person at great risk from falls.

Next, the feet are inspected for cleanliness and lesions such as corns, bunions, blisters, plantar warts, and evidence of fungal infections. Deformities, hallux valgus (a medial deviation of the great toe which affects the second toe as well), and the raised "hammer toe" are noted. The nails are inspected to see whether they are overgrown, ingrown, thickened, infected with fungi, or discolored. The skin is inspected for redness or blisters, fissures between the toes, a shiny, thin appearance, and the disappearance of hair on the toes which is a sensitive indicator of even mild degrees of ischemia.

The absence of the dorsalis pedis and posterior tibial pulses is not uncommon in the elderly, even without other evidence of claudication or ischemia. If these cannot be detected, check for the presence of the popliteal and femoral pulses, and feel with the back of the hand for a temperature gradient to help establish the status of the peripheral circulation.

The rest of the leg is then inspected for equality, which may be checked (if there is any doubt) by measuring and comparing the length of each extremity and the width of each thigh and calf. Varicosities are noted along with "varicose ulcers" or the bronze pigmentation called "stasis dermatitis" which may accompany them. Firm pressure along the dorsal aspect of the foot and up the shin, to locate the level and degree of pitting edema which may be present, is done systematically and then compared bilaterally when edema is found. Bruises on the legs or knees often point to evidence of recent falls or even abuse of the subject by another person.

Palpation of the legs is undertaken methodically, by compressing the muscle bodies gently and paying attention both to muscle tone and to any areas of tenderness. A venous thrombosis should be suspected when unilateral tenderness is found in the area of the calf, especially when the overlying skin temperature is also increased and the superficial veins on the front of the calf

are dilated. Homans' sign in the elderly is less frequently present as an indicator of this condition.

The joints are examined as they were in the upper extremities, with particular attention given to the internal and external rotation of the hip. The earliest sign of hip disease, especially osteoarthritis, is limitation of internal rotation. The strength of the muscle bodies and mobility of the joints are likewise tested by passive and active pressure, movement of the toes, plantar flexion and dorsiflexion of the ankle, flexion and extension of the knee, flexion of the hip, the ability to get up out of a chair (the iliopsoas and quadriceps), and the ability to stand on tiptoe. Testing of the reflexes and sensory testing are usually carried out in the course of the neurological examination.

Clinical Considerations

Back pain is a common complaint of elderly people, and once again, the history of this symptom is often an excellent indicator of the nature of the problem. If the person has suffered for years from this pain, it is probably more likely due to a degenerative process such as osteoarthritis of the spine or to osteomalacia (a deficiency of vitamin D and, thus, easily treated) than to a more ominous cause. Pain of sudden onset, such as that developing after a fall, more often indicates a sprain, fracture, or metastatic deposit. The nurse's task is to determine the history as precisely as possible and to pinpoint the location and nature of the symptom, if it radiates or is present on twisting the trunk or coughing. She should also note muscle spasm and look for sensory changes along nerve pathways.

In the upper extremities, pain and the loss of function are the most common complaints. Pain resulting from joint disease is usually accompanied by other signs such as localized erythema, restriction of movement, and local tenderness, while pain which is referred, such as the pain of angina, does not affect function.

Pain in the proximal interphalangeal and metacarpophalangeal joints of the fingers, wrists, elbows, and shoulders, usually bilateral with pain especially on moving but also at rest, is most often due to rheumatoid arthritis. Stiffness after

inactivity and upon awakening is also characteristic of this disease, which may affect the ankles,
hips, and temporomandibular joints as well.
Rheumatoid arthritis is usually polyarticular
and symmetrical, and it should be remembered
that it can begin for the first time in an elderly
person with either an insidious or an acutely
inflammatory onset.

Shoulder pain is not uncommon in the
elderly, and it is often arthritic in origin.
"Frozen shoulder," however, is a chronic
tenosynovitis of unknown cause which produces
severe pain (especially at night) and is characterized by a notable limitation of movement,
especially abduction. Giant cell arteritis and
polymyalgia rheumatica are both diseases which
affect the shoulder area and cause local tenderness, but do not involve the joint capsule and
thus do not limit movement of the shoulder
joint.

Problems in the lower extremities involving
the hips or knees are assessed by the same
criteria as those symptoms involving the major
joint areas of the upper extremities. The
duration of the problem, the nature of its
onset, and its relation to movement, especially
walking and sitting, are the most useful points
to establish. Pain of sudden onset affecting the
hip is most likely due to a fracture or to acute
arthritis. Pain which appears gradually in this
region is probably caused by a chronic, degenerative process (osteoarthritis), although an
unidentified fracture is also possible. The
degree of pain on movement with any of
these conditions will limit the person's desire
and ability to walk, of course.

Pain referred to the hip from the back does
not ordinarily make its initial appearance in the
elderly. If these symptoms are present, they
have generally occurred before. More often,
pain from acute or chronic arthritis in the hip is
referred to the knee, confusing the examiner
who looks no further as to its source. As a
general rule of thumb, acute knee pain is
attributed to the knee joint itself only when an
effusion is present or when there is tenderness
along the joint line.

Many elderly adults complain of discomfort
of the lower legs, which takes a variety of
forms. Painful cramping of a single muscle

group in the leg or foot, usually developing at
night, can occur at any time but often becomes
increasingly bothersome with age. While underlying conditions may be at fault, such as
peripheral vascular insufficiency, sodium or
calcium deficiency, or hypoglycemia, generally
the cause is unknown. This night cramping can
usually be relieved by gentle but firm hyperextension of the foot during an episode, by
exercises which stretch the calf muscles during
the day, and sometimes by the administration
of calcium or quinine.

Other strange sensations which afflict older
people are a burning and tingling sensation
involving the soles of the feet which again
seems to occur primarily at night, a jerking of
the legs as a person relaxes and begins to fall
asleep, and a tingling sensation occurring night
or day called the "restless legs syndrome." In

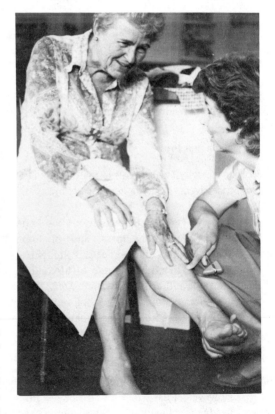

Figure 20-2. The lower legs seem to be a site of frequent
discomfort in the elderly. Night cramping, tingling or
burning sensations and the irritating "restless legs
syndrome" are just a few of the forms these problems
assume.

this latter condition, the irritating sensation occurs when the legs have been still for a period of time. Movement dispells the tingling, so that the individual tends to keep his legs in motion.

Intermittent claudication, a more serious problem, is usually fairly easy to identify because it is a cramping sensation in the calf area which occurs with exercise and which is relieved by rest. Because the cramping is produced by vascular spasms and underlying arteriosclerosis, the distance the individual can walk before the discomfort begins tends to be relatively consistent and, thus, predictable.

THE NERVOUS SYSTEM

The nervous system is primarily a network of stimulus-response relationships, the intricate switchboard of the body. It is a dynamic system, a system which matures late and which has a remarkable capacity for adaptation. Like many other parts of the body, it also has an enormous reserve which makes possible a wide variety of responses to a single event, highly complex and varied behavior in a single individual, and even a fairly large loss of mass without marked alterations in the individual's functioning.

Normal Changes

Morphologically, we see three major degenerative processes in the aging nervous system.

- There is generalized atrophy of the brain surface, of brain mass, and of brain cells. Atrophy of brain cells is thought to begin by the third decade of life and to continue rather steadily thereafter. Probably because of the huge total number of brain cells, some of which may serve as a reserve supply, the brain usually functions well throughout an individual's lifetime, despite great numerical losses, without any major signs of intellectual disability. However, this structural shrinkage may produce behavioral changes, diminished emotional responses, confusion or disorientation, a narrowing of interests, memory impairment, and a reduced ability to learn new materials. Yet there are also

psychological components of defenses and energy-conserving mechanisms which produce similar results with or without generalized atrophy.
- An atrophy of the tendon reflexes occurs, resulting in stimulus-response changes which are especially notable in diminished tactile discrimination and a raised pain threshold. These changes may be due more to the atrophy of muscles and tendons, however, then to changes in the reflex arc.
- There is neuron pigmentation which diminishes the control of the nervous system over the circulation. This change increases the elderly individual's susceptibility to shock.

Physical Examination

All of the previous portions of the examination process provide the broad base necessary for accurately assessing the function of the subject's nervous system in all its complexity. In fact, many of the steps which constitute the "routine neurologic examination" have already been incorporated in earlier parts of the exam, as the nurse proceeds with this head-to-toe investigation. The older person's speech and language function, emotional status, memory, judgment, and behavior have all been repeatedly demonstrated throughout the history-taking process and in all the interpersonal interactions up to this point. Some of the cranial nerves were assessed with the head and neck, and the peripheral vascular and musculoskeletal systems were evaluated when the extremities were inspected. At this point, however, the remaining portions of the examination are carried out, and the findings are organized and described for the neurological system as a whole.

The neurologic examination involves the same steps for the elderly as for any adult subject; it consists of the following items:

- Assessment of the person's mental status and speech, including a description of his state of consciousness and mood as well as his orientation to time, person, and place

- Testing the 12 cranial nerves
- Observation of the subject's motor function
- Assessment of the sensory mechanisms (light touch, pain, vibration, and proprioception)
- Testing of the tendon reflexes and the plantar response

Mental Status. With any subject who is not entirely responsive, a precise description of his level of consciousness and the stimuli to which he does or does not react is always much more useful than a classification such as "stuporous" or "semicomatose." Since a person's mental state may also be altered by fatigue or in response to certain individuals or situations, the changes and factors which seem to precipitate them should be noted.

When the older person is alert, the author has found that using one of the simple, standard tools as a guide for assessing depression, anxiety states, and organic brain disorders is extremely helpful when employed in conjunction with the examiner's ongoing observations (Kahn et al., 1960). These brief series of quantifiable questions prevent arbitrary judgments and serve as rather sensitive indices of mild to moderate problems of mood or intellectual impairment, which might otherwise easily be missed or discounted in a person who is pleasant and in whom social behavior is well preserved.

A simple introductory explanation should be offered when such a tool is used. For example, the examiner might say, "I'm going to ask you a few standard questions about your memory and concentration now. As you've gotten older, have you noticed any difference in how you think?" or "The questions I'm going to ask you have to do with how you're feeling within yourself."

Many questions relevant to memory can be incorporated in the history-taking process, provided the information can be checked against other reliable sources. An evaluation of the subject's ability to calculate and his judgment can also be included deliberately in obtaining the history, while the person's general

appearance and his behavior throughout the interaction provide a wealth of information for the observant nurse.

Once again, change from the person's previous behavior or from his intellectual or personality pattern is more important than any particular characteristic or group of characteristics. Equally indicative is the speed with which this change has occurred. A rapid deterioration suggests a vascular episode, an acute response to medications, a fever, physical illness, a sudden emotional shock, or a metabolic disorder, and may well be remediable. Investigation of the cause must be immediate and thorough to minimize the chance of permanent damage occurring.

Deterioration which has developed gradually over a period of months or years is more likely due to a chronic, progressive process such as cerebral arteriosclerosis, a tumor, or an undetected condition such as hypothyroidism, a low grade drug toxicity, or a gradual sensory loss. Many of the causes of chronic deterioration can also be corrected or arrested if they are sought and recognized. Mild to severe anxiety or depression may overlie any of the acute or chronic conditions afflicting an elderly person, of course, which complicates the picture still further.

The Cranial Nerves. Examination of the cranial nerves proceeds as for any adult patient. Only the areas in which some differences may be commonly noted for this particular age group are summarized (the number of the cranial nerve appears in parentheses):

- *Olfactory nerve* (first). The progressive bilateral loss of the sense of smell may occur in later years, especially in people with a history of chronic rhinitis.
- *Optic nerve* (second). The decreased visual acuity for near objects (presbyopia) commonly found in the older adult is due to the impaired elasticity of the lens rather than to deterioration of the optic nerve.
- *Oculomotor nerve* (third). Defects in conjugate upward gaze and convergence of the eyes occur normally in some older

people, but they may also occur in individuals with Parkinson's disease and in those with severe brain dysfunction.

The pupils of old people may display a slightly irregular margin bilaterally and may be smaller, with a slower, less marked response to direct and consensual stimulation and to accommodation. Still, the pupils should be equal in size and should constrict visibly when stimulated.

- *Trigeminal nerve* (fifth). Three important reflexes, which are present in infancy and then suppressed early in life, may be released again in later years as the result of cerebral cortical atrophy and other diffuse disorders of the cerebral hemispheres.

1. The snout reflex consists of a quick pursing of the lips and may be seen occurring spontaneously in some elderly people. It may be elicited by a light tap beneath the nose with the examiner's finger.

2. The blink reflex consists of the forced closure of the eyes when the examiner, standing behind the subject with the tapping finger coming over the subject's forehead, lightly percusses the bony prominence on the frontal bone joining the supraorbital ridges (i.e., the glabella). This reflex is present in patients with parkinsonism and in those with generalized brain disease, and occasionally is found in otherwise normal older people.

3. The snout reflex is often accompanied by the sucking reflex, which is tested for by gently stroking the lips from the center laterally with a tongue blade. If the reflex is present, the lips will protrude and close around the blade, or if very pronounced, the tongue, head, and lips will follow the blade and attempt to take hold of it. The first two reflexes are pathologic but cannot be ascribed to lesions in any specific region of the brain. They are elicited in the area supplied by the fifth nerve. The sucking reflex is due

to destruction of the medial premotor portions of the frontal lobe (Prior and Silberstein, 1977).

- *Facial nerve* (seventh) *and glossopharyngeal nerve* (ninth). The sense of taste is frequently diminished in the elderly, with the sensation of sour and bitterness tending to be lost last. The seventh nerve transmits taste sensations on the anterior two-thirds of the tongue (sweet at the tip, salt at the tip and sides, and sour on the sides), while the ninth nerve registers the sensations (primarily bitter tastes) on the posterior third of the tongue.

- *Acoustic nerve* (eighth). Presbycusis, the sensorineural hearing loss caused by the involution of the cochlea and neurons of the higher auditory pathways, produces a progressive loss first of high frequency sounds and then of midfrequency sounds; eventually, low frequencies may be lost as well.

Motor Activity. Examination of gross motor activity begins with the critical assessment of the individual's gait. Standing and walking are actually very complex and revealing action which require muscle strength and coordination, proprioception, vestibular function, and vision.

The subject, wearing shoes for maximum security and support, is given the Romberg test, with the nurse standing near enough to protect him if he should lose his balance. A person with cerebellar disease will have difficulty maintaining a normal stance even with his eyes open and will automatically broaden his stance to stabilize himself. If proprioception is impaired, the subject will show increased swaying and unsteadiness when he closes his eyes. In a situation where there is acute, unilateral vestibular dysfunction, the person tends to fall to the affected side.

Next, the subject is asked to step out freely at his normal pace, and the examiner carefully notes the onset of walking, whether the stride, however distorted, looks stable enough to be safe, and how the individual turns. If the examiner senses a subtle deficit, heel-toe walking in a straight line may exaggerate the gait abnormality so that it can be more easily analyzed. If possible, it is also desirable to watch the person ascend and descend a short flight of stairs and demonstrate how he manipulates any walking aids he normally uses.

Some commonly observed gaits which are suggestive of important underlying muscular, joint-related, or neurological problems may be recognized by an alert examiner. The "propulsive gait" of parkinsonism begins with short, shuffling steps, with the person leaning forward as if in pursuit, yet with rigid arms which move very slightly and mechanically. The individual may have difficulty checking his gait and will turn clumsily, again with short, shuffling steps. A person with severe brain disease often walks with a tottery, shuffling gait and tiny steps similar to the individual with parkinsonism, but the former is able to turn without difficulty. The lateral reeling and wide-based stagger of a person with cerebellar disease appear drunken and totally ataxic, while a person with a pyramidal tract disorder steps out with obviously unequal lengths of steps, the unaffected leg carrying him further with each step than the affected one (Caird and Judge, 1979).

The abnormal elevation of a hip suggests pain or stiffness in that area, while a less marked degree of elevation in the moving leg may point to a stiff knee as the source of trouble. People with bilateral hip disease, obesity, or proximal muscle wasting demonstrate a characteristic side-to-side waddle. Bilateral spastic paresis produces scissoring of the knees, while the legs are moved forward in a jerky manner, accompanied by extreme, compensatory movements of the trunk; in the hemiplegic gait, there is circumduction of the spastic leg and the foot moves in an arc during forward movement. A person with foot drop often shows some circumduction accompanied by an abnormal elevation of the limb (Prior and Silberstein, 1977).

The inspection of muscle bodies for atrophy, fasciculations, involuntary movements of other kinds, or abnormalities of position, and the assessment of muscle tone, tenderness, and strength have already been included in the evaluation of the musculoskeletal system. Now, having the subject hold his arms straight in front,

palms up, with his eyes closed for 30 or 40 seconds, provides a sensitive test for early neurological problems in the upper extremities. The drifting or falling away of an arm or the tendency to pronation suggests a mild pyramidal tract disorder.

Coordination of arms, hands, and legs is tested in the usual way with rapid, rhythmic alternating movements and point-to-point testing. Cerebellar disease results in poor coordination, awkwardness, and inaccuracy, while inaccuracy only when the eyes are closed indicates a loss of position sense.

Any tremors which are noticed during this evaluation should be described, along with any other characteristics that accompany them. For example, the pill-rolling tremor of parkinsonism occurs at rest and is temporarily decreased by movement. Typically, general slow movement (bradykinesia) and cogwheel rigidity will also be present. The common "familial" or "essential" tremor, by contrast, involves a side-to-side or fine-bobbing, resting tremor of the head and an irregular, lateral deviation of the individual's fingers, which is accentuated by voluntary movement and emotional stress.

Cerebellar tremors too are action tremors, becoming more obvious when repetitive movements are performed, such as patting the thigh or finger-nose-finger touching. These actions will seem awkward, will vary in force, and will not all land at the same point. Muscle tone is usually diminished in this condition, and nystagmus may also be present. The coarse tremor of metabolic disease, which results in the flapping action of the hands, occurs in very sick patients with chronic hepatic disease ("liver flap") or chronic respiratory failure.

The apraxias are worthy of special note in dealing with the elderly. In these disorders, muscle function is normal, but when given verbal instructions to perform "as if" acts (i.e., "Act as if you were blowing out a match, combing your hair, drinking from a cup . . ."), the subject seems to have forgotten how to comply. If a real match, comb, or cup is given to the person, however, his performance often improves because of the additional tactile and visual cues. The apraxias occur with lesions of the hemisphere which is dominant for the particular function that is requested, producing a bilateral motor disorder.

Sensory Mechanism. The occurrence of general sensory changes due specifically to the processes of aging is a subject which is still under investigation. Although opinions vary on the subject, in this author's experience, a decrease in sensory acuity to light touch and vibration, and a raised threshold to certain kinds of pain, are frequent findings in otherwise neurologically intact older people.

Sensory testing is tiring, so a general survey should be conducted as efficiently as possible to serve as a screening device. Testing for hot and cold sensory perception may be omitted if pain sensation is found to be normal in the arms, trunk, and legs, for example. If vibration is perceived in distal portions of the extremity, testing the more proximal areas of the limb may be omitted. Each area tested is compared with the corresponding area on the opposite side of the body, and any area of sensory loss to pain, temperature, light touch, or vibration is mapped out with care by the examiner, moving from the area of reduced sensation to areas of accurate perception.

Testing for position sense of an arm can be done by grasping the sleeve of the extremity, in order to minimize gross sensory cues, and by asking the subject to catch the thumb of his suspended hand. After rehearsing this maneuver with the eyes open, the subject should be instructed to repeat the process with his eyes closed. When he shuts his eyes, the limb should be moved to a new position before the person is again prompted to reach for his thumb. Normally, he should be able to move toward and grasp the thumb precisely. With a minor proprioceptive impairment he may catch his hand instead, while with a severe deficit he will either miss the limb entirely or, locating some part of it, will feel his way up the arm until he arrives at the thumb (Caird and Judge, 1979).

When the foregoing tests for sensory acuity and position sense are intact, testing for stereognosis is useful to determine posterior column function. If arthritis or motor impairment makes it difficult for the elderly person to manipulate familiar objects (a key, a coin,

cotton, etc.), the examiner can use the blunt end of a pen or pencil to draw a large number in the person's palm. Most normal older people can identify these numerals accurately.

Two-point discrimination is tested in the usual way on the finger pads. Touching the subject, whose eyes are closed, at a single point on his trunk or legs and then having him open his eyes and point to the place which was touched ("point localization") constitute another useful test for evaluating the sensory cortex, especially when this is given in conjunction with the "extinction" test. In this latter movement, two corresponding points on the body (cheek and cheek, hand and hand, etc.) are touched simultaneously and the subject is asked where he feels the touch. Ordinarily he should identify both points of contact.

Nurse examiners need to be aware of a common disorder seen in some stroke victims with lesions affecting the dominant parietal and temporal cortex. In this situation, the patient may neglect his hemiparetic side, failing to recognize his own left hand, paying little attention to any stimulus approaching from the left, and generally rejecting the existence of his left side in spite of a good return of strength. This problem must be identified early since it poses very real difficulties for self-care and for the rehabilitation process. This person, suffering from a right parietal lesion, will fail the test for position sense, often grasping the examiner's thumb instead and insisting that it is his own. He may also leave his left side unclothed and omit the details on the left of simple geometric figures (a star, a triangle, or a clock) that he is asked to draw.

Reflexes. Examination of the reflexes of the elderly may show a decrease in the briskness of these responses in general, with only the ankle jerk and the abdominal reflexes frequently unobtainable. Still, the biceps, triceps, brachioradialis, and knee reflexes should be present and symmetrical in neurologically normal older people. Severe arthritis in the knees, which can cause the knee jerk to be depressed or absent, may be an exception to this rule. Identification of abnormally brisk knee jerks is frequently aided by the presence of a marked adduction of the hips bilaterally when the reflex is elicited. When hyperactive reflexes exist, the examiner must test — gently — for ankle clonus. Sustained clonus indicates upper neuron disease. The elderly should respond to the test for the plantar response with the normal flexion of the toes.

All areas of functioning echo, to some degree, the impact of any neurological insult on the system. The nature of the problem, the older person's resources, and the aging process itself — all help to shape reasonable treatment goals. Thus, neurological problems in the elderly generally require not only all the skill nursing can supply, but also the concerted and coordinated efforts of medicine, physical therapy, and social services.

REFERENCES

Aloia, J.F. Exercise and skeletal health. *Journal of the American Geriatrics Society* **29**(3):104-107 (1981).

Caird, F.I. and Judge, T.G. *Assessment of the Elderly Patient* (2nd ed.). London: Pitman Medical Publishing, 1979, pp. 56-61, 86, 77-116, 100-101.

Chase, Stuart. Our Amazing Network of Nerves. In *Power of Words*. New York: Harcourt Brace Jovanovick, Inc., 1954, p. 56.

Kahn, R.L. et al. Brief objective measures for the determination of mental status in the aged. *American Journal of Psychiatry* **117**:326 (1960).

Prior, J.A. and Silberstein, J.S. *Physical Diagnosis, the History and Examination of the Patient* (5th ed.). St. Louis: C.V. Mosby, 1977, pp. 400-401, 405-407.

Part V
Clinical Conditions in the Elderly and Implications for Nursing

21
Cardiovascular Conditions in Older Adults

Frances S. Knudsen

Heart disease related to ischemia causes one-third of the nation's total mortality. Moreover, age-specific death rates from heart disease increase sharply with advancing years for both men and women (Recent Trends, 1979). Heart disease remains the major cause of disability and death in our aged population. Educational efforts in health maintenance have made a significant impact, but still more can be achieved in rehabilitating and maintaining cardiac wellness in older individuals.

From 1969 through 1977, age-adjusted death rates for ischemic and related heart disease decreased 19% among white men and 24% among white women (Recent Trends, 1979). Many factors are believed to have contributed to this decline: reduced smoking, diets lower in fats and calories, better understanding of heart-related disorders, more reliable diagnostic tools, better emergency medical care (paramedic rescue teams and coronary care units), and earlier detection and treatment of hypertension. By and large, it is believed that these tremendous strides are due to health education and its resultant public awareness of risk factors in heart disease and changes in life-styles (Recent Trends, 1979). The aged population, already victimized by cardiovascular problems, is in need of preventive and maintenance measures (secondary and tertiary prevention). Older individuals are generally very receptive to health education when approached individually.

Anatomical changes in the heart are few after age 25. The heart size remains unchanged or becomes smaller due to decreased activity. Accumulations of pigment (lipofuscin granules) and subpericardial fat increase with age. Sclerosis and fibrosis cause the valves to thicken and become rigid (Timiras, 1972).

Functionally the heart becomes a less effective pump due to cellular changes in myocardial metabolism, loss of muscle fibers, decreased cardiac output, increased irritability of the myocardium, reduced strength and efficiency of contraction, changes in the conduction system, and other biochemical, anatomical, and physiological changes (Harris, 1978). The aged heart is able to maintain the normal activities of daily living, but tachycardia and/or hypertension may be prolonged during occasions of stress.

Vascular changes throughout the body become quite evident with increasing age. Arteries become less elastic as calcium and plaques accumulate in the intima. Valves in veins become less efficient, and varicose veins or ulcers may develop. Blood vessels may become occluded or rupture, and tissues normally nourished by those vessels suffer ischemia from the compromised circulation.

Certain specific cardiovascular problems occur with more frequency than others in the geriatric patient. Those involving the heart include ischemic heart disease, hypertension, congestive heart failure, endocarditis, arrhythmias, and conduction disruptions.

The most common problems of arteries and veins in older individuals are chronic and acute arterial occlusions, aneurysms, transient ischemic attacks, cerebrovascular accidents, phlebitis, and varicosities. Raynaud's disease and Buerger's disease will not be discussed in this book. Older adults may have these two conditions, but the onset usually occurs in young adulthood.

CARDIAC PROBLEMS

Ischemic Heart Disease
(Coronary Artery Disease)

The most frequently occurring heart pathology in old age is ischemic heart disease which may lead to coronary occlusion (Kannel, McGee, and Gordon, 1976). Its prevalence and severity increase with age. The coronary arteries become narrowed due to atherosclerosis or thrombosis, and the supply of blood and oxygen to the myocardium is inadequate.

Unlike younger adults with ischemia, the aged usually do not suffer cardiac pain. Instead they complain of dyspnea, substernal pressure, or pain from a digestive, bladder, or tooth problem. Exertion, overeating, emotional upset, or exposure to inclement weather may precipitate the complaint which is frequently relieved with a few minutes of rest. Nightmares and Cheyne-Stokes respirations may cause the patient to awaken with dyspnea from a sound sleep. As ischemia increases, greater severity or persistence of symptoms results.

The patient with ischemia severe enough to cause tissue necrosis or a myocardial infarction (coronary occlusion) usually appears more ill. His chest pain or pressure is severe; he becomes cold, clammy, and cyanotic; his blood pressure falls; his pulse becomes weak and thready; and his urinary output is reduced or absent.

Nearly one-fourth of those with myocardial infarction have "silent" or atypical attacks and go undiagnosed. The possibility of a myocardial infarction should be explored whenever older patients experience a sudden change in appearance, behavior, and/or mental processes, or whenever they experience hiccups or vomiting (Harris, 1978; Kart, Metress, and Metress, 1978).

Nursing Implications. Sublingual nitroglycerin is frequently used to control cardiac ischemia in aged individuals. A range in dosage is usually prescribed. Nurses can encourage patients to try the lowest dosage in the prescribed range. This minimal dosage frequently relieves symptoms without causing the undesirable and uncomfort-able side effects of headache, flushing, and hypotension. Since nitroglycerin reduces blood pressure, patients should be cautioned to sit or lie down after taking it. After using sublingual nitroglycerin, patients should be advised not to swallow for a few minutes in order to promote maximal absorption of the medication through the oral mucosa.

In aged individuals, pulmonary edema and congestive heart failure may develop quickly. The nurse should watch for and report any significant changes that develop, and should be prepared for necessary resuscitative efforts.

Bypass surgery may be resorted to if the medical regime is ineffectual. Generally, treatment of severe ischemic heart disease includes rest until the injured heart heals, relief of pain and emotional stress, and maintenance of homeostasis. Prolonged bed rest is inadvisable for older patients. Chair rest is preferable since it increases circulation and respiratory ventilation. Chair rest also reduces the incidence of thrombophlebitis, decubiti, hypostatic pneumonia, pulmonary embolism, urinary incontinence, constipation, and psychological deterioration. The older cardiac patient can and should return to his usual physical and social activities while taking care to guard against emotional and physical stress (Dehn, 1980; Devney, 1980; Harris, 1978; Hoepfel-Harris, 1980; Winslow and Weber, 1980).

Although older individuals usually adapt their activity to their physical limitations, most might benefit from counseling about avoiding strenuous outbursts of activity, especially in extreme temperatures or strong winds, and about the use of relaxation techniques to minimize emotional stress. Patients should be encouraged to keep physically active with walking, bicycling, dancing, and/or swimming.

A prudent diet should be maintained. Excessive fat, salt or sodium, and sugar should be avoided. Patients need to be taught to read labels to determine the sodium content of food, beverages, and over-the-counter drugs. Many need to be cautioned to avoid water that is high in sodium because it has been processed with a water softener or conditioner. Lifetime habits pose a challenge in counseling older people to reduce their intake of foods high in sodium and to alter the use of salt in food preparation and at the table. Individualized dietary plans need to be developed with individual patients and their families. Patients may find it helpful to keep a diary to record dietary and other health problems for review and discussion with the health team members. The health team members' individualized interest in the patient is a highly motivating factor for compliance of older persons.

Printed educational materials are usually helpful. Materials can be obtained from the American Heart Association, or they can be developed by the health team members (Ketchum, 1980). The older person usually adheres to individualized health care plans better than a younger person. This is especially true if the older person lives with someone who assists him in remembering to take his medicine, follow his diet, or exercise (Knudsen, 1979). Therefore, health personnel should include significant others in educational programs for patients.

Congestive Heart Failure

Congestive heart failure (CHF) results when the myocardium can no longer pump blood efficiently and the body's circulation becomes congested. It is a frequent complication in those with organic heart disease or atherosclerosis, especially in the elderly. The symptoms of CHF are exertional dyspnea, paroxysmal nocturnal dyspnea (PND), coughing, wheezing, and hemoptysis. Nausea and vomiting with abdominal pain may be present. Disruptions in fluid balance may cause edema and oliguria. Unusual weakness and fatigue may also be present. Often the patient needs guidance in reporting his symptoms. He may have limited his activities to avoid dyspnea on exertion. Exploration of his sleeping habits may reveal the PND or the need for sleeping on several pillows or in a recliner. He may have nocturia although his urinary output during the day is decreased. He may experience gastrointestinal symptoms due to inadequate perfusion or congestion of the digestive organs (Atwood, 1979).

Cardiac signs of CHF may be present. These include abnormal sounds, sternal lifts or heaves, and displacement of the apical impulse below

Table 21-1. Assessment of Edema.

I.   Keep a daily weight record.
II. Keep a record of fluid intake and output.
III. Make periodic measurements of the circumference of the extremities.
IV. Periodically estimate pitting (the depth tissue is able to be depressed over bony surfaces) – record this in millimeters and specify the sites. (The examiner who has measured the nail width of her index finger can use it for comparison in approximating the depth of the depression.)

the fifth intercostal space to the left of the midclavicular line. Rales that do not clear with coughing, Cheyne-Stokes respirations, and wheezing are often the signs of respiratory involvement in CHF. Careful observation is essential because pulmonary edema may be occurring if the patient has diaphoresis or cyanosis of the nail beds and around the lips, and uses the accessory muscles for breathing. Edema is frequently present in CHF. Although edema may be due to other causes such as varicose veins, salt intake, or prolonged sitting, it is usually cardiac related if it is bilateral, nontender, pitting, and occurring in dependent areas. Edema of this nature does not occur until at least ten pounds of fluid have been retained (Atwood, 1979). With daily monitoring of weight, fluid retention may be assessed before edema develops (see Table 21-1).

Nursing Implications. Prevention is the main consideration in CHF. CHF can best be prevented by early treatment of acute health problems and by helping the older patient to implement and maintain his prescribed medical regimen and his general health promotional activities. The treatment of CHF has three goals: reducing the demand for cardiac output, increasing cardiac output, and reducing congestion (sodium and water retention).

As stated earlier, chair rest is preferable to bed rest. Sodium restriction and diuretics are usually preferable to digitalis because of possible toxicity. Potassium, in the form of fruit, juices, or medication, helps maintain electrolyte balance in patients with adequate renal function. Shock must be detected promptly and treated, usually with vasopressors. The combination of edema, poorly nourished tissue, and the fragile skin of the elderly provides a challenge in maintenance of skin integrity. While administering physical care, the nurse should also remember to give psychological support to patients and families (Bramoweth, 1983).

Hypertension

Both systolic and diastolic blood pressure increase with advancing years. Forty percent of all Americans between the ages of 75 and 79 have hypertension, and more than three-quarters of these have hypertensive heart disease (Harris, 1978). Although there is no universal definition of hypertension, the World Health Organization defines it as a persistent elevation of systolic blood pressure above 140 mm Hg and of diastolic pressure above 90 mm Hg. The etiology of most hypertension is unknown, although heredity, obesity, and stress are related to its development.

Despite the lack of agreement about the definition of hypertension and its cause, the effects of prolonged hypertension are well known. The heart, vascular system, brain, kidneys, and eyes can be affected, resulting in heart and kidney failure, blindness, and cardiovascular accidents. Early pathological changes in blood vessels throughout the body cause varying symptoms — dull headache on awakening, impaired memory, nausea and vomiting, epistaxis, and a slow tremor (Eliopoulos, 1979).

There are wide fluctuations in everyone's blood pressure. Activity, stress, or anxiety may cause temporary elevations. A reliable determination of hypertension can only be made by taking blood pressure readings on both arms and one leg in sitting, standing, and supine positions repeatedly over time, such as every 1–2 hours for 1–2 days. Accurate blood pressure readings require correct technique, proper equipment, and an awareness of the auscultatory gap; see Table 21-2 (Hill, 1980; Malasanos, Barkauskas, Moss, and Stoltenberg-Allen, 1981).

Treatment is usually instituted for the patient who has a persistently elevated blood pressure and related symptoms. The goal is to increase the patient's comfort and working capacity by gradually reducing his blood pressure to a level that prevents complications

Table 21-2. Blood Pressure Procedure to Avoid the Auscultatory Gap.

Equipment:

Bell stethoscope is more effective in transmission of low frequency Korotkoff sounds than diaphragm.
Cuff width should be 20–25% wider than diameter of extremity used (covering approximately 2/3 of upper arm).
Inflatable bladder should extend completely (or at least halfway) around extremity.

Procedure:

Have person relax completely for at least 5 minutes.
Place equipment so meniscus of mercury manometer will be viewed at eye level. (Aneroid manometers are placed for unobscured viewing.)
Support flexed arm on surface at heart level.
Place center of bladder with bottom edge 1–2 inches above antecubital space.
Apply cuff snugly and smoothly.
Palpate brachial artery below the cuff.
Inflate cuff until palpable pulse disappears, and note level.*
Deflate cuff.
Place stethoscope eartips directed forward in ears.
Palpate artery. Place bell stethoscope firmly over artery. Do not lose the bell's effectiveness by applying so firmly that the skin becomes indented.
Inflate bladder to approximately 30 mm Hg above where palpated pulse disappeared.
Deflate bladder slowly and steadily 2–3 mm Hg per heartbeat or second until approximately 30 mm Hg of silence. Bladder can then be deflated rapidly.

*Estimating the systolic pressure by the disappearance of the palpable pulse avoids errors due to the auscultatory gap (temporary disappearance of sounds lasting from 30 to 40 mm Hg).

but does not cause hypotensive reactions. Hypotensive reactions are caused by cerebral, coronary, or renal insufficiency, and the symptoms include dizziness, light-headedness, drowsiness, syncope, decline in intellectual functioning, restlessness, nausea, and/or a rising blood urea nitrogen (Moser, 1980; *Special Report on Aging,* 1979).

Conservative treatment of hypertension includes rest, mild regular activity and recreation, stress reduction, salt restriction, and if the patient is obese, weight reduction. If hypertension persists, tranquilizing and/or antihypertensive medications are prescribed.

Nursing Implications. Nursing care for the older patient with hypertension includes:

1. Promoting a restful and stress-free environment; explaining procedures and policies to hospitalized patients; discussing with the patient and family his daily activities and helping plan modifications to reduce stress.
2. Explaining dietary measures and facilitating adaptation to them; discussing food preferences that are compatible with the patient's dietary regime, sociocultural background, and lifelong habits; discussing the use of food, spices, and seasonings that are low in sodium and can be used freely; cautioning about drinking water that has been softened or conditioned (this adds sodium); teaching patient and family to read labels of foods and over-the-counter drugs to determine sodium content.
3. Administering medications, and monitoring their subjective and objective effects.
4. Educating patients to minimize hypotensive reactions to antihypertensive drugs by:
   a) Moving slowly from sitting or lying position, allowing time for the vascular system to adjust to changes.
   b) Avoiding (1) immobility following exercise, (2) standing motionless, (3) hot baths, or (4) excessive alcohol (these cause vasodilation and possible fainting).
   c) Using caution if driving or operating equipment within two hours after taking an antihypertensive drug (acute hypotension may cause fainting).
   d) Lying down with feet elevated to promote cerebral blood flow if hypotension should develop.
5. Helping the patient and his family learn that hypertension is a chronic condition that is controlled but not cured by medication, diet, exercise, rest, and control of stress (Daniels and Gifford, 1980; Filson and Morris, 1980; Wyka, Levesque, Ryan, and Mattea, 1980).

Cor Pulmonale

Cor pulmonale is the chronic or acute enlargement of the right ventricle of the heart superimposed on disorders of respiration or pulmonary circulation. Usually, it is a persistent condition secondary to obstructive pulmonary disease, such as chronic bronchitis or emphysema. Acute cor pulmonale may be precipitated by a massive pulmonary embolism or infection; frequently the patient already has congestive heart failure and/or atrial fibrillation (Rodstein, 1971).

Indications of cor pulmonale include cough, substernal pain, dyspnea, cyanosis, syncope with exertion, a precordial systolic lift, and a loud pulmonic second sound (Luckmann and Sorensen, 1980). Progression to heart failure is indicated by peripheral edema, distended jugular veins, and orthopnea. Treatment may include diuretics, digitalis, oxygen, rest, and sodium restriction.

Nursing Implications. Nursing care for cor pulmonale includes implementation of the therapeutic medical regimen, ongoing assessment of the patient, and education and emotional support for the patient and family. Teaching should emphasize nutrition, hydration, breathing exercises, planning activities to prevent fatigue and to promote rest, and avoidance of smoking, constipation, and medications that depress respirations (Luckmann and Sorensen, 1980).

Arrhythmias and Conduction Disorders

Arrhythmias and conduction disturbances increase with age. Degenerative changes accompanying aging cause fibrosis, loss of muscle, increased collagen, calcification, and occlusion of coronary arteries with resultant interference in conduction or heart block. Ischemia, hypokalemia, infection, blood loss, and digitalis toxicity may also be precipitating factors (Harris, 1978).

Arrhythmias and conduction disorders are more serious in older persons because vital organs already impaired by aging cannot tolerate reduced cardiac output. Patients with arrhythmias and conduction problems may have dyspnea or be symptom free. Diagnosis is usually made by electrocardiograms. Since carotid sinus massage is hazardous in the aged and may result in cerebral insufficiency with hemiplegia, it is not used for differential diagnosis. In the aged, digitalization is preferable to direct-current electrical conversion. Prescribed therapy may also include tranquilizers and potassium. Artificial pacemakers are used to stimulate a regular heartbeat for bradycardia with syncope or partial or complete heart block (Harris, 1978).

Nursing Implications. The care of older patients with potentially life-threatening arrhythmias and conduction problems includes:

- Implementation of prescribed medical plan of care (the nurse needs to be knowledgeable and able to assess and make judgments about drugs, drug interactions, and side effects in her administration of drugs such as digitalis)
- Careful periodic monitoring of patients
- Early detection of problems or complications
- Preparedness for possible resuscitative activities
- Emotional support of the patient and family
- Patient education related to medicine, diet, activity regimen, and stopping or reducing smoking

ARTERIAL PROBLEMS

Arterial insufficiency may be due to atherosclerosis, trauma, thrombosis, or embolism. Arteries may develop aneurysms and rupture. Arteries may occlude and cause transient ischemic attacks, cerebrovascular accidents, or gangrene. An embolus may lodge in the pulmonary circulation and become life threatening.

Atherosclerosis

The leading cause of death in the United States and northern Europe is arterial insufficiency. The culprit is arteriosclerosis or any progressive thickening and loss of resilience in the arteries. The most common type of arteriosclerosis is atherosclerosis, which is the development of plaques or fatty accumulations in the intima and increased connective tissue in the subintima of the arterial walls. It is considered universal to all animals and is so progressive with age that it is considered an inevitable aspect of aging (Timiras, 1972).

According to Timiras (1972), atherosclerosis interferes with normally functioning arteries by:

- Corroding the walls so that they suddenly yield to the blood's pressure and explode in a hemorrhage
- Causing a proliferation of tissue leading to a narrowing or closing of the lumen
- Producing clots that may impede blood flow

Various measures are currently believed to minimize the development and threat of atherosclerosis:

- Limit the intake of sugar, salt, and saturated fats.
- Engage in a routine exercise program (this will also facilitate the development of collateral circulation).
- Stop smoking (the nicotine in cigarettes causes vasoconstriction).

Acute Arterial Occlusion

Acute occlusion, or sudden complete obstruction, of an artery may be due to trauma, thrombosis, or embolism. The first symptom is usually sudden burning or aching pain in tissues distal to the site of the occlusion. Movement aggravates the pain. Numbness, pallor, coldness, weakness, or paresthesia may be present. The pulse is weak or absent. The site of the occlusion is usually tender.

Nursing Implications. Treatment of acute arterial occlusion consists of protecting the limb, keeping it straight and at room temperature, and probably elevating it slightly. Anticoagulation therapy is usually instituted immediately — beginning with heparin and then changing to an oral anticoagulant for an indefinitely long period. In some cases an embolectomy may be performed (Atwood, 1979; Luckmann and Sorensen, 1980).

Nursing implications include periodically assessing the patient's status, implementing the therapeutic regimen, and discussing the plan of care with the patient and family. Frequent assessment of the affected part includes observations of color and temperature and, perhaps, use of an ultrasound (Doppler) stethoscope or amplifier to assess the area's circulation (Disch, 1979; Kurth, 1983).

Chronic Arterial Occlusion

The older patient with chronic partial obstruction of an artery will usually complain of pain in the legs precipitated by exercise and relieved by rest. This symptom is called intermittent claudication. He may also complain of rest pain, coldness, or numbness. Alterations in skin temperature and color, thick nails, thin skin, absence of hair, bruits, weak or absent pulses, ulcerations, and gangrene may also be present. Marked rubor of the foot and toes on dependency and rapid blanching on elevation are evidence of inadequate collateral circulation.

Nursing Implications. Intermittent claudication can frequently be relieved by the patient's walking increasing amounts daily to establish collateral circulation. Since nicotine causes vasoconstriction, the patient should be advised to stop smoking. If analgesics or narcotics do not afford relief of pain at rest, surgical intervention may be needed.

Treatment of lesions which may develop from ischemia includes protection from trauma and control of infection and pain. Muscle strength and motion must be maintained in order to resume maximal activity after the lesions have healed. Education of the patient is a vital nursing responsibility. Preventive foot care is also essential.

Aneurysms

Aneurysms are dilatations in arteries caused by weakness and stretching of the arterial wall. Aneurysms may be classified as saccular (saclike), fusiform (spindle shaped), or dissecting (blood is being forced between the coats of the artery), as shown in Figure 21-1. Aneurysms usually develop after age 60. Males are ten times more prone to aneurysms than women. Most persons who develop aneurysms have hypertension (Luckmann and Sorensen, 1980). Approximately half of the patients with aneurysms experience pain. A pulsating mass in the umbilical area is the most frequent sign of an abdominal arterial aneurysm. Assessment of an abdominal aneurysm is facilitated by taking the blood pressure in the arm and leg of the patient in the supine position. Usually the blood pressure in the thigh is 15 mm higher than that in the arm. However, with an aneurysm, the systolic pressure may be much lower in the thigh than in the arm. Sometimes normal variations in blood pressure persist even in the presence of an aneurysm. Aneurysm is best diagnosed with x-ray. The treatment consists of surgical resection and grafting, especially when the patient is symptomatic. Pain may indicate a rapid, progressive enlargement and possible impending rupture. A rupture causes death due to hemorrhage and shock.

The thoracic aorta is the most common site of a dissecting aneurysm. Approximately 2000 cases of dissecting aneurysm are diagnosed annually in the United States, but it is estimated that 60,000 Americans develop this life-threatening condition annually. Without treatment for a dissecting aneurysm, death occurs within 15 minutes for over one-third of the cases and within a week for three-fourths of cases (Robbins and Cotran, 1979).

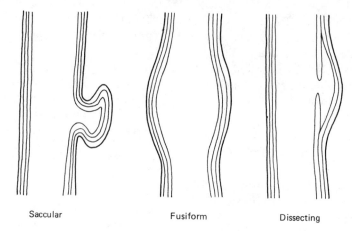

Saccular   Fusiform   Dissecting

Figure 21-1. The three common classifications of aneurysms are: saccular — sac-like outpouching; fusiform — spindle-like outpouching, usually encircling the artery; dissecting — blood is being forced between the coats of the artery.

The onset of a dissecting aneurysm is heralded by sudden, severe, persistent pain usually described as "ripping" or "tearing." The pain may be in the anterior chest or reflected to other areas such as the neck or face. Because of the diaphoresis, pallor, shock, and elevated blood pressure that are the early symptoms, diagnostic errors may occur. Aortograms, x-ray, and ultrasound assist with diagnosis.

In addition to aneurysms occurring in the abdominal and thoracic aorta, they may also occur in the extremities. The most common sites are the femoral and popliteal arteries. Assessment of peripheral aneurysms can be made by palpation. Surgical treatment is usually instituted promptly to prevent thrombosis of the aneurysm and the distal circulation, with the resultant need for amputation (Haimovici, 1971).

Nursing Implications. The diagnosis of aneurysms is sometimes missed. Therefore, older persons who have acute or severe pain must be carefully evaluated, with the possibility of an aneurysm kept in mind. Although prognosis for an aneurysm is poor, prompt assessment and surgical resection may be lifesaving.

Transient Ischemic Attacks

A transient ischemic attack (TIA), also called a "little stroke," is a sudden disruption in neurological functioning caused by an interruption or reduction in circulation of blood to the brain. The signs and symptoms may last from a few minutes to 24 hours, with spontaneous, rapid recovery. The impaired blood flow is caused by atherosclerosis, emboli, or spasm of the blood vessels. Frequently the attack may be precipitated by temporary vasoconstriction such as that caused by smoking, flexing or extending the head when one falls asleep in a chair, or suddenly rising from a sitting position. Drugs such as antihypertensives and diuretics may contribute to the development of postural hypotension. Symptoms are determined by the specific area and number of neurons which have temporarily been deprived of an adequate supply of blood. These transient signs and symptoms are listed in Table 21-3.

Table 21-3. Signs and Symptoms of Transient Ischemic Attacks.

Amnesia
Speech disturbances
Personality changes
Vertigo
Blackouts
Falling
Motor weakness
Unilateral loss of vision
Diplopia
Nausea/vomiting
Hemianesthesia
Hemiparesis
Failure to recognize familiar persons or objects

Since TIAs often serve as a warning before a major stroke, diagnostic measures and treatment should be instituted promptly. Patients with TIAs should be admitted to hospitals for a day or two for close observations and studies which may include auscultation for bruits, angiograms, ophthalmodynamometry (indirect measurement of retina arterial pressure), skull x-rays, brain scans, echoencephalography, and computerized axial tomography (CAT scan).

Treatment consists of surgical intervention (bypass of occluded vessel or endarterectomy of vessel with atherosclerosis) and/or drug therapy (anticoagulants or aspirin) in an effort to prevent progression to a stroke. Aspirin appears to prevent thrombosis by inhibiting adhesion of blood platelets. Recent studies indicate that 1300 mg of aspirin daily reduces the risk of recurrent TIAs or strokes in men who have had TIAs, especially in men without diabetes who have had no myocardial infarctions. Aspirin does not appear to be of value in preventing TIAs in women or in treating completed strokes (Aspirin for Transient Ischemic Attacks, 1980).

Nursing Implications. The nurse's responsibility with individuals who have experienced TIAs is encouragement to report transitory signs and symptoms which they considered to be insignificant neurological problems of short duration. Such symptoms may be a warning of more serious problems such as a true cerebrovascular accident, so they should be urged to seek prompt evaluation. These persons should be advised to change to standing positions slowly and to wear antiembolic hose if they experience postural hypotension. They should be advised to post emergency numbers on their telephone to facilitate quick summoning of help if an emergency occurs. Someone should maintain daily telephone contact with them. Safety in their homes should be emphasized (e.g., safety strips and support bars in tub and shower, no obstructions in traffic patterns, and no dangling cords or scatter rugs).

If anticoagulants are prescribed, the patient and his family should be educated to watch for bleeding gums, increased bruising, smoky urine, and/or bloody or black stools. Caution should be taken to evaluate the possible interaction with other medications being taken which may potentiate or inhibit the anticoagulant therapy. Physicians and pharmacists should be reminded of other medications prescribed for the patient and consulted before over-the-counter drugs are taken.

Cerebral Vascular Accident

A cerebral vascular accident (CVA) or stroke may occur with or without the previous warning of a transient ischemic attack or attacks. Stroke and its consequences constitute the greatest fear of older individuals. More than 1,800,000 Americans annually realize they have had a stroke as they awaken from sleep or are "struck down" in the course of their daily activities (*Fact Sheet,* 1980). Fortunately, the number of stroke victims is not increasing as our population becomes proportionately older. Perhaps public education has had an impact.

A CVA is a neurological dysfunction caused by an inadequate supply of blood to the brain. The cerebral circulation is interrupted by a spasm, occlusion, or hemorrhage of a blood vessel. The symptoms persist more than 24 hours, perhaps permanently, in contrast to those of TIAs which last less than 24 hours. Symptoms depend on the location and the extent of the neurons experiencing the ischemia. Usually the blood vessels have become less patent due to the development of atherosclerotic plaques. With vascular constriction or spasm, the development or extension of a clot or thrombus, or the arrival of an embolus or other foreign body in the bloodstream, circulation beyond a specific point becomes inadequate or nonexistent. Hemorrhages also cause CVAs, but they are less likely in older persons. The exceptions are subdural hematomas resulting from falls.

The specific cause of a CVA is determined by studies which may include brain scans, angiograms, x-rays, and computerized axial tomography (CAT scan). The specific cause determines the treatment and prognosis:

1. If thrombosis or embolism has caused the CVA, the following nursing interven-

tions are instituted to maintain circulation to the brain: keeping the head flat or lower than the body, maintaining blood pressure, preventing shock, preventing pooling of blood in leg veins with anti-embolic hose, avoiding sudden postural changes, and giving prescribed medications – anticoagulants, vasodilators, etc.

2. If hemorrhage has caused the CVA, nursing measures usually include controlling hyperthermia, convulsive seizures, hypertension, intracranial pressure, headache, and restlessness. Oral intake may be withheld for 24-48 hours in order to prevent aspiration and vomiting. After a day or two of clear liquids, a soft diet is given. The patient is usually kept in bed until his headache and stiff neck are relieved.

In order to plan total integrated care, the type and degree of dysfunctions resulting from a CVA must be carefully identified. Communication, including aspects of both comprehension and expression, should be evaluated. Either one or both may be affected. Rehabilitation after stroke is probably the most neglected treatment of older adults; it should begin immediately (see Chapter 32).

Certain conditions predispose to CVAs. Individuals with diabetes, cardiac disorders, hypertension, atherosclerosis, or anemia are more apt to develop CVAs. After menopause, females are as CVA prone as males. Being a smoker, being black, or having a family history of CVAs also increases the risk of a stroke.

The signs and symptoms of a stroke may be drastic or subtle. A stroke's onset may be signaled by sudden minor disruptions such as lapses of memory, numbness, inability to speak or swallow, or falling. Family members, neighbors, or friends can help to confirm these subtle changes. More often a stroke is heralded by major disruptions. Involvement may be unilateral, bilateral, or quadriplegic depending on the location of the circulation disruption. Signs and symptoms may be unlimited. Classically, the patient has generalized symptoms such as convulsions, coma, fever, vomiting, headache, hypertension, and confusion. Focal

symptoms depend on the specific neurons involved. Focal symptoms may be hemiplegia, aphasia, hemianopia, dysphagia, and incontinence. Evaluation of CVAs may utilize x-rays; brain scans; arteriograms; laboratory examination of blood, urine, and cerebrospinal fluid; ophthalmodynamometry; and various encephalograms.

Nursing Implications. Nursing assessments contribute much to determining the extent and progression of the dysfunction in CVAs. In the acute phase immediately following a CVA, nursing care focuses on lifesaving measures.

The nurse must not forget the patient's significant others while administering to the CVA patient. They need information about the patient's condition and care and, if they indicate an interest, should be allowed to participate in meeting the patient's physical needs.

Sensory and motor loss, and the individual's adaptation to them, must be assessed (for further discussion of rehabilitation, see Chapter 32). After a stroke, emotional lability may cause the patient to laugh or cry inappropriately. In addition, he is grieving for the loss of the more functional person he was prior to his CVA. His mood may vacillate among anger, depression, denial, or bargaining before he finally resigns himself to coping with life after a CVA. His rehabilitation depends on his personality and resources (Wolanin and Putt, 1980). The patient's condition should be discussed in detail with his family or with significant others who are his support system. Understanding the patient's dysfunction may not make him easier to live with, but it will help his family to work with him in maximizing his potential for high level wellness.

Pulmonary Emboli

Pulmonary emboli are caused by thrombi, fat, air, or neoplasms in the circulating blood. Their incidence is high in the aged, and diagnosis is difficult. The older patient may not report chest pain because of altered pain sensations or attributing the pain to previously existing problems. The dyspnea may be either gasping and deep, or rapid and shallow, depending on whether the main problem is hypoxia or hypercapnia, respectively (Luckmann and Sorensen, 1980). Hemoptysis, shock, slight jaundice, slight temperature elevation, and cyanosis may also be present. Diagnosis of pulmonary embolism is made by pulmonary angiograms, lung scans, blood gases, enzyme studies, and x-rays.

Nursing Implications. Treatment of pulmonary emboli includes anticoagulant therapy and treatment of the shock and respiratory distress. Nursing intervention also focuses on allaying the patient's anxiety and apprehension. The patient experiencing inability to breathe and a realistic fear of possible sudden death needs emotional support as well as efficient, intensive nursing care.

Prevention of pulmonary emboli is facilitated by adequate nutrition, early ambulation, range of motion exercises, turning, coughing, deep breathing, and using elastic hose. These measures are especially important in the care of all hospitalized or bedridden elderly. Because pulmonary emboli are a frequent complication of hip fractures, anticoagulation therapy may be instituted soon after the injury.

VENOUS PROBLEMS

The main problems of venous circulation in the elderly are venous insufficiency and phlebitis. There is a positive correlation between age and these two venous problems (Haimovici, 1971).

Thrombophlebitis and Phlebothrombosis

It is difficult to distinguish between thrombophlebitis and phlebothrombosis. In the latter, inflammation of the vein may not be present initially and pulmonary embolism may develop without warning. Usually after several days however, both the thrombus and the inflammation are present. For this reason, both conditions will be discussed as one, and the term thrombophlebitis will be used.

Thrombophlebitis and its frequent complication, pulmonary embolism, are common in older patients. As people age, they become

prone to injuries because of visual problems, unsteadiness due to arthritis and neurological disorders, dizziness due to ischemia, and/or osteoporosis. Also at high risk are patients with hypercoagulability, venous stasis, and/or injury to a vein. Hypercoagulability may develop from dehydration, medication (especially hormones), clotting factors, and increased platelets and/or viscosity. Varicose veins, surgery, obesity, and prolonged inactivity contribute to venous stasis. Veins may be injured by trauma such as fractures and intravenous injections, especially of antibiotics and radiopaque dyes (Atwood, 1979; Luckmann and Sorensen, 1980; Wright, 1978).

Thrombophlebitis is characterized by a tender, red, warm area over a hard string-like vein. Pain may occur in the calf with dorsiflexion of the foot (Homans' sign) or with other movement. Edema may be present and determined by measuring and comparing the circumferences of both legs. Tests which assist in the diagnosis of thrombophlebitis are phlebograms, isotope studies, and examination with a Doppler flowmeter.

Nursing Implications. Care for thrombophlebitis focuses on preventing the formation of new thrombi and preventing those present from becoming larger or dislodged and circulating as emboli. Aspects of care which are especially important for older patients include:

- Bed rest for 4-7 days until the thrombus becomes adherent to vessel walls
- Elevating the foot higher than the knee and the knee higher than the heart (best done by elevating the foot of the bed 6-8 inches on blocks); this decreases edema and pain, and minimizes the formation of new thrombi
- Wearing properly fitted elastic hose or bandages when ambulating to compress the veins and promote venous return
- Avoidance of prolonged sitting or standing still which increases pressure in the capillaries
- Applying warm moist packs to promote analgesia and to relieve vasospasm and inflammation

- After the thrombus has become adherent (4–7 days), walking or exercising in bed by dorsiflexing the feet, "drawing" circles with the toes, and making bicycling movements
- Wearing elastic bandages or hose for at least 6–8 weeks

Although prompt treatment of thrombophlebitis usually prevents pulmonary embolism, early symptoms may not be present or may not be correctly interpreted. Sometimes the attention of health personnel is focused on the primary disease, trauma, or surgery. Therefore, the nurse should watch for the signs and symptoms of pulmonary embolism and, if they are present, promptly notify the physician. Diagnosis is usually made by a lung scan (Wright, 1978).

Anticoagulants are used if the phlebitis is becoming, or threatens to become, more extensive. Fibrinolytic drugs may be used to dissolve thrombi; dextran may be used to reduce coagulation and improve circulation. Surgical procedures to retain the emboli distal to the surgical site include vein ligation and the insertion of a grid, sieve, or umbrella-like appliance (Atwood, 1979; Luckmann and Sorensen, 1980; Wright, 1978).

Primary prevention is the most desirable approach. Nursing measures especially important to prevent thrombophlebitis in older person include:

- Educating the patient and family about preventive measures
- Avoiding pressure in the antecubital space
- Avoiding tight clothes on trunk and legs
- Range of motion exercises
- Early ambulation after surgery or illnesses
- Properly fitted elastic support hose
- Deep breathing and coughing every two hours
- Adequate hydration

SUMMARY

With aging and its accompanying slower metabolic rate, the prevention and control of obesity while maintaining adequate nutrition become increasingly difficult. The nurse's role in dietary counseling requires specific knowledge of nutrition, as well as skill in understanding the feelings and behavior of old people (see Chapters 5 and 33).

Case finding and getting the person to early diagnosis and treatment are crucial in cardiovascular disease. Nursing care and patient education are essential to the patient's survival, recovery, and achievement of maximum health. Observations and communication with the patient's family can facilitate gathering a more complete objective and subjective data base. Comments such as "I awakened and felt short of breath" or "I can only walk one block before I get too tired to walk further" are significant and need to be explored further. The nurse assesses, evaluates, interprets, and educates.

Tertiary prevention, that is, rehabilitation and the limitation of disabilities, is probably the most neglected aspect of gerontological nursing. Patients and families often need help in identifying community resources to assist with rehabilitation and retraining. The efforts of many health professionals, family, and significant others may be needed to assist the older person with cardiovascular problems in maintaining and maximizing his highest possible level of wellness.

REFERENCES

Aspirin for transient ischemic attacks. *FDA Drug Bulletin* 10(1) (February 1980).

Atwood, J. Cardiovascular problems. In Carnevali, D.L. and Patrick, M. (Eds.) *Nursing Management for the Elderly*. Philadelphia: J.B. Lippincott, 1979.

Bramoweth, E.R., Psychologic considerations. In Sanderson, R.G. and Kurth, C.L. (Eds.), *The Cardiac Patient: A Comprehensive Approach* (2nd ed.), Philadelphia: W.B. Saunders, 1983.

Daniels, L. and Gifford, R.W. Therapy for older adults who are hypertensive. *Geriatric Nursing* 1(1):37–39 (1980).

Dehn, M.M. The effects of exercise. *American Journal of Nursing* 80:435–440 (1980).

Devney, A.M. Bridging the gap between inhospital and outpatient care. *American Journal of Nursing* 80:446–449 (1980).

Disch, J.M. *Diagnostic Procedures for Cardiovascular Disease* (Unit 1). New York: Appleton-Century-Crofts, 1979.

Eliopoulos, C. *Gerontological Nursing.* New York: Harper & Row, 1979.

Fact Sheet on Heart Attacks, Stroke and Risk Factors. Dallas: American Heart Association Communications Division, 1980.

Filson, D. and Morris, D.T. Guidelines to educating the patient with hypertension. In Czerwinski, B.S. (Ed.) *Manual of Patient Education for Cardiopulmonary Dysfunctions.* St. Louis: C.V. Mosby, 1980.

Haimovici, H. The peripheral vascular system. In Rossman, I. (Ed.) *Clinical Geriatrics.* Philadelphia: J.B. Lippincott, 1971.

Harris R. Special problems of geriatric patients with heart disease. In Reichel, W. (Ed.) *Clinical Aspects of Aging.* Baltimore: Williams and Wilkins, 1978.

Hill, M.N. What can go wrong when you measure blood pressure. *American Journal of Nursing* 80: 942–946 (1980).

Hoepfel-Harris, J.A. Improving compliance with an exercise program. *American Journal of Nursing* 80:449–450 (1980).

Kannel, W.B., McGee, D., and Gordon, T. A general cardiovascular risk profile: the Framingham study. *American Journal of Cardiology* 38:46–51 (1976).

Kart, C.S., Metress, E.S., and Metress, J.F. *Aging and Health: Biologic and Social Perspectives.* Menlo Park, Calif.: Addison-Wesley, 1978.

Ketchum, P.P. Coronary artery disease: overall view. In Czerwinski, B.S. (Ed.) *Manual of Patient Education for Cardiopulmonary Dysfunctions.* St. Louis: C.V. Mosby, 1980.

Knudsen, F.S. Comparison of structured and unstructured teaching of cardiac patients (doctoral dissertation, Arizona State University, 1979). *Dissertation Abstracts International* 40:1213-A (1979) (University Microfilms No. 7920501).

Kurth, C.L., Hemodynamic monitoring and specialized equipment. In Sanderson, R.G., and Kurth, C.L., (Eds.) *The Cardiac Patient: A Comprehensive Approach* (2nd ed.), Philadelphia: W.B. Saunders, 1983.

Luckmann, J. and Sorensen, K.C. *Medical-Surgical Nursing: A Psychophysiologic Approach* (2nd ed.). Philadelphia: W.B. Saunders, 1980.

Malasanos, L., Barkauskas, V., Moss, M., and Stoltenberg-Allen, K. *Health Assessment.* (2nd ed.), St. Louis: C.V. Mosby, 1981.

Moser, M. Hypertension: how therapy works. *American Journal of Nursing* 80:937–941 (1980).

Recent trends in mortality from cardiovascular diseases. *Statistical Bulletin* 60(2):2–8 (1979).

Robbins, S.L. and Cotran, R.S. *Pathologic Basis of Disease* (2nd ed.). Philadelphia: W.B. Saunders, 1979.

Rodstein, M. Heart disease in the aged. In Rossman, I. (Ed.) *Clinical Geriatrics.* Philadelphia: J.B. Lippincott, 1971.

Special Report on Aging (NIH Publication No. 79-1907). Washington, D.C.: U.S. Department of Health, Education and Welfare, September 1979.

Timiras, P.S. *Developmental Physiology and Aging.* New York: Macmillan, 1972.

Winslow, E.H. and Weber, T.M. Progressive exercise to combat the hazards of bed rest. *American Journal of Nursing* 80:440–445 (1980).

Wolanin, H.J. and Putt, A.M. The long road back from stroke. *Geriatric Nursing* 1(1):34-36 (1980).

Wright, I.S. Venous thrombosis and pulmonary embolism in the elderly. In Reichel, W. (Ed.) *Clinical Aspects of Aging.* Baltimore: Williams and Wilkins, 1978.

Wyka, C.A., Levesque, P.G., Ryan, S.L., and Mattea, E.J. Group education for the hypertensive. *Cardio-Vascular Nursing* 16(1):1-5 (1980).

22
Gastrointestinal and Metabolic Problems in Older Adults

Frances S. Knudsen

The gastrointestinal tract stands the test of time better than all the other systems. It has been said that no one ever dies because of a digestive organ wearing out. Although there are age-related changes which affect gastrointestinal functioning, they do not seem to significantly affect the nutritional state of the older individual. These alterations with aging include decreases in motility, secretions, muscular tone, neurosensory feedback, and response to pain and internal sensations. However, nutritional problems are frequently related more to pathology and social functioning. For example, poorly fitting dentures may limit dietary intake and variety. The loss of teeth is not necessarily due to age, but is usually caused by chronic gum disease, which in turn developed from improper dental care.

Although the gastrointestinal tract continues its function of digestion, absorption, and elimination throughout life, it often causes chronic distress. Common complaints include constipation, indigestion, flatulence, and heartburn. These symptoms frequently occur in the absence of organic problems (Sklar, 1978), but steps must be taken to eliminate the possibility of underlying pathology. The problems of older persons will be discussed in sequence by following the gastrointestinal tract through the body, beginning with the mouth and continuing through to the common condition of hemorrhoids. Because the older person may need to receive hyperalimentation due to gastrointestinal infection or malabsorption, an overview of this topic is also included.

GASTROINTESTINAL PROBLEMS

Oral and Dental Conditions

One-half of all Americans age 65 or older have no natural teeth (Yellowitz, Portnoy, and Smith, 1979). In older persons, dental loss is most often due to periodontal disease, but many older adults may have lost their teeth from dental caries when they were younger. Dental care has changed greatly during the lifetime of most older persons. A philosophy of maintaining one's natural teeth at all costs has replaced the expectation of previous generations who anticipated being edentulous or having dentures in later life. Fluoride, nutritious diet, and dental hygiene have been recognized as measures to prevent dental caries in old and young alike. In addition to those who benefit from topical fluoride applications, the drinking water of nearly 60% of the population is now fluoridated (U.S. Department of Health, Education and Welfare, 1978).

Plaque, the main cause of periodontal disease, can be prevented or removed by dental flossing and brushing with a soft toothbrush. Older people are not always able to do this and are not always convinced of the value if they are able. Assistance with this kind of care is grossly lacking in acute care settings and long term care facilities.

Denture wearers have many problems. They fear loss of bridgework, and they experience troubles such as a sore mouth and difficulty chewing because their gums shrink and their dentures become loose. Mandibular (lower) plates are especially difficult to fit and are easily dislodged in speaking, swallowing, or coughing. Therefore, some of the lower natural teeth, particularly the cuspids, should be preserved as long as possible to anchor partial plates. Relining or replacement of dentures must be done periodically because of changes in the tissues of the mouth.

Nursing Implications. If the patient has dentures, their fit should be observed before their removal for inspection of the mouth tissues. If the patient is unable to remove them himself, the nurse should see that they are removed daily for cleaning. The upper dentures are removed by gently breaking the suction seal. Removing the lower denture is most easily done by grasping the plate toward the front and lifting. After dentures are removed, inspect them carefully for breaks, cracks, plaque, and calculus, then place them in a denture cup or a safe container. Every acute care and long term care facility should have stringent protocols about the care and storage of dentures. The number of dentures reported damaged and lost in hospitals and nursing homes is tragic.

Assessment of the mouth is prerequisite to planning comprehensive care. The tools needed are a tongue blade, an adequate source of light, and a glove to prevent bacteria in the patient's mouth from becoming resident flora on the nurse's hand. If the patient is unconscious or irrational, the nurse uses a padded tongue blade to keep his mouth open and to protect herself from being bitten inadvertently. The nurse observes and palpates every surface of the mouth (see Chapters 18 and 38). Any lesions should be palpated, especially if they are unilateral. Suspicious lesions require immediate evaluation by a physician or dentist. Biopsy may be needed to assure that there is no malignancy. More than 90% of all oral cancer occurs in persons over 45 years of age (Yellowitz et al., 1979).

Frequently, older persons have leukoplakia or whitish patches due to chronic irritation or systemic conditions. These should be evaluated immediately because these lesions are frequently precancerous. A biopsy should be done if they persist. Changes in oral tissue may also be caused by drugs such as aspirin and dilantin, and by diabetes and other hormonal imbalances. Special equipment may be purchased or improvised to facilitate dental care for the handicapped or helpless. A toothbrush can be made more easy to hold by attaching a strip of plastic or hard rubber tubing to its handle or by inserting the handle into a bicycle handlebar grip or into a Styrofoam or soft rubber ball

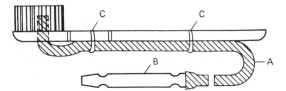

Figure 22-1. Soft toothbrush with suction attachment for care of the helpless patient: (A) plastic tubing, (B) adapter for attachment of tubing to aspirator or suction outlet, (C) rubber bands to attach tubing to toothbrush handle. Plastic tube is inserted through a hole in the head of the brush and extended to a level slightly below the brushing plane. [Source: Wilkins, E.M. *Clinical Practice of Dental Hygienist* (4th ed.). Philadelphia: Lea and Febiger, 1976, p. 585.]

(Ramos, 1981). Mouth care for a helpless patient is facilitated by use of a toothbrush with suction attachments (Wilkins, 1976); see Figure 22-1.

Keeping the patient hydrated, the mouth clean, and the lips lubricated is the main goal in oral hygiene. When patients are drowsy or unconscious, precautions need to be taken to avoid aspiration.

Dysphagia

The older person may experience difficulty in swallowing due to less efficient esophageal peristalsis and changes in the lower esophageal sphincter (Bartol and Heitkemper, 1979). Other causes include stroke, motor neuron disease, pseudobulbar palsy, pressure from an aneurysm or carcinoma, or pathology of the esophagus itself, such as diverticuli, carcinoma, reflex esophagitis, achalasia (constricted muscle fibers), and moniliasis (Brocklehurst and Hanley, 1976). Liquids may be as difficult to swallow as solids. Acidic foods such as tomatoes and citrus seem to precipitate abnormal motility (Bartol and Heitkemper, 1979). These symptoms are usually intermittent rather than continuous. Diagnostic measures usually include a barium swallow and esophagoscopy. Sometimes nutrition needs to be maintained by means of nasogastric, gastroscopy, or jejunostomy tubes. The patient needs a liquid intake of 2500-3000 cc daily.

The very frail elderly are less able to achieve anabolism or positive nitrogen balance because of gastrointestinal inflammation, infection, malabsorption, etc. These people will probably receive hyperalimentation or total parenteral alimentation, which is the administration of a hypertonic solution (glucose, amino acids, and polypeptides) through a central vein. The hypertonic solution that would cause phlebitis and occlusion if perfused into a smaller peripheral vein is diluted by the large volume of blood circulating through a central vein, such as the superior vena cava. Because the older person has increased susceptibility to infection and electrolyte imbalance, expert care during hyperalimentation is essential.

Esophageal Diverticuli

Esophageal diverticuli are not uncommon in older persons. Food collects in the diverticular pouch, causing dysphagia. Frequently older persons gag and regurgitate undigested food hours after its ingestion. Foul breath results when the food begins to decompose. The threat of aspiration is constantly present. Diagnosis is usually made by means of a barium swallow. Treatment is surgical. Postoperative nursing care includes nasogastric feedings.

Hiatal Hernia

A hiatal hernia results from a weakness in the diaphragm, causing the proximal portion of the stomach to slip through the esophageal opening in the diaphragm. Hiatal hernias, which occur with increasing frequency with aging, occur in at least 40-60% of those over 60 years of age (Sklar, 1978). The incidence is greater in women than in men (Leeming and Dymock, 1978). Hiatal hernias are so common that some people believe they should be considered a normal finding in old age (Winsberg, 1979). Most hiatal hernias do not cause symptoms, but patients may suffer mild to severe heartburn, sour stomach, or vise-like pain. Dysphagia or belching may occur. Activities that increase intra-abdominal pressure, such as overeating, coughing, or a reclining position, may precipitate or increase discomfort. Walking and elevating the head of the bed may relieve the pain

(Sodeman and Sodeman, 1974). Since surgery is not always effective, it is resorted to only when symptoms are severe, or when bleeding or ulceration occurs.

Nursing Implications. Patients are usually taught to live with hiatal hernias. Eating slowly should be advised as a method of decreasing episodic substernal discomfort. If liquids are difficult to swallow, they can be thickened or soaked up with bread, crackers, or cookies. Sometimes increasing neural stimulation with very cold liquids, sherbets, or ice cream facilitates swallowing.

Epigastric distress or pain during or after meals occurs due to esophageal reflux of gastric contents. This problem may be minimized by small, frequent feedings of a low fat, decreased cholesterol diet. Coffee, tea, alcohol, chocolate, orange juice, or cola should be limited or avoided. Walking about or remaining upright is encouraged after meals. Restricting fluids and food 1-2 hours before bedtime and having the head of the bed elevated at approximately 30° or with 4- to 6-inch pads or blocks usually promote comfort. The symptoms may be minimized by avoiding increased abdominal pressure, such as coughing, bending forward, lifting, straining, and wearing tight clothing. Weight reduction may be helpful in the obese. Antacids may be taken for symptomatic relief (Bartol and Heitkemper, 1979; Leeming and Dymock, 1978; Sklar, 1978).

If surgical intervention is necessary, the care is similar to that of any postoperative patient. Consideration should be given to the special needs of the older adult, including adequate respiratory exchange, maintenance of hydration and circulation, promotion of skin integrity, and compensating for sensory losses.

Ulcers

Ulcers, especially those in the duodenum, occur more frequently in men than in women. In the general population, duodenal ulcers are ten times as frequent as gastric ulcers. The highest incidence of gastric ulcers is in those aged 45 to

55 (Luckmann and Sorensen, 1980). Deaths from gastric ulcers are increasing among the elderly (Bartol and Heitkemper, 1979).

Heredity may play a factor in the development of ulcers, but other influencing factors, such as diet, emotional reactions, and socioeconomics, are also family characteristics. The elderly, those who are poorly nourished, and those from impoverished social groups are considered to be especially prone to gastric ulcers. Ulcers frequently accompany other health problems of the aged, such as chronic obstructive pulmonary disease and other stress-producing conditions. Drugs may also produce or reactivate gastric ulcers. These include aspirin, reserpine, tolbutamide, colchicine, phenylbutazone, and corticosteroids (Bartol and Heitkemper, 1979; Straus, 1979).

In a study of 40 subjects with ulcers and 40 control subjects, aged 50–78 years, matched for economic status and age, the physical strength and maximum breathing capacity of the subjects with ulcers were significantly lower than those of the controls. The individuals with ulcers also showed a more rapid decline in intellectual capabilities; more neurotic disturbances, anxiety, and depression; more stress in childhood, marriage, and occupation; and a less satisfactory adaptation to the problems of aging. From this it was concluded that stress and inability to cope not only precipitate ulcers but also accelerate the aging process (Bouliere, 1978).

The symptoms of ulcers may be atypical or absent in the older person. Generalized abdominal pain, vomiting, and decreases in appetite, energy, and weight may occur. Diagnosis is made by upper gastrointestinal x-rays. The treatment is conservative but flexible in terms of diet and activity. Immobility of older persons does more harm than good, and any advantage of a bland diet may be counteracted by the psychological stress it creates.

Gastrointestinal bleeding is more serious in the older person. If bleeding continues or recurs, surgery is needed. Management of gastrointestinal bleeding has been markedly improved due to the advent of angiography and fiberoptic endoscopy, which permit visualization, photography, and biopsy or removal of lesions. By means of gastroscopic, cytologic, and radiologic examinations, malignant changes can readily be detected (Sklar, 1978).

Nursing Implications. The nurse's role is to assist the patient in symptom control through diet, medication, and stress management. Measures aimed at decreased production of hydrochloric acid include avoiding smoking, alcohol, strong spices, and caffeine in coffee, tea, chocolate, or cola. Low fat or skim milk has replaced the traditional whole milk regimen which caused rebound acid production (Bartol and Heitkemper, 1979) and probably increased the development of atherosclerosis. Small frequent meals help to control gastric acidity and thus relieve pain. Relaxed mealtimes should be encouraged, with consideration given to how one eats as well as to what one eats (Meyers, 1981).

Prescribed medications may be anticholinergics which decrease acid output and hypermotility, antacids which neutralize acidity, and/or cimetidine (Tagamet) which blocks histamine stimulation of gastric secretions. However, despite the usefulness of medications, their side effects can cause problems for older persons. Anticholinergics may become intolerable due to the development of blurred vision, urinary retention, constipation, a feeling of stomach fullness, and dry mouth. Some antacids precipitate diarrhea, while others cause constipation.

Cholelithiasis

The incidence of cholelithiasis increases with age. Gallstones are found in 30% of those over age 70 and in 40% of those in their eighties (Goldman, 1979). Women are twice as likely as men to have cholelithiasis. The treatment is usually conservative, including weight reduction, antacids, and a low fat diet. Surgery may be indicated if symptoms are recurrent or if complications such as acute cholecystitis, perforation, or an obstruction are present (Sklar, 1978; Straus, 1979). Nursing care of older persons with cholelithiasis is essentially no different from those who are younger. However, nurses need to understand that recovery may be slower, and that the older person is at greater risk of developing complications due to infection and the hazards of immobility.

Acute Pancreatitis

There is no known direct cause for many cases of pancreatitis. Some pancreatitis is precipitated by biliary tract disease in all age groups. In the elderly, for some unexplained reason, there is an increased incidence of postoperative pancreatitis. Alcohol is frequently considered a cause, but less commonly in older adults (Webster, 1978). However, the consumption of alcohol in the elderly may be underestimated.

One-third of older adults who develop pancreatitis experience nausea and vomiting as early symptoms. Pain, when it occurs, develops suddenly. It is usually epigastric, radiating into the back in half of the cases. Nearly one-fourth of those over 50 years of age lose consciousness, and of these, nearly one-half die (Hoffman, Perez, and Somera, 1959). It is thought that the hypokalemia accompanying the acute attack contributes to impaired function of the cerebrum. Older adults are more prone to "silent" attacks than younger adults. These attacks, while pain free, nevertheless may be fatal. Diagnosis is made on autopsy (Webster, 1978).

The most useful test in diagnosing acute pancreatitis is a grossly elevated serum amylase level. However, impaired renal function and other abdominal problems may also produce elevations (Webster, 1978).

Nursing Implications. Mortality is probably highest in the elderly with pancreatitis because of their sensitivity to dehydration. Therefore, fluid and electrolyte replacement is the main goal of care. Measures of central venous pressure monitor changes in blood volume and facilitate maintenance of proper hydration. Potent analgesics are needed to control the pain, but the older adult is especially prone to their side effects. Nasogastric suction, which is used frequently, has two purposes: (1) to reduce intestinal distension and, therefore, nausea and vomiting, and (2) to prevent gastric secretions from stimulating secretion of pancreatic juice (Bonaparte, 1981; Webster, 1978).

Blood glucose levels should be carefully monitored because of the role of the pancreas in insulin production.

Chronic Pancreatitis

Chronic pancreatitis usually results from repeated attacks of acute pancreatitis due either to biliary tract disease or to alcohol abuse. Pain, the most common symptom, may be precipitated by alcohol ingestion. Half of those with chronic pancreatitis experience nausea and vomiting, compared to one-third of those with acute pancreatitis. Weight loss and anorexia occur, probably due to the pain, nausea and vomiting, and faulty absorption of fats and fat-soluble vitamins. The expected steatorrhea occurs, but constipation is twice as likely to occur as diarrhea in older adults. Older adults with chronic pancreatitis are twice as likely as younger ones to have elevated blood sugar. Jaundice and elevated bilirubin levels are common (Webster, 1978).

Nursing Implications. Preventing stimulus to the pancreas may be achieved by various dietary measures: small meals, low fat diet, and abstinence from alcohol and caffeine. Oral antacids may control gastric acidity and, in turn, the production and secretion of pancreatic juice. When steatorrhea is a problem, pancreatic extracts are usually prescribed to be taken with each meal. This may improve bowel function and the absorption of fats and fat-soluble vitamins. Anticholinergic drugs may also be part of the medical regime (Webster, 1978). Blood glucose levels must be carefully monitored in order to assess the altered insulin production resulting from the pancreatitis.

Appendicitis

Appendicitis is not a common problem in older adults; however, its identification is. The beginning signs and symptoms may be absent or atypical, but a rapid, severe course may follow. Although there may be little or no fever, tachycardia and leukocytosis are usually present. The area over the appendix is hypertensive and demonstrates rebound tenderness when a distal area is pressed and suddenly released. The usual nausea, vomiting, constipation, and/or anorexia may be present (Villaverde and MacMillan, 1980). Peritonitis readily develops, causing a mortality rate of 12% in those over 60 and 30% in those over 70 years of age (Charlesworth and Baker, 1978).

Diverticulosis and Diverticulitis

Diverticuli are pouch- or sac-like herniations of mucous membrane through the muscular coat of the colonic membrane. They usually are multiple and involve the left colon (Straus, 1979). They begin to develop at about the age of 50, and increase in size and number with advancing age. It is thought that more than 40% of individuals over 70 years of age have diverticulosis. Contributors to its development appear to be a low residue diet, constipation, obesity, and emotional tension (Bartol and Heitkemper, 1979). Pain in the left lower abdomen may occur after meals and be relieved after a bowel movement, although many with deverticulosis have no symptoms. Slight rectal bleeding may also be present (Bartol and Heitkemper, 1979; Burakoff, 1981; Sklar, 1978).

Occasionally the diverticuli become inflamed. Diverticulitis occurs more often in males. Irritating foods, alcohol, straining at defecation, or coughing may precipitate the inflammation. Complications include intestinal perforation, severe bleeding, peritonitis, abscesses, and obstruction (Bartol and Heitkemper, 1979; Burakoff, 1981; Maasdam and Anuras, 1981; Yurick, Robb, Spier, and Ebert, 1980).

Nursing Implications. Management of diverticulosis includes a diet of nonspicy foods and the control of constipation and weight. A high residue diet is thought to be the best means of preventing and treating diverticulosis (Arnold, 1980; Burakoff, 1981; Mondal and Topley, 1981). Bran, whole grain cereals and bread, fruits, vegetables, and peanut butter should be used freely. Harsh laxatives should be avoided; those providing bulk such as Metamucil are recommended (Bartol and Heitkemper, 1979). With education and guidelines, older individuals can usually effectively control their own stress factors and dietary regimens.

Diarrhea

Diarrhea is more serious in older patients than in the young because dehydration and electrolyte imbalance occur more quickly. Since fecal impaction may be the precipitating factor, its presence should be ruled out before other causes are explored (this will be discussed later in this chapter). Additional factors may include laxative abuse, intestinal infections, food poisoning, medication, food allergy, diverticulitis, and malignancy. Assessment is usually made by taking a careful history and by visualization of the lower gastrointestinal tract through fiberoptic endoscopy and/or radiological studies (Bartol and Heitkemper, 1979).

Nursing Implications. Maintaining adequate hydration, restoring electrolyte balance, and providing a nonirritating diet are measures to promote recovery from diarrhea. Antidiarrheal medication may be prescribed, but identification and removal of the cause are more important. If antibiotics have been administered, fermented dairy products such as yogurt and buttermilk can assist in replacing the normal intestinal flora (Bartol and Heitkemper, 1979). The nurse who sees each older person as an individual with his own unique life-style, strengths, and problems can develop specific educational programs to maximize wellness. Persons of all ages usually respond to significant others who communicate that they care and want to help, and that there is hope.

Constipation

Constipation is one of the most common complaints of older people. Contributing factors are decreased peristalsis and elasticity of the bowels and atrophy of the mucous glands in the colon that lubricate the feces. Habits may also cause constipation: inadequate intake of bulk and fluids, physical inactivity, chronic use of laxatives and/or enemas, and ignoring the urge to defecate (Hull, Greco, and Brooks, 1980; Williams and Shaffer, 1980). Medication, prescribed bed rest, and depression also contribute to constipation (Bowles, Portnoi, and Kenney, 1981; Straus, 1979; Tucker, 1980). Since this problem can also be due to pathology, every older person should have careful medical evaluation, including rectal and sigmoid examination, every 1-2 years (see Chapter 29 on bowel and bladder control).

Irritable Bowel Syndrome

Irritable bowel syndrome or functional bowel distress is frequently referred to as "colitis" by older persons. Either constipation or diarrhea is present and accompanied by abdominal pain. Sometimes bouts of diarrhea are interspersed with periods of constipation. Frequently, mucus is passed with or in the stool. Bleeding rarely occurs except from anal fissures or hemorrhoids. Hyperactive bowel sounds and left abdominal tenderness are usually present. Other symptoms include flatulence, belching, heartburn, and nausea. Frequently stress and tension seem to precipitate the problem (Straus, 1979).

Nursing Implications. Older persons need guidelines to effectively control their "colitis." Activity that is enjoyed, rest, and relaxation should be planned into daily schedules in an effort to control stress and anxiety. Spicy and fried foods should be avoided, as well as any other foods usually not tolerated. Increased dietary fiber has proved to be more beneficial than the traditional low residue diet in controlling this syndrome (Manning, Heaton, Harvey, and Uglow, 1977; Straus, 1979).

Fecal Impaction and Fecal Incontinence

The severest form of constipation is fecal impaction. With prolonged retention in the bowel, the fecal mass gradually loses water. This dehydrated mass then irritates the mucosa and causes increased mucous secretions. The mucus dissolves some of the fecal mass, resulting in leakage of liquid stool and diarrhea (Caldwell and Hegner, 1975). Examination of the rectum

with a gloved, lubricated finger validates the presence of hard, impacted feces. Warm oil retention enemas, followed by cleansing detergent or soapsuds enemas, usually resolve the problem. If the fecal mass is large, digital breakdown may be required before it can be passed (Bartol and Heitkemper, 1979; Brocklehurst and Hanley, 1976; Cefalu, McKnight, and Pike, 1981; Straus, 1979). Small amounts of hydrogen peroxide may be instilled to encourage breakage of the impaction (Eliopoulos, 1979; also see Chapter 29 for fecal incontinence).

Hemorrhoids

Hemorrhoids or piles are dilated, swollen terminal veins in the anal area. Older persons may have developed them earlier in life, or they may be a recent occurrence. They tend to occur in women who have been pregnant, anyone who has stood for long periods of time, and those who are chronically constipated. Hemorrhoids cause perianal itching and pain, and sometimes blood-streaked stools. Careful examination should be made of anyone with rectal bleeding because it is one of the earliest signs of colon and rectal cancer, and hemorrhoids do not rule out the presence of cancer (Bartol and Heitkemper, 1979; Cox, 1969). Hemorrhoids are usually treated conservatively. Since hemorrhoids may recur, surgical excision, elastic band ligation, or sclerosing injection therapy is only resorted to when itching or pain is severe or bleeding has caused anemia (Abramson, 1981).

Nursing Implications. Patients with hemorrhoids should be cautioned to avoid constipation and straining with elimination. The pain and itching may be relieved with sitz baths, witch hazel soaks, or ointments containing anesthetic agents, emollients, and/or corticosteroids applied to the perianal area. Relief from prolapsed hemorrhoids can sometimes be achieved by pushing them back into the rectum, and extreme discomfort may be alleviated by standing and by elevating the legs when lying or sitting (Bartol and Heitkemper, 1979; Cox, 1969).

METABOLIC PROBLEMS

Impaired metabolism is the villain of aging. This culprit sneaks up upon the older body and diminishes its efficiency until at the end, the body is devoid of the energy necessary to sustain life.

Metabolism is the sum total of the physical and chemical processes by which body tissue is produced, maintained, and transformed into energy. With age, each and every body cell, organ, and system is changed. Some of these changes are easily seen. There are others which become apparent only in times of stress, when the aging body lacks the reserve to cope as rapidly and successfully as it once did. Some of the more frequently occurring metabolic problems in older adults include diabetes, osteoporosis, and gout.

Diabetes

Diabetes is probably the most common metabolic disease among older people. It is believed that one-fifth or more of those over 65 have diabetes. The incidence appears to be increasing, but perhaps this is because people are living longer, obesity is becoming more prevalent, and diagnostic techniques for its detection are used more frequently (Williams, 1978). Although diabetes is prevalent in older persons, it may not be as common as previously thought (Tobin and Andreas, 1979). While on the whole, concentrations of glucose during a tolerance test tend to increase with advancement of age, there is much variation in individuals of the same age. There seems to be little doubt that as one's body grows older, the ability to handle glucose decreases. For this reason, it is recommended that a nomogram (see Figure 22-2) be used to evaluate the glucose test of the older person. In using the nomogram, a straight line is drawn from the scale for the patient's age, through his glucose level, and continued to the percentile rank. In this manner, the person's glucose tolerance can be compared to others of his age group. If he is in the sixtieth percentile,

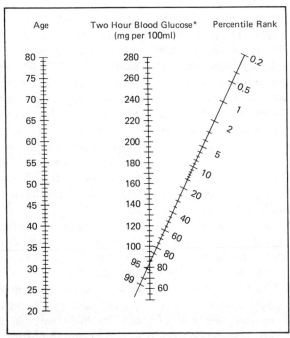

*The oral glucose dose was 1.75g per kilogram (kg) of body weight.

Figure 22-2. Glucose tolerance test nomogram. A straight line is drawn from the scale for the patient's age, through his glucose level, and continued to the percentile rank to compare his glucose tolerance with others of his age group. [Source: Tobin, J. and Andreas, R. *Diabetes and Aging* (NIH Publication No. 79-1408). Washington, D.C.: U.S. Government Printing Office, 1979.]

he performs better than 60% of those his age, but less efficiently than the other 40%. This schematic in assessment serves as a useful, but perhaps imperfect, guide to detection of diabetes in older adults.

Caution is urged in labeling the older person as diabetic. Careful follow-up must be conducted (Denham, 1981; Williams, 1978). The diagnosis of diabetes on the basis of glucose intolerance is difficult and the severity of the disease is sometimes misjudged. This calls for further investigation of what may appear to be borderline cases. Since fasting glucose levels rise slightly with age, elevated concentrations must be found repeatedly before the older adult is considered diabetic. Another method of establishing positive diagnosis is on the basis of repeatedly elevated two-hour postprandial glucose levels or when diabetic complications, such as neuropathy or retinopathy, are associated with slightly elevated glucose levels (Williams, 1978).

Since the threshold for urinary glucose secretion becomes elevated with age, there may be a markedly elevated serum glucose before there is glucosuria. Without glucosuria, the three P's that usually signal the presence of diabetes are absent in the elderly. Rather than polyuria, polydipsia, and polyphagia, the first symptoms may be fatigue, infection, or indications of neuropathy, such as sensory changes. Diabetes may also lead to sexual dysfunctioning in the form of vaginitis in females and chronic impotence in males (see Chapter 36, Sexuality and Aging).

Nursing Implications. The goal of nursing is to assist the older person with diabetes in modifying his life-style in order to control the disease and its effect on his body. The nurse needs to make comprehensive assessments to determine what knowledge, skills, and needs the patient has (Miller and White, 1980).

Insulin and oral hypoglycemic agents may be unnecessary and may increase the risk of hypoglycemia. Many adults who develop diabetes achieve considerable control with exercise and diet alone. Regular exercise improves metabolic control, controls weight, promotes collateral circulation, and maintains morale and fitness (Cusack, 1981; Koivisto, 1981). Dietary guidelines encompass these goals: reduction to, and maintenance of, ideal weight; avoidance of refined sugar; and adequate nutrition and satiation (Podolsky and El-Beheri, 1980). Recently, dietary fiber has been advocated. The fiber aids dietary control by reducing glucose absorption (Anderson and Sieling, 1981; Cusack, 1981). Having a written dietary plan assists the patient in following the guidelines and facilitates periodic modification.

Although older persons with diabetes have elevated urinary glucose thresholds, they are encouraged to test their urine daily in order to promptly detect any change in their status or control (Palumbo, 1977). The rationale for, and correct methods of, obtaining and testing specimens need to be understood and practiced. The first voided specimen of urine which has been stored in the bladder for hours should be discarded. The urine voided one-half hour later is a more valid indication of glucose in the bloodstream and excreted by the kidneys in the last 30 minutes. Urine test results should be recorded and periodically reviewed with members of the health team.

Especially important and difficult in aged persons with diabetes is the maintenance of healthy skin. The skin needs to be protected from trauma or infection. Perception of extreme temperatures may be altered due to peripheral neurological changes in old age. Temperatures of bath water and of water for washing dishes and doing other cleaning chores should be tested with the individual's elbow. Padded oven mitts should be used to remove articles from the freezer. Any breaks in the skin should promptly receive first aid in an effort to minimize infection.

Because of peripheral neuropathy, the feet are especially prone to trauma, infection, and gangrene. Proper care of the feet needs to be understood by persons with diabetes. Older people find it hard to remember to observe and care for body parts if discomfort does not remind them. If obesity and arthritic joints physically prevent the person with diabetes from viewing and caring for his own feet, significant others may need to help with foot care. The feet should be bathed daily with mild soap and lukewarm water, and should be patted dry (rubbing should be avoided because it may damage the skin). Lotions or oils should be applied gently and without massage to maintain soft, smooth skin. Dry brittle toenails, which are a common hazard, should be softened by soaking for 20-30 minutes before clipping. The nail corners should not be clipped. Podiatrists may prove especially valuable to the older person with diabetes. Finally, the shoes of the older adult with diabetes should fit well, without pressure or rubbing. High heels should be avoided. New shoes should be broken in carefully.

Factors which impair circulation should be discussed with the diabetic patient. The following advice should be given:

- Avoid smoking (nicotine is a vasoconstrictor).

- Dress warmly when in a cold environment (cold also constricts blood vessels).
- Avoid tight clothing such as knee-length hose.
- Avoid furniture that presses against the back of the knee or calf of the leg.
- Avoid crossing the legs.
- Avoid tight bedcovers.

In addition, such persons should not apply any irritating substances or external heat. The loss of sensation and already compromised circulation may cause serious injury to the skin. Activities that increase circulation should become a part of the daily routine of the person with diabetes.

Those with diabetes and their significant others need to know two major complications of diabetes: diabetic coma (hyperglycemia) and insulin shock (hypoglycemia); see Table 22-1. Knowledge of these two serious disrup-

Table 22-1. Comparison of Hyperglycemia and Hypoglycemia.

| DISRUPTION | HYPERGLYCEMIA | | HYPOGLYCEMIA |
	KETOACIDOSIS	HYPEROSMOLAR NONKETOTIC COMA	
Symptoms	Polyuria Thirst Nausea and vomiting Dry skin and mucous membranes Weight loss Abdominal pain Kussmaul respirations (deep rapid respirations) Sluggish reflexes Acetone breath Weakness and/or paralysis Soft eyeballs Hypotension	Like ketoacidosis except: No Kussmaul respirations No acetone breath	Moist skin Perspiring Normal or increased blood pressure Nausea Anorexia Visual disturbances Confusion Seizures

Lab findings
  Blood glucose
  Urine glucose
	300-1500 mg/100 ml
	Elevated
		600-3000 mg/100 ml
		Elevated
			60 mg or less/100 ml
			Normal

Onset	Slow (hours to days)	Slow (hours to days)	Rapid (minutes to hours)
Precipitating factors	Infection, stress, lack of diagnosis or treatment	Infections, stress, medications	Delayed or omitted meals; excessive insulin or exercise
Treatment	Insulin, IV fluids, sodium bicarbonate, or potassium if indicated	Insulin, IV fluids	Glucose in the form of grape or orange juice or candy; glucagon; 50% dextrose

tions in blood sugar and of the resultant necessity for prompt medical care is essential. A variation of hyperglycemia is hyperosmolar nonketotic coma. It occurs most frequently in people over 50 in whom diabetes is mild or even undiagnosed. Approximately half of those developing this coma die. Treatment consists of intravenous fluids, electrolytes, and insulin.

Hypoglycemic shock is more serious than hyperglycemia. Without adequate blood glucose, the brain may suffer irreversible damage. For this reason, some physicians prefer that patients spill a little sugar into their urine rather than experience insulin reactions. This is also the rationale for administering glucose as an emergency measure when diabetic patients are found unconscious.

Older people with diabetes are prone to other problems, especially those of the eye and the genitourinary tract. Early retinopathy may be treated successfully with laser treatment or photocoagulation (Cusack, 1981; Guthrie and Guthrie, 1977). If the bladder is not completely emptied, urinary tract infections are likely. Drinking two quarts of liquid daily and using external pressure to facilitate emptying the bladder may be advocated. Poorly controlled diabetes may cause vaginitis and female sexual dysfunction. Diabetes may cause histologic changes in penile tissue resulting in chronic impotence. Counseling, sex education, and therapy are especially important for middle-aged and elderly diabetics with sexual problems (Krosnick and Podolsky, 1981).

The older person with diabetes needs to understand the rationale for early identification, intervention, and management of problems. He should not think, "This ulcer will heal in a few days" or "They'll amputate if I show them this area." He should know that early treatment of problems may minimize their severity and reduce complications. The nurse's educative and supportive role and skills are especially important in helping the older person with diabetes achieve maximal health.

Osteoporosis

Osteoporosis is a metabolic malefactor in older adults. Although this condition may occur in relationship to other diseases, thereby affecting all age groups, in older adults it usually occurs as an independent problem. Approximately 11 million persons in the United States are affected. Women are four times more likely than men to experience osteoporosis. Not only does bone loss begin earlier in women, but the rate of loss is faster than that in men, especially after menopause. Women lose approximately 25% of their bone mass; men, only 12%. Caucasians and those of northern European descent are particularly prone to the development of osteoporosis (Barzel, 1978).

Bone density is related to physical activity. This has been demonstrated by astronauts' significant loss of calcium from their wrist bones after 72 hours of space travel. Also, studies have shown that in right-handed people, the bone density of the right hand is 8–12% greater than that of the left hand. The relationship is reversed in left-handed people (Albanese, Edelson, Lorenze, and Wein, 1978). In a cross-sectional study of marathon runners, the usual decrease of total body calcium with increasing age was not observed. Research has demonstrated an increase in bone mass after an exercise program (Aloia, 1981).

Most studies indicate the effectiveness of specific measures to assist aging adults in maintaining positive calcium balance and decreasing skeletal demineralization: increase dietary calcium (greater than 1.2 grams daily); maintain the correct calcium-phosphorus balance by avoiding excessive protein and phosphorus intake; and ingest adequate vitamin D (Seeman and Riggs, 1981). Additional nutrients considered essential for the development and maintenance of bone matrix are fluoride and vitamins C and K (Jowsey, 1977; Pinel, 1976; Raper, 1977; U.S. Department of Health, Education and Welfare, 1979; Whedon, 1978; Wolff, 1979). Three hundred milligrams of calcium are found in the normal daily adult diet, excluding dairy products. A quart of milk would add nearly 1 gram of calcium. Supplementary calcium may also be supplied by medicinal tablets such as calcium carbonate, calcium lactate, or calcium gluconate, in order to achieve the daily calcium intake of greater than 1.2 grams recommended for prevention of bone loss (Seeman and Riggs, 1981); see Chapter 33 on nutrition.

Not only do inactivity and deficient nutrients adversely affect bone metabolism in older adults, but hormone alterations and intestinal malabsorption are also serious factors. Excessive secretions by the parathyroids, thyroid, and adrenal cortex may cause excessive bone loss. Absorption of calcium in the gastrointestinal tract decreases with age to the extent that equivalent dietary intake provides less calcium to an older man than to a younger one (Barzel, 1978; Exton-Smith, 1978).

A careful history and various laboratory studies are used to diagnose osteoporosis. Other metabolic abnormalities related to decreased bone density must be excluded. X-rays of those with osteoporosis usually show uniform progressive changes.

Fractures of the wrist and hip may occur, but those of the vertebrae are most common. Treatment of vertebral fractures includes analgesics and two weeks of complete bed rest. High fluid intake and stool softeners are used to prevent the constipation related to bed rest. Straining at stool increases the pain and should be avoided. Ambulation begins the third week with the patient using a brace for the next eight weeks. Normal functions are then resumed. Usually there are recurrent fractures, although 7-10 years may intervene between episodes. Eventually, recurrent fractures cause kyphosis and forward bending to the extent that the rib cage comes to rest on the iliac crest (dowager's hump). Usually the accompanying change in weight distribution prevents further fractures (Barzel, 1978; Exton-Smith, 1978). Women especially are surprised to learn that their height has decreased 3-4 inches or more.

Nursing Implications. Treatment for osteoporosis is nonspecific because there is no certain way to increase bone formation and slow resorption. The effectiveness of estrogen replacement is controversial (Albanese et al., 1978; Jowsey, 1977; Vaughan, 1976). In order to minimize the risks of hormone therapy, women receiving estrogen should be taught to do monthly breast examination, should have annual pelvic examination and Pap smears, and should be alert for signs of phlebitis.

Older persons should be informed of measures that minimize or slow the development of osteoporosis. These include: engaging in some regular exercise such as walking, bicycling, dancing, and swimming (Richards, 1982); drinking fluoridated water; and having a dietary calcium intake greater than 1.2 grams daily (Seeman and Riggs, 1981). It is thought that drinking milk at bedtime, and during the night if awakened, may help decrease nocturnal calcium loss (Soika, 1973) as well as act as a sedative. Since vitamin C is involved in calcium metabolism and excreted from the body within eight hours, ideally a good source of vitamin C, such as fruits, citrus juices, and tomatoes, should be ingested approximately every eight hours. Inadequate amounts of vitamin D may also be a risk factor in homebound patients (Seeman and Riggs, 1981).

Pain and discomfort should be relieved with analgesics. The possibility of drug dependence is of decreasing concern after age 70 (Wolff, 1979). Warm packs, gentle massage, and various "deep heat" preparations may promote comfort. Braces, splints, and other kinds of immobilizing apparatus should be used cautiously. They may cause breakdown of the older person's thin skin, and the restriction of activity may actually increase bone demineralization. Prescribed bed rest for other conditions may also accelerate osteoporosis. Isometric or range of motion exercises should be utilized every 4-5 hours unless contraindicated. Ambulation should be resumed as soon as possible (Wolff, 1979).

Frequently, an older person with osteoporosis has had a spontaneous fracture, such as when turning over in bed or stepping off a curb, which caused him to fall, rather than the fall causing the bone to break. These persons may become fearful of getting out of bed, or even turning over in it, and rightfully so. Caution must be exercised in all aspects of care to prevent spontaneous fractures.

Gout

Gout is a systemic disease in which there are recurrent severe pain and joint inflammation, with urate crystals being deposited in the synovial fluid. Many individuals develop tophi (chalky deposits of urates) in the ears, joints, and kidneys. Gout is caused by overproduction, retention, or both, of uric acid, resulting in hyperuricemia. Primary gout is due to hereditary error in metabolism. Gout may also develop secondary to obesity, acidosis, psoriasis, myocardial infarction, leukemia, polycythemia, multiple myeloma, or lymphoma (Grob, 1978).

The incidence of gout increases with age. Primary gout occurs most often in men in their fifth decade; the incidence in women increases postmenopause. Frequently, joint trauma or surgery precipitates gout. Usually only one, two, or three joints are involved. Most often the big toe, especially the first metatarsophalangeal joint, is involved. Often ankles, knees, fingers, wrists, and elbows are also involved. The affected joint or joints suddenly become tender, painful, red, and swollen. Without treatment, the attack lasts several days to several weeks, disappears, and recurs again and again, often with increasing frequency and severity. Those persons with gout are also more apt to have hypertension, renal insufficiency, cardiac and cerebral atherosclerosis, hypertriglyceridemia, and diabetes (Grob, 1978).

Serum urate levels are sensitive to stress and to many medications such as aspirin, corticosteroids, probenecid, phenylbutazone, allopurinol, sulfinpyrazone, pyrazinamide, and diuretics, including thiazides and ethacrynic acid. For this reason, patients should avoid unusual stress and abstain from the mentioned medications for at least three days before a blood specimen is drawn for uric acid determination (Grob, 1978).

Treatment focuses on prevention and control of acute attacks and reduction of hyperuricemia. The hyperuricemia is usually treated either with allopurinol (Zyloprim) or with probenecid (Benemid). Since these medications may initially precipitate acute attacks, medications such as colchicine, indomethacin (Indocin), phenylbutazone (Butazolidin), and corticosteroids are also used initially and temporarily during the acute attack (Grahame, 1978; Grob, 1978).

Nursing Implications. Persons with gout and their significant others need to be educated about the signs and symptoms of acute attacks,

and about the lifelong necessity of taking the prescribed medicine to control hyperuricemia and prevent acute recurrences. Information should also be given about any possible side effects from the prescribed medication.

Although medication to control hyperuricemia is thought by many authorities to negate the need for a special diet (Luckmann and Sorensen, 1980), avoidance of foods high in purine, such as shellfish and organ meats, and moderation in the use of alcohol are considered by other authorities to be of value (Currie, 1980; Grob, 1978; Wolff, 1979).

Osteoarthritis

Osteoarthritis is virtually universal in older adults (Habermann, 1979). Almost all persons over age 45 have some form of this degenerative joint disease, and the degree increases with age. Women are affected more often than men. Predisposing factors include aging, joint trauma, obesity, and a familial tendency (Grahame, 1978; Grob, 1978; Habermann, 1979; Luckmann and Sorensen, 1980; Wolff, 1979).

Unlike rheumatoid arthritis which is a systemic disease, osteoarthritis is a local joint disorder and is frequently referred to as degenerative joint disease. Most commonly affected are one or several of the weight-bearing joints (lumbar spine, hips, knees), cervical spine, shoulders, and terminal interphalangeal finger joints. The latter frequently develop hypertrophic spurs called Heberden's nodes. Spurs also occur on the proximal interphalangeal joint and are then called Bouchard's nodes. The main symptom is an aching pain which occurs with motion or weight bearing and is relieved by rest. The ache may forewarn of changes in the weather. Stiffness after inactivity persists for only a few minutes, compared to that of rheumatoid arthritis which may last for several hours (Grob, 1978). Diagnosis is confirmed by x-ray observation of the characteristic changes — narrowed joint space, hypertrophied bone, near destruction of cartilage, and extensive spurs (Grahame, 1978; Luckmann and Sorensen, 1980; Pathy, 1978; Troup, 1980). However, the degree of degenerative joint changes and the severity of the symptoms are often not correlated. Someone with minor changes may be quite uncomfortable, while another person may have few symptoms with radical changes.

Although osteoarthritis cannot be cured, its progression is slow. Joint mobility can be retained better than with other forms of arthritis. For some patients, weight reduction, physical therapy, orthopedic procedures, and medications completely relieve their symptoms of osteoarthritis. Antispasmodic or anti-inflammatory drugs may be beneficial. Physical therapy in the form of heat, traction, massage, and exercises helps relieve aching and stiffness. Traction or a cervical collar may relieve nerve root pressure in the neck. Walkers or canes may reduce the strain on weight-bearing joints (Hart, 1980; Luckmann and Sorensen, 1980; Wolff, 1979); see Chapter 30 for rehabilitation in arthropathy.

When symptoms are not relieved by other measures, total joint replacement may be considered. Antibiotics and topical cleansing of the operative site are initiated 72 hours before surgery (see Chapter 26 for surgical care).

Nursing Implications. The nurse's role in working with the patient with osteoarthritis is mainly that of a counselor/educator. The patient may need help in learning to live with osteoarthritis. Weight reduction may be advised but is difficult in older adults because of their decreased caloric requirements, basal metabolic rates, and activities; because of the eating habits acquired over a lifetime; and perhaps because of a limited food budget.

Overuse of involved joints is not recommended; however, total rest should be avoided since it causes muscle atrophy and weakness. Heat, massage, and exercise relieve aching and stiffness, and relax the involved muscles. Rest, especially in the afternoon, is beneficial.

Osteoarthritis of the legs seriously impairs motility; going up or down stairs, rising from a low chair or commode, and getting in or out of the bathtub pose problems (Grahame, 1978). Maintenance of maximal range of motion is encouraged by daily exercise.

Radicular symptoms such as paresthesia, pain, and numbness or weakness of the arms usually respond to wearing a cervical collar. The immobilization of the cervical spine by the collar is particularly helpful at night when radicular symptoms are especially troublesome.

When symptoms subside, usually in a few weeks, the collar may be left off (Gilmore, 1980; Grahame, 1978).

Osteomalacia

Osteomalacia is another metabolic bone disease which is much like osteoporosis. However, its etiology and treatment are known, and complete recovery is possible. The cause is vitamin D deficiency.

In the absence of vitamin D, the absorption of calcium will be deficient, and newly deposited bone matrix will not calcify. Generalized, persistent bone pain results, accompanied by muscle weakness. A careful history is essential since deficiency of vitamin D is rare in the United States where milk and bread are fortified with vitamin D. However, osteomalacia may occur if the elderly person does not have any exposure to sunlight and has a poor diet. Early diagnosis is made by high alkaline phosphatase and low urinary calcium levels. Later hypophosphatemia and hypocalcemia develop to complete the pathognomonic composite of osteomalacia symptoms. Pseudofractures occur in more advanced cases (Barzel, 1978; Corless, 1980; Exton-Smith, 1978; Spencer and Lender, 1979).

Upon maintenance of adequate intake of vitamin D, serum calcium and phosphorus usually return to normal in two weeks, and alkaline phosphatase in several more. Pseudofractures heal; bone pain and muscle weakness are relieved.

Nursing Implications. In osteomalacia, the importance of an adequate diet must be stressed in interactions with patients and their significant others. Consideration should be given to the individual's income and food preferences in adapting the diet to his needs. Outdoor activities should be encouraged, and the role of vitamin D from sunshine in health maintenance should be discussed.

Measures that can be taken to relieve or minimize pain are gentle handling, proper positioning, warm baths, and analgesics. Diversional activities may be especially helpful for the first few weeks until the symptoms are relieved. The prevention of complications is most important.

Paget's Disease

Paget's disease, or osteitis deformans, is a metabolic bone disease which causes excessive bone resorption and deposits. The incidence begins after 40 and increases with age until, at the age of 80, one out of nine persons has Paget's disease. The ratio of male to female incidence is 4:3 (Barzel, 1978; Spencer and Lender, 1979).

This slowly developing, chronic disease is characterized by rapid bone metabolism, perhaps 20–40 times the normal rate. One or more of the bones may be involved. The new bone is structurally abnormal. Roentgenograms may reveal typical pagetic lesions such as a "cotton wool" skull, cortical thickening, and/or wide, "bowed" long bones (Gilmore, 1980; Lender and Menczel, 1981; Subbarae, 1979). Approximately one-fifth of those with Paget's disease are symptom free, and diagnosis is made by roentgenograms done for other pathology (Spencer and Lender, 1979). The most common symptoms are areas hot to the touch and bone pain, their locations dependent on the site of the pathology (Caird and Dall, 1978). Spontaneous fractures can occur. Symptoms such as hearing loss, blindness, paralysis, or pain can result from increased bone tissue causing nerve compression. Hearing loss or deafness, facial palsy, and generalized headache are common due to pressure on the seventh and eighth cranial nerves (Barzel, 1978; Carter, 1979). Due to the rapid changes in the bone tissue, the serum alkaline phosphatase may be highly elevated, sometimes 10–20 times normal. Urinary hydroxyproline is also increased (Barzel, 1978).

Calcitonin has been found to be effective in the treatment of Paget's disease. Pain is usually relieved in 2–6 weeks (Barzel, 1978; Brocklehurst and Hanley, 1976; How, 1980). Neurological symptoms may improve, with the exception of hearing loss. Alkaline phosphatase and urinary hydroxyproline fall to half their initial values. Skin testing for sensitivity is recommended before calcitonin is used (Barzel, 1978). The value of other medications is being explored. Emphasis at present is placed on symptomatic treatment and health maintenance measures.

Osteogenic sarcoma develops in 5–14% of those with Paget's disease, in a male to female ratio of 2:1 (Spencer and Lender, 1979). Peri-odic observation is necessary in order to make an early assessment of malignant changes, usually indicated by sharply elevated alkaline phosphatase and pain of a more continuous nature (Barzel, 1978).

Nursing Implications. In severe Paget's disease, nursing care focuses on minimizing the effects and complications of the condition. Periodic assessments are essential to evaluate the effectiveness of nursing measures and medications to control the pain and other symptoms.

Thyroid Disorders

As persons age, their thyroid glands decrease in mass, and their thyroxine turnover decreases. However, since older thyroid glands are found to be able to respond normally to stress, medical scientists think that their normally decreased activity is related to decreased need (Goldman, 1979). Others think that 40% of the older population have undiagnosed hypothyroid problems. Many consider hypothyroidism to be a major contributing factor to many chronic problems of older individuals, including easy fatigability, joint pain, and mental depression (Hamdy, 1980; Tunbridge, 1981). The two most common thyroid disorders are thyrotoxicosis and myxedema (Gilbert, 1981; Irvine and Hodkinson, 1978).

The symptoms of thyrotoxicosis are not typical in the older individual. Exophthalmos and an elevated basal metabolic rate may not be present. Cardiac fibrillation and failure, weight loss, and apathy may be the symptoms (Rodstein, 1979; Schultz, 1978).

Extreme hypothyroidism or myxedema may be diagnosed, but for those with less obvious symptoms the changes may be attributed to aging. Since older persons are more sensitive to medications than those who are younger, when therapy is initiated they need to be observed for effects of overdosage, such as tachycardia, nervousness, weight loss, and diarrhea (Irvine and Hodkinson, 1978).

REFERENCES

Abramson, D.S. Hemorrhoidal banding: Which patients are apt to obtain relief? *Geriatrics* 36(1):122, 124 (1981).

Albanese, A.A., Edelson, A.H., Lorenze, E.N., and Wein, E.H. *Calcium throughout the Life Cycle.* Rosemont, Ill.: National Dairy Council, 1978.

Aloia, J.F. Exercise and skeletal health. *Journal of the American Geriatrics Society* 29:104–107 (1981).

Anderson, J.W. and Sieling, B. High-fiber diets for diabetics: unconventional but effective. *Geriatrics* 36(5):64–72 (1981).

Arnold, K. Gastro-intestinal diseases: the benefits of fibre. *Geriatric Medicine* 10(11):60, 63–64, 67 (1980).

Bartol, M.A. and Heitkemper, M. Gastrointestinal problems. In Carnevali, D.L. and Patrick, M. (Eds.) *Nursing Management for the Elderly.* Philadelphia: J.B. Lippincott, 1979.

Barzel, U.S. Common metabolic disorders of the skeleton in aging. In Reichel, W. (Ed.) *Clinical Aspects of Aging.* Baltimore: Williams and Wilkins, 1978.

Bonaparte, B.H. Teaching patients with biliary and pancreatic disorders. In Bonaparte, B.H. (Ed.) *Gastro-intestinal Care: A Guide for Patient Education.* New York: Appleton-Century-Crofts, 1981.

Bouliere, F. Ecology of human senescence. In Brocklehurst, J.C. (Ed.) *Textbook of Geriatric Medicine and Gerontology* (2nd ed.). New York: Churchill Livingstone, 1978.

Bowles, L.T., Portnoi, V., and Kenney, R. Wear and tear: common biologic changes of aging. *Geriatrics* 36(4):77–80, 83, 86 (1981).

Brocklehurst, J.C. and Hanley, T. *Geriatric Medicine for Students.* New York: Churchill Livingstone, 1976.

Burakoff, R. An updated look at diverticular disease. *Geriatrics* 36(3):83–87, 90–91 (1981).

Caird, F.I. and Dall, J.L.C. The cardiovascular system. In Brocklehurst, J.C. (Ed.) *Textbook of Geriatric Medicine and Gerontology* (2nd ed.). New York: Churchill Livingstone, 1978.

Caldwell, E. and Hegner, B.R. *Geriatrics: A Study of Maturity.* New York: Delmar, 1975.

Carter, A.B. The neurologic aspects of aging. In Rossman, I. (Ed.) *Clinical Geriatrics* (2nd ed.). Philadelphia: J.B. Lippincott, 1979.

Cefalu, C.A., McKnight, G.T., and Pike, J.I. Treating impaction: a practical approach to an unpleasant problem. *Geriatrics* 36(5):143–146 (1981).

Charlesworth, D. and Baker, R.H. Surgery in old age. In Brocklehurst, J.C. (Ed.) *Textbook of Geriatric Medicine and Gerontology* (2nd ed.). New York: Churchill Livingstone, 1978.

Corless, D. One way to prevent fracture of the hip. *Geriatric Medicine* 10(4):32–36 (1980).

Cox, E.A. *Bottoms up with a Rear Admiral.* Durham, N.C.: Moore, 1969.

Currie, W.J.C. Gout and its management. *Geriatric Medicine* 10(12):11–14 (1980).

Cusack, B. Diabetes mellitus: the management. *Geriatric Medicine* 11(3):88, 91, 92, 95 (1981).

Denham, M.J. Diabetes mellitus: the diagnosis. *Geriatric Medicine* 11(2):45–47 (1981).

Eliopoulos, C. *Gerontological Nursing.* New York: Harper & Row, 1979.

Exton-Smith, A.N. Bone aging and metabolic bone disease. In Brocklehurst, J.C. (Ed.) *Textbook of Geriatric Medicine and Gerontology* (2nd ed.). New York: Churchill Livingstone, 1978.

Gilbert, P.D. Thyroid function and disease. In Libow, L.S. and Sherman, F.T. (Eds.) *The Core of Geriatric Medicine.* St. Louis: C.V. Mosby, 1981.

Gilmore, R.L. Recognizing problems of the aging spine. *Geriatrics* 35(11):83–92 (1980).

Goldman, R. Aging changes in structure and function. In Carnevali, D.L. and Patrick, M. (Eds.) *Nursing Management for the Elderly.* Philadelphia: J.B. Lippincott, 1979.

Grahame, R. Diseases of the joints. In Brocklehurst, J.C. (Ed.) *Textbook of Geriatric Medicine and Gerontology* (2nd ed.). New York: Churchill Livingstone, 1978.

Grob, D. Prevalent joint diseases in older persons. In Reichel, W. (Ed.) *Clinical Aspects of Aging.* Baltimore: Williams and Wilkins, 1978.

Guthrie, D.W. and Guthrie, R.A. (Eds.). *Nursing Management of Diabetes Mellitus.* Saint Louis: C.V. Mosby, 1977.

Habermann, E.T. Orthopaedic aspects of the lower extremities. In Rossman, I. (Ed.) *Clinical Geriatrics* (2nd ed.). Philadelphia: J.B. Lippincott, 1979.

Hamdy, R.C. Easy fatigability. *Geriatric Medicine* 10(9):47–48 (1980).

Hart, F.D. Managing osteoarthritis without drugs. *Geriatric Medicine* 10(2):69–72 (1980).

Hoffman, E., Perez, E., and Somera, V. Acute pancreatitis in the upper age groups. *Gastroenterology* 36:675–685 (1959).

How, N.M. Managing Paget's disease. *Geriatric Medicine* 10(7):64 (1980).

Hull, C., Greco, R.S., and Brooks, D.L. Alleviation of constipation in the elderly by dietary fiber supplementation. *Journal of the American Geriatrics Society* 28:410–414 (1980).

Irvine, R.E. and Hodkinson, H.M. Thyroid disease in old age. In Brocklehurst, J.C. (Ed.) *Textbook of Geriatric Medicine and Gerontology* (2nd ed.). New York: Churchill Livingstone, 1978.

Jowsey, J. Osteoporosis: dealing with a crippling bone disease of the elderly. *Geriatrics* 32:41–50 (1977).

Koivisto, V.A. Diabetes in the elderly: What role for exercise? *Geriatrics* 36(6):74–83 (1981).

Krosnick, A. and Podolsky, S. Diabetes and sexual dysfunction: restoring normal ability. *Geriatrics* 36(3):92–95, 99–100 (1981).

Leeming, J.T. and Dymock, I.W. The upper gastrointestinal tract. In Brocklehurst, J.C. (Ed.) *Textbook of Geriatric Medicine and Gerontology* (2nd ed.). New York: Churchill Livingstone, 1978.

Lender, M. and Menczel, J. Office management of Paget's disease. *Geriatrics* 36(5):105–112 (1981).

Luckmann, J. and Sorensen, K.C. *Medical-Surgical Nursing: A Psychophysiologic Approach* (2nd ed.). Philadelphia: W.B. Saunders, 1980.

Maasdam, C.F. and Anuras, S. Are you overlooking GI infections in your elderly patients? *Geriatrics* 36(2):127–134 (1981).

Manning, A.P., Heaton, K.W., Harvey, R.F., and Uglow, P. Wheat fiber and irritable bowel syndrome. *Lancet* 2:417 (1977).

Meyers, J. Teaching the patient with a peptic ulcer. In Bonaparte, B.H. (Ed.) *Gastro-intestinal Care: A Guide for Patient Education.* New York: Appleton-Century-Crofts, 1981.

Miller, B.K. and White, N.E. Diabetes assessment guide. *American Journal of Nursing* 80:1314–1316 (1980).

Mondal, B.K. and Topley, E.M. Complications of diverticulosis. *Geriatric Medicine* 11(6):27 (1981).

Palumbo, P.J. How to treat maturity-onset diabetes. *Geriatrics* 32(12):57–63 (1977).

Pathy, M.S. Clinical presentation and management of neurological disorders in old age. In Brocklehurst, J.C. (Ed.) *Textbook of Geriatric Medicine and Gerontology* (2nd ed.). New York: Churchill Livingstone, 1978.

Pinel, C. Metabolic bone disease in the elderly. *Nursing Times* 72:1046–1048 (1976).

Podolsky, S. and El-Beheri, B. The principles of a diabetic diet. *Geriatrics* 35(12):73–78 (1980).

Ramos, L.Y. Oral hygiene for the elderly. *American Journal of Nursing* 81:1468–1469 (1981).

Raper, N.R. Calcium and phosphorus – dietary concerns. *Nutrition Program News.* Washington, D.C.: U.S. Department of Agriculture, January–April 1977.

Richards, M.L. Osteporosis. *Geriatric Nursing* 1(2):98–102, (1982).

Rodstein, M. Heart disease in the aged. In Rossman, I. (Ed.) *Clinical Geriatrics* (2nd ed.). Philadelphia: J.B. Lippincott, 1979.

Schultz, A.L. Diagnosing and managing hyperthyroidism. *Geriatrics* 33(2):77–81 (1978).

Seeman, E. and Riggs, B.L. Dietary prevention of bone loss in the elderly. *Geriatrics* 36(9):71–73, 75, 79 (1981).

Sklar, M. Gastrointestinal diseases in the aged. In Reichel, W. (Ed.) *Clinical Aspects of Aging.* Baltimore: Williams and Wilkins, 1978.

Sodeman, W.A., Jr. and Sodeman, W. *Pathologic Physiology: Mechanisms of Disease* (5th ed.). Philadelphia: W.B. Saunders, 1974.

Soika, C.V. Combatting osteoporosis. *American Journal of Nursing* 73:1193–1197 (1973).

Spencer, H. and Lender, M. The skeletal system. In Rossman, I. (Ed.) *Clinical Geriatrics* (2nd ed.). Philadelphia: J.B. Lippincott, 1979.

Straus, B. Disorders of the digestive system. In Rossman, I. (Ed.) *Clinical Geriatrics* (2nd ed.). Philadelphia: J.B. Lippincott, 1979.

Subbarae, K. Radiological aspects of aging. In Rossman, I. (Ed.) *Clinical Geriatrics* (2nd ed.). Philadelphia: J.B. Lippincott, 1979.

Tobin, J. and Andres, R. *Diabetes and Aging* (DHEW Public Health Service NIH Publication No. 79-1408). Washington, D.C.: U.S. Government Printing Office, 1979.

Troup, J.D.G. The management plan. *Geriatric Medicine* 10(7):33–38 (1980).

Tucker, J. When patients complain of "stubborn bowels." *Geriatric Medicine* 10(4):48 (1980).

Tunbridge, W.M.G. Is hypothyroidism causing your patient's lethargy? *Geriatrics* 36(5):79–80, 82, 87–88 (1981).

U.S. Department of Health, Education and Welfare. *Health: United States 1978* (DHEW Publication No. PHS 78-1232). Washington, D.C.: U.S. Government Printing Office, 1978.

U.S. Department of Health, Education and Welfare. *Special Report on Aging: 1979* (NIH Publication No. 79-1907). Washington, D.C.: U.S. Government Printing Office, 1979.

Vaughan, C.C. Rehabilitation in postmenopausal osteoporosis. *Israel Journal of Medical Sciences* 12:652–657 (1976).

Villaverde, M.M. and MacMillan, C.W. *Ailments of Aging: From Symptom to Treatment.* New York: Van Nostrand Reinhold, 1980.

Webster, S.G.P. The pancreas and small bowel. In Brocklehurst, J.C. (Ed.) *Textbook of Geriatric Medicine and Gerontology* (2nd ed.). New York: Churchill Livingstone, 1978.

Whedon, G.D. Osteoarthritis, osteoporosis, and benign prostatic hyperplasia: a prognosis. *Geriatrics* 33:27, 31 (1978).

Wilkins, E.M. *Clinical Practice of Dental Hygienist* (4th ed.). Philadelphia: Lea and Febiger, 1976.

Williams, I. and Shaffer, J.L. Gastrointestinal disorders: treatment without drugs. *Geriatric Medicine* 10(9): 20, 23–24, 27 (1980).

Williams, T.F. Diabetes mellitus in older people. In Reichel, W. (Ed.) *Clinical Aspects of Aging.* Baltimore: Williams and Wilkins, 1978.

Winsberg, F. Roentgenographic aspects of aging. In Rossman, I. (Ed.) *Clinical Geriatrics* (2nd ed.). Philadelphia: J.B. Lippincott, 1979.

Wolff, H. Musculoskeletal problems. In Carnevali, D.L. and Patrick, M. (Eds.) *Nursing Management for the Elderly.* Philadelphia: J.B. Lippincott, 1979.

Yellowitz, J., Portnoy, R., and Smith, B. *Did You Know: You Can Save Your Teeth for Old Age.* St. Paul, Minn.: Pilot Dental Care Program for Senior Citizens, Minnesota Department of Public Welfare, Minnesota Board on Aging, 1979.

Yurick, A.G., Robb, S.S., Spier, B.E., and Ebert, N.J. *The Aged Person and the Nursing Process.* New York: Appleton-Century-Crofts, 1980.

23
Respiratory Conditions in Older Adults

Frances S. Knudsen

The elderly individual is subject to a host of pulmonary problems related not only to the biologic processes of aging per se but also to the prolonged exposure in a polluted urban and/or occupational environment.

J.R. Wright (1978, p. 78)

As one grows older, respiratory problems become more common and more life threatening. Even with today's chemotherapeutic agents and machines to assist respiratory ventilation, influenza and pneumonia remain the fourth leading cause of death in those 70 years and older. Bronchitis, emphysema, and asthma rank sixth as the cause of death in those 65–74 years of age (U.S. Department of Health, Education and Welfare, 1979b).

The respiratory system becomes less efficient with age. Older lungs have decreased vital capacity and elasticity. Chest capacity is reduced because of ossified cartilage, stooped posture, and arthritic changes in joints. In addition, the reduction in immunity that accompanies aging causes increased susceptibility to infections (Timiras, 1972). The most serious respiratory problems of older adults are pneumonia, chronic obstructive pulmonary disease, and tuberculosis.

PNEUMONIA

Pneumonia has been known for generations as the friendly killer of the elderly. It still is often the presenting cause of death, although some other chronic condition or situation, such as malnutrition, is the real reason that the older adult succumbs to pneumonia.

Pneumonia is an acute inflammation of the lung alveoli which causes exudate formation, tissue consolidation, and interference with respiratory exchange of gases. Bronchopneu-

monia, to which older persons are especially prone, occurs in scattered areas in the lungs but only in those alveoli in contact with the bronchi. Bacteria and viruses are the leading causative agents of pneumonia. The majority of pneumonias found in older people are bacterial in origin (Bither, 1979). The pneumococcus is the most common cause of bacterial pneumonia, but other forms of pneumonia are caused by *Klebsiella, Hemophilus influenzae,* streptococcus, and staphylococcus (Futrell, Brovender, McKinnon-Mullet, and Brower, 1980; Reichel, 1978; Villaverde and MacMillan, 1980; Wynne, 1979).

Pneumonia is best prevented by promoting optimal health, especially in the area of respiratory function. Individual health habits, especially avoidance of smoking, are important. Those persons with existing respiratory problems are more likely to develop bronchopneumonia (Luckmann and Sorensen, 1980). Prevention of pneumonia is also an important consideration in the care of institutionalized older patients. Measures include: adequate hydration; frequent turning, coughing, and deep breathing; positioning to avoid aspiration of secretions; avoiding respiratory depression due to sedatives, narcotics, etc.; and avoiding administration of oral fluids to those who are unconscious or semiconscious.

The classic signs and symptoms of pneumonia — chest pain, fever, cough, and pink- or rust-colored sputum — may be absent due to altered responses in the older person. A general deterioration with an increase in pulse and respiration, may herald the onset of pneumonia. Occasionally, a shaking chill indicates its presence (Bither, 1979; Reichel, 1978). The diagnosis is frequently made by x-ray. Culture and sensitivity tests of the sputum assist in planning the chemotherapy.

Nursing Implications

Bed rest is utilized in caring for older persons with pneumonia in order to decrease the need for oxygen. However, it should be modified to prevent the hazards of immobility. Periodic turning, deep breathing, and coughing are used to keep the airway patent. Spirometers may stimulate the patient's interest in this activity. Fluid intake should be maintained at 2000–3000 ml daily in order to keep mucus thin and readily expectorated. Fluid output is monitored to assess if intake is adequate and to provide one indication of renal failure. Productive coughing is encouraged, but an unproductive cough is treated with cough suppressants to promote needed rest. Postural drainage may be used to facilitate removal of secretions. Auscultation before and after drainage assesses the degree of necessity and effectiveness of postural drainage.

Hypoxia is indicated by restlessness, confusion, extreme personality changes, and renal failure. Arterial blood gas studies assist in assessing the need for, and amount of, oxygen to administer. Persons whose pathology causes retention of carbon dioxide receive temporary stimulation for breathing from low oxygen levels. Consequently, oxygen administered at flow rates above 2 liters per minute may cause further depression of respirations and apnea (Bither, 1979).

Although pneumonia is not usually treated as a communicable disease, patients should be taught that pneumonia is spread through airborne droplets which are expelled during talking, coughing, and sneezing. Tissues must be readily accessible. Soiled tissues should be placed in paper bags and removed at least 2–3 times a day for burning. Frequent handwashing by staff is also essential in preventing the spread of infection.

Within 2–3 days of the initiation of therapy, the patient begins to improve. However, full recovery and return to pre-illness energy level may take much longer than the older patient would like. Frequent rest periods, avoidance of overexertion, and deep breathing exercises should be continued for 6–8 weeks (Luckmann and Sorensen, 1980). Since pneumonia tends to recur, patients should be encouraged to main-tain a healthy life-style and to seek early evaluation of respiratory problems. Vaccination for influenza is recommended in those over 65. The injections need 2–3 weeks to be effective and are probably most effective if taken in the early fall (Bither, 1979; Influenza Vaccine, 1980).

CHRONIC OBSTRUCTIVE PULMONARY DISEASE

Chronic obstructive pulmonary disease (COPD) is the term commonly used to describe a respiratory dysfunction in which there is a persistent, chronic obstruction to bronchial air flow that continues to worsen (see the profile of the typical older adult with COPD). COPD most commonly includes two respiratory problems, chronic bronchitis and emphysema (Wright, 1978); these are also discussed in Chapter 31. Although asthma causes obstruction that is intermittent, it is usually classified as COPD (Luckmann and Sorensen, 1980). Bronchiectasis, tuberculosis, pulmonary fibrosis, bronchiolitis, silicosis, and small airways disease are also associated with and often considered COPD (Luckmann and Sorensen, 1980; Reichel, 1978). Each of these respiratory disorders causes similar pathophysiological changes and symptoms. Each can occur alone or in combination with another. The two that coexist most often are emphysema and bronchitis. The trend is to focus on the commonalities of COPD rather than on a specific diagnosis.

PROFILE

Typical Older Adult with Chronic Obstructive Pulmonary Disease

Anxiety and exhaustion deepen the lines that time has etched on his face. His color becomes more cyanotic as he talks — stopping frequently to rest and concentrate on his breathing. The effort to push out his breath is now the focus of his whole life. His chest is barrel shaped; the transverse chest diameter is no longer larger than his anterior-posterior measurements. His ribs are now horizontal instead of sloping normally downward. He tries to rest in his favorite sitting position but must lean forward with his arms braced against his knees, a chair, or the bed, struggling for any means to force the air from his lungs. This additional leverage allows his neck, and his intercostal and abdominal muscles, to assist in the all-important task of forcing his breath out. His lips are pursed in a whistle-like position. By exhaling against a narrow opening of pursed lips, with painstaking deliberateness, he maintains positive pressure in the bronchial tree and prevents collapse of his airway. This struggle to breathe continues night and day for the patient with chronic obstructive pulmonary disease (COPD).

COPD has been identified as the most rapidly increasing health problem in the United States. As a cause of death, it has increased 224% in the past 20 years. It is thought that there are at least 15 million Americans with this condition (Shapiro, Harrison, and Trout, 1975). The increased occurrence is attributed to better diagnostic measures, an increasingly older population, increasing survival from other pathology, and increased smoking among women (Luckmann and Sorensen, 1980). The incidence of COPD increases with age (Reichel, 1978). The main cause appears to be smoking, although other predisposing factors are recurrent respiratory infections, changes in the lung due to aging, air pollution, allergies, and genetic factors (Bither, 1979; Van Lancker, 1977). Prevention focuses on avoidance of pulmonary irritants and on prompt investigation and treatment of respiratory problems, especially a persistent cough.

The three main symptoms of COPD are intermittent productive cough and dyspnea and fatigue upon exertion. At first these symptoms are mild, but they worsen insidiously with time. Forced expiration is a common symptom. General debilitation, weight loss, and wheezing also occur. Diagnosis is based on history, physical examination, chest x-rays, pulmonary function tests, and arterial blood gas studies.

Nursing Implications

COPD is frequently present in elderly patients institutionalized for other problems. A diagnosis of COPD may not appear on the care plan or chart since it may not be the admitting or primary diagnosis. For this reason, the nurse needs to be able to assess COPD in elderly patients. Besides the symptoms already discussed, the nurse should observe the following: use of accessory muscles of respiration especially in expiration, prolonged expiration, wheeze or rhonchi at end of expiration, decreased breath sounds, restlessness, twitching, increased anterior-posterior chest diameter (barrel chest), hyperemia of hands, and cyanotic or clubbed fingers (Bither, 1979; Luckmann and Sorensen, 1980).

Care of the older patient with COPD includes assisting with respiration; promoting bronchial drainage; controlling present infection; preventing superimposed infection; observing progress and watching for possible complications such as ulcers, cor pulmonale, and heart failure; and educating the patient.

Upon diagnosis of COPD, patients need to be prepared to assume responsibility for their own care. Education will be instrumental in helping them to achieve not only their maximal health potential but also, and especially important for older adults, maximal feelings of independence, self-worth, and ability to adapt to a changed life-style (Shamansky and Hamilton, 1979). Patients need to learn about their pathophysiology, symptoms of exacerbation and complications, and goals and specifics of the plan of care. Family and significant others also need education in order to assist intelligently with the health care plan (Blomefield, 1980). The planning begins with gathering data about the older patient's life-style in order to help him to learn to adapt to his limitations and conserve energy. Educational programs should include information about medications; how to effectively rest, breathe, cough, and use steam to loosen secretions; ingesting enough liquids to keep sputum thin and easy to expectorate (i.e., usually enough fluids to keep urine pale); exercise; postural drainage; and observation of sputum for increased thickness, unpleasant odors, and changed color (Bither, 1979; Blomefield, 1980; Luckmann and Sorensen, 1980). Printed educational materials such as those developed by Blomefield (1980) and by McDowell and Galbraith (1975) should be given to patients and significant others for later reference and review. Drug management of COPD includes bronchodilators, steroids, antibiotics, and oxygen. In addition to knowing the name, purpose, and side effects of each prescribed drug, older adults should plan their medication taking to fit their daily schedule.

Although not generally considered as such, oxygen is a drug. Older adults may resist its use unless they can be helped to consider it as a medication that will give them greater freedom from shortness of breath and increased ability for activities. As a medication, it also has its disadvantages. Oxygen is expensive and has unique hazards because it is a gas under pressure. Also, once patients with COPD begin to use oxygen, they can seldom do without it. Then, too, the balance between optimal dosage and the level that causes depression of the respiratory center is delicate. In the patient with chronic retention of carbon dioxide, as in COPD, the stimulus for respiration no longer is an elevated carbon dioxide level but has become a diminished oxygen level in the blood. Administration of oxygen may eradicate this secondary stimulus to respiration, causing hypoventilation and respiratory failure. Generally, those with COPD are given no more than 1-2 liters of oxygen per minute in order to prevent carbon dioxide narcosis, unless their arterial blood gases have been checked. Consequently, neither older adults nor others should change their oxygen dosages without consulting their physician (Bither, 1979; Luckmann and Sorensen, 1980).

Older patients with COPD who are receiving oxygen can increase their mobility by attaching 50-90 feet of tubing to the oxygen reservoir. They also have the alternative of placing the tanks on carriers and pulling them or having someone else carry them as they get their daily exercise. Travel can also be arranged for those receiving oxygen.

Because it is a gas under high pressure, oxygen has some unique hazards. It can become a torpedo-like missile if the valve should break. To prevent the possibility of its flying through the air or crashing through walls, it should be firmly fastened to a carrier or structure to prevent its falling over. Since gases expand with heat, tank oxygen should be kept away from sources of heat. Grease, oil, or other combustibles should not come in contact with the oxygen equipment. Patients and others should be reminded to wash their hands before touching the oxygen setup. Smoking should be prohibited around oxygen (Bither, 1979; Luckmann and Sorensen, 1980).

Older patients with COPD benefit from assistance in planning to manage their life-styles. A workable schedule is needed so patients can remain adequately hydrated. They need to thin and raise secretions, thus clearing air spaces for ventilation and decreasing the risk of infection. Some patients find it beneficial to fill a two-quart container with water every morning and drink from it throughout the 24 hours. Additional fluids such as coffee and juices are taken ad lib.

Some patients may find it helpful to have periods of increased humidity to help liquefy and expectorate secretions. These may be achieved by standing near running hot water in the sink, tub, or shower. Older adults with COPD and their families need to explore and discover acceptable ways for the patient to cough and spit. Considerable adaptation may be necessary after a lifetime of repressing these behaviors and considering them socially unacceptable.

Older adults without health problems are frequently unhappy with their sleep patterns; the elderly with COPD may be especially concerned. Their need to rest frequently during the day and concern that their breathing and coughing may disturb the sleep of others may cause them to seek a separate room. A call system should be devised to alert others if an emergency arises. A bedtime snack may promote sleep. Diuretics and stimulants such as tea, soft drinks containing caffeine, coffee, and chocolate should be avoided in the evening.

Those with COPD are especially sensitive to humidity, temperature extremes, and air pollution. Sometimes a change of geographic location is considered, but a trial of 2-3 months should precede a permanent move. Mates of those with COPD need to discuss and help make decisions about treatment options. There should also be opportunity for both partners to discuss sexual activity separately and together. Sometimes providing reading material in these areas will suggest questions to begin the needed discussions.

Respiratory hygiene may include nebulizers, postural drainage, and percussion. Breathing exercises and learning to conserve energy to climb stairs may also benefit patients with COPD. The open, sensitive nurse can often help patients manage their life-styles with their chronicity and declining activities. The patients and their significant others should feel free to discuss problems as they arise. Together they can plan and test approaches, some of which may be innovative. For example, a patient afraid of inhaling while showering may breathe more freely by using an underwater snorkle in the shower (Creative Care Unit, 1981).

In addition to the physiological effects of COPD, the nurse also must consider the psychological aspects. COPD usually causes disabling effects in those aged 45-55, normally the most economically productive individuals in American society. Gradually the respiratory impairment leads to a decrease in energy to such an extent that employment must be curtailed, altered, or discontinued. This in turn results in changes in roles, style of living, self-esteem, and intrafamily and social relationships (Barstow, 1974).

The adaptation of the older person to COPD is similar to the grieving process described by Engel (1964). During the initial disbelief or denial stage, medicines may be "forgotten," old age or lack of exercise blamed for the shortness of breath, and smoking continued. With gradual awareness of the reality of increasing disability, anger may be turned outward to family and friends or inward on self with resultant depression. Anxiety, overdependence, emotional lability, and/or withdrawal may be demonstrated. As relationships with significant others are reorganized, family and friends also go through the grieving process. Gradually, as they assume additional responsibility, they begin to see the patient as someone with an increasingly debilitating disability. Finally, older patients with COPD resolve their loss and accept their identity change. They become able to live with their illness, treatment, and dependence (Bither, 1979).

TUBERCULOSIS

The death rate for tuberculosis has dropped dramatically in the lifetime of most of today's elderly population. Many can recall when "consumption" was rampant and a leading killer, especially of the young. Public health control measures and the introduction of isoniazid in the 1940s have changed the course of history in regard to the epidemiology of tuberculosis.

Approximately 30,000 new cases of tuberculosis are diagnosed each year (U.S. Department of Health, Education and Welfare, 1979c). The incidence is 13 cases per 100,000 population (U.S. Department of Health and Human Services, 1980a). However, these figures are somewhat misleading because they are national averages and do not reveal the very high incidence rates of some areas, especially among native Americans (Shrout, 1980).

The incidence rate is disproportionately high for the geriatric population: 32 cases per 100,000 population in those aged 65 and over. Those aged 45-64 have a case rate of 21 cases per 100,000 population (U.S. Department of Health and Human Services, 1980a). These older persons probably had a primary infection in their youth before modern prophylactic treatment, and the organisms have lain dormant in their lungs for many years. Their reactivitated disease, if untreated, makes them a primary reservoir of infection for young people, particularly their grandchildren.

Finding the new or reactivated case of tuberculosis requires an epidemiological approach, including history, signs and symptoms, skin (Mantoux) test, and laboratory and radiological findings. Because antibody reaction tends to weaken in older individuals, those over age 50 with a suspicious reaction require additional testing. The primed immune system may be restimulated by repeated skin tests or by the use of second strength purified protein derivative (PPD; Wynne, 1979). A second PPD given any time from one week to a year after the initial test will cause the true reaction to appear. This is known as the booster phenomenon (Farer and Atkinson, 1979). This second PPD only boosts the delayed hypersensitivity in a previously infected person. In the noninfected person, numerous and frequent PPDs will not produce a positive reaction. Skin tests using PPD are usually read in 48-72 hours, although evidence of a positive reaction will persist for one week. Therefore, the following recommendations (Farer and Atkinson, 1979) are made for those age 50 and over:

1. The initial PPD is given and read in seven days.
2. The second PPD is given at that time if the reading is less than 10 mm.
3. The second reading is made in 48–72 hours.
4. A 14 × 17 inch chest x-ray should be ordered on all those with a PPD of 10 mm or more.

Because of the potential for the transmission of tuberculosis among patients and employees in nursing homes (U.S. Department of Health, Education and Welfare, 1979c; U.S. Department of Health and Human Services, 1980b), patients should have both a chest x-ray and a two-step tuberculin skin test upon admission. Thorough evaluation is necessary to exclude current disease, determine who should have a course of isoniazid (INH) preventive therapy, and decide who should be monitored for symptoms suggesting tuberculosis.

Employees should be screened using the two-step skin test when they are hired. Those who have been tuberculin negative should be retested if exposed to a case of tuberculosis. Annual retesting is desirable if tuberculosis is prevalent in the community or if exposure in the nursing home is likely (U.S. Department of Health and Human Services, 1980b).

The physical symptoms of tuberculosis usually include fatigue, evening fever, sweating, cough, and weight loss. The individual may suspect he has influenza, but the symptoms persist and increase in severity. Finally, chest pain and hemoptysis develop. Radiographic studies reveal necrosis and cavities, with later development of calcification and fibrosis. In older adults, tuberculosis may take an atypical form. This, combined with the altered immune response, causes problems in diagnosis.

Nursing Implications

Nurses should always be alert to the possibility of reactivated tuberculosis infection in older individuals, especially those with long term

deteriorating disease and/or alcoholism. Prophylactic regimes and even treatment of active cases have been modernized to require very little, if any, hospitalization. In an effort to prevent the emergence of drug-resistant organisms and increase the effectiveness of chemotherapy, combinations of three medications are usually given. Among the most common combination of primary or first line drugs is isoniazid, ethambutol, and rifampin; para-aminosalicylic acid (PAS) and streptomycin are also used as first line drugs in some cases. If necessary, secondary drugs, which are also effective but more toxic, are prescribed. These second line drugs include viomycin, capreomycin, kanamycin, ethionamide, and pyrazinamide (Barlow, 1976).

The treatment of tuberculosis usually requires 12–36 months; however, most health departments are currently evaluating the effectiveness of a shorter 9-month period of chemotherapy. Education of patients and families should emphasize the need for periodic medical evaluation and an uninterrupted drug regime. Many patients want to stop taking their drugs when they feel better. Patients must be monitored closely for effectiveness of treatment, early detection of drug toxicity, and development of drug-resistant organisms (Bergersen, 1979).

Tuberculosis is not the scourge it once was, but it has not been eradicated as was hoped in the 1960s. Persistent surveillance is still needed to control tuberculosis.

SUMMARY

The normal changes of aging in the respiratory system increase the older person's susceptibility to severe pathophysiology. Homeostasis becomes more precarious with age, and a minor respiratory problem may precipitate a chain of events leading to serious respiratory problems, cardiac decompensation (Groer and Shekleton, 1979), and a life-threatening situation.

As with all pathology, the prevention of respiratory problems is far superior to any treatment. Education of the public is needed in order to minimize the hazards of respiratory problems for everyone, but especially for the older person. The control of air pollution, and especially that of one's own immediate surroundings by the avoidance of smoking, will help to decrease the prevalence of respiratory problems (Bither, 1979; Van Lancker, 1977). The majority of those with COPD are cigarette smokers. Cellular adaptations in bronchi and alveoli are in direct proportion to the amount of smoke inhaled (Van Lancker, 1977). Changing behavior is difficult for anyone, but the elderly smoker finds it especially hard to alter lifelong habits. Although he may be aware of the consequences of smoking, his efforts to stop are compounded by withdrawal symptoms and depression.

Nonsmokers are becoming increasingly aware of their exposure to sidestream smoke which goes directly into the air from a burning cigarette, as well as their exposure to the smoker's exhaled mainstream smoke (*Second-Hand Smoke*, 1980; U.S. Department of Health, Education and Welfare, 1979b). Sidestream smoke has higher concentrations than mainstream smoke of hazardous compounds such as tar, nicotine, carbon monoxide, ammonia, and cadmium. These substances cause alveolar and bronchial changes which precipitate and exacerbate COPD. Nonsmokers are taking political and social action to restrict smoking in public places. A decrease in atmospheric pollution will undoubtedly contribute to a reduction in respiratory problems.

REFERENCES

Barlow, P.B. Treatment of tuberculosis. *Basics of Respiratory Disease* 5(1):1-6 (1976).

Barstow, R.E. Coping with emphysema. *Nursing Clinics of North America* 9:140 (1974).

Bergersen, B.S. Pharmacology in Nursing (14th ed.). St. Louis: C.V. Mosby, 1979.

Bither, S. Respiratory problems. In Carnevali, D.L. and Patrick, M. (Eds.) *Nursing Management for the Elderly*. Philadelphia: J.B. Lippincott, 1979.

Blomefield, J. Living with chronic obstructive pulmonary disease. In Czerwinski, B.S. (Ed.) *Manual of Patient Education for Cardiopulmonary Dysfunctions*. St. Louis: C.V. Mosby, 1980.

Creative care unit. *American Journal of Nursing* 81:539 (1981).

Engel, G.L. Grief and grieving. *American Journal of Nursing* 64:93-98 (1964).

Farer, L.S. and Atkinson, M.L. Recommendations for skin testing. *Hospital Infection Control* 6:1-16 (1979).

Futrell, M., Brovender, S., McKinnon-Mullett, E., and Brower, H.T. *Primary Health Care of the Older Adult*. North Scituate, Mass.: Duxbury Press, 1980.

Groer, M.E. and Shekleton, M.E. *Basic Pathophysiology: A Conceptual Framework*. St. Louis: C.V. Mosby, 1979.

Influenza vaccine 1980-81. *Arizona Morbidity* 5(6): 16-18 (1980).

Luckmann, J. and Sorensen, K.C. *Medical-Surgical Nursing: A Psychophysiologic Approach* (2nd ed.). Philadelphia: W.B. Saunders, 1980.

McDowell, D. and Galbraith, A. *Chronic Lung Disease: Save Your Breath for Tomorrow*. Phoenix: St. Luke's Hospital Medical Center, 1975.

Reichel, J. Pulmonary problems in the elderly. In Reichel, W. (Ed.) *Clinical Aspects of Aging*. Baltimore: Williams and Wilkins, 1978.

Second-Hand Smoke: Take a Look at the Facts. New York: American Lung Association, 1980.

Shamansky, S.L. and Hamilton, W.M. The health behavior awareness test: self-care education for the elderly. *Journal of Gerontological Nursing* 5(1):29-32 (1979).

Shapiro, B.A., Harrison, R.A., and Trout, C.A. *Clinical Application of Respiratory Care*. Chicago: Year Book Medical Publishers, 1975.

Shrout, L. Personal communication (Tuberculosis Control, Arizona Department of Health Services, Phoenix, September 8, 1980).

Timiras, P.S. *Developmental Physiology and Aging*. New York: Macmillan, 1972.

U.S. Department of Health, Education and Welfare. *Healthy People: The Surgeon General's Report on Health Promotion and Disease Prevention* (DHEW PHS Publication No. 79-55071). Washington, D.C.: U.S. Government Printing Office, 1979.(a)

U.S. Department of Health, Education and Welfare. *Leading Causes of Death and Probabilities of Dying, United States, 1975 and 1976*. Washington, D.C.: U.S. Government Printing Office, 1979.(b)

U.S. Department of Health, Education and Welfare, Centers for Disease Control. *Morbidity and Mortality Weekly Report* 27:523-526 (1979).(c)

U.S. Department of Health and Human Services, Centers for Disease Control. *Morbidity and Mortality Weekly Report* 28:88 (1980).(a)

U.S. Department of Health and Human Services, Centers for Disease Control. *Morbidity and Mortality Weekly Report* 29:465-467 (1980).(b)

Van Lancker, J. Smoking and disease. In Jarvik, M.E., Cullen, J.W., Gritz, E.R., Vogt, T.M., and West, L.S. (Eds.) *Research on Smoking Behavior*

(NIDA Research Monograph 17). Washington, D.C.: U. S. Government Printing Office, 1977.

Villaverde, M.M. and MacMillan, C.W. *Ailments of Aging: From Symptom to Treatment.* New York: Van Nostrand Reinhold, 1980.

Wright, J.R. Cardiovascular and pulmonary pathology of the aged. In Reichel, W. (Ed.) *Clinical Aspects of Aging.* Baltimore: Williams and Wilkins, 1978.

Wynne, J.W. Pulmonary disease in the elderly. In Rossman, I. (Ed.) *Clinical Geriatrics* (2nd ed.). Philadelphia: J.B. Lippincott, 1979.

24
Genitourinary and Gynecological Problems of Older Adults

Frances S. Knudsen

Older persons are at high risk for developing genitourinary and gynecological problems. Because of their anatomical location, there is a reluctance to discuss and seek help for such problems. Since they are closely associated with one's sexuality, there is a justifiable concern when all is not well.

Only the main genitourinary and gynecological problems common to older adults will be discussed in this chapter. These are: benign prostatic hypertrophy, menopause, problems resulting from muscle weakness in the pelvic floor, vaginitis, vulvitis, and urinary tract infection. Urinary incontinence is discussed in Chapter 29.

BENIGN PROSTATIC HYPERTROPHY

PROFILE 1

Typical Patient with
Benign Prostatic Hypertrophy

The typical individual presenting with Benign Prostatic Hypertrophy is in his 60s or 70s, though the problem began much earlier. The onset of symptoms is so insidious that he does not realize he has a problem till he becomes aware of a full bladder and yet is able to produce only a diminished stream of urine. He has difficulty getting the stream started and may have episodes of complete inability to empty the bladder. Catheterization relieves the symptoms, and he forgets or denies the problem until he has another attack. All too frequently, early signs and symptoms and even physicians' warnings about recurrence and probable need for surgery are ignored or denied till the problem becomes acute. From interviewing these individuals and from follow-up study, one learns that many equate a prostate problem with cancer, undesirable old age, and loss of ability to perform sexually. Most are not counseled adequately by physicians or care givers.

The prostate gland is the only organ to add functioning glandular and stromal tissue with aging (Jaffe, 1978). About 30% of white males over 50 have benign prostatic hypertrophy (BPH). This hyperplasia surrounding the urethra may continue to progress until eventually symptoms appear. In men who are 80 of age, 30% experience impaired renal flow (Moore-Smith, 1973).

BPH is thought to develop because of the gradually decreasing ratio of testosterone to estrogen that occurs with aging. Since Western white males show the greatest incidence and black males are seldom affected, race appears to be a factor (Basso, 1974). The four separate periurethral glands that comprise the prostate continue to enlarge and develop into adenomas that increase in size and number. Their location causes them to compress the posterior urethra and the urinary bladder outlet as well as compressing the true prostate toward the fibrous capsule (see Figure 24-1 and 24-2). The enlarged prostate may cause any of a number of complications (Luckmann and Sorensen, 1980):

- Thickened, hypertrophied urinary bladder
- Diverticuli or herniations between muscle layers of bladder
- Bladder infection (cystitis)
- Formation of urinary stones (calculi)
- Reflux or backward flow of urine into the ureters because of increased bladder pressure

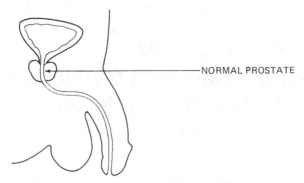

Figure 24-1. The prostate gland lies below the bladder and surrounds the first inch of the urethra. It is a solid organ and normally the size of a chestnut.

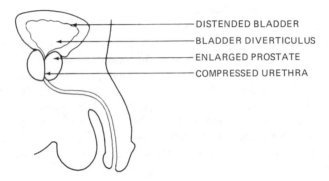

Figure 24-2. In benign prostatic hypertrophy the enlarged prostate constricts and compresses the urethra and the urinary bladder outlet, causing the bladder to form diverticuli where urine collects and infection may develop.

- Distended ureter (hydroureter)
- Distended pelvis and calices of kidneys (hydronephrosis), causing atrophy of functional kidney tissue (renal insufficiency)

Symptoms develop so gradually that the older male considers them just part of aging. The increased frequency of urination and nocturia may result from the physiological changes accompanying aging. However, changes not due to aging include the reduced force and size of the urinary stream, hesitancy and interruption of the urinary stream during voiding, straining to urinate, and dribbling. These are signs of obstructive prostatism. Obstruction can become complete, especially if the man is drinking alcohol or becomes chilled. This is a painful emergency necessitating gradual bladder decompression.

Sometimes the prostate enlarges but the man is symptom free. This is called silent prostatism. Silent prostatism can progress to urinary obstruction with stasis and retention of urine, altered kidney function, kidney damage, and uremia. The "sleepy grandfather" syndrome characterized by nausea and vomiting, poor appetite, weight loss, apathy, and stupor is, in reality, unrecognized uremia (Ehrlich, 1976). Various approaches are used in making the diagnosis. These include:

- Rectal examination
- Laboratory examination of renal function, urine, and blood
- Catheterization, cystourethroscopy, and biopsy
- X-ray studies, such as intravenous pyelogram and voiding cystogram

Evidence of infection includes alkaline urine rather than the normally acid urine and the presence of albumin, bacteria, and red or white blood cells in the urine. The urine specimen should be taken before the rectal examination. During the rectal examination, massage of the prostate produces secretions which, if infection is present, contain pus.

Conservative treatment of BPH (Luckmann and Sorensen, 1980; Tobiason, 1979) includes:

- Prostatic massage and hot sitz baths (which cause secretion of some prostatic fluid and reduction of the edema)
- Chemotherapy (specifically determined by culture and sensitivity tests)
- Androgen therapy (which increases bladder tone and excretion of urine)

The patient needs to be encouraged to void whenever he has the urge and to avoid bladder distention from drinking alcohol or large amounts of fluids in a short time. If the older noninstitutionalized person has an indwelling urinary catheter, he and his significant others must be taught its care and maintenance. The risk of infection should be discussed, along with the rationale for a closed urinary drainage system, a daily fluid intake of 3000 cc, and catheter and meatal care. It is educationally sound to use written guidelines and illustrations and have the person who is learning meatal and catheter care demonstrate the procedure.

Surgery may become necessary if residual urine exceeds 60 cc, or if hematuria or urinary tract infections persist. The procedure is called a prostatectomy, but in actuality only the adenomas are removed and the true prostate and its capsule remain (except in the case of cancer). The most frequent technique is a transurethral resection or TUR, although the alternative approaches used for the prostatectomy may be retropubic, suprapubic, or perineal. In the TUR, a resectoscope with a light and tungsten loop for cutting tissue is inserted through the urethra and the enlarged tissue is scraped out.

Since mild symptoms of prostatic hyperplasia may remain stable during a man's lifetime, a prostatectomy is not done as prophylactic surgery. However, men with symptoms of urinary obstruction should not delay having a prostatectomy. Data demonstrate that mortality increases if the surgery is delayed or if complications such as uremia, infection, or acute retention are present (Tolley, 1981; Whitmore, 1981).

Nursing Implications

Preoperatively, the older patient and his significant others need accurate information about how the surgery or any complication may affect sexual activity or incontinence. This is primarily the doctor's responsibility, but the patient or significant others may want further discussion with the nurse. Some authorities advocate that the term impotence be avoided, as the mere suggestion may contribute to its later occurrence (Luckmann and Sorensen, 1980). Many patients are concerned about their "manhood" being reduced. If the patient does not initiate discussion in this area, the health professional should. The TUR does not cause impotence, but neither does it cause magical rejuvenation. Patients can be reassured that sexual activity is usually related to general health status, and a TUR may prove to be rehabilitating (Jaffe, 1978).

Health professionals vary in the degree to which they think the counselor's optimistic attitude has a positive effect on resolution of sexual problems. However, they agree that during emotionally vulnerable periods for the patient, an encouraging, interested counselor is needed. Urologic counseling should be essentially aimed at reassuring the patient and reinstating his self-esteem (Finkle and Finkle, 1977; Finkle and Thompson, 1972); see Chapters 25 and 36.

Preoperative care is focused on:

- Allaying anxiety
- Establishing optimal nutritional status
- Encouraging adequate hydration (2500–3000 cc intake per 24 hours)
- Promoting optimal urinary flow (gradual bladder decompression may be necessary; if more than 700 cc are in the bladder, after the initial removal of that amount,

the catheter should be clamped and 200–300 cc should be removed every 30–60 minutes to prevent shock)

- Assessing adequacy of patient's cardiovascular and respiratory system for surgery
- Preparing the patient and significant others for the postoperative period

An indwelling catheter is routine after a prostatectomy. Bleeding is expected during the first postoperative day, with a gradual decrease in amount. A closed irrigation will probably be in place to flush out clots. Traction may be used on the catheter balloon to apply pressure to denuded areas and reduce bleeding. This traction may produce bladder spasms which can be relieved with antispasmodic drugs. To allay the anxiety of patients and families, they should be carefully counseled and prepared for the bloody irrigation returns and bladder spasms (Bridges, 1980; Shaw, 1981; Twinam, 1980).

When the urine draining from the catheter is no longer bloody, the catheter is removed. This usually occurs, 2–3 days postoperatively. After removal of the catheter, the patient must be observed for indications of urethral stricture, e.g., straining, dysuria, or small urinary stream. The patient should be encouraged to void as soon as he. feels the urge. He should be told that urinary frequency and incontinence may occur. In fact, it may be reassuring for the patient to be told that a rapid return to urinary control is not anticipated and dribbling will probably occur. Upon discharge, the patient should be cautioned to avoid strenuous exercise or long automobile rides for several weeks to minimize the possibility of bleeding.

Perineal exercises should be taught to the patient to help him gain urinary sphincter control. He may begin on the second or third postoperative day to contract his perineal, gluteal, and abdominal muscles about 12–25 times an hour. He should be advised to contract these muscles as if he urgently needed to urinate and no facilities were readily available. He should also squeeze the rectal sphincters. The remainder of the body's muscles should be relaxed. Concentration on the exercises may be

helped by saying aloud, "Relax — squeeze." The patient can be taught awareness of tense muscles by placing his hands on and feeling his abdomen. Perineal exercises should not be discontinued before urinary control is achieved (Luckmann and Sorensen, 1980).

Postsurgically the patient should again be given the opportunity to discuss his sexual activity. Impotence should not result from the TUR (Pfeiffer, 1979). When it does occur, previous problems should be suspected, and counseling should be encouraged and provided (Specht and Cordes, 1979).

MALE MENOPAUSE

Although there is no physical evidence of a male menopause because there is no male equivalent of menstruation, middle age frequently brings disconcerting changes for males. Many experience marked decrease in their sexual drive and activity, recurrent impotence with identity crises, fatigability, insomnia, and lessened self-confidence. Emotional problems, business failures, and divorce frequently accompany these changes. A decrease in testosterone or "andropause" does occur in most men, but replacement therapy is still questionable (Asch and Greenblatt, 1978; Crilly and Nordin, 1980; Lamb, 1973; Reuben, 1974); see Chapter 36 on sexuality.

MENOPAUSE

Menopause, or the gradual or sudden cessation of menstruation, marks the end of a woman's reproductive life. It is the counterpart of menarche, which identifies the beginning of fertility. Conventionally, menopause is defined as beginning one year after a woman's last menstrual period, not related to gestation (Glowacki, 1978).

The climacteric, or "change of life," refers to the years when there are definite morphological and physiological body changes which, in women, result from estrogen deprivation (Timiras, 1972). The symptoms of the climacteric are variable, but three are found universally and have a physiological basis: (1) disruptions in the menstrual cycle, (2) hot flushes and sweats, and (3) atrophy of the tissues of the vulva and vagina. Other symptoms that occur in our culture but have not been demonstrated either to occur in other cultures or to have a physiological basis are psychosomatic complaints of insomnia, headaches, lower back pain, changed libido, and palpitations; and psychological symptoms of depression, anxiety, mood swings, and irritability (Speroff, Glass, and Kase, 1975).

The nature of the climacteric or menopausal syndrome has been quite controversial over the past ten years. Critics, many of them feminist scholars, have challenged Western physicians who have identified various physical and psychosocial complaints as part of the climacteric (Townsend and Carbone, 1980). These critics contend that most symptoms of menopausal syndrome are related to psychosocial factors. Their view is that some of the behavior is due to role conditioning, loss of status, and lack of role alternatives. In cultures where menopause contributes to an improvement in role, with more social freedom and privileges, there are few problems with the climacteric other than changes in the menstrual cycle (Flint, 1975; Fuchs, 1977; Griffin, 1977; Seaman and Seaman, 1977). Moreover, in a study of 448 Swiss women, those who reported more functional and recreational activities also had fewer menopausal complaints and vice versa (Van Keep and Kellerhals, 1974).

It is thought that 85% of women have symptoms during their climacteric. However, only about 20% consider their symptoms serious enough to consult a physician. Help is most often sought for the vasomotor symptoms. Lowered estrogen levels cause changes in the subcutaneous capillaries, precipitating hot flushes of the head, neck, and thorax, and excessive perspiration, especially at night.

Estrogen deficiency causes some changes which occur many years after the climacteric. These are usually reversals of the changes that occurred at puberty: decreased elasticity of skin, and atrophy of breasts and genitalia. Osteoporosis, hypothyroidism, arthralgia, atherosclerotic vascular disease, and tendency to easily gain weight may also occur.

Sedatives, tranquilizers, and/or estrogen replacement therapy may be prescribed. Estrogen deficiency can be verified by a "maturation index" done on cells scraped from the vaginal wall. Usually estrogen replacement therapy (ERT) is used for a period of a few weeks to a few years for relief of symptoms. ERT should be discontinued gradually after the transitional stage of the climacteric, although it is sometimes used indefinitely for problems of late climacteric, osteoporosis, or atrophic vaginitis (Glowacki, 1978). Usually a short course of estrogen therapy causes reepithelialization of the vaginal mucosa with subsequent relief from symptoms of itching, burning, and discharge due to atrophic vaginitis.

Women who have a hysterectomy before menopause experience a surgical cessation of menses. Since they no longer have a uterus which sheds its lining monthly, they have no periods. Usually their ovaries continue to function until the women are of menopausal age. Then the changes their bodies undergo are those of the typical climacteric, with the exception of the gradual cessation of menses; their menses were surgically and suddenly disrupted years ago. These women may also be candidates for ERT at their climacteric.

Currently, patient package inserts must be dispensed with all drugs that contain estrogen. Women need an opportunity to discuss the information on the patient package inserts with a health professional (Kutzner, Guzzetti, and Land, 1981). After reading the information, they may be frightened, confused, and unsure about using ERT.

The Controversy Over Estrogen Replacement Therapy

Menopause is often considered a deficiency disease, like diabetes (Seaman and Seaman, 1977). Consequently, the logical treatment has been thought to be estrogen replacement therapy. In January 1966, a physician named Robert Wilson published a book *Feminine Forever* which promised that ERT would alleviate menopause and postpone aging. Within seven months, 100,000 copies had been sold, and excerpts appeared in *Time, Look, Vogue,* and many newspapers. Women by the thousands demanded the "youth pill" and wanted to have their estrogen levels checked (Seaman and Seaman, 1977).

Articles in the *Washington Post* and the *New Republic,* along with a book *The Pill, an Alarming Report* (Mintz, 1969), called attention to the fact that in 1964, Wilson had been accepting money from three drug companies who produced estrogen while conducting research on the "youth pill." In November 1966, the Food and Drug Administration (FDA) notified Wilson's research sponsor, one of the drug companies, that he was an unacceptable investigator because he was making promotional claims that had not been proved. To this day, the FDA has not approved Premarin or any other hormone as a means of preventing aging (Seaman and Seaman, 1977).

As early as December 1947, the *American Journal of Obstetrics and Gynecology* carried an alarm by S.B. Gusberg along with six full pages of advertisements for ERT (Seaman and Seaman, 1977). This gynecologist and cancer researcher pointed out that long term use of ERT stimulates the endometrium, causing bleeding and the need for diagnostic curettage. Other gynecologists who read the article, as well as the advertisements in their medical journals, began to see ERT in a different light. In December 1975, the *New England Journal of Medicine* published two studies which demonstrated the association of exogenous estrogen and endometrial carcinoma (Smith, Prentice, Thompson, and Herrmann, 1975; Zieh and Finkle, 1975); another study appeared in 1979 (Antunes et al., 1979).

Finally, more and more physicians and women patients became aware that the benefits of ERT had to be carefully weighed against the risks (Gambrell and Greenblatt, 1981; Gambrell, Massey, Tristan, and Boddie, 1980; Greenblatt, 1977). On October 18, 1977, FDA regulation mandated that patient package inserts be dispensed with all estrogen-containing drugs (*Federal Register,* 1977). Now every woman has the facts that may assist her in deciding whether or not to have estrogen replacement therapy.

Alington-MacKinnon and Troll (1981) espoused the devil's advocate position that menopause is an adaptive process which may be related to the female's superior longevity and not a symptom of physiological decline.

Nursing Implications

Women who are experiencing a difficult or uncomfortable menopause are often made to feel guilty for verbalizing their discomfort. They think that friends and relatives are annoyed or alienated by their complaints and that they are expected to cope in silence. In addition, middle-aged husbands and wives may believe the myth of marital problems at the time of menopause and make it a self-fulfilling prophecy.

Menopause is a significant "passage" in female maturation and warrants the consideration and time of professionals, perhaps sex counselors, to assist some women with a transition which can be fulfilling and self-actualizing. Nurses are in a unique position to pick up cues indicating a need for "girl talk" with older women. Older women are much less reticent to discuss sexuality than many younger women and are perhaps more comfortable with the topic in some instances than the nurse or doctor!

RELAXED PELVIC SUPPORT

In normal aging there is general loss of muscle fiber, resulting in decreased muscle elasticity and contractility (Timiras, 1972). Muscles of the abdomen, perineum, and pelvic area also are altered. These changes occur in the absence of disease; however, definite health problems related to these changes, such as uterine prolapse, cystoceles, urethroceles, rectoceles, and enteroceles, appear to be more prevalent in those women who have had multiple pregnancies or have led lives in which frequent heavy lifting was required (see the profile of a woman with cystocele). Figure 24-3 illustrates the stages of uterine prolapse. Figures 24-4 illustrates the gynecological problems resulting from diminished muscle tone.

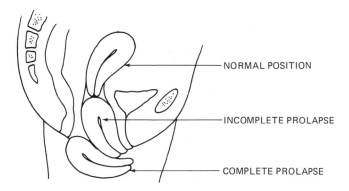

Figure 24-3. Stages of uterine prolapse. During incomplete prolapse, the uterus is still within the vagina, but the cervix may protrude beyond it. With complete prolapse, the entire uterus protrudes from the vagina and has caused it to become inverted.

PROFILE 2

Woman with Cystocele

The typical female patient with urinary retention problems due to cystocele or other muscle weaknesses in the region of the pelvic floor is in her 60s. The condition may have existed for many years, but it becomes a problem in the late 50s and increases with age. Bladder capacity is dimished, and her greatest complaint (and greatest annoyance) is a dribbling of urine upon coughing, sneezing, exercise, or even laughing. She is not able to walk or jog far without wearing a protective pad. The tissue of the vaginal area is fragile and vulnerable. Backaches and bladder infections are not infrequent. Because the urethra is less protected at this stage of life, infections are easily introduced from wet pads, ointments and creams, tight nylon panty hose, etc. With these frequent and rapidly occurring infections, she complains of urgency to urinate which results in severe painful spasms radiating throughout the pelvic area and the body. Most of the time the patient tolerates the problem for years and lives in fear of wetting the bed or having a social accident in public.

The symptoms of uterine prolapse do not necessarily correlate with the degree of the prolapse, but most women have a feeling of "something coming down in there." In addition, they may have vague pelvic feelings of heaviness or pressure, dyspareunia, and backaches. If a cystocele or urethrocele is present, there may be urinary incontinence (often stress), urgency, frequency, and urinary tract infections. The difficulty in emptying the bladder is lessened by pushing on the anterior vaginal wall. Those with a rectocele or enterocele may have inadequate control of the passage of gas or feces, and may have difficulty passing feces, sometimes requiring pressure on the posterior vaginal wall.

Exercises to strengthen the pelvic floor (Mandelstam, 1980) or a pessary may help mild problems. Surgical repair of a cystocele or urethrocele is an anterior colporrhaphy; of a rectocele or enterocele, a posterior colporrhaphy. Usually uterine prolapse is corrected with a vaginal hysterectomy and, as necessary, either type of colporrhaphy or both of them (Kenney and Moncrieff, 1981). Research has found that postmenopausal women who undergo vaginal hysterectomies run a lesser risk of developing postoperative infections than women of reproductive age. This has been attributed to the fact that postmenopausal women have relatively fewer vaginal microorganisms. The practical implication of this finding is that antibiotics are not usually necessary preoperatively, thus avoiding the hazard of drug toxicity to which this age group is especially prone (Galask and Larsen, 1981).

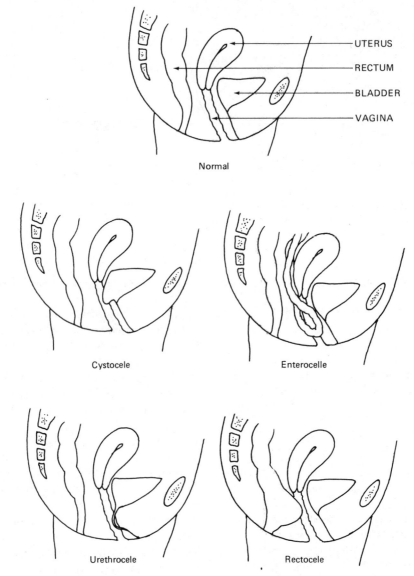

Figure 24-4. Gynecological problems resulting from diminished muscle tone (sagittal views of the normal pelvis and effects of weakened pelvic support): a cystocele occurs when the bladder is displaced downward into the vagina; a urethrocele is a herniation of the urethra into the vagina; an enterocele is a herniation of the vagina by the small bowel; a rectocele is caused by the rectum herniating into the vagina.

Nursing Implications

The nurse's role in working with women who have relaxed pelvic support consists mainly of assessment and education. By listening to the woman describe her symptoms, the nurse can identify a potential problem. Direct observation can provide further confirmation. Although the woman should be referred to her physician for diagnosis and prescribed treatment, the nurse can make valuable contributions. She can assure the woman that there is a definite physical problem and that measures to minimize it may be available. Sometimes women think they are imagining or exaggerating their symptoms. They may be reluctant or embarrassed to discuss such problems because of their anatomic location. Moreover, they sometimes recall older relatives having similar problems without any relief and think that, in turn, little or nothing can be done for them.

Frequent rest periods, especially with the hips elevated, may help to minimize the symptoms. The woman can be taught to use Kegel's exercises and encouraged to practice them frequently during the day and whenever she voids. Adequate liquids should be encouraged to decrease the possibility of urinary tract infection. A minimum of eight 8-ounce glasses of fluids should be the goal for every 24 hours. Liquids may be limited in the evening to allow for longer periods of sleep.

Using digital pressure on the anterior wall of the vagina and leaning forward on the commode during voiding should assist the woman with a cystocele in emptying her bladder. Adequate fluids and roughage in the diet should help allay difficulty with bowel movements. Digital pressure to the posterior vaginal wall may also be helpful.

If a pessary is prescribed, education should focus on its correct usage and care of surrounding tissues in an effort to prevent complications such as discomfort, fistulas, leukorrhea, ulceration, and malignancy. When surgical repairs are made, postoperative care focuses on preventing infection and pressure on the suture line. A patent catheter and closed urinary drainage must be maintained. The urinary meatus and 3-4 inches of the proximal part of the catheter should be cleansed with an antiseptic solution such as Betadine every eight hours. After the catheter is removed, careful monitoring and recording of time and amount of output are essential. Adequate fluid intake, appropriate diet, and perhaps stool softeners and mild laxatives have their role in preventing straining at defecation. Perineal care is essential in promoting comfort as well as preventing infection.

Routine postoperative care should be individualized to the special needs of the older adult, such as compensating for sensory losses. Measures should be instituted to maintain adequate respiration, circulation, and skin integrity. Turning and deep breathing every hour, using antiembolic hose, and applying lotion to areas of dry skin periodically speed convalescence.

VAGINITIS

Vaginitis or inflammation of the vagina occurs when the pH becomes more alkaline, the normal flora changes, or invasion by a virulent organism occurs. It is such a common problem that it is thought most women experience it at some time in their lives. It frequently occurs after treatment with antibiotics or steroids.

During and after the climacteric, atrophic or senile vaginitis may become a problem. The vaginal mucosa has become thin and atrophic, and the secretions have become thin and more alkaline. With these changes, inflammation is common, and resistance to infection is lowered. Older institutionalized women, especially those cognitively impaired, may have vaginitis and never be diagnosed or treated.

Symptoms of infection include an odoriferous discharge that may be streaked with blood, itching and burning of the vagina, and dyspareunia. Vulvar excoriation and burning with urination may occur. Diagnosis is made by pelvic examination. A Pap smear may be done to rule out malignancy; a culture may be done to determine/rule out infectious organisms. Treatment for senile vaginitis usually consists of estrogen creams or suppositories. If there is a secondary infection, additional therapy is prescribed (Brown, 1978; Glowacki, 1978; Goldfarb, 1979; Luckmann and Sorensen, 1980). Local application of a mild disinfectant such as Betadine may occasionally replace antibiotic therapy (Henriques, 1976).

Nursing Implications

The nurse should clarify with the patient that all cleansing of the perineum is done from the front of the perineum toward the rectum, in an effort to protect the urinary meatus and vagina from fecal contamination. Some older women may not know this, and because of the loss of the fatty cushion in the genital area, the urethral meatus is more vulnerable to irritation and infection. The patient may find sitz baths helpful in relieving the local irritation. Maintenance of a clean, dry perineum helps to prevent vaginitis.

Contemporary clothing does not contribute to maintenance of a dry perineum. Panty girdles, nylon panties and panty hose, and polyester slacks prevent evaporation of perspiration and secretions, and thus may contribute to vaginitis. Cotton panties, girdles, stockings and loose clothing are preferable. Careful laundering with hot water is essential to prevent autoinfection (Specht and Cordes, 1979). The additional problems of obese women in maintaining a clean, dry perineum may act as a stimulus to weight control.

Older women may consider douching an integral part of their hygiene. Since douching is of questionable value and may cause trauma, it should be discouraged. If the woman is reluctant to stop douching, the nurse can help to minimize its effects by reinforcing the use of the following: mild acid solution (1 tablespoon of vinegar to a quart of water), clean equipment, gentle insertion, and pressure.

If the woman is having problems with dyspareunia, estrogen therapy may be indicated and supplemental lubrication may be needed (Felstein, 1981).

VULVITIS

The older woman is especially susceptible to vulvitis. With the loss of hormonal stimulation, the vulva shrinks and decreases in size. There is loss of subcutaneous fat, thinning of the epidermis, and decreased circulation. These changes make the area especially susceptible to irritation either directly or by extension from the vagina. The most common symptom is local discomfort — itching, pain, burning — although there may be no symptoms.

Common types of vulvitis in postmenopausal women include leukoplakic vulvitis and kraurosis vulvae (Kenney, 1981; Luckmann and Sorensen, 1980). Painful herpetic rash is also sometimes seen in the elderly (Pearson and Kotthoff, 1979). In leukoplakic vulvitis or premalignant vulvitis there are scattered, thickened gray patches. These may crack and become infected, ulcerated, or macerated. Since they may become malignant, a biopsy should be done.

Kraurosis is identified by its smooth, nearly transparent, bright red epithelium. It too can become secondarily infected. Systemic antibiotics constitute the treatment for secondary infections of both conditions; the symptoms are treated palliatively. Persistent or chronic vulvitis may occur in diabetes. Control of the diabetes usually improves the vulvar condition (Goldfarb, 1979).

Nursing Implications

Education is the main role of the nurse in interacting with the older woman with vulvitis. Sometimes the nurse can help the woman recall or learn some concepts to promote comfort or hygiene. Hot compresses or sitz baths, as well as application of cornstarch, lotions, or ointments, may provide local relief. Careful hygiene after each elimination promotes comfort. Cotton, light, nonrestrictive clothing is preferable to clothes that are synthetic and tight. Feminine hygiene sprays, bath salts, bath oils, talcum powder, and perfumed or medicated soaps should be avoided (Kenney, 1981).

URINARY TRACT INFECTION

The prevalence of urinary tract infections (UTI) increases with age. Seneca (1981) considered them iatrogenic, a biological pollution of humans. Until middle age, women are more prone to UTI because of the anatomy of the female perineum. However, older men are more at risk of developing UTI than older women because of the obstructive nature of prostatic hypertrophy (Freeman, 1975; Moore-Smith, 1973).

The incidence of bacteriuria increases with hospitalization or residence in a nursing home (Sherman, Tucci, Libow, and Isenberg, 1980). Bacteriuria was found in 30% of the women and 70% of the men in one city hospital (Freeman, 1975). An incidence as high as 65% was found in hospitalized elderly in another study (Moore-Smith, 1973). Furthermore, bacteriuria in older institutionalized adults was found to be related to a reduced survival rate of 30–50% (Dontas, Kasviki-Charvati, Papanayiotou, and Marketos, 1981).

There is an increased incidence of UTI in those with diabetes or renal failure. Hypertension is also associated with UTI, although which causes which has yet to be determined (Freeman,

1975). Sexual activity predisposes women of all ages to UTI. Trauma to the urethra and bladder during sexual intercourse is thought to predispose to a bruise-like inflammatory process that develops into bacterial cystitis (O'Donnell, 1980). In addition, postmenopausal estrogenic changes in the genital tissues make them especially sensitive to mechanical irritation. Extended foreplay is also thought to introduce bacteria into the paraurethral glands (Kent, 1975).

Instrumentation and catheterization usually precipitate UTI (Hadfield, 1981; Kurtz, 1980; Romano and Kaye, 1981; Seneca, 1981). Even the systemic administration of antibiotics is not fail-safe because they cannot clear a stagnant pool of residual urine. Also resistant bacteria may persist.

In the presence of any obstruction to the outward flow of urine, upward invasion of bacteria is highly probable. The elderly have numerous conditions that can cause urinary stasis, retention, or obstruction. The most frequent cause in females is cystocele; in males, prostatic hypertrophy. Both sexes are prone to stenosis, strictures, calculi, contractures, and neoplasms (Jaffe, 1978). Neurological changes from strokes of hemiplegia also frequently cause urinary stasis and thus UTI in the elderly.

The symptoms of UTI are frequency and urgency or urination, dysuria, lower abdominal discomfort, and turbid urine. Fever, chills, hematuria, and vomiting may also indicate a UTI. Diagnosis may often be made on the basis of symptoms alone. A clean-catch urine specimen may confirm the diagnosis. However, the possibility of the specimen having been contaminated must be considered, especially with obese or elderly women. Contamination is also suspected if multiple organisms are cultured rather than a single species of bacteria indicating bacteriuria.

Elderly patients with bacteriuria are frequently treated with sulfonamides because gram-negative infections, especially *Escherichia coli*, are sensitive to sulfa drugs. Findings from the culture and sensitivity studies guide the therapy for the sulfa-resistant organisms.

If the symptoms do not subside in 4-5 days, oral suppressive therapy may be implemented to prevent acute attacks. These drugs have no systemic effect and do not change the normal flora. The methenamine salts liberate formaldehyde in acidic urine to suppress the growth of organisms.

Nursing Implications

Any older adult who demonstrates a change in general health status or voiding patterns should be checked carefully for the presence of UTI. Accurate recording of intake and output and collecting a urine specimen should be performed whenever a possible UTI is suspected. Adequacy of hydration (2500-3000 cc per 24 hours) and output (1500 cc per 24 hours) can readily be assessed. Retention with overflow may be detected. Voiding every 2-3 hours during the day and 1-2 times at night can be encouraged to avoid distension. Adequate intake promotes the washout effect of high urine flow and decreased reproduction of bacteria. Since pathogens grow poorly in acid urine, an acid-ash diet or administration of vitamin C may prove beneficial. Prunes, plums, cranberries, grains, meat, eggs, cheese, and fish produce an acid urine. Other fruits, most vegetables, carbonated beverages and nuts produce alkaline urine (Specht and Cordes, 1979). Because milk produces an alkaline ash, its ingestion is usually restricted to a pint daily during the presence of urinary tract infections.

Since immobility increases the possibility of a UTI as well as other complications in the institutionalized elderly, the nurse should promote periodic activity of all her older patients. Bathroom facilities should be readily available, day or night. Betadine cleansing and absorbent pads appear to be the best option. Diapers and perineal pads cause perineal irritation and shatter dignity.

Since catheters precipitate UTI, they should only be used when bladder training and other approaches have failed. Penile sheaths may be used for incontinent males. Meticulous catheter care should be done every eight hours.

The nurse can counsel the sexually active older female in measures to prevent UTI. Bathing before and after coitus, voiding after coitus, and increasing fluid intake, especially after coitus, may be of assistance. Alternative positions may be tried, thus reducing the stress produced on the urethra by the male superior position (Kent, 1975).

REFERENCES

Alington-MacKinnon, D. and Troll, L.E. The adaptive function of the menopause: a devil's advocate position. *Journal of the American Geriatrics Society* 29:349-353 (1981).

Antunes, C.M.F., Stolley, P.D., Rosenshein, N.B., Davies, J.L., Tonascia, J.A., Brown, C., Burnett, L., Rutledge, A., Pokempner, M., and Garcia, R. Endometrial cancer and estrogen use: report of a large case-control study. *New England Journal of Medicine* 300:9-13 (1979).

Asch, R.H. and Greenblatt, R.B. Geriatric endocrinology. In Reichel, W. (Ed.) *Clinical Aspects of Aging.* Baltimore: Williams and Wilkins, 1978.

Basso, A. Genitourinary tract problems of the aged male. *Journal of the American Geriatrics Society* 21:352-354 (1974).

Bridges, M. Transurethral resection of the benign enlarged prostate. *Nursing Times* 76:2098-2107 (1980).

Brown, A.D.G. Gynaecological disorders in the elderly. In Brocklehurst, J.C. (Ed.) *Textbook of Geriatric Medicine and Gerontology* (2nd ed.). New York: Churchill Livingstone, 1978.

Crilly, R.G. and Nordin, B.E.C. Aging and sex steroids. *Geriatric Medicine* 10(7):21-22, 24, 26 (1980).

Dontas, A.S., Kasviki-Charvati, P., Papanayiotou, P.C., and Marketos, S.G. Bacteriuria and survival in old age. *New England Journal of Medicine* 304:939-943 (1981).

Ehrlich, R.M. Benign prostatic hypertrophy. In Conn, H. (Ed.) *Current Therapy.* Philadelphia: W.B. Saunders, 1976.

Federal Register 42:141 (July 22, 1977).

Felstein, I. Aging and sexual problems: 2 – mixed dyspareunia. *Geriatric Medicine* 11(5):84-85 (1981).

Finkle, A.L. and Finkle, P.S. How counseling may solve sexual problems of aging men. *Geriatrics* 32(11):84-89 (1977).

Finkle, A.L. and Thompson, R. Urologic counseling in male sexual impotence. *Geriatrics* 27(12):67-72 (1972).

Flint, M. The menopause: reward or punishment? *Psychosomatics* 16:161-163 (1975).

Freeman, J. Urinary tract infections: prevention, diagnosis, and treatment. In Schwartz, A. (Ed.) *Nephrology for the Practicing Physician.* New York: Grune and Stratton, 1975.

Fuchs, E. *The Second Season: Life, Love, and Sex – Women in the Middle Years.* Garden City, N.Y.: Anchor Press, 1977.

Galask, R.P. and Larsen, B. Identifying and treating genital tract infections in postmenopausal women. *Geriatrics* 36(3):69-70, 75-77, 79 (1981).

Gambrell, R.D. and Greenblatt, R.B. Hormone therapy for the menopause. *Geriatrics* 36(7):53-56, 59-61 (1981).

Gambrell, R.D., Jr., Massey, F.M., Tristan, A.C., and Boddie, A.W. Estrogen therapy and breast cancer in post-menopausal women. *Journal of the American Geriatrics Society* 28:251-257 (1980).

Glowacki, G. Geriatric gynecology. In Reichel, W. (Ed.) *Clinical Aspects of Aging.* Baltimore: Williams and Wilkins, 1978.

Golfarb, A.F. Geriatric gynecology. In Rossman, I. (Ed.) *Clinical Geriatrics.* Philadelphia: J.B. Lippincott, 1979.

Greenblatt, R.B. Estrogen and endometrial cancer - gross exaggeration or fact? *Geriatrics* 32(11):60-64 69-72 (1977).

Griffin, J. A cross-cultural investigation of behavioral changes at menopause. *Social Science Journal* 14. 49-55 (1977).

Gusberg, S.B. Precursors of corpus carcinoma estrogens and adenomatous hyperplasia. *American Journal of Obstetrics and Gynecology* 54:905-926 (1947).

Hadfield, J. Urinary tract infection. *Nursing Mirror* 152(4):ii-v (1981).

Henriques, E. Vaginitis. In Conn, H. (Ed.) *Current Therapy.* Philadelphia: W.B. Saunders, 1976.

Jaffe, J.W. Common lower urinary tract problems in older persons. In Reichel, W. (Ed.) *Clinical Aspects of Aging.* Baltimore: Williams and Wilkins, 1978.

Kenney, A. The vulval dystrophies. *Geriatric Medicine* 11(2):24, 27 (1981).

Kenney, A. and Moncrieff, D. Prolapse of the female genital tract. *Geriatric Medicine* 11(5):32, 35-37 (1981).

Kent, S. Urinary tract problems in women are linked to sexual activity. *Geriatrics* 30:145-146 (1975).

Kurtz, S.B. UTI in the elderly: seeking solutions for special problems. *Geriatrics* 35(10):97-99, 102 (1980).

Kutzner, S.K., Guzzetti, P.J., and Land, M.J. Facts and opinion: estrogens + patient package insert = confused patients. *Journal of Obstetric, Gynecologic, and Neonatal Nursing* 8:220-223 (1981).

Lamb, L.E. *Dear Doctor: It's about Sex.* New York: Dell, 1973.

Luckmann J. and Sorensen, K.C. *Medical-Surgical Nursing: A Psychophysiologic Approach* (2nd ed). Philadelphia: W.B. Saunders, 1980.

Mandelstam, D. Special techniques: strengthening pelvic floor muscles. *Geriatric Nursing* 1:251-252 (1980).

Mintz, M. *The Pill, An Alarming Report.* New York: Fawcett, 1969.

Moore-Smith, B. Medicine in old age: urinary tract disease. *British Medical Journal* 29:686–688 (1973).

O'Donnell, R.P. Acute urethral syndrome in women. *New England Journal of Medicine* 303:1531 (1980).

Pearson, L.J. and Kotthoff, M.E. *Geriatric Clinical Protocols.* Philadelphia: J.B. Lippincott, 1979.

Pfeiffer, E. Sexuality and aging. In Rossman, I. (Ed.) *Clinical Geriatrics* (2nd ed.). Philadelphia: J.B. Lippincott, 1979.

Reuben, D. *How to Get More out of Sex.* New York: Bantam Books, 1974.

Romano, J.M. and Kaye, D. UTI in the elderly: common yet atypical. *Geriatrics* 36(6):113–115, 120 (1981).

Seaman, B. and Seaman, G. *Women and the Crisis in Sex Hormones.* New York: Rawson Associates, 1977.

Seneca, H. Urinary-tract infections: etiology, microbiology, pathophysiology, diagnosis and management. *Journal of the American Geriatrics Society* 29:359–369 (1981).

Shaw, L.M. A teaching plan for TURP. *Association of Operating Room Nurses' Journal* 33(2):240–245 (1981).

Sherman, F.T., Tucci, V., Libow, L.S., and Isenberg, H.D. Nosocomial urinary-tract infections in a skilled nursing facility. *Journal of the American Geriatrics Society* 28:456–461 (1980).

Smith, D.C., Prentice, R., Thompson, D.J., and Herrmann, W.L. Association of exogenous estrogen and endometrial carcinoma. *New England Journal of Medicine* 293:1164–1167 (1975).

Specht, J. and Cordes, A. Genitourinary problems. In Carnevali, D.L. and Patrick, M. (Eds.) *Nursing Management for the Elderly.* Philadelphia: J.B. Lippincott, 1979.

Speroff, L.R., Glass, R., and Kase, N. *Clinical Gynecologic Endocrinology and Infertility.* Baltimore: Williams and Wilkins, 1975.

Timiras, P.S. *Developmental Physiology and Aging.* New York: Macmillan, 1972.

Tobiason, S.J. Benign prostatic hypertrophy. *American Journal of Nursing* 79:286–290 (1979).

Tolley, D. Problems of the prostate. *Geriatric Medicine* 11(6):19, 22, 25 (1981).

Townsend, J.M. and Carbone, C.L. Meopausal syndrome: illness or social role — a transcultural analysis. *Culture, Medicine, and Psychiatry* 4:229–248 (1980).

Twinam, J. Transurethral resection of the prostate gland. *Nursing Times* 76:2094–2097 (1980).

Van Keep, P. and Kellerhals, J. The impact of sociocultural factors on symptom formation. *Psychotherapy and Psychosomatics* 23:251–263 (1974).

Whitmore, W.F. Benign prostatic hyperplasia: widespread and sometimes worrisome. *Geriatrics* 36(4):119–122, 127, 131, 136 (1981).

Wilson, R. *Feminine Forever.* New York: M. Evans, 1966.

Zieh, H.K. and Finkle, W.D. Increased risk of endometrial carcinoma among users of conjugated estrogens. *New England Journal of Medicine* 293:1167–1170 (1975).

25
Common Cancer Problems of the Elderly

Marjorie Vander Linden Albert

This chapter provides information about cancer, its causes, and treatment common to older persons. Emphasis is on the aged patient — his individual strengths and weaknesses during an acute, chronic, or limiting disease process. A general discussion of diagnosis and common therapies is followed by specific information on the most common cancers diagnosed in aged persons.

INCIDENCE

The risk of a cancer diagnosis increases with age especially in the areas of the stomach, colorectum, skin, lung, prostate, breast, uterus, pancreas, and esophagus. The malignancies which significantly result in death in the population over 75 are cancer of the digestive and respiratory systems, prostate, and breast (Gunn, 1980; Lew, 1978). Other frequently reported malignancies include cancer of the bladder and kidney, myeloma, and chronic leukemias. Skin cancer is a common finding in the aged, but it is rarely associated with death. Overall, there is a significant risk in the incidence of cancer with age and an even greater occurrence than mortality figures show due to the phenomenon of death *with cancer*, but not *of cancer* (American Cancer Society, Facts and Figures for 1979). The malignancies which result in two-thirds of the cancer deaths in the aged are found in five tumor locations: lung, colorectum, prostate, stomach, and breast.

The etiology of increased malignancy in the aged may be explained by several factors. First, a decrease in the immunological defense system during aging has been suggested. This lowers the aged body's ability to protect against abnormal growths. Another factor is the increased length of exposure to carcinogens due to occupation, diet, and social habits. Also to be considered is the lack of sufficient DNA (genetic coding) for the increased repair needs of the aging body, which allows defective cells to grow in body structures (Jarvik, 1979).

The diagnostic protocols and procedures for cancer are similar for all ages, with consideration given to the developmental stage of the individuals involved. Therefore, the total scope of diagnostic procedures is not addressed here, but clarification of diagnostic grading and staging protocols will be reviewed briefly because of the direct relevance to gerontological nursing.

The pathologist evaluates the microscopic appearance of a tumor by histologic grading. Grading of the tumor allows some guidelines as to the prognosis and treatment of the malignancy. The tissue (tumor) biopsy is done by frozen section and permanent paraffin section. Grading is reported in tissue variation from normal (see Table 25-1).

Table 25-1. Histologic Grading of Tumors.

	DEFINITION	DESCRIPTION
Grade I	Resembles parent tissue	Well differentiated
Grade II	Like parent tissue with some difference	Moderately differentiated
Grade III	Abnormal cell with some parent tissue similarities	Poorly differentiated
Grade IV	Highly malignant with little likeness to parent tissue	Undifferentiated

Adapted from Lew (1978) and Rubin (1978).

Table 25-2. Cancer Stage Grouping.

| CLINCIAL STAGE | TUMOR SIZE | ANATOMIC GROWTH | |
		NODAL INVOLVEMENT	METASTATIC GROWTH
Stage I	T1a	N0 or N1a	
	T1b	N0 or N1a	M0
Stage II	T0	N1b	
	T2a	N0 or N1a or N1b	
	T2b	N0 or N1a or N1b	M0
Stage III	Any T3	N1 or N2	M0
Stage IV	T4	Any N	Any M
	Any T	N3	Any M
	Any T	Any N	M1

NOTE: The numbers 0–4 and letters a and b show the amount of growth and the current state of symptoms; T = tumor, N = node, M = metastases [adapted from Rubin (1978) and Savlov (1978)].

After diagnosis, the patient undergoes further examination to determine the extent of the disease. This procedure is called staging and is used to determine treatment protocols and prognosis. As the disease progresses and staging changes, optimal therapy regimes will be altered according to research findings and new developments in treatment. Each type of malignancy will be staged according to specific growth characteristics, but the overall model of staging is presented in Table 25-2.

COMMON MODES OF CANCER TREATMENT

Surgery

Surgery for patients with cancer is utilized to achieve diagnosis, staging, cure, control, and palliation (Patterson, 1978; Shiplacoff, 1981). Diagnosis and staging of the extent of the cancer by biopsy require special preparation of the elderly who are usually at higher surgical risk than younger patients. There is a good curative rate in surgical treatment of long cycle cell cancers (slow) typically seen in gastrointestinal neoplastic growths. Examples of surgery for control are removal of metastatic sites or reduction of tumor mass for better treatment. Surgery for palliation is to relieve pain, remove obstruction, or control hemorrhage or infection (Baldonado and Stahl, 1978; Shiplacoff, 1981). While undergoing treatment for cancer, the aged individual will require special attention to previous and/or chronic disease states which increase surgical complications. Health professionals should be sensitive to the fact that older individuals may have sensory deficits, chronic disease(s), and limited mobility. The patient's coping ability may be reduced with this added stress.

Chemotherapy

Chemotherapy is utilized in treating cancer with the goal of cure or treatment of disseminated disease, or it can be used in adjunct with other therapies to achieve better response. The cancer cells continue dividing with a smaller portion of cells being in the resting phase during the growth cycle. Chemotherapeutic drugs are effective in stopping cell growth by interfering with protein needed for metabolism or by combining with the cell in a way which prevents its future growth (Sarna, 1981). The reader should consult an oncology text for in-depth information about chemotherapeutic agents, their actions, side effects, and suggested nursing interventions. Table 25-3 lists common categories of chemotherapeutic agents.

Radiation

Radiation is used as the primary treatment of cancer or in combination with other modalities for cure, control, and/or relief of pain or com-

Table 25-3. Cancer Drugs and Patient Care.

CHEMOTHERAPEUTIC AGENTS	SIDE EFFECTS	THERAPEUTIC MEASURES
Alkylating agents Busulfan Chlorambucil Cyclophosphamide Dibromodulcitol Mechlorethamine	Nausea and vomiting, bone marrow depression for all Bleeding Hair loss, bladder irritation	*FOR ALL: PREMEDICATE WITH ANTIEMETIC AS NEEDED AND PROTECT FROM INFECTIONS* Nausea more severe if fasting during administration. Check urine and stools for blood. Give fluids to 2000 cc daily. Patient may need wig.
Melphalan Triethylenethiophosphoramide	Bone marrow depression, nausea and vomiting Bone marrow depression, nausea and vomiting Bone marrow depression, nausea and vomiting	Check lab work for marrow depression.
Antimetabolites Cytosine arabinoside 5-Fluorouracil 6-Mercaptopurine Methotrexate Thioguanine	Decreased platelets, liver toxicity GI ulceration, stomatitis, diarrhea Bone marrow depression, vomiting GI ulceration, fibrosis of lung	Watch for bleeding and hepatic symptoms. Use local antiseptic after diluted mouthwash. Give Kaopectate for diarrhea. Assess lung sounds; watch for pneumothorax.
Plant alkaloids Vinblastine Vincristine	Bone marrow depression, nausea and vomiting, stomatitis, headache, alopecia Bone marrow depression, constipation, paresthesia, paralytic ileus, headache	Check for bleeding and infection; use wig for hair loss. Assess for sensory loss and decreased peristalsis; give stool softener or laxative.
Antibiotics Dactinomycin Doxorubicin Bleomycin sulfate Daunomycin Mithramycin Mitomycin C Adriamycin	Nausea and vomiting, bone marrow depression, GI irritation, stomatitis, diarrhea, hair loss, local tissue necrosis, phlebitis Chills, elevated temperature, pneumonia, GI ulcerations, hair loss, pulmonary fibrosis Nausea and vomiting, phlebitis, tissue necrosis, cardiac toxicity at high doses Nausea and vomiting, bone marrow depression, decrease in platelets, calcium elevation, liver toxicity GI disturbance, bone marrow depression, hair loss, cardiac toxicity with total doses over 600 mg/m^2	Assess for ulcerations and infections Intake and Output. Watch for excessive fluid loss; may reactive radiation site. Assess vital signs every 4 hours, use antipyretic; assess lung sounds and respiratory difficulty. Check infusion site; assess cardiac rhythm; urine is red. Watch for bleeding or bruising; check liver function studies. Watch for bleeding and ulceration; do baseline cardiac studies.
Miscellaneous synthetics Dacarbazine (may be alkylating agent) Hexamethylmelamine (may be alkylating agent)	Severe nausea and vomiting	Premedicate with antiemetic; keep patient still; instruct to breath through mouth; patient must avoid food for 2 hours after treatment; give nonspicy, nonirritating, nutritional diet.
Hydroxyurea Procarbazine	Bone marrow depression, anorexia, diarrhea, anemia Bone marrow depression, nausea and vomiting, skin reaction, CNS symptoms	Assess for skin and neurological changes.

Table 25-3. Cancer Drugs and Patient Care. (continued)

CHEMOTHERAPEUTIC AGENTS	SIDE EFFECTS	THERAPEUTIC MEASURES
Nitrosoureas Carmustine Lomustine Semustine Streptozotocin	Nausea and vomiting, bone marrow depression, renal toxicity, flushing of blush area, pain along infusion vessel Nausea and vomiting, kidney damage, GI ulceration, abdominal pain, alteration in urine glucose, vessel infusion irritation	Assess intake and output; do kidney function studies; give medication for pain. Clinitest urine; watch for hypoglycemia.
Enzymes L-Asparaginase	Renal and liver toxicity, hyperglycemia, elevated temperature, allergic response	Check lab work for liver and kidney function; check urine for glucosuria; give antipyretic for fever.
Hormones Adrenocorticosteroids Dexamethasone Prednisone	Fluid retention, steroid-induced diabetes, hypertension, impaired immune response GI bleeding, mood changes, osteoporosis, hypokalemia, CHF	Assess vital signs every 4 hours, intake and output; check weight and edema daily. Check for bleeding; support during psychological stress; protect from bone fractures; watch for cardiac arrhythmias, dyspnea, and edema.
Adrogens Testosterone propionate	Fluid retention, masculinization changes, increased sexual desire	Monitor intake and output; weigh daily; check blood pressure; explain masculinization.
Estrogens Diethylstilbestrol Ethynylestradiol	Nausea and vomiting, vaginal bleeding, feminization, fluid retention Nausea and vomiting, vaginal bleeding, femization, fluid retention	Assess for bleeding; limit salt intake. Weigh daily. Monitor intake and output; assess for edema.
Antiestrogens Tamoxifen	Hot flushes, mild nausea and vomiting, bone pain, possible dermititis	Explain side effects; assess skin. Medicate for severe pain. Assess for skin condition.
Progesterons Hydroxyprogesterone caproate Medroxyprogesterone acetate Megestrol acetate	Nausea and vomiting, fluid changes, back pain, elevated serum calcium, breast enlargement, increased sexual desire Bone marrow depression	Monitor intake and output, weight changes, and edema. Accept variable moods. Assess for physical changes.

NOTE: This table lists only some of the most common therapeutic agents (drugs) used in cancer chemotherapy. The side effects listed are generalized for each group. The therapeutic measures listed are necessary nursing assessments and interventions for optimum outcomes of treatment and care.

pression. The aged tolerate radiation therapy less well than younger patients. The tolerance of normal tissue is 10–15% less in the elderly, and the physically exhausted older patient may consider withdrawing from treatment prematurely because of side effects (Gunn, 1980). Therefore, the nurse should explain radiation goals and supportive care to older patients and their families.

The radiation bean is delivered in prescribed amounts to the specific area by a cobalt-60 unit, which contains a radioactive material, or by a linear accelerator, which superspeeds electrical charges. The dividing cancer cell is damaged so that it can no longer reproduce and it eventually dies (Baldonado and Stahl, 1978). The course of radiation treatment will vary from approximately 3 to 5 weeks, with a dosage of 3500 to 7000 RADS (radiation absorbed dose) depending on the desired total dose as determined by the radiation oncologist (Rubin and Poulter, 1978).

During radiation there is increased metabolism of both tumor and normal cells which compete for available nutrients (Marino, 1981). Aging slows the recovery and proliferation of normal cells. The nutritional status of the aged person requires particular attention to calories and proteins to meet both tumor and body demands. Dietary management during radiation is especially important in the elderly because of dental problems, reduced enzyme secretion, and slowed peristalsis (Shils, 1978). Five small meals spaced throughout the day, so that food is not taken immediately prior to treatment or for three hours after, will protect the gastrointestinal tract and still provide adequate nutrition. Remaining at home where culturally preferred foods are served is a nutritional advantage.

Problems with anorexia, nausea and vomiting, and bone marrow depression may cause serious obstacles during radiation (see Table 25-4). An alternative may be to give the planned therapy in a "split-dose" schedule. This type of scheduling permits a 2–6 week rest period between divided treatment courses. This brief respite can be beneficial for the aged patient by allowing recovery and repair of normal tissues (Gunn, 1980); see Table 25-5.

Table 25-4. Common Patient Problems during Radiation Therapy.

COMMON MANIFESTATIONS	THERAPY
Nausea and vomiting	Avoid eating before treatment. Medicate for nausea 1/2 hour prior to treatment and prn. Provide small meals spaced away from treatment time and late in the day.
Loss of appetite	Provide low fat, high calorie, low residue diet. Liquid diets or supplements may be used. Check for preferred foods.
Fatigue	Encourage rest periods daily, as well as adequate fluids and protein intake.
Alopecia	Use head covering to protect skin and maintain body image. When head is treated, hair will be temporarily lost 3 weeks after initial therapy. If dosage is under 6000 rads, hair will return after a few months, thinner and perhaps a redder shade. American Cancer Society has wigs to loan.
Insomnia	Explore for depression. A safe sleep mixture high in tryptophane is: one cup milk (whole or skim), 2 t. vegetable oil, and one sliced banana (should be prepared in blender and given 20 minutes before bedtime).
Bone marrow depression	Protect from viral infection and bacterial contamination. Assess for bleeding and anemia. Use soft tooth brush, good oral hygiene.

METASTASIS

Metastasis indicates disease progression. It means that there is self-sustaining growth in another part of the body. The most common sites of metastasis are lymph nodes which drain the primary tumor site, lung, liver, bone, and brain. The malignant cell will break off from the primary site and travel by lymph, blood, direct tissue invasion, or gravity to grow in the secondary site. The microscopic appearance of the cell will be the same as the primary even

Table 25-5. External Radiation and Skin Care.

RADIATION REACTION	MANIFESTATION	THERAPY
Radiodermatitis	Reddened skin	Wash gently with lukewarm water and pat dry. Expose to air. Patient should avoid sun or heat.
Radioepithelitis	Dry peeling of skin	Wash gently; apply vegetable shortening or oil; do not use perfumed creams.
Radioinjury	Moist desquamation of skin	Wash gently; apply steroid cream. Avoid powders or lotions containing alcohol or mineral oil. Apply mild vegetable oil. Inspect exit site.

though the cells are within different tissue. The metastatic growth will result in a less favorable prognosis (Sugarbaker and Ketcham, 1979).

SKIN CANCER

Skin cancer is the most common of all malignancies, most frequently occurring after age 50. Carcinoma of the skin is also the most frequent second cancer found in patients who have another cancer diagnosis. The sun's ultraviolet rays damage the skin, causing it to wrinkle and to lose its elasticity and static melanin property. Overexposure during sunbathing, gardening, or over prolonged episodes is considered to be a carcinogenic. Education about overexposure and the beneficial use of sunscreen agents is paramount in the prevention of skin cancer. Other skin irritants include arsenic preparation, x-rays, petroleum products, or thermal burns (Baldonado and Stahl, 1978). There are three types of skin cancer: (1) basal cell carcinoma, which is highly curable; (2) squamous cell carcinoma, with limited metastasis and curability; and (3) malignant melanoma, with high metastatic rate, which is less common and will not be discussed in depth here.

Skin cancer usually appears in exposed areas, especially the "T zone" area of the face (lips, nose, cheeks, eyelids, and forehead) and the back of the hands. Malignant melanoma occurs most often in the midline of the body, on the sole of the foot, or near the fingernails (Gumport, Harris and Kopf, 1974).

Treatment of Skin Cancer

Lesions and some surrounding tissue are surgically excised and examined. The patient must be informed of the importance of follow-up. In basal cell and squamous cell carcinoma, local recurrence is common, but the disease is controllable by continued surveillance and excision of new growths. Regional nodes are usually removed when involved. Surface radiation is utilized in areas where surgery is avoided. A local chemotherapy application may control and prevent recurrence of malignant lesions (Burkhalter and Donley, 1978).

Nursing Implications

A common and prevailing concern in the treatment of skin cancer is body image because physical appearance is such an important factor in social acceptance in our society. The aging person may be experiencing loss of positive body image due to normal aging changes; then as malignant skin growths appear, he may view himself even more negatively and less acceptably. The nurse must be able to assess this as a problem during treatment and should support adaptation toward regaining a healthy self (body) image. Body image is a fluid and changing self-awareness. Individuals can be helped to adjust to physical changes when personal strengths are recognized and emphasized, and when significant others around them react in a constructive manner (Donovan and Pierce, 1976).

CANCER OF THE GASTROINTESTINAL TRACT IN THE AGED

Cancer of the gastrointestinal tract is the second most frequent type of cancer occurring in both the older male and the older female (Morton, 1978). The symptoms vary according to the location of the malignancy along the alimentary canal. As erosion of the lining occurs; bleeding is common and will appear fresh bright red or dark and tarry, according to the proximity to an external orifice and action by digestive enzymes (Kennedy, 1981).

Causative factors include dietary regimes characteristic of certain cultures. *Esophageal cancer* is higher in people who drink home-brewed alcohol, are alcoholics, or have suffered chemical damage to the esophagus. *Gastric carcinomas* are of higher incidence in areas where smoked or salted food or talc-treated rice is a mainstay of the diet. It is found more often in lower socioeconomic groups who have high starch intake with low amounts of fruits and vegetables. *Colorectal cancer* is much more common where there is high use of refined carbohydrates and lack of cellulose or bran (Morton, 1978).

Early diagnosis is important but may be delayed because of the insidious onset of symptoms in the aged. Indigestion and abdominal pain are frequently treated symptomatically at home, and medical care is not sought until late. Early detection of rectal cancer is more likely when digital exam or sigmoidoscopy is performed as part of the routine exam for anyone over 45 years of age (Morton, 1978). When digital exam is done a quaiac test of stool can be obtained by the practitioner in minutes (Kennedy, 1981). The older patient may avoid examination because of associated discomfort. Current development of laboratory screening tests such as carcinoembryonic antigen (CEA) may assist future diagnosis for the aged. This test is already useful in determing the presence of metastasis after surgery (Dhar et al., 1972).

Surgical Treatment of Gastrointestinal Cancer

Preoperative instructions should be based on the previous surgical experiences of the elderly and on helping them to understand the routine of care in the preoperative, recovery room, and postoperative units (Eliopoulous, 1979). The patient and family should be informed of the surgical findings in terms they understand. Information about a malignancy is given with plans for later referral and always with hope. Hope

fosters a positive attitude and cooperation with required adjustments (Werner-Beland, 1980).

After radical alimentary tract surgery, the patient is maintained on hyperalimentation until gastric activity is resumed. Then an elementary diet mixture can be given by tube or by mouth to supplement nutritional intake. Both of these temporary nutritional supportive measures are especially valuable when caring for the aged.

Elemental diets contain nutrients that are less complex and composed of small molecules which are easily digested. Elemental diet mixtures are bland in taste and may be flavored or mixed with sherbet. The advantage of elemental mixtures is that they may be taken by mouth or given by tube. Any solution started by tube feeding should be initially diluted, and the patient should be assessed for absorption; then the concentration can be increased gradually. These types of nutritional support are also beneficial for the aged patient who is receiving chemotherapy.

Colostomy Care

For the aged patient who has a colostomy, it is important to learn how to manage his own care at home and with limited financial resources. Detailed step-by-step instructions should be written for the patient before discharge. Discharge planning includes referrals for home health care, as well as access to the stoma therapist at the hospital. A significant other person should receive instruction about colostomy care as a backup. Facilitating a question-and-answer session and encouraging a significant other to take part in colostomy care will initiate the adjustment between the patient and this important person.

Rehabilitation after colostomy is both a physical and a psychosocial process. The first social outing is a challenge for any patient but especially so for the aged person with other physical limitations. Colostomy clubs which exist in most cities help in sharing experiences and providing peer support. These groups aid in recognizing and appreciating coping abilities gained in previous life experiences and try to capitalize on strengths.

LUNG CANCER IN THE AGED

Cancer of the lung is the leading cause of cancer deaths and is four times more common in men than in women. The average age for persons newly diagnosed with lung cancer is 60 years. When diagnosed, the aged person who has lived with a lifetime fear of cancer may immediately resign himself to death. The health care team may write him off because of his age (Gunn, 1980). The prognosis for cancer of the lung continues to be poor. The mortality rate for lung cancer patients over 65 is twice that of younger patients (Kennedy, 1981).

Surgical lobectomy is the primary therapy for operable tumors. A portion of the lung is removed, and chest tubes are placed for drainage. Chest surgery is anxiety producing because it interferes with an organ essential to breathing and life. Clear explanations and sensitivity to the aged person's needs will aid in recovery. See Table 25-6 for a specific plan of nursing care.

Intravenous chemotherapy studies have shown that there are some responses to treatment of oat cell carcinoma by certain alkylating and antimetabolite agents (Emerson, Phillips, and Rubin, 1978). Chemotherapy may also be administered by drug instillation into the pleural cavity. Atabrine or nitrogen mustard may be instilled to treat recurrent pleural effusions (Dorr and Fritz, 1977).

PROSTATE CANCER

Prostate cancer is primarily a disease of older men. It is the most common type of cancer for men aged 50–70. Undiagnosed prostatic cancer is a common finding on pathologic exam at autopsy (Frank, 1978). Early detection before subjective symptoms are noticed depends on palpation of a prostate nodule through rectal examination. Rectal exam is simple, with only mild discomfort, and should be part of the routine physical for all males over age 45.

Table 25-6. Standard Care Plan for Patient with Lung Surgery.

PATIENT PROBLEM	EXPECTED OUTCOME	NURSING INTERVENTIONS
Possible surgical infection (the older person may be at greater risk for infections)	To recover from surgery without infection	Assess lung sounds. Turn, cough, and deep breathe with splintering. Record temperature every 4 hr. Give fluid to 2000 cc daily. The older person who needs assistance may be in jeopardy.
Postoperative pain	To have minimal pain with decreasing amounts of medication	Reposition every 2 hr. Give pain medication every 4 hrs. as needed. Allow rest periods between activity and ambulation.
Decreased oxygen-exchanging ability	To be able to perform self-care activities without dyspnea.	Use incentive spirometry. Turn, cough, and deep breathe with splinting. Give oxygen at 4 liters by nasal prongs. Assess pulse rate for exertion during activity.
Surgically collapsed lung	To reexpand lung by closed chest drainage	Provide chest tube care. Assess lung sounds and movement. Mark amount of drainage and note character. Milk and strip chest tubes.

NOTE: The nurse must consider and adapt the care plan to meet the special needs of the frail elderly, such as maintaining activity, adequate diet, and sufficient fluid intake.

Elderly males frequently have benign prostatic enlargement with insidious onset first noted with urinary frequency and dribbling. An enlarged prostate may be caused by either benign or malignant growths. Because symptoms evolve slowly and are associated with advancing age, men who deny aging avoid seeking health care. This hesitancy is a crucial factor in delaying diagnosis of carcinoma. Symptoms of advanced growth include complete outlet obstruction with urinary retention. Diagnosis is confirmed by histologic examination of a surgically removed specimen from an enlarged gland. Other assessment measures to determine the extent of the disease include laboratory studies of serum acid phosphatase and alkaline phosphatase levels. These levels are elevated above normal when bony metastatic growth has occured. (Rectal palpation of the prostate can cause transient elevation of phosphatases.) The most frequent sites of bone metastases are the pelvis and the vertebrae (Frank, 1978; Tilkian and Conover, 1975). A bone scan with radioisotope ^{99}Tc will indicate where malignant lesions have invaded the skeleton. A lymphangiogram is also used to determine the extent of disease: a dye is injected which flows through the lymph channels and outlines suspicious areas. The extent of disease determines the treatment protocol.

Surgery

The prostate gland is removed by one of three different surgical routes: perineal, suprapubic, or transurethral. The transurethral approach is most preferred, but more radical procedures are necessary for very large tumors (Frank, 1978). Surgical procedures and treatments should always be described to patients; however, patients frequently report having received little or no preparation for this surgery, which is frequently brushed off by professionals as minor surgery when, indeed, to the patient it has devastating implications. Older men often see prostate problems as "the end" (see Chapter 24 for a description of transurethral surgery and Chapter 36 for a discussion of sexuality.

When the suprapubic approach is used, the patient returns to the room with a second drainage catheter placed into the bladder through an abdominal incision. The urethral catheter remains in place after the suprapubic catheter has been removed and until the bladder wall is well healed.

In a perineal prostatectomy, the surgical incision is made just anterior to the anus. This route also allows easy removal of a very large prostate, weighing over 50 grams. It is important to change drainage dressings frequently and to use a T binder or similar supportive dressing belt so that activity can be encouraged (Murphy, 1974). Incontinence (temporary or permanent) may be a problem in up to 15% of the patients who have this radical surgery. The patient can be taught to overcome temporary incontinence with perineal exercises. He is instructed to alternately contract and relax the perineal, gluteus maximus, and abdominal muscles five times for three seconds each while breathing normally. These exercises should begin on the second day postoperatively and should continue until the catheter is removed and normal excretion has been established for at least five days (Vredevoe, 1981).

During postoperative recovery from the radical prostatectomy procedures, the patient has a potential for hemorrhage because of lysis of fibrinogen. The pharmacotherapeutic agent ε-aminocaproic acid (Amicar) may be administered to counteract this problem (Falconer et al., 1978).

The most common pain during the postoperative period is associated with bladder spasms. Belladonna and opium suppositories continue to be the best treatment for this pain (Falconer et al., 1978). Since this is not a common route for administration of pain medication, it is important to explain and reinforce its purpose (the associated relief usually reinforces its use). Adequate hydration, along with a diet high in protein and in vitamins B and C for tissue repair, is recommended.

The incidence of impotence is lower in less radical surgeries which do not interrupt parasympathetic innervation and higher in radical surgeries and radiation (Zinman et al., 1978). Counseling is a determining factor in adjustment and in the resolution of problems (Houston and Rodriguez, 1981).

Retrograde ejaculation may result when innervation is lost due to a tumor and/or the surgical procedure. The lack of a regular ejaculation appears to be a significant loss, but if the patient and his partner understand that a retrograde ejaculation should not interfere with coital climax, rehabilitation will be encouraged. Unfortunately, many nurses and physicians seem uncomfortable in this situation, or they do not perceive this as important to the older man or to the couple. So, frequently, the counseling begins with the care giver after surgery (Leiber et al., 1976). The following is a rather typical statement (see Chapter 36 on sexuality):

When I asked the doc about my sex life after the operation, he said, "Hell, George, what do you expect at your age?"

Radiation for Prostatic Cancer

The purpose of radiation for the aged patient with prostatic cancer is to cure or control the radiosensitive cell. Radiation is also effective in palliative treatment of bone metastasis from prostate cancer, which is a source of severe pain (Frank, 1978); see Table 25-4 on care of the patient during radiation. It is important to note that when the prostate is treated by radiation, the exit point will be over the sacrum and gluteal fold. In the aged person with poor skin resilience, there will be increased surface desquamation. Irritation by bed linens, dampness, and limited nutrition cause this area to break down quickly and heal slowly (Baldonado and Stahl, 1978).

BREAST CANCER

Cancer of the breast is the most common type of cancer in women, the leading cause of cancer death in women, and the leading cause of death from all causes for women aged 40–44 years. It occurs more frequently in the mature woman, with 83% of all detection in the 40-year-old group and 66% clinically detectable in the over-50 age group. The median age for breast cancer in the male is 60. There is an increase in incidence throughout the life span, with the highest peak in patients over 85 years of age (Baldonado and Stahl, 1978).

The causative factors of breast cancer have been thought to be: genetic predisposition, impaired immunological response, viruses, and estrogens which are believed to act as promoters of carcinogenesis (Leis, 1977). More recently, breast cancer has been considered to be a multifocal disease with no known causative factor (Savlov, 1978).

Early diagnosis and treatment are aimed at cure. The most important aspect of early diagnosis is breast self-examination. A lump or mass found by the woman herself has been primary in case finding of about 90% of women with breast cancer. All women can be instructed in routine self-examination of their breasts. Ideally, this should begin in the teenage years and should become a monthly habit on the last day of the menstrual flow. The postmenopausal woman should continue a regular examination on a specific day of the month. Other screening methods include mammograms for women over the age of 50 or in high risk groups, or the use of xeromammography or thermography. The mammogram remains an important diagnostic aid. Mammography has been found to be less hazardous for high risk groups than is the danger of having a breast cancer which is not detected at a curable stage (*Breast Cancer Digest*, 1980).

Malignant breast tumors are most frequently found by the woman herself as a painless lump. The most common breast tumors are located in the upper outer quadrants of the breast and are associated with late child bearing, nulliparity, a positive family history, and late menopause.

A biopsy is done on suspicious tumors by needle aspiration or surgical incision. Recent laboratory methods provide for the determination of hormonal influence on biopsied tissue. Malignant cells are tested by estrogen receptor assay (ERA) to determine whether estrogen receptors are present. If so the growth of the tumor may be controlled by using estrogens as the primary therapy or as an adjunct to other forms of therapy to enhance their effect.

The older woman's fears as she approaches surgery for a breast tumor are compounded. She fears surgery and disfigurement, and is at higher risk for developing complications and dying.

Types of Surgery

The older woman will have heard of many types of breast surgery from radicals to "lumpectomies" (where only the lump is removed). The Halstead radical mastectomy procedure is the most traditional. Currently, many surgeons are comparing the prognosis and results of this procedure with those of procedures which leave an extra skin flap for later breast reconstruction. The later reconstruction permits a silicone prosthesis to be placed over the chest wall, which allows a fairly "normal" appearing breast. The woman who elects this type of internal prosthesis has many advantages. Reconstructive surgery should be available for any woman, at any age. The older patient may hesitate to request information or referral for this, but her needs and desires should be recognized and acknowledged.

Nursing Implications

It is wise to remember that any surgery results in body image changes. The nurse's emotional support during the first dressing change after mastectomy will facilitate a positive self-image. Even years later a woman may avoid exposure of the scar to others to protect her weak self-concept if she has not resolved the initial conflict. Effective rehabilitation may be enhanced by referral to Reach for Recovery, which is a successful group of postmastectomy women, sponsored by the American Cancer Society, whose goal is helping other mastectomy patients. A trained volunteer visits the new patient and shares experiences of physical and emotional adjustment which assist with rehabilitation.

The aged female will experience grief at the loss of a breast just as a younger woman does. Because of other current losses, her grief may be even more acute. She may be a widow with sagging breasts, but her body image and self-concept are more important than ever. She may ask fewer questions about the procedure and yet need repetitive explanations for preparation and recovery. The nurse can assist the patient with limited financial resources by referring her to the American Cancer Society for assistance in obtaining a breast prothesis free of charge and in adapting clothing she already has to regain a positive body image. The need for follow-up exams and self-examination of the other breast should be stressed.

Radiation

Radiation may be used with or without mastectomy to stop malignant growth; it may be given before or after surgery, depending on the preferred therapy for the current stage of the disease. Currently, clinical study groups are researching the statistical rate of cure using radiation alone. Radiation alone or with limited surgery may be preferred for the male with breast cancer (Robison, 1980). The aged woman may be referred for radiation to treat metastatic sites. When bone metastasis occurs, the patient will experience continual persistent pain which can be an overwhelming problem in an already aggravated situation. When radiation is given, the patient will require continued pain medication into the week of surgery. The first 2–3 days of radiation therapy may result in increased pain due to the local inflammatory response, but this will subside soon. Because a woman may develop additional or new problems, each episode of pain should be assessed; one should never assume the cause is the same (see nursing implications for radiation elsewhere in this chapter for more interventions regarding skin care and diet).

LEUKEMIA IN THE AGED

Leukemia, which means "white blood," is the abnormal proliferation of immature leukocytes. It is a malignant disease which affects both young and old. Acute lymphocytic leukemia is a malignancy common to children. Chronic lymphocytic leukemia is a malignancy common to adults over age 45, which occurs more frequently in males. The incidence of chronic lymphocytic leukemia increases with each decade of life (Bates and Orton, 1981).

It has been difficult even with research to determine the cause of leukemia in the aged. A number of factors have been identified as contributory causative agents, including radiation; drugs and chemicals such as chloromycetin, benzene, and arsenic; environmental interactions; genetic and chromosomal abnormalities; and viral and immunological factors (Baldonado and Stahl, 1978). The onset of symptoms is slow and nonspecific, with the disease often diagnosed by laboratory tests while treatment is being sought for other medical problems (Lichtman and Klemperer, 1978).

The aged person with leukemia will probably have limiting debilitation due to arthritis, diabetes, or hypertension. A new diagnosis of chronic leukemia will produce additional fears. If chronic lymphocytic leukemia is not active or is in remission, it does not require treatment. When there is anemia, thrombocytopenia, hypermetabolism, or lymph and spleen enlargement, treatment should be initiated. The most successful treatment has been chemotherapy with the use of alkylating agents (Weinstein and Rosenthal, 1978). The patient may receive treatment in the hospital or as an outpatient. The outpatient protocol is preferred for the aged so that the individual can maintain contact with a familiar environment and significant persons. Alkalyting agents such as chlorambucil (Leukeran) and cyclophosphamide (Cytoxan) are commonly used in the treatment of chronic lymphocytic leukemia (See-Lasley and Ignoffo, 1981). These agents interfere with the DNA (genetic coding) of the cell during division and result in the destruction of some tumor cells. The regularity of administration of the drug is important so that more tumor cells are killed, while normal tissues repair and proliferate (Dorr and Fritz, 1977).

Nursing Implications

Currently cancer nurses are given increasing responsibility in the administration of chemotherapeutic agents. Information and literature available from drug companies should be studied for correct mixing, administration, and potential side effects. The most critical universal side effect of all cancer chemotherapy drugs is bone marrow depression. In addition to intense nursing care, the nurse must be vigilant in assessment for bleeding, bruising, and impaired resistance to infection. The appropriate laboratory reports (hemoglobin, leukocytes, and platelets, typically) aid in recognition of specific blood deficiencies and should be closely monitored (Marino, 1981); see Table 25-3.

SUMMARY

The most common cancers of older adults, and related therapies, have been presented here. This does not represent an inclusive list. Older patients also suffer from other types of cancer which are more common to younger persons and have not been covered here.

Caring for the elderly cancer patient is a challenging opportunity for nurses to demonstrate their professional skill. Nurses have a key role in maximizing treatment so that older patients can live with a diagnosis of cancer. The emphasis in care should be on maintenance of physical and mental capabilities and helping the person to "live till they die."

REFERENCES

American Cancer Society, *Facts and Figures for 1979.* A Cancer Report from the American Cancer Society, New York, 1979.

Baldonado, A. and Stahl, D. *Cancer Nursing.* Garden City, New York: Medical Examination Publishing Company, 1978.

Bates, M. and Orton, M. Infection control in clients with acute leukemia. In Marino, L. (Ed.) *Cancer Nursing.* St. Louis: C.V. Mosby, 1981, pp. 524–546.

Breast Cancer Digest. National Cancer Institute Publication No. 80-1691 (1980).

Burkhalter, P. and Donley, D. *Dynamics of Oncology Nursing.* New York: McGraw-Hill, 1978.

Dhar, P., Moore, T., Zamcheck, N., and Kupchik, H. C.E.A. in colonic cancer. *Journal of the American Medical Association* 221:31–35 (June 1972).

Donovan, M.I. and Pierce, S.G. *Cancer Care Nursing.* New York: Appleton-Century-Crofts, 1976.

Dorr, R.T. and Fritz, W.L. *Cancer Chemotherapy Manual.* New York: American Elsevier, 1977.

Eliopoulos, C. *Gerontological Nursing.* New York: Harper & Row, 1979, pp. 274–279.

Emerson, G., Phillips, C., and Rubin, P. Lung cancer. In *Clinical Oncology for Medical Students and Physicians.* New York: American Cancer Society, 1978.

Falconer, M. Sheridan, E., Patterson, H.R., and Gustafson, E.A. *The Drug, the Nurse, the Patient.* Philadelphia: W.B. Saunders, 1978.

Frank, I.N. Urologic and male genital cancers. In *Clinical Oncology for Medical Students and Physicians.* New York: American Cancer Society, 1978.

Gumport, S.L., Harris, M.N., and Kopf, A.W. Diagnosis and management of common skin cancers. *Ca: A Cancer Journal for Clinicians* 24(4):27 (1974).

Gunn, W.G. Radiation therapy for the aging patient. *Ca: A Cancer Journal for Clinicians* 30(6):63 (1980).

Houston, G. and Rodriguez, D. Male sexuality and genitourinary cancer. In Marino, L. (Ed.) *Cancer Nursing.* St. Louis: C.V. Mosby, 1981, pp. 595–613.

Jarvik, L. Genetic aspects of aging. *Clinical Geriatrics.* Philadelphia: J.B. Lippincott, 1979.

Kennedy, B.J. Cancer and the aging. *The Clinical Aspects of Aging* 2–11 (January-February 1981).

Leiber, L., Plumb, M., Gerstenzang, M., and Holland, J. The communication of affection between cancer patients and their spouses. *Psychosomatic Medicine* 38(6):121 (1976).

Leis, H. The diagnosis of breast cancer. *Ca: A Cancer Journal for Clinicians,* 27(4):209 (1977).

Lew, E.A. Cancer in old age. *Ca: A Cancer Journal for Clinicians* 28(1):2–6 (1978).

Lichtman, M.A. and Klemperer, M.R. The leukemias. In *Clinical Oncology for Medical Students and Physicians.* New York: American Cancer Society, 1978, pp. 245–258.

Marino, L.B. *Cancer Nursing.* St. Louis: C.V. Mosby, 1981.

Morton, J.H. Alimentary tract cancer. In *Clinical Oncology for Medical Students and Physicians.* New York: American Cancer Society, 1978, pp. 85–99.

Murphy, G. *Prostate Cancer.* New York: American Cancer Society, 1974.

Patterson, W.B. Principles of surgical oncology. In *Clinical Oncology for Medical Students and Physicians.* New York: American Cancer Society, 1978.

Robison, R. Treatment Procols for Cancer, Paper presented at American Society of Therapeutic Radiologists, Houston, Texas, October 24, 1980.

Rubin, P. Statement of the clinical oncologic problem. In *Clinical Oncology for Medical Students and Physicians.* New York: American Cancer Society, 1978, pp. 1–10.

Rubin, P. and Poulter, C. Principles of radiation oncology and cancer radiotherapy. In *Clinical Oncology for Medical Students and Physicians.* New York: American Cancer Society, 1978, pp. 29–41.

Sarna, L.P. Concepts in the nursing management of patients receiving cancer chemotherapy and immunotherapy. In *Concepts of Oncology Nursing.* Englewood Cliffs, N.J.: Prentice-Hall, 1981, pp. 81–153.

Savlov, E. Breast cancer. In *Clinical Oncology for Medical Students and Physicians.* New York: American Cancer Society, 1978.

See-Lasley, K. and Ignoffo, R. *Manual of Oncology Therapeutics.* St. Louis: C.V. Mosby, 1981.

Shils, M. Eternal nutritional management of the cancer patient. *The Cancer Bulletin* 30:98–101 (1978).

Shiplacoff, J. Concepts in surgical oncology. In *Concepts of Oncology Nursing.* Englewood Cliffs, N.J.: Prentice-Hall, 1981, pp. 206–226.

Sugarbaker, P.H. and Ketcham, R.E. The Treatment of Metastatic Disease. *Annuals of Internal Medicine* 84:149–154 (1976).

Tilkian, S. and Conover, M. *Clinical Implications of Laboratory Tests.* St. Louis: C.V. Mosby, 1975.

Vredevoe, D. *Concepts of Oncology Nursing.* Englewood Cliffs, N.J.: Prentice-Hall, 1981.

Weinstein, H. and Rosenthal, D. Leukemia. In *Cancer* (5th ed.). Mass.: American Cancer Society, 1978.

Werner-Beland, J.A. Nursing and the concept of hope. In *Grief Responses to Long-term Illness and Disability.* Englewood Cliff, N.J.: Prentice-Hall, 1980.

Zinman, L., Friedell, G., Schwartz, J., and Shipley, W. Carcinoma of the prostate and bladder. *Cancer: A Manual for Practitioners.* Mass.: American Cancer Society, 1978, pp. 217–230.

BIBLIOGRAPHY

Adams, J.T. Cancer of the major digestive glands. In *Clinical Oncology for Medical Students and Physicians.* New York: American Cancer Society, 1978, pp. 100–106.

Blumberg, B. Evaluating patient education programs. *Oncology Nursing Forum* 8(2):29–31 (1981).

Boyer, M. Treating invasive lung cancer. *American Journal of Nursing* 1916–1923 (December 1977).

Cancer Facts and Figures 1981. New York: American Cancer Society, 1981.

Ebersole, P. and Hess, P. *Toward Healthy Aging.* St. Louis: C.V. Mosby, 1981.

Elliott, S.C. Radiation: a focused assault. *Helping Cancer Patients Effectively.* Springfield, Ill.: Intermed Communications, 1977.

Gertman, S. (Ed.). *Working with Older People,* Vol. 1. Washington, D.C.: U.S. Department of Health, Education and Welfare, 1974.

Goldstein, S.E. Depression in the elderly. *Journal of the American Geriatrics Society* 27(1):305–307 (1979).

Holland, J. *Cancer Medicine.* Philadelphia: Lea & Febiger, 1980.

Kennerly, S.L. Breast cancer confronting one's changed image. *American Journal of Nursing* 1430–1432 (September 1977).

Levene, M.B. A new role for radiation therapy. *American Journal of Nursing* 1443–1446 (September 1977).

Meissner, W.A. Pathologic evaluation and classification of tumors. *Cancer: A Manual for Practitioners.* Mass.: American Cancer Society, 1978, pp. 30–38.

Murphy, G.P. *Prostate Cancer: Progress and Change.* New York: American Cancer Society, 1978.

Paroni, A. Women and cancer. *Cancer News* 34(1):268 (1980).

Rogers, J. and Fergusson, J. Oncology articles. *Clinical Nursing* 2(4): (1981).

Ruckdeschel, J. Small cell anaplastic carcinoma of the lung: changing concepts and emerging problems. *Ca: A Cancer Journal for Clinicians* 29(2):28–34 (1979).

Thomas, S.B. and Yates, M.M. Breast reconstruction after mastectomy. *American Journal of Nursing* 11(9):1438–1442 (1977).

Tulley, J. and Wagner, B. Helping the mastectomy patient live life fully. *Nursing '78* 8(1):18–25 (1978).

Welch, D.A. Waiting, worry and the cancer experience. *Oncology Nursing Forum* 8(2):14–18 (1981).

Wise, T.N. Sexual functioning in neoplastic disease. *Medical Aspects of Human Sexuality* 16–31 (March 1978).

Woods, N.F. *Human Sexuality in Health and Illness.* St. Louis: C.V. Mosby, 1975, pp. 219–232.

26
Surgical Conditions in the Elderly

Nancy E. White

Gerontological nurses can expect an increasing number of geriatric surgical patients in hospitals, in long term care facilities, and in home health care. Gerontological nursing will require greater emphasis on the surgical aspects of patient care. In previous years, surgery was often withheld from the elderly because of anticipated risks and complications. Because of improvements in surgical procedures, better pre- and post-operative management, and more persons living to old age, more surgeries are currently performed on the elderly then ever before.

This chapter focuses on the surgical conditions which are experienced by the elderly population. Included are the general considerations and nursing care during the preoperative and postoperative periods for the elderly surgical patient. There is an emphasis on those particular surgeries that the older person might be more likely to require because of his age.

The presence of unrelated chronic medical conditions and the narrowed margins of physiological reserve will ultimately increase the risk of surgery for the aged. The postoperative mortality rate for patients with heart disease is twice that of a control population, and 50% of patients over age 70 have significant cardiovascular disease (Schein, 1979). However, surgical intervention not only has added years to the life of aged persons, but also has added functional years (Eliopoulos, 1979).

The decision to accept surgery is not arrived at lightly but, rather, after careful consideration. Realistically, older people have a right to more fear and apprehension because they are at higher risk. However, they usually do well and have in fact already demonstrated their coping ability by reaching old age. By strengthening their capacities preoperatively, maintaining these capacities postoperatively, and assessing for complications, the nurse can help reduce the risk of surgery (Eliopoulos, 1979).

PREOPERATIVE CONSIDERATIONS

Nursing care of the hospitalized elderly person requires special consideration and understanding. The older person may, because of prior experience of his peers, associate hospitalization with death. At the very least, it involves a change in environment and an alteration in long established routines. Hospitalization means separation from loved ones and often a change in role. The aged person who was once the provider and decision maker of the family often reacts with regressive childlike behavior. Nurses must recognize that this is a form of temporary coping which is not pathological (Lore, 1979).

Clear introduction to staff and an orientation to the unit are essential if the elderly person is to adjust to hospitalization. The patient should be permitted to keep personal articles at the bedside and within easy reach. The nurse must explain the use of the call bell and the routines of the hospital schedule. Manipulating the hospital environment to suit the patient may be a more viable alternative than asking the elderly patient to adjust. This includes assessing the patient's level of anxiety, sensory loss, and perception of the environment and changing the environment to enhance the adaptive potential of the elderly patient (Bagwell and Ludlow, 1980). Unfortunately, most nurses do not perceive themselves as being able to manipulate the environment. Perhaps the most important aspect of care is to listen to the patient and allow him every opportunity to express his fears and concerns.

Preoperative physical assessment is essential for obtaining baseline data against which postoperative comparisons are made. An evaluation of the effects of aging on organ systems and the patient's general nutritional status alerts the nurse to potential postoperative complications. Particular attention is directed to those organs that can affect or be affected by surgery, specifically the cardiac, respiratory, gastrointestinal, and renal systems (Sheehy, 1979). It is also imperative to identify all medications the patient is taking for chronic conditions as it may be necessary to continue their administration throughout the pre- and postoperative period.

Elderly patients will require frequent reassurance regarding the successful outcome of their surgery because they know they are at high risk. It is often helpful if they can meet someone who has recovered from similar surgery. Patients and their families should receive adequate teaching regarding expected reactions to anesthesia, the length of the surgery, and (with a brief description) the management of pain (Eliopoulos, 1979). A tour of the recovery room or intensive care unit and an introduction to the staff help to decrease anxiety and possible disorientation. Patients and families should be familiarized with equipment, such as intermittent positive pressure breathing (IPPB) machines, monitors, etc., and with routine pro-cedures, such as turning, coughing, deep breathing, and dressing changes, to which they will be exposed during the postoperative phase.

POSTOPERATIVE CONSIDERATIONS

The most common immediate complications of surgery are shock, hemorrhage, pulmonary atelectasis, cardiovascular disturbance, infection, and gastrointestinal ileus (Glenn, 1979). These are directly related to the narrow margin of cardiac, pulmonary, and renal reserve in even the healthiest aged patient (Howells, 1977). Prevention of complications is the key to nursing care; however, when this is not possible, early detection should be emphasized. It is, of course, essential that the nurse recognize the signs and symptoms indicating a change in the postoperative status of the patient which may require prompt treatment. See Table 26-1 for common postoperative complications.

Routing postoperative nursing care of the elderly is similar to that of all patients. Understanding the special feelings, behaviors, and reactions of old people is as important as the special knowledge and skills required for other age groups such as infants or adolescents. Vital signs and urine output are carefully assessed,

Table 26-1. Common Postoperative Complications.

CONDITION	MANIFESTATION	THERAPY
1. Shock	Decreased blood pressure, increased pulse rate, increased respiratory rate, pallor, clammy skin, and decreased urine output	Fluid replacement (plasma and whole blood), vasopressor, increased oxygen
2. Hemorrhage	Same as above	Control of bleeding and restoration of blood loss
3. Pulmonary atelectasis	Cyanosis, decreased breath sounds, diminished chest expansion, and dyspnea	Maintaining patient airway, positioning to maximize chest expansion, breathing exercises, early ambulation, and cautious use of narcotics
4. Phlebitis and emboli	Swelling, pain, redness, and positive Homans' sign	Compression stockings or ace wraps, early mobilization, adequate hydration, anticoagulant therapy
5. Infection	Variable depending on site; wound infection characterized by redness, tenderness, heat, and drainage	Drainage of the source, antibiotic therapy, and asepsis
6. Gastrointestinal ileus	Absence of bowel sounds, flatus, or bowel movement	Gastric decompression until return of bowel sounds, cautious use of narcotics, progressive diet (clear liquids to regular diet)

pulmonary hygiene is maintained, and ambulation is encouraged as soon as possible. The administration of pain medication requires special consideration because the elderly patient may not require as large a dose of analgesics or as frequent administration as the younger adult. The relief of chronic pain brought about as a result of surgery may negate the need for potent analgesics. When narcotics are required for pain relief, they should be administered in small doses in order not to depress the already compromised respiratory system.

Conditions related to the aging process and age-related disease predispose elderly patients to infections and may result in a higher mortality in elderly surgical patients (Polly and Sanders, 1977). Antibiotic therapy is indicated when wound infection is present; however, it is not a substitute for meticulous wound care. The development of a urinary tract infection (UTI) is closely related to the use of indwelling catheters. Prevention of UTI is dependent on aseptic insertion, meticulous care, and early removal of the catheter. Removal of the catheter is encouraged even if other methods of bladder control have to be implemented.

The calorie demand is increased in the elderly surgical patient, and nutritional support must provide sufficient calories and nitrogen to meet the metabolic requirements (Organ and Finn, 1977). Parenteral hyperalimentation may be required to meet the patient's nutritional needs; however, there are risks involved in this, such as hyperglycemia and infection. An alternative is the use of the gastrointestinal route with a nasogastric or gastrostomy tube. The first choice, of course, is to assist the patient in eating. This requires that the nurse be patient and not hurry the aged person during mealtime, but rather assist in preparing the tray and in feeding. Small frequent feedings may be more easily tolerated. It is also helpful to assess the patient's likes and dislikes, and communicate this information to the dietitian.

Efforts at mobilization of the elderly should be initiated as soon as possible following surgery. Debilitation occurs quickly as a result of immobility, and the complications of immobility are more easily prevented than treated in the elderly. Early activity prohibits the development of potential complications such as atelectasis and phlebitis.

The care of elderly patients undergoing surgery is challenging but not without rewards. It is exciting and gratifying to work with patients who were once debilitated and are now experiencing a new lease on life. The following sections deal with some special considerations in some of the more common surgeries performed on elderly patients. The writer assumes that readers will have general medical and surgical nursing backgrounds and, therefore, will concentrate only on the gerontological aspects of surgical nursing. The medical and rehabilitative aspects of most of the conditions described here are also addressed in other chapters of this book.

EYE SURGERY

Age-related vision problems have become more prevalent with the growing number of aging individuals. When these problems reach the point of interfering with an individual's daily activity, surgery should be considered as a possible alternative. The techniques of microscopic eye surgery have become increasingly successful interventions for pathological eye conditions in the aged.

Cataract Surgery

Senile cataract formation is the clouding of the normally transparent crystalline lens. It is present, to variable degrees, in most individuals over 70. With aging, the lens becomes opaque and more dense; it loses elasticity and accom-

Table 26-2. Stages of Cataract Development.

STAGE	DESCRIPTION
Incipient	Cloudlike opacities of cortex or nucleus
Immature	Swelling of lens
Mature	Shrinkage of lens; lens becomes opaque
Hypermature	Lens becomes solid and shrinks, or becomes soft and liquid

modation, which results in a loss of visual acuity. Senile cataracts usually develop bilaterally. However, they progress at different rates in each eye and may be classified by stage of development (Luckmann and Sorensen, 1980); see Table 26-2.

In the past, surgical removal of the lens was delayed until the cataract was "ripe" or matured. However, this is no longer necessary (Boyd-Monk, 1977). Currently, lens extraction is performed when vision is sufficiently impaired so as to interfere with the individual's activities of daily living; it is a successful treatment for 95–98% of all cases (Kornzweig, 1979). The elderly may equate a diagnosis of cataracts with blindness and should be made to understand that relatively few cataracts progress to the point of requiring surgical intervention. In addition, they need to know that they have done nothing to cause the cataract to develop.

Surgical removal of the senile cataract lens is generally accomplished by intracapsular extraction. In this procedure, the lens and its capsule are removed through an incision at the junction of the cornea and sclera. An enzyme which is injected into the anterior chamber prior to extraction results in lysis of the fibers holding the lens. This technique in conjunction with the use of a freezing probe (cryoextraction) permits a safer and easier removal of the intact lens (see Figure 26-1).

Other methods of extraction may be utilized for different kinds of cataracts and circumstances. Extracapsular extraction (removal of the anterior capsule and lens) may be recommended for congenital or traumatic cataracts. Phacoemulsification is the use of an ultrasonic probe to break up and aspirate the lens contents through a small incision. Implantation of an intraocular lens at the time of extraction leaving the lens capsule intact has become more popular in the United States over the last decade (see Figure 26-2). The prosthetic lens, which is made of methyl methacrylate, a type of plastic, aids in focusing and accommodation in much the same way as the patient's normal lens (Smith, 1978). This may be the most promising procedure for the older individual with a unilateral cataract as it maintains binocular vision for that individual.

Nursing Implications. Preoperative teaching is extremely important because most extractions are performed under local anesthesia and require patient cooperation. Because this surgery may also be done on an outpatient basis, the family may be providing postoperative care and should be included in teaching sessions (Low, 1978). The patient must understand what the surgery will accomplish and what life-style may occur as a result of the lens removal. The patient is usually hospitalized for a period of 3–4 days, and the recovery period lasts 6–8 weeks (Boyer, 1979). Much of this recovery is an adjustment period.

Following surgery, the operative eye is dressed, patched, and protected by a shield. The patient is advised to continue wearing the protective shield during the night for one month or longer. This protects the eye from accidental injury or damage from contact with bed linens.

The extreme limitations of movements required several years ago are no longer necessary. However, during convalescence, the patient is instructed to avoid activities which would result in an increase in intraocular pressure and strain on the suture line. Patients are told not to strain on the toilet and to avoid stooping and heavy lifting. In addition, they are asked to avoid rubbing their eyes and lying on the operative side.

Complications of cataract extraction occur in less than 4% of the cases (Kasper, 1978). Because these complications may be serious, it is essential that the nurse be familiar with the manifestations and be able to discriminate normal postoperative discomfort from the pain of pathologic conditions (see Table 26-3).

The aphakic (without lens) patient will require a replacement lens to focus light rays and reestablish visual acuity. Unless an intraocular lens implant was employed the patient will use either cataract spectacles or contact lenses to restore vision. The spectacles may be made of glass or of a plastic material which is two-thirds lighter than the glass but more expensive.

The spectacles restore adequate central vision; however, images are magnified about 30% and peripheral vision is distorted. Until

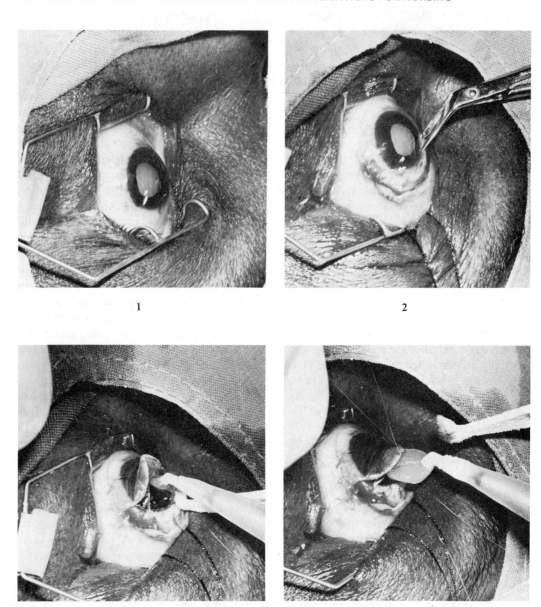

Figure 26-1. Cataract extraction by cryosurgery: (1) retraction of eyelids immediately before the operation to reveal mature cataract; (2) making a 120–180° arc at the limbus to prepare for insertion of cryoprobe (3) applying the cryoprobe to the cataractous lens; (4) easy removal of the intact, cooled lens and capsule. From Boyd-Monk, H.: "Cataract Surgery" from June issue of *Nursing '77,* Copyright © 1977. Photographs courtesy of Wills Eye Hospital, Philadelphia, Pennsylvania.)

the other lens is extracted, binocular vision is impossible because of the different sized images from each eye. Visual accommodation is best if patients are taught to use one eye at a time, look through the center portion of the glasses where distortion is least, and turn their head rather than shift their gaze.

The corneal contact lens has several advantages over spectacles. The image size is more normal, with magnification being only 5–10%, and full visual field with no peripheral distortion is obtained (Kwitko, 1978). Unfortunately many elderly people do not have sufficient manual dexterity to insert the contact lens, particularly with one or both eyes being aphakic. Current research is working to eliminate this problem with the development of an extended-wear or continuous-wear contact lens (Stark and Kracher, 1979).

Glaucoma

Glaucoma is the elevation of intraocular pressure which may result in visual impairment; it is responsible for 12% of the blindness in the United States (Luckmann and Sorensen, 1980). The incidence increases rapidly between the ages of 45 and 65 and with a positive family history (Kornzweig, 1979). The most common form, chronic open-angle glaucoma, develops insidiously and usually bilaterally. Narrow-angle glaucoma is the acute condition which may require immediate surgery in order to prevent blindness.

The pathophysiology of glaucoma is an interference with the normal outflow of aqueous humor from the anterior chamber. The increase in intraocular pressure eventually damages the retina and optic nerve and, if untreated, results in blindness.

The individual with wide-angle glaucoma may complain of a morning headache which disappears after arising or of a nondescript aching in the eyes. The loss of peripheral vision occurs gradually over a period of years. The patient often attributes the generalized symptoms to a need for change of glasses.

Medical management of glaucoma is the first line of defense and consists of drugs to constrict the pupil, increase the angle, and increase the outflow. In addition, diuretics such as Diamox may be prescribed to inhibit the production of aqueous humor. Surgical treatment is withheld unless there is visual fluid loss or an inability to

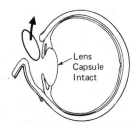
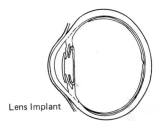

Figure 26-2. A current and highly successful procedure for implantation of an intraocular lens is to remove the old lens leaving the lens capsule intact. The optic of the prosthetic lens (the part we see through) is implanted behind the iris; loops extend horizontally into the capsule to help fixate the implant. The prosthetic lens is not visible with the naked eye. (Diagrams reprinted with the permission and courtesy of David Dulaney, M.D.)

Table 26-3. Complications of Cataract Extraction.

CONDITION	MANIFESTATION	CAUSE	TREATMENT
1. Iris prolapse	Bulging wound; pear-shaped pupil	Wound rupture or pressure	Prolapsed portion excised and sutured
2. Hyphema	Sharp eye pain up to 5 days postoperatively; may be precipitated by strain on eye	Hemorrhage into anterior chamber	Bedrest; keep pupil dilated; Diamox if ↑ intraocular pressure
3. Pupillary block glaucoma	Pain, high intraocular pressure, iris bombé (iris looks like windswept awning)	Air, blood, lens material, or vitreous body blocks circulation between anterior and posterior chamber	Turn patient and change position to reopen circulation; keep pupil mobile – alternate constriction/ dilation
4. Uveitis	Fine, white, half-moon cells in lower part of anterior chamber	Inflammation of iris	Hourly corticosteroids

control intraocular pressure with medical treatment (Boyer, 1979).

Although there are several ways to accomplish it, the objective of surgery for glaucoma is to establish an alternate pathway for circulation of the aqueous humor. Postoperative nursing care is similar to that discussed under cataract surgery, and relatively few restrictions on activity are indicated.

EAR SURGERY

Otosclerosis is a genetic disease which affects the meddle ear of middle-aged persons or youths. This condition results in the fixing of the stapes and may not be discovered until the hearing impairment is compounded by a sensorineural loss in the later years. Reconstructive surgery of the middle ear may restore sufficient hearing to enable the individual to use a hearing aid with considerable success. Reconstructive surgery may also benefit the person with hearing loss as the result of middle ear infections. These surgeries are minor, can be performed under local anesthesia, and do not present a significant risk to the patient (see Chapter 6 on sensory deprivation).

ORTHOPEDIC SURGERY

Caring for elderly persons who have sustained orthopedic injury or require surgery for other reasons demands a great deal of empathy and patience. The experience, although frightening for the individual, need not be envisioned in terms of permanent disability and loss of independence. Advances in surgical corrective techniques have significantly reduced mortality and morbidity of the elderly despite chronologic age (Habermann, 1979). Techniques in elbow replacement are emerging but will not be covered here.

Hip Fractures

Fractures of the proximal end of the femur constitute one of the most common orthopedic conditions encountered by the elderly. They occur most frequently in postmenopausal women with diminished bone mass as a result of osteoporosis (Hagberg and Nilsson, 1977). Although these injuries generally occur as the result of a fall, in some instances the fracture occurs initially and results in the fall (Dunnery, 1979). The brittleness of the elderly persons' bone structure allows them little reserve against even minor insult. For this reason, a hip fracture should be suspected however minor the accident is. There are many factors which contribute to accidental falls in the aged — vertigo, muscle weakness, decreased vision, urinary urgency, unsteady gait, mental confusion, depression, and agitation (Feist, 1978; Lipner and Sherman, 1975).

The damage to the hip joint most often occurs in either the head or the neck of the femur (intracapsular) or the intertrochanteric area (extracapsular); see Figure 26-3. If the fracture results in displacement, the individual will experience extreme pain and inability to bear weight. The injured extremity will appear shortened, adducted, and externally rotated. Fractures of this type may result in hemorrhage and shock, deformities, or secondary arthritis. Since the head of the femur normally has a reduced vascular supply, fracture and displacement in this area may result in avascular necrosis and delayed healing (Bonner, 1974). For these reasons, reduction and/or surgical repair should commence quickly unless contraindicated because of poor health.

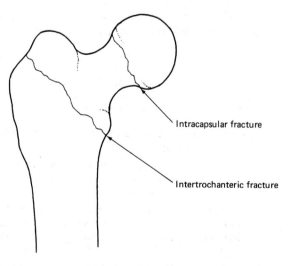

Figure 26-3. Common fracture sites in the hips of the elderly.

The choice of treatment for hip fractures depends on the location and severity of the fracture, as well as on the general health of the individual. Conservative management by means of traction may be acceptable in certain situations (impacted fractures); however, the lengthy immobilization period is quite hazardous to the individual. Therefore, surgical intervention is preferable and, in fact, has resulted in a decrease in morbidity and mortality for victims of fractured hips (Habermann, 1979).

The reparative surgery for hip fractures is internal fixation or implantation of a partial prosthesis to replace the head and neck of the femur. Although controversy exists, it is generally believed that the prosthetic implant may be more suitable for the very elderly person as it allows for early mobilization and weight bearing without the complications experiences with internal fixations (Freehafer, 1978); see Table 26-4.

Nursing Implications. Because of the extensive treatment involved, imposed immobility, and potential complications, hip fractures may be both physically and psychologically devastating to the elderly. The aged person may recall a friend or relative hospitalized for the same condition 20 years ago who either expired in the hospital or was left crippled. Thus, ventilation of anxiety, psychological support, and reinforcement of the technological advances are essential components of care for the patient and family. Introducing the patient to someone who has undergone successful rehabilitation is beneficial.

The nurse who cares for the elderly postoperative hip reduction patient must have knowledge of the type of surgery performed, the patient's previous medical history, and the physician's orders and preferences (Luckmann and Sorensen, 1980); see Table 26-5.

In nursing care, emphasis is placed on positioning, exercising, and early mobilization. The nursing goal for positioning is to maintain proper body alignment, while preventing adduction and rotation of the leg and acute hip flexion in order to prevent dislocation of the prosthesis. Maintenance of alignment is assisted by the use of pillows, sandbags, trochanter rolls, and careful and repeated explanations to the patient. Elevation of the head of the bed is usually restricted to less than 30–45° in order to prevent hip flexion. Patients should be cautioned not to reach for things, and the call bell *must* be placed within convenient access.

The physician's orders regarding the turning of the patient will vary depending on the physician and the type of surgery (internal fixation or partial prosthetic replacement). Exercises are started on the first postoperative day to prepare the patient for early mobilization. Isometric exercises of the quadriceps and gluteal muscles strengthen the muscles for ambulation,

Table 26-4. Comparison of Surgical Corrections for Hip Fractures.

	INTERNAL FIXATION (NAIL OR SCREW)	PARTIAL PROSTHETIC IMPLANT
1. Description	Insertion of pins or nails through the trochanter and femoral neck and into the head of the femur; fixated along femoral shaft with side screwplate	Excision of femoral head; replaced with metal ball, and intramedullary stem inserted into femoral shaft
2. Uses	Intertrochanteric and some femoral shaft fractures	Femoral head or neck fractures (intracapsular)
3. Candidates	Younger patients able to tolerate prolonged non–weight bearing	Elderly patients who would experience difficulty non–weight bearing
4. Mobilization	Early mobilization to non–weight bearing ambulation with walker (2–3 months) to independence in 4–6 weeks	Early mobilization and partial weight bearing within one week
5. Complications	Avascular necrosis Nonunion	Displacement of prosthetic device with abduction or hip flexion during turning

Table 26-5. Postoperative Complications of
Surgical Reduction of the Hip.

CONDITION	OBJECTIVE AND SUBJECTIVE FINDINGS
Shock and hemorrhage	Excessive blood on dressing or linen Alteration in vital signs
Dislocation of hip joint	Sharp hip pain or abnormal positioning
Avascular necrosis	Pain or muscle spasm
Fat embolism	Disorientation; increased pulse, temperature, respirations; dyspnea; decreased pO_2; potential presence of rash
Infection (wound or other source)	Increased temperature
Thrombophlebitis	Calf tenderness

while upper extremity exercises prepare the patient for the use of a walker or crutches.

The patient is allowed out of bed on the first postoperative day to minimize the potential for problems of immobility. With the prosthetic implant, no weight bearing is permitted for the first 96 hours. The patient gradually progresses to ambulation with a walker and minimal weight bearing by the end of a week. Patients who have had internal fixation devices are restricted from bearing weight for a considerably longer time.

Getting out of bed for the first time after injury is extremely frightening to the elderly patient. Directions should be carefully explained, patients should be moved in stages, and they should never be rushed. Two nurses should be on hand to help the patient accomplish the task.

Thorough investigation and evaluation are required to determine the feasibility of discharge to home or the need for an extended care facility for the individual with reparative hip surgery. Rehabilitation and restoration of independence for the individual are not complete at discharge from the hospital, but may take several weeks to months to accomplish (see Chapter 30). Patients are taught to use an elevated toilet seat, a long handled shoehorn, a dressing stick, a sock cone, and other adaptive devices to assist them in their daily activities after discharge (Meyers, McNelly, and Nelson, 1978).

Total Hip Replacement

Osteoarthritis is a degenerative joint disease which affects the majority of elderly people to a variable extent and may require surgical intervention (Grahame, 1978). The weight-bearing joints of the hips and knees are primarily affected, and this may occur unilaterally or bilaterally. In the past, surgical treatment was withheld until severe joint destruction had occurred. At that time, the surgical correction generally consisted of an osteotomy (cutting the bone to correct deformities) or fusion of the joint (Habermann, 1979). Currently, total hip replacement, also called hip arthroplasty, has become a successful procedure for patients with severe pain or limitation of motion.

The total hip arthroplasty involves reconstruction of both the head of the femur and the acetabulum. The head is replaced by a metal ball cemented into the shaft of the femur with methyl methacrylate (dental filling material), and the acetabulum is replaced with a polyethylene cup; see Figure 26-4.

Nursing Implications. Preoperative teaching and preparation of the patient for total hip arthroplasty are essential factors in maximizing patient cooperation and minimizing the length of hospitalization (Meyers et al., 1978). The teaching, often done on an outpatient basis, emphasizes exercise to strengthen muscles and learning to ambulate with crutches or a walker.

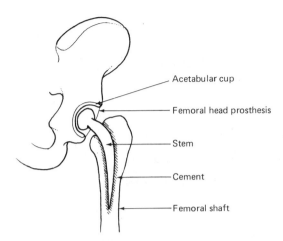

Acetabular cup

Femoral head prosthesis

Stem

Cement

Femoral shaft

Figure 26-4. Total hip arthroplasty.

The presence of any infection is a major contraindication for surgery (Feinstein and Habermann, 1977). Patients must be carefully evaluated to rule out the possibility of any infection, regardless of the source or of how minor it appears. For this reason, most patients receive prophylactic antibiotics for several days.

The postoperative care is similar to that of the patient who has surgical reduction of a hip fracture. Bed rest, with elevation of the head of the bed less than 60°, is permitted. The patient alternates between lying on his back and turning to the unaffected side, at the same time preventing adduction, rotation, or acute hip flexion. Ambulation may be started on the second or third day; the patient progresses from crutches or walker to cane, with weight bearing encouraged to the point of tolerance.

The nurse should be aware that patients may cough up pink-tinged sputum postoperatively. Although alarming to the patient, this is not dangerous. It is thought to be the result of the cement being excreted through the alveoli (Luckmann and Sorensen, 1980). The two major postoperative complications are infection and dislocation. Sepsis is extremely hazardous and may necessitate removal of the prosthesis. Dislocation can generally be prevented by adhering to position restrictions.

Discharge planning, referrals, and continuation of rehabilitation are much the same as for the patient with repair of a hip fracture. Patients are cautioned not to cross their legs for three

months and not to sit for periods longer than one hour without standing and walking a few steps (Wolff, 1979). The majority of patients who undergo total hip replacement experience relief of pain, restoration of range of motion, and return to a more normal level of activity (Habermann, 1979). The long term results of prosthetic joint use are not known; however, the change in the quality of life for the elderly long term sufferer is extremely dramatic and worthwhile.

Total Knee Replacement

Total knee replacement may be indicated for the patient with severe osteoarthritis of the knee joint when more conservative measures of management have been unsuccessful. It is indicated primarily to relieve pain, provide joint stability, and allow motion. There are numerous prosthetic devices available. The choice of which is to be used depends upon the amount of destruction, the stability of the ligaments, and the preference of the surgeon (Habermann, 1979). One example of knee arthroplasty consists of a metallic replacement for the distal femur and a polyethylene prosthetic plateau to replace the superior surface of the tibia; see Figure 26-5.

Nursing Implications. Postoperatively, the knee joint is protected from flexion by either a dressing or an immobilizer (not necessarily a cast). This provides the support required for progressive ambulation and early weight bearing. Postoperative discomfort and swelling may be diminished by the application of ice packs and by elevating the leg with a pillow under the ankle. The immobilizer remains on until active flexion-extension exercises are initiated (usually within the first week). Complete rehabilitation is variable and may take as long as 12 months. However, most people are discharged from the hospital bearing full weight without supportive aid.

CARDIAC AND VASCULAR SURGERY

At least 40% of individuals over age 65 will die of cardiac disease, 15% of cerebrovascular

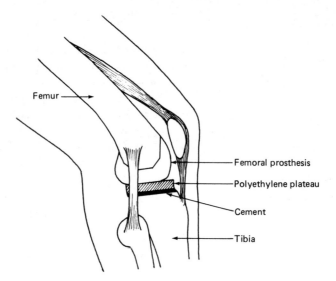

Figure 26-5. Total knee arthroplasty.

disease, and possibly another 5% of related vascular impairment (Goldman, 1979). The statistics are frightening, but the decreasing reluctance of surgeons to operate on the elderly and advances in perioperative management may soon affect an improvement.

Cardiac Pacemakers

Pacemakers are electrical devices which may be permanently implanted to provide electrical stimulation to the patient's heart. The average age of the pacemaker population is between 70 and 72 years of age, with an overwhelming majority of implants occurring between 60 and 90 years of age (Furman, 1978). The indications for permanent pacemaker implantation include bradycardia, complete heart block with a slow ventricular response, or asystole. Regardless of the particular pathology, the result is a severely compromised cardiac output causing syncope, convulsions, or death. Most patients experience warning signs such as blackouts, fatigue, or dizziness, or they are aware that their pulse has slowed (Rossel and Alyn, 1977). The mortality rate for patients with untreated symptomatic heart block is 50% at the end of one year, while the rate for the pacemaker population is 14% (Furman, 1978).

The pacemaker is composed of a pulse generator and a lead wire which transmits the electrical stimulation to the heart muscle. There are many different types of pacemakers currently available. They may be fixed rate or demand, ventricular or atrial, bipolar or unipolar lead, and powered by mercury zinc batteries or by nuclear power. Regardless of the specifics, the nursing care of patients with pacemaker implants is fairly standard.

Most often the pacemaker is surgically implanted under local anesthesia and with the with the aid of fluroscopy. The lead wire is inserted via a right cephalic vein cut down and threaded transvenously into the apex of the right ventricle (see Figure 26-6). The pulse generator is implanted in a subcutaneous pocket in the region of the pectoral muscle and connected by tunneling the lead wire to it. Although scientific advances in power generators have extended the life of batteries, it is likely that the elderly patient will have a mercury zinc model which requires changing the battery every 3–5 years. Lead wires are not routinely replaced.

Nursing Implications. It is important for the elderly patient to understand that pacemaker

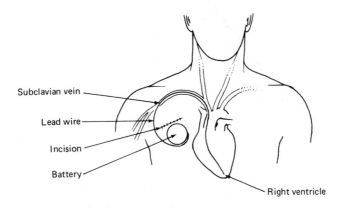

Subclavian vein

Lead wire

Incision

Battery

Right ventricle

Figure 26-6. Insertion of a permanent pacemaker.

implantation is not open heart surgery, but a relatively minor procedure performed under local anesthesia. Postoperatively the use of the right arm is restricted in order to prevent displacement of the lead wire. The patient's heart is monitored continuously for a period of time to insure that the pacemaker is functioning adequately.

With the use of a demand-type pacemaker, the nurse must look for the pacer artifact and appropriate ventricular response to the EKG tracing, indicating that the pacemaker is firing when the patient's inherent heart rate drops below the predetermined rate (usually 70 beats per minute). Ventricular premature beats (VPBs) may occur as a result of irritation to the ventricles and usually subside without treatment, but they require close observation by the nurse. Abnormal pacemaker stimulation resulting in chest wall twitching or hiccups should be reported to the physician immediately as it may indicate lead displacement (Winslow and Marino, 1975).

The dressing and incision area must be carefully inspected for signs of infection because of the danger of transmitting the bacteria directly into the heart. Prior to discharge, the patient (or significant other) is taught to check his pulse daily for one minute. The patient should know the normal pulse rate, the rate at which the pacemaker is set, and when to call the physician (Manwaring, 1977). A pulse rate decrease may occur for a variety of reasons (battery failure, presence of VPBs), all

of which will require the physician's attention. If the patient's pulse speeds up for no apparent reason (exercise or stress), the patient should contact his physician.

Patients should be informed about possible electromagnetic interference from such appliances as microwave ovens and automobile generators. Newer pacemakers are built with protective shielding to prevent interference, but patients should recognize that if they feel dizzy or unusual in the presence of these devices they should simply move 5–10 feet away and check their pulse (Manwaring, 1977).

It is now possible for pacemaker patients to have their pacemaker function evaluated by a special telephone monitor. Patients are instructed to call in at regular intervals or if they experience any symptoms of malfunction. Generators that are more than two years old are evaluated every two weeks. Telephone monitoring reduces the number of follow-up office appointments and assists with the detection of such problems as battery failure, electrode displacement, and malfunctioning generator (Czerwinski, 1977).

The mortality rate of patients with implanted pacemakers is at least as good as, or perhaps better than, that of the general population of the same age (Furman, 1978). Most patients who receive implants describe positive changes in life-style, an increase in activity level, and a decrease in previously experienced symptoms (Rossel and Alyn, 1977).

Open Heart Surgery

As discussed in Chapter 21, the aged person is extremely likely to develop one or several cardiovascular pathologies. In many situations, medical management and behavior modification are sufficient to control symptoms and extend life. If, however, the patient deteriorates rapidly, the symptoms become incapacitating, or death becomes imminent, the patient may be faced with the alternative of surgical intervention (Alam, Hutchinson, and Schwartz, 1977). Patients with severe cardiovascular disease are poor risks for general surgery. Therefore, it may be recommended that the elderly patient undergo open heart surgery in order to become a better risk for some other surgical procedure (Sketch and Mohiuddin, 1977).

Two types of open heart surgery commonly performed on the aged are coronary bypass surgery and prosthetic valve replacement. In coronary bypass surgery, the saphenous leg vein is removed and anastomosed to the ascending aorta and to the coronary artery distal to the blockage. Valvular damage (most often the mitral valve) resulting in insufficiency or regurgitation is often treated by surgical excision of the valve and prosthetic valve replacement.

The ultimate decision of whether or not to have surgery rests with the patient and the family. The individual must possess a clear understanding of the procedure, the risks involved (which certainly increase with age), the postoperative course, and expect rehabilitation. The aged person must carefully weigh the quality of life and life expectancy with the without surgical intervention. The patient who consents to surgery with full knowledge and cooperation stands the best chance of surviving the surgery.

Nursing Implications. The nursing care of the immediate post–open heart surgical patient has developed into a nursing specialty within the cardiovascular intensive care unit. Since most gerontological nurses will not be caring for clients during this critical phase of recovery, this section will deal with preoperative preparation and early rehabilitation with emphasis on psychological adjustments.

Patients anticipating open heart surgery are likely to experience overwhelming fear and depression which may adversely affect their physical and emotional recovery. This is even more likely to occur in the elderly client with decreased physical and emotional reserves. It is imperative for surgical candidates to receive adequate preoperative information and encouragement to express themselves freely in order to reduce their anxiety.

In many hospitals a cardiovascular nurse specialist is responsible for patient teaching and acts as a liaison between the patients and their families during and after surgery. Patients receive a tour of the intensive care unit, including introduction of the nursing staff and an explanation of the equipment which will be used. They should be told what to expect when they regain consciousness. They will have a chest tube to reexpand the lungs and an endotracheal tube which will prevent them from talking; they will be connected to a monitor and may have several intravenous lines. In addition, patients are taught coughing, deep breathing, and how to use the IPPB machine. It should be noted that individuals have variable learning needs; some desire to know everything in depth, while others prefer only minimal information. It takes an intuitive nurse to establish teaching goals derived from the patient's needs.

For an excellent account of a patient's personal experience with this surgery, the reader is referred to the article by Derrick (1979) in the *American Journal of Nursing,* "How Open Heart Surgery Feels." Research indicates that patients go through psychological and physical phases of recovery from open heart surgery (Jillings, 1978). An awareness of the phases and accompanying behaviors provides a focus for assessment, guidance, and teaching as the patient moves toward discharge. The somatic phase, beginning postanesthesia, lasts about three days and involves an egocentric focus. During this period, the nurse must provide pain relief, a restful environment, and reassurance that the patient is progressing. The second phase is a transition, which occurs from the fourth to the ninth day postoperatively and embodies an emotional "sorting out" period.

Patients should be encouraged to express anxieties, fears, or unpleasant memories. During the resolution phase, three days prior to discharge, patients show the greatest physical and emotional recovery and are extremely receptive to planned teaching sessions. Therefore, predischarge teaching for necessary changes in patient behavior and life style should begin at this time.

Peripheral Vascular Reconstruction

Atherosclerosis is the most common disease in the elderly and the probable cause of peripheral arterial insufficiency. Intermittent claudication is the typical symptom described by the patient. Because of the elderly person's decreased physical activity, claudication may not be present, but the patient may still require surgery. Medical research indicates that withholding vascular reconstruction may lead to the development of ischemic legs and, ultimately, to amputation. Thus, it should be emphasized that the surgical risk of amputation may be as hazardous to the patient's life as reconstruction surgery and that the prognosis for success is as good in elderly patients as in the young (Margolis and Hayes, 1977).

Lesions of the femoropopliteal area are the most common, especially in patients over 70 years of age. Surgical correction involves anastomosing a bypass above, and distal to, the obstruction. A saphenous vein bypass is generally preferred; however, plastic, Dacron, and bovine grafts may also be used. Advances in surgical techniques and postoperative management have led to the wide acceptance of peripheral vascular reconstruction for the geriatric patient.

Nursing Implications.
Following vascular reconstruction, special attention is directed to assessing blood flow to the extremities. All peripheral pulses are determined by palpation, or if necessary the Doppler flowmeter to emplify sounds of blood flow and marked for subsequent reference. Many patients have no distal pulses for the first 6–12 hours because of vascular spasms or trapped air bubbles (Atchison and Murray, 1978). Additional information may be obtained by assessing skin color, temperature, and capillary refill of the foot.

Positioning is maintained to avoid kinking the graft, and patients should be instructed not to cross their legs. If the vascular graft does not cross a joint, ambulation may be started on the first postoperative day. However, patients with an aortofemoral bypass may be maintained on bed rest for several days. Prior to discharge, patients are instructed in foot care, signs of vascular insufficiency, and the need to avoid sitting for long periods with knees and hips flexed.

Aortic Aneurysm Resection

Aneurysms may occur in the descending thoracic aorta or the lower abdominal aorta. Typically the patient with an aortic aneurysm is a man between the ages of 60 and 70 (Long, 1978). The thoracic aorta is the most common site of a dissecting aneurysm, while rupture of the abdominal aorta is the most deadly complication (Luckmann and Sorensen, 1980). Surgery usually involves resection of the aneurysm and replacement with a graft. The likelihood of rupture and the resulting mortality in patients with untreated abdominal aortic aneurysms indicate the necessity of surgical intervention on an elective basis (Margolis and Hayes, 1977); see diagrams of aneurysms in Chapter 21.

Nursing Implications.
Postoperative care of the patient with aortic aneurysm resection is similar to that of peripheral vascular reconstruction. Renal function is carefully monitored because the renal arteries branch off from the descending aorta. Because of the massive retroperitoneal dissection, paralytic ileus can easily occur (Long, 1978). Gastric decompression is maintained until bowel sounds are heard and the patient is passing flatus.

Usually the head of the bed is limited to 30–40° elevation. The ambulation schedule is determined by the physician, but generally the patient walks with assistance by the second postoperative day. If the patient's recovery is free of complications, he can expect to be discharged about ten days after surgery.

Carotid Endarterectomy

Cardiovascular accidents (CVAs) rank third in the United States as a cause of death. Those fortunate enough to survive them face the physical, mental, and financial burdens of rehabilitation. Atherosclerosis of the carotid arteries may account for as many as 80% of all strokes (Groteboer, 1978).

The presence of transient ischemic attacks or asymptomatic carotid bruits is sufficient evidence that surgical intervention is required if a stroke is to be prevented (White, 1980). Carotid endarterectomy is the removal of the atheromatous plaque from the intima of the carotid artery through a small incision parallel to the sternocleidomastoid muscle (Butler, 1980). Bilateral endarterectomies are performed in two stages. Because of the potential aggravation of neurological deficits, the patient must be fully recovered from the first surgery before the second is scheduled. Complications which may result from the surgery include stroke, cranial nerve paresis, blood pressure deviations, and hematoma (Szaflarski, 1980).

Nursing Implications. Standard nursing care for carotid endarterectomy requires a well-documented preoperative and postoperative neurological assessment. In addition to the level of consciousness, pupil reaction, and motor response, it is essential to assess cranial nerve function. Cranial nerve paresis, which is usually temporary, is the result of traction on the nerve during the surgical procedure. The seventh, tenth, eleventh and twelfth cranial nerves are most commonly affected, and may result in difficulty swallowing, loss of the gag reflex, hoarseness, or the inability to speak.

GENERAL SURGERY

Earlier sections in this chapter covered surgical procedures frequently required by older people because of the physical changes of aging. Surgery required because of malignancies of the lung, prostate, and gastrointestinal tract has not been included because it has been covered in Chapter 25.

The aged person is just as likely as the younger individual to require surgery for non-age-related disorders. Advancing age does not give the individual immunity against appendicitis, cholecystitis, hernias, hemorrhoids, ulcers, or gynecological problems. The list is potentially endless, and all of these conditions may necessitate surgical intervention.

In most instances, conservative nonsurgical treatments are initially attempted. When symptoms persist or if the condition is likely to require emergency surgery at a later time, then surgery is usually scheduled on an elective basis. Nursing care of patients requiring surgery for these conditions is no different because of their age, other than the fact that allowance must be made for sensory losses and metabolic changes which have an effect on medication.

SUMMARY

The gerontological nurse can expect to care for increasing numbers of clients who need or have undergone surgery. Advances in the technology of the procedures and improvements in perioperative management have made surgical intervention an increasingly acceptable and feasible treatment modality for the elderly. Often the immediate postoperative care is provided by highly specialized nurses in the recovery room or intensive care unit. The nursing challenge is to be aware of and prevent complications, and to provide good long term care.

As patients become more knowledgeable about illness and treatment modalities, they are assuming more responsibility for their own self-management. Nurses have the responsibility of providing patients with information relevant to their own care. If the patient is elderly, the teaching-learning process is facilitated by the nurse with a background in gerontology.

REFERENCES

Alam, S.E., Hutchinson, J.E., and Schwartz, M.J. Replacing the aortic valve during the ninth decade of life. *Geriatrics* 100–101 (January 1977).

Atchison, J.S. and Murray, J. Post-vascular surgery — when happiness can be a warm foot. *Nursing '78* 8:36–39 (December 1978).

Bagwell, M. and Ludlow, E. The elderly patient in the hospital. *Supervisor Nurse* **11**:32–35 (February 1980).

Bonner, C.D. *Hamburger and Bonner's Medical Care and the Rehabilitation of the Aged and Chronically Ill.* Boston: Little, Brown, 1974, pp. 77–84.

Boyd-Monk, H. Cataract surgery. *Nursing '77* 56–61 (June 1977).

Boyer, G.G. Vision problems. In Carnevali, D.L. and Patrick, M. (Eds.) *Nursing Management for the Elderly.* Philadelphia: J.B. Lippincott, 1979, pp. 479–496.

Butler, S. Carotid endarterectomy: care in the OR. *AORN Journal* **32**:42–47 (July 1980).

Czerwinski, B. Trans-telephonic surveillance for pacemaker patients. *American Journal of Nursing* 828–829 (May 1977).

Derrick, H.F. How open heart surgery feels. *American Journal of Nursing* 276–285 (February 1979).

Dulaney, D.D., M.D., Personal Communication, 4530 No. 40th St., Phoenix, Az. 85018, Feb. 20, 1983.

Dunnery, E. Fractured hip – how to position and mobilize patients – without undoing their surgery. *RN* 45–57 (June 1979).

Eliopoulos, C. *Gerontological Nursing.* New York: Harper & Row, 1979, pp. 275–279.

Feinstein, P.A. and Habermann, E.T. Selecting and preparing patients for total hip replacement. *Geriatrics* 91–96 (July 1977).

Feist, R. A survey of accidental falls in a small home for the aged. *Journal of Gerontological Nursing* **4**:15–17 (December 1978).

Freehafer, A.A. Injuries to the skeletal system of older persons. In Reichel, W. (Ed.) *Clinical Aspects of Aging.* Baltimore: Williams and Wilkins, 1978, p. 297.

Furman, S. Recent developments in cardiac pacing. *Heart and Lung* **7**(5):813–826 (1978).

Glenn, F. Surgical principles for the aged patient. In Reichel, W. (Ed.) *Clinical Aspects of Aging.* Baltimore: Williams and Wilkins, 1978, pp. 367–381.

Goldman, R. Aging changes in structure and function. In Carnevali, D.L. and Patrick, M. (Eds.) *Nursing Management for the Elderly.* Philadelphia: J.B. Lippincott, 1979, p. 55.

Grahame, R. Diseases of the joints. In Brocklehurst, J.C. (Ed.) *Textbook of Geriatric Medicine and Gerontology.* Edinburgh: Churchill Livingstone, 1978, pp. 528–531.

Groteboer, J. Stroke, carotid endarterectomy, and the neurosurgeon. *Journal of Neurosurgical Nursing* **10**:52–59 (June 1978).

Habermann, E.T. Orthopedic aspects of the lower extremities. In Rossman, I. (Ed.) *Clinical Geriatrics.* Philadelphia: J.B. Lippincott, 1979, p. 479.

Hagberg, L. and Nilsson, B.E. Can fracture of the femoral neck be predicted? *Geriatrics* 55–61 (April 1977).

Howells, E.M. Managing fluids and electrolytes in surgical patients. *Geriatrics* 100–101 (May 1977).

Jillings, C.R. Phases of recovery from open heart surgery. *Heart and Lung* **7**(6):987–994 (1978).

Kasper, R.L. Eye problems of the aged. In Reichel, W. (Ed.) *Clinical Aspects of Aging.* Baltimore: Williams and Wilkins, 1978, p. 396.

Kornzweig, A.L. The eye in old age. In Rossman, I. (Ed.) *Clinical Geriatrics.* Philadelphia: J.B. Lippincott, 1979, pp. 369–392.

Kwitko, M.L. Artificial lens implantation. *AORN* **28**:47–53 (July 1978).

Lipner, J. and Sherman, E. Hip fractures in the elderly – a psychodynamic approach. *Social Casework* 97–103 (February 1975).

Long, G.D. Managing the patient with abdominal aortic aneurysm. *Nursing '78* **8**:21–27 (August 1978).

Lore, A. Supporting the hospitalized elderly person. *American Journal of Nursing* 496–499 (March 1979).

Low, C.R. Outpatient cataract surgery. *AORN* **28**:35–40 (July 1978).

Luckmann, J. and Sorensen, K. *Medical-Surgical Nursing.* Philadelphia: W.B. Saunders, 1980.

Manwaring, M. What patients need to know about pacemakers. *American Journal of Nursing* 825–827 (May 1977).

Margolis, I.B. and Hayes, D.F. Managing peripheral vascular disease secondary to arteriosclerosis. *Geriatrics* **32**:79–87 (June 1977).

Meyers, M.H., McNelly, D.B., and Nelson, K. Total hip replacement – a team effort. *American Journal of Nursing* 1485–1488 (September 1978).

Organ, C.H., Jr. and Finn, M.P. The importance of nutritional support for the geriatric surgical patient. *Geriatrics* 77–83 (May 1977).

Polly, S.M. and Sanders, W.E., Jr. Surgical infections in the elderly: prevention, diagnosis, and treatment. *Geriatrics* 88–97 (May 1977).

Rossel, C.L. and Alyn, I.B. Living with a permanent cardiac pacemaker. *Heart and Lung* **6**(2):273–278 (1977).

Schein, C.J. A selective approach to surgical problems in the aged. In Rossman, I. (Ed.) *Clinical Geriatrics.* Philadelphia: J.B. Lippincott, 1979, pp. 410–427.

Sheehy, T.W. Preoperative examination of the elderly patient. *Resident and Staff Physician* 63–67 (September 1979).

Sketch, M.H. and Mohiuddin, S.M. Care of the patient with cardiovascular disease undergoing general surgery. *Geriatrics* 61–64 (May 1977).

Smith, J. Focusing your care for the patient with an intraocular lens implant. *RN* **41**:46–50 (March 1978).

Stark, W.J. and Kracher, G.P. Extended-wear contact lenses and intraocular lenses for aphakic correction. *American Journal of Ophthalmology* **88**:535–542 (September 1979).

Szaflarski, N. Carotid endarterectomy: after surgery. *AORN Journal* **32**:48–54 (July 1980).

Townley, C. and Hill, L. Total knee replacement. *Amer-

ican Journal of Nursing 1612–1617 (September 1974).

White, N. Carotid endarterectomy: before surgery. *AORN Journal* **32**:35–41 (July 1980).

Winslow, E.H. and Marino, L.B. Temporary cardiac pacemakers. *American Journal of Nursing* 586–591 (April 1975).

Wolff, H. Musculoskeletal problems. In Carnevali, D.L. and Patrick, M. (Eds.) *Nursing Management for the Elderly*. Philadelphia: J.B. Lippincott, 1979, pp. 399–425.

27
Neurological Disorders of the Elderly

Mary Opal Wolanin
Bernita M. Steffl

To enter the country of old age is a new experience, different from what you supposed it to be.

Malcolm Cowley (1982)

Neurological disorders of the aged are interrelated and often dependent upon other physical conditions and trauma such as stroke; they may also be associated with loss of brain substance and with changes in the neurons, and synaptic functions. Considerable progress has been made in the past decade in the study of changes in neuronal structure and function which are presumed to be age related. This is due in part to the expanded fund of neurobiological knowledge (Bondareff, 1977). The focus of a great deal of current study is directed toward the neurotransmitters and their implications in such conditions as Parkinson's disease and Alzheimer's disease.

In this chapter only the most common neurological disorders affecting the older individual are discussed. A broad range of neurological problems is included, but the focus is on these problems which affect communication, mobility, the ability to know reality, or one's level of pain. Cerebrovascular accidents (CVAs — strokes), Alzheimer's disease, diabetic neuropathy, sexual impotence, incontinence, and certain drug behavior — all of which are neurological problems to some extent — are discussed in Chapters 12, 21, 29, and 36 of this book.

Almost all problems which affect human beings have neurological overtones especially if a person is older; for example, incontinence is as much a neurological problem as a urological one (Wells, 1980). The skin, ears, eyes, taste buds, joints, and tendons are all end organs which tell an individual what the world is and where he is in his environment. There are impairments to these end organs that are accepted as normal in aging, and there are those which result from the insults of years of living. The nervous system has remarkable capacity for adaptation, for making a broad selection of responses and variations of behavior, and even for loss of substance without great alteration of function (Locke, 1971).

The integrative functions of the nervous system are depended upon to make suitable responses to the social and physical environment. Communication with others can be impaired by aphasia and by mechanical or motor problems; also, the lack of coordination of the many muscles which are necessary for movement impedes communication and results in reduced mobility and space. These integrative functions all may be interrupted in conditions such as cerebrovascular accidents, Parkinson's disease, or tardive dyskinesia. There may be loss of brain substance or changes in the synaptic functions especially in relation to neurotransmitters. There may also be problems with integrating knowledge of the environment with appropriate actions (mental confusion), which are associated with any of the factors that can interfere with brain cell function (e.g., fever, dehydration, electrolyte imbalance, drug toxicities, or hypoxia).

Finally, there are problems with the automatic responses that are regulatory, such as temperature control, and with feedback responses from the autonomic nervous system that controls body organ function. If it is true that there is little that can be said about the older human without implicating the nervous system to some degree, then all aging must be looked at in relation to changes in neurological function.

EXTENT OF THE PROBLEM

An attempt was made to measure the extent of neurological loss in normal aging persons in a study of 100 individuals over age 70 who did not have neurological disease, diabetes, or peripheral vascular disease. Eighty percent of the 100 patients showed some abnormality such as irregular pupillary outline, loss of tone in the musculature of the face or neck, loss of ankle jerks, and some loss of position sense of the toes. There was cervical spondylitis with universal wasting of the interosseous musculature such as that observed in the dorsum of the hand in half of the people over 70 (Carter, 1979). These neurological losses occur gradually and are usually compensated for as older persons adapt their life-styles and energy needs to decreased ability to perform. *Older persons usually do not complain of loss of function until it interferes with their ability to act independently, to communicate, to maintain mobility, or to control personal affairs. Older individuals often accept reduced levels of performance until there is an irreducible level that is obvious to everyone and can no longer be denied.*

THE NEUROLOGICAL ASSESSMENT

A gross neurological assessment can be made by observing an individual function in his own environment in terms of his level of response in motor coordination, sensoriperceptual challenges, and communication ability. Every baseline assessment, without fail, should include the level of function in these three areas. A much more specialized assessment should be done for intense and/or long term care. This should include testing the cranial nerves for motor strength, sensory ability, and coordination, and testing the limbs for strength and function. Orientation and the ability to remember, to make simple computations, and to follow directions should also be matters of record.

The highly specialized examination which is given by the neurologist to determine pathology is still another level of assessment which the older person should have if there has been any question in the more general assessment. Then there should be a precise record which indicates pupil response, tongue strength, grip, coordinated efforts, etc. (Wolanin and Phillips, 1981). Basic to every assessment, of course, is such basic information as blood pressure, quality and rate of pulse, rate and nature of respiration, height, weight, general appearance, temperature at various times of the day with activity and lack of activity, drugs taken, kinds of food eaten, and patterns of sleep, rest, and activity. With these baseline data, changes can be detected which indicate neurologic problems at a vulnerable or pathologic level.

The diversity of physical states found in the elderly is such that what may seem to be a critical difficulty may be a well-compensated chronic problem which is perceived by the older person not as a disability, but merely as one of the inconveniences of aging. This does not mean that all aged people should be expected to have untreatable problems, but it does mean that perspective must be used in making clinical judgments. The incontinent, elderly, confused person (Wells, 1980) is just as far from the norm as the 90-year-old mountain climber. The range includes both, however, for there is no average older person.

CLASSIFICATION OF NEUROLOGICAL PROBLEMS OF THE AGED

It would be convenient and useful to be able to classify neurologic problems of the elderly by some simple system or categories such as loss of consciousness, immobility, pain, or aphasia. However, these problems often do not separate themselves neatly but are all found in the same neurologic difficulty. The authors found that looking at disabling neurological conditions in the rather loose scheme of categories which follows, facilitates nursing assessment and intervention (see Table 27-1).

Parkinsonism; Parkinson's Disease (Paralysis Agitans)

Parkinson's disease is a slowly progressive, disabling disease of the central nervous system which affects the brain centers that control movement; it is one of the major causes of

Table 27-1. Categories of Disabling Neurological Disorders.

DISABLING CATEGORY	COMMON CONDITIONS IN CATEGORY
Impaired mobility	CVA; stroke; Parkinson's Disease;
Infection	Encephalitis; herpes zoster
Pain	Herpetic lesions
Communication problems	Parkinson's disease; tardive dyskinesia; CVA; stroke
Trauma	Subdural hematoma
Anemias	Pernicious anemia; folic acid deficiency

neurologic disability in individuals over 60 years of age. Its true incidence is not known because parkinsonism is not a reportable disease; however, it is estimated as 100-150 cases per 100,000 population or roughly 1% of the population over age 50, and there are 20,000-40,000 new cases each year. The incidence increases with age. Symptoms are rare under age 40 and occur most frequently after age 60. It occurs in all parts of the world and more often in men than in women (Hull, 1970; Parkinson's Disease Foundation, 1980).

Parkinson's disease is a degenerative disease of unknown origin. Pathological findings include destruction of nerve cells in the basal ganglia (central nuclei of the brain). Increased knowledge of the regional biochemistry of the brain shows a selective neural cell depletion of dopamine, a neurotransmitter, creating an imbalance between depleted dopamine and acetylcholine (Kinney, 1979). A deficiency results in interruption of the smooth passage of nerve messages. It may follow encephalitis, or carbon monoxide or metallic poisoning, and is often spoken of as idiopathic parkinsonism. It seems to be associated with the 1918 influenza which many older people had in their youth. It appears to be caused by a lethargic encephalitis virus (Moore, 1977; Poskanzer and Schwab, 1961). See Table 27-2 for common symptoms of parkinsonism and Figure 27-1 for Myerson's sign. The cardinal signs are tremor, bradykinesia,

Table 27-2. Common Symptoms of Parkinson's Disease.

Rigidity	May be unilateral or bilateral Fixed, "masked" facial expression Spasms of eyelid and eye muscle Speech disturbance – lips freeze Interferes with articulation Gait disturbances – propulsive, shuffling gait with head down Muscle contracture deformities may occur
Tremors	Most characteristic is a resting tremor with "pill rolling" movement of fingers and shaking head Often first seen in upper extremities; worsen with emotional stress Disappear with full relaxation and sleep Minor tremors: mild, inconstant, affected by emotions Major tremors: severe, constant, day and night; unable to sleep, physically exhausted
Bradykinesia	Slowness of movement, body restlessness, faulty body balance, difficulty in turning, attacks of "legs freezing"
Sluggish swallowing	Excessive salivation and drooling accompany sluggish swallowing; usually found with speech disturbances; swallowing ability should be tested if speech is hard to understand
Lethargy	Drowsiness, uninterested in activities of living
Mobility	Loss of automatic movement and learned skills
Depression	Embarrassment, sadness, anger, intractable flat affect
Communication problems	Related to lack of facial expression and use of gestures, as well as to deep voice or loss of voice and slurred words; talking takes great effort

NOTE: Adapted from Butler and Lewis (1982), Duvoisin (1978), Luckmann and Sorensen (1974), and Rossman (1979).

and rigidity; two of these normally must be present to confirm a diagnosis (see Figure 27-2 and 27-3).

Parkinson's disease does not constitute a direct threat to life. For the patient who is well managed medically and who has good emotional support from his family or care givers, there may be 10-30 years of productive life from the time of diagnosis. The patient with Parkinson's disease is more likely to die of complications of invalidism, falls, or even suicide than from the disease itself (Haber, 1969).

There is no sure cure for Parkinson's disease at this time. Currently the treatment focuses on medication to relieve symptoms and to prevent symptoms from progressing to stages of severe disability, on physical therapy, and on measures to assist afflicted persons in coping because they are often depressed. The medical treatment consists of antiparkinsonism drugs, most commonly levodopa and levodopa combined with carbidopa (Sinemet). Other drugs used are anticholinergics such as Artane and Cogentin, antihistimines, and antiviral agents.

Levodopa, an amino acid which is the precursor of the neurotransmitter dopamine, is used to replace the depleted supply. It is introduced slowly over a period of weeks or months. Side effects which are often encountered decrease with continued use and decreased dosage. These include nausea and vomiting, orthostatic hypotension, insomnia, agitation, and mental confusion. Levodopa may enhance libido and activate sexual behavior in some individuals. Nurses should be aware of this so that they do not misinterpret the behaviors of their patients. There may also be a need to counsel the staff and the patient's

Myerson's sign

— a practical clue to facilitate differential diagnosis

The patient shows a certain lack of facial expression and decreased blinking, but blepharospasm can be induced by tapping the frontalis muscle. This positive glabellar tap test is also known as Myerson's sign, which is often present in Parkinson's disease.

the technique:

Tap the patient's forehead or glabella slowly with the finger.

• The patient with Parkinson's disease blinks repetitively and synchronously with the tapping.

• The normal person stops blinking after the first few taps.

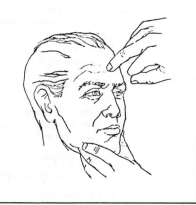

Figure 27-1. (Reprinted with permission of Merck Sharp & Dohme from a Clinical Notebook on Sinemet, 1979, pp. 8–9.

Cardinal Signs

TREMOR —
rhythmic tremor at rest when the muscles are relaxed. This may first be seen in one limb but eventually involves others, and even the head and tongue.

BRADYKINESIA —
slow, deliberate, thoughtful movement, often interspersed with freezing of motion (akinesia). Bradykinesia produces a reduced blinking rate and the so-called reptilian stare. ("Weakness" may be a "precursor.")

RIGIDITY —
in the limbs and trunk; an abnormal taffylike resistance to passive movement. (Rigidity and bradykinesia of the vocal cords produces a low, monotonous voice.)

Two of these normally must be present to confirm a diagnosis.

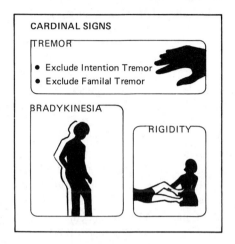

CARDINAL SIGNS

TREMOR
- Exclude Intention Tremor
- Exclude Familal Tremor

BRADYKINESIA

RIGIDITY

Figure 27-2. Cardinal signs of parkinsonism. (Reprinted with permission of Merck and Co. Inc. from a Monograph — A Question of Time: Toward Earlier Diagnosis of Parkinson's Disease by Joel Brumlik, 1978.)

Secondary Signs

GAIT DISTURBANCES —
lack of purposeful stride, shuffling with arms flexed and unswinging; walking on tiptoes; often propulsive (retropulsion may occur)

POSTURAL DISTURBANCES —
stopped and flexed posture, and freezing during postural adjustments

AUTONOMIC NERVOUS SYSTEM DISORDERS —
sweating, seborrhea, glazed skin, swallowing difficulties that cause drooling

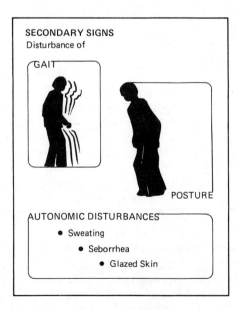

SECONDARY SIGNS
Disturbance of

GAIT

POSTURE

AUTONOMIC DISTURBANCES
- Sweating
- Seborrhea
- Glazed Skin

Figure 27-3. Secondary signs of parkinsonism. (Reprinted with permission of Merck and Co. Inc. from a Monograph — A Question of Time: Toward Earlier Diagnosis of Parkinson's Disease by Joel Brumlik, 1978.)

spouse and/or family so that the patient is not punished when indeed there may be an opportunity to enhance the expression of human sexuality (Costello, 1975); see Chapter 36.

Carbidopa-levodopa (Sinemet), commonly used in neurological practice, is levodopa combined with an inhibitor of the enzyme dopa decarboxylase. This limits the metabolism of levodopa peripherally and reduces the side effects of levodopa seen at higher doses. Anticholinergic alkaloids such as hyoscyamine act against the cholinergic excitatory effects and have been used for over a century. Synthetic drugs such as Artane, Cogentin, Kemadrin, and Akineton which are now used have the disadvantage of side effects such as blurred vision, dry mouth, urinary retention, and constipation. There are no easy answers, and treatment must be continuous. It is important to know that there are some very specific contraindications for the levodopa-carbidopa drugs such as Sinemet. Patients receiving monoamine oxidase inhibitors should be instructed that these inhibitors must be discontinued at least two weeks prior to initiating therapy. Patients with known narrow-angle glaucoma should not take the drugs, and those with chronic wide-angle glaucoma should be treated cautiously. Parkinson's patients with suspicious undiagnosed lesions or a history of melanoma should not receive the drugs.

The newest drug for treatment of Parkinson's disease, bromocriptine, was approved by the FDA in November 1981. This drug has received extensive testing over the past few years. It is usually prescribed as an adjunct to levodopa or Sinemet. It is an antiparkinsonism drug itself and, when given in combination, allows the total dose of standard drugs to be reduced and longer acting. In combination, it also reduces the side effects of Parkinson's disease drugs. Fifty to seventy percent of the patients respond. The greatest improvement has been noted in the early stages. Ten percent of the patients do not respond to the drug, and a considerable number have serious side effects such as nausea, vomiting, visual disturbance, and mental disturbance (e.g., hallucinations). The drug is also still very expensive (Hoehn, 1981; Parkinson's Disease Foundation, 1982).

Many patients with Parkinson's disease also suffer from concomitant depression which is associated with their poor physical condition and the ensuing interruption to a normal social and emotional life. Antidepressive drugs are given, and recently, electroconvulsive therapy (ECT) has been given to those persons whose depressions have not responded to drugs. One case report of a severely impaired man's depression being mitigated by ten ECT treatments found that his physical symptoms responded to anticholinergic drugs for two years following ECT. It is suggested that possibly ECT not only increases the dopamine available at the relevant receptor sites but also renders these sites in the basal ganglia more receptive to dopamine (Yudotsky, 1979).

Assessment. Parkinson's disease is a chronic progressive and deteriorating condition which demands a true understanding of the disease and an ability to assess the devastating consequences for its victims. The mask-like face is misleading in that it hides the "hurting" person who is mentally intact and longing to be treated as he has always been. We have a firm conviction that the mentality is intact and that intelligence is not changed by Parkinson's disease. However, the person with parkinsonism is subjected to the same medical, social, and emotional stresses as any older person plus those which derive from the disease. Often "confusion" is listed as one of the symptoms of parkinsonism. If there is confusion, it is likely to be from another cause. All the social, emotional, environmental, and drug factors which lead to confusion in everyone do not exempt the person with Parkinson's disease. When levodopa was first used with such success in treating parkinsonism, families were startled when patients who had been passive, docile, and apparently not in touch with reality suddenly showed that every slight, every insult, and every neglect had been noted and remembered. When rigidity no longer inhibited action or speech, the person with Parkinson's disease demonstrated that he was intact and a fully feeling person who had felt rejected and bitter about the interaction with, and reaction from, his family and friends (see Figure 27-4 for examination hints).

Nursing Implications. Nursing care goals should focus on the following:

1. *Control of symptoms with medication.* This implies being knowledgeable about treatment regimes and side effects of drugs. Popular magazines which carry sensational articles about new treatments for Parkinson's disease often arouse unjustified hopes. The patient and family are uncritical and eager for any help, and may need professional guidance in

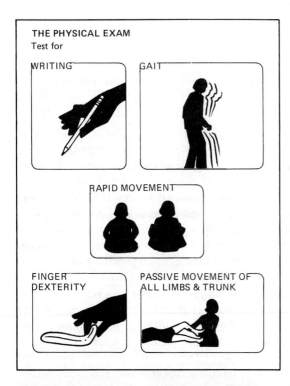

Figure 27-4. Assessment techniques for Parkinson's disease include asking the patient to perform various skills and testing the passive status of muscles for rigidity. (Reprinted with permission of Merck and Co. Inc. from a Monograph — A Question of Time: Toward Earlier Diagnosis of Parkinson's Disease by Joel Brumlik, 1978.)

assessment of these claims and in seeking the best care.

2. *Activity.* Activity should be promoted and maintained. Vigilant effort should be directed at preventing the stooping forward posture which is characteristic of parkinsonism. The trunk is out of line with the center of gravity and can lead to falls. Sleep should be on a firm mattress without a pillow or in the prone position. When walking, the hands should be held behind the back to keep the spine erect, or the arms should be swung vigorously in time with the gait to prevent spasticity at the shoulders and elbows. Fingers should be kept busy with repetitive tasks — typing, playing a piano, jingling or stacking coins, tearing paper. If the feet become "glued" to the floor, lift the toes to break the muscle spasm. Often raising the arms at the same time helps to get moving again. See Table 27-3 for ten basic exercises for the individual with Parkinson's disease.

3. *Speaking and swallowing.* The problem of swallowing can be inferred from the difficulty with speaking. If the person with parkinsonism has a difficult time being understood, he is also having trouble swallowing and frequently with drooling. Speaking should be practiced in front of a mirror and with a tape recorder. Listening to sound can lead to practicing better phonation. Patience on the part of the listener is necessary. Spastic muscles of the face can often be loosened by rubbing with a rough washcloth and by taking quick strokes with an ice cube around the mouth. The ice helps to tighten up the muscles around the mouth to prevent drooling, and aids in swallowing and speaking. The ice stroking (three strokes over all parts of the lip area) before meals is especially important. The patient can do it for himself. Shirts and jackets should have huge pockets for tissues in case of drooling. Aspiration can be a problem when swallowing becomes difficult. Thick liquids are easier to swallow than thin ones: heavy milk

Table 27-3. Ten Basic Exercises for the Parkinson Patient.

1. Bring the toes up with every step you take. In Parkinson's disease, "you never make a move" without lifting the toes.

2. Spread the legs (10 inches) when walking or turning, to provide a wide base, a better stance, and to prevent falling. It may not look "beautiful," but neither does falling.

3. For greater safety in turning, use small steps, with feet widely separated. Never cross one leg over the other when turning. Practice walking a few yards and turn. Walk in the opposite direction and turn. Do so 15 minutes a day.

4. Practice walking into tight corners of a room, to overcome fear of close places.

5. To insure good body balance, practice rapid excursions of the body, backward, forward, and to the right and left, five minutes, several times a day. Don't look for a wall when you think you are falling. It may not be there. Your body will always be there to protect you, if you will practice balance daily.

6. When the legs feel frozen or "glued" to the floor, a lift of the toes eliminates muscle spasm and the fear of falling. You are free to walk again.

7. Swing the arms freely when walking. It helps to take body weight off the legs, lessens fatigue, and loosens the arms and shoulders.

8. If getting out of a chair is difficult, rise with "lightning speed," to overcome the "pull of gravity." Sitting down should be done slowly, with body bent sharply forward, until one touches the seat. Practice this at least a dozen times a day.

9. If the body lists to one side, carry a shopping bag loaded with books or other weights in the opposite hand to decrease the bend.

10. Any task that is difficult, such as buttoning a shirt or getting out of bed, if practiced 20 times a day, becomes easier the 21st time.

NOTE: Reprinted with permission from *Exercises for the Parkinson Patient*, distributed by the Parkinson Disease Foundation, Columbia University, William Black Medical Research Building, 640 West 168th Street, New York, NY 10032.

shakes, creamy soups, thin cooked cereals, and purees are the foods of choice. Milk toast with eggs can usually be swallowed without choking.

4. *Promotion of independence and prevention of premature institutionalization.* Often an occupational therapist can assess the life-style of the person with Parkinson's disease in a short consultation and make recommendations to remove barriers to independence. Also professionals should ask the patient himself what gets in his way. Planning with the patient leads to adaptations that foster independence and self-esteem. The family needs support just as the patient does. Families have isolated the persons with parkinsonism because of the messy eating, choking, and drooling which interfere with family meals. Very frequently, a change in eating arrangements, icing and stroking around the mouth before meals, and a change in food consistency can lead to more esthetic eating so that the patient no longer needs to be isolated and treated like a prisoner in his own room. Think of the patient as a person with the same needs and drives as yourself, but one who has Parkinson's disease and depends on you to help him remain a whole person instead of a partial person or a nonperson.

5. *Safety measures in the environment.* The environment should be looked at through the eyes and mobility of the person with Parkinson's disease, never through the eyes and mobility status of the care giver. Time is one of the social and human components of the environment. The neurologically impaired patient should never be hurried. One task should be done at a time, and directions should be given one at a time (Erb, 1973; Gresh, 1980; Haber, 1969; Robinson, 1974; Rosal, 1978). Assets should be counted,

rather than impairments. How can the person's assets be used and potentiated? The answer requires imagination and a willingness to go beyond the routine. Families are valuable adjuncts to therapy when they care and are involved. The nurse works with the entire family. Often the family can benefit from group work or therapy sessions where ideas and feelings can be exchanged.

6. *Monitoring health.* The person with Parkinson's disease has a very visible, apparent, and devastating disorder. Professionals and others may forget that this person can have additional problems. The older person with parkinsonism is as likely to have cancer, hypertension, cardiac or renal problems, and reactions to drugs as any other older person. He is even more likely to have pulmonary problems and later on gastric disturbances because of breathing, chewing, and swallowing difficulties. These are not necessarily complications, but they are frequently associated with parkinsonism. Also, the problems in maintaining the physiologic status for health after spasticity are so severe that self-care often becomes impossible. Adequate fluids, good elimination, activity, and nutrition are dependent activities, and the patient is at the mercy of his care givers. If speech is difficult for him, he may not be able to make himself understood so that pain and discomfort are not relieved. Therefore the care giver must monitor the patient's needs by looking for and listening to what may not necessarily be articulated or heard.

Though the disease has been known for 140 years, little research was done till 1957 when William Black established the Parkinson's Disease Foundation. In 1960 the Foundation established the only brain bank in the world. Numerous donated brains have been studied anatomically and chemically. A vast fund of knowledge and information has been published in medical journals from these studies (Parkinson's Disease Foundation, 1980). Two very

helpful booklets available from the foundation are: *Exercises for the Parkinson Patient* and the *Parkinson Patient at Home,* William Black Research Building, 640 West 168th Street, New York, NY 10032.

Tardive Dyskinesia

Tardive refers to late appearing or tardy, and dyskinesia refers to movement. The whole refers to the rhythmic and involuntary movements of the mouth, tongue, face, and limbs of persons who have been using neuroleptic drugs, particularly those of the phenothiazine family. The overall prevalence rate of tardive dyskinesia for 17 studies conducted between 1971 and 1980 was 23.3% (Jeste and Wyatt, 1981).

The etiology of this disorder is not certain although it is always associated with and follows the use of neuroleptics. A study of outpatients at Mount Sinai Medical Center (New York) reported that 40% of the patients on neuroleptic drugs had tardive dyskinesia, although some represented subtle and barely detectable symptoms (Horowitz, 1978).

All the signs and symptoms of tardive dyskinesia are related to involuntary use of the muscles. There is a great variation in the extent and degree of the condition among individuals. The facial muscles show tics and grimaces; the ocular muscles, blinking and blepharospasm; the masticatory muscles, chewing and lateral jaw movements; the oral musculature, lip smacking, puckering, sucking, pouting, cheek puffing; and the tongue protrudes with choreoathetoid movements. The trunk and limbs show torticollis and retrocollis of the neck, shoulder shrugging, pelvic thrusting, and rotation and rocking. The hands show athetoid movements of the fingers and wrist flexion. The feet indicate toe movement and foot tapping. There is generalized rigidity and involuntary swallowing. The overall picture is that of lack of control over any or part of the body (see Figure 27-5). The disease resembles Parkinson's syndrome in many ways.

Early detection and discontinuing drug therapy or using a drug holiday regime whenever possible may resolve or reduce the problem, but at this time there is no treatment for the

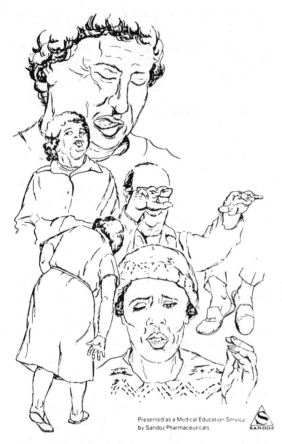

Presented as a Medical Education Service
by Sandoz Pharmaceuticals

Figure 27-5. Signs and symptoms of tardive dyskinesia. (Reprinted with permission of Sandoz Pharmaceuticals, Division of Sandoz, Inc.)

condition when it persists even after medication
is discontinued. In fact, the symptoms may
begin after the medication has been discontinued. Symptomatic treatment with antispasmodic drugs is given, and experiments are being
conducted with choline-rich foods as a preventive measure when neuroleptics are given
(Wolanin and Phillips, 1981).

Nursing Implications. Communication is difficult because the distracting facial movements of
tardive dyskinesia interfere with meaning. The
goal is to maintain the self-esteem and confidence of the person behind the grimacing
uncontrolled movement. It is important for the
nurse to keep in mind that the person behind
that mask is the same one who has always been
there — no less intelligent and just as in need of
reinforcement as an adequate human being. In

the most extreme cases, the involuntary movements may prevent the patient from assisting
with any self-care. There will be loss of weight
and weariness from constant movement. Self-
care requires special adaptations just as for the
person with Parkinson's disease. Socialization
is very important (Wolanin and Phillips, 1981).
Complications of tardive dyskinesia include
difficulty in wearing dentures, fractures due to
the unsteady gait, loosening of the temporomandibular joint, and mucosal ulcerations from
the constant movements of the tongue and
mouth.

The person with tardive dyskinesia will be
embarrassed at his inability to control facial
and limb movements; he will be depressed and
often suicidal. Families must be helped to
understand that the movements are drug caused
and completely involuntary. The nursing care
of the person with Parkinson's disease applies
to the person with tardive dyskinesia, that is,
maintenance of mobility, communication, and
socialization.

NEUROLOGICAL CONDITIONS
DUE TO INFECTIONS

Encephalitis

Encephalitic infections are usually pyogenic,
such as bacterial endocarditis, urinary tract
infections, pulmonary infections, and others.
The usual symptoms are a slight headache,
disorientation, confusion, malaise, a lack of
desire to be up and about, drowsiness, and loss
of interest in surroundings. The universality of
cervical spondylitis in the elderly makes the
finding of neck stiffness less than significant,
but the stiffness will be on rotation rather than
flexion. There may be a slight elevation of
temperature, and if the older person has been ill
long, there is usually dehydration and vomiting;
however, fever, leukocytosis, and neck stiffness
may be absent in the elderly. Diagnostic
measures include lumbar puncture, blood
culture, history of infection, and a search for
the primary infection. If an organism is cultured,
the treatment is specific. If not, antibiotics are
administered and good nursing care is required.

Nursing Implications. The first goal is to maintain the older person's physiological status during a period when drowsiness and inertia prevent adequate self-care. A slightly darkened room will prevent discomfort from glare. The room should be warm enough to prevent use of heavy bedcovers. Fluid intake and output should be regulated in relation to the pulse to prevent either dehydration or overload. Adequate mobility should be insured by frequent changes of position including sitting at the side of the bed opposite the care giver in order to maintain eye contact, and to observe the visual environmental cues in their proper perspective and relationships.

It is necessary to observe for urinary or pulmonary infection and/or endocarditis by careful assessment of chest, pulse, activity challenges, urinary frequency, and character of the urine. The sensorium is clouded and responses are often ineffective. The nurse should give information of the surroundings and self. Reality testing is done daily, but quietly and matter of factly. Correct information should always be offered. Touching and massage with warm hands and solutions help maintain contact with distal portions of the body (Copstead, 1980; Hollinger, 1980). The drowsy person should have programmed relationships with his feet, knees, hips, and back during some period of each day. Arthritic joints should be moved through a complete range of motion by the patient if possible, otherwise by the nurse. Transfer to a chair and the act of combing the hair form two excellent normal ranges of motion.

Herpes Zoster (Shingles)

Herpes zoster is an infection of the nerve root with varicella virus. It is common in the elderly who apparently lose their resistance to viral infection. It is often found in connection with chickenpox epidemics of children. (Chickenpox is also caused by a varicella virus.) The elderly should be protected from children with chickenpox, and children from the elderly with herpes zoster. During the early days of the infection during vesicle formation and breaking, the patient should be isolated.

The herpetic lesions first occur as a stinging or burning sensation under the skin over the nerve trunk. This is followed by redness, swelling, vesicle formation, and breaking, with a coalescing of lesions into one huge draining area which may become purulent before crusting. Healing is a long process, taking weeks or months while the band of lesions reaches from the spine to the anterior midline of the chest. If the trigeminal nerve is involved, lesions may spread over the face. The ophthalmic branch may be involved with lesions over the eye, forehead, nose, and cheek (see Figure 27-6). The geniculate branch will involve the auditory meatus, the soft palate, the inside of the cheek, and the jawline. Orbital edema will be severe and painful, and the patient may be unable to open the eye on the affected side. The crusting and healing may take ten days to a month or longer.

Treatment is aimed at three goals: relief of pain, prevention of secondary infection, and specific treatment such as swabbing with 5% idoxuridine which often appears to promote healing.

Nursing Implications. The patient with herpes zoster is extremely ill with pain. The elderly in particular tend to become exhausted with the discomfort and to neglect maintaining their physiological status for health. The nurse's goal should be to provide freedom from pain, adequate nutrition, fluids, activity, and rest. The second and equally important goal is to prevent secondary infection by maintaining an environment free from infections. Not only do the elderly have pain during the visible part of the disease, but postherpetic pain occurs for weeks and years along the nerve trunk. This often makes the choice of analgesics dependent upon the personality of the patient. Drugs with addictive qualities should be used judiciously and with the knowledge that postherpetic pain persists. The use of pain clinics with pain control options that do not include drugs should be part of the course of postherpetic pain treatment if available. The pain is real and totally absorbing.

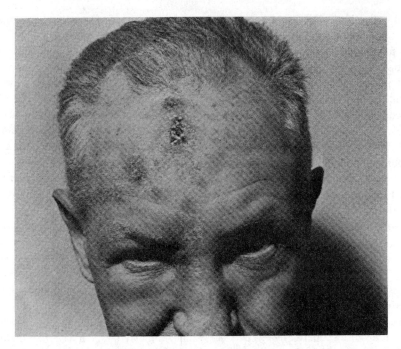

Figure 27-6. This type of herpes zoster affects the first branch of the trigeminal nerve, a most important type because of the possibility of the involvement of the eye. (Photo reprinted with permission from *A Manual of Dermatology* by Donald M. Pillsbury, M.D. Philadelphia: W.B. Saunders Company, 1971, p. 93.

Herpetic Keratitis

This condition is fairly common and quite distressing to older individuals. A lesion on the cornea forms an ulcer with an infection of herpes simplex. The ulcer can be dormant over a long period of time, then become activated with stress conditions such as the dry eyes of the elderly. The lesion cannot be seen with the naked eye, but must be treated with a fluorescent dye and observed with a slit lamp. The treatment consists of drops of ophthalmic solution of trifluorothymidine given every two hours for two weeks. Prevention is then attempted by frequent use of special lubricants for the eyes or artificial tears. A lubricant in an oil base is available for use at night to keep the eye lubricated in the absence of normal lachrymal secretions.

Pernicious Anemia
(Macrocytic, Normochromic Anemia)

Over one half of those who have pernicious anemia develop symptoms after the age of 60. It is a disease of older people and more particularly of blue-eyed, fair-haired people who gray prematurely (Barrowclough and Pinel, 1979).

Pernicious anemia occurs in the absence of an intrinsic factor which is normally produced by the parietal cells of the stomach, resulting in an inability to absorb vitamin B_{12}. Pernicious anemia is described by the blood picture which includes abnormally large and bizarre shaped red blood cells, but it is more often brought to the physician's attention by neurological signs and symptoms such as confusion, paresthesias, numbness, loss of vibratory sense in the lower extremities, and loss of coordination and fine hand movements (Alpers and Mancall, 1971). There may be incontinence. Later this is followed by the presence of the Babinski reflex, the loss of position sense, spasticity, and increased or decreased reflexes. Other signs and symptoms include yellowing skin, glossitis, tachycardia, and enlargement of the liver and spleen with slight icterus of the sclera. Treatment consists of parenteral injection of vitamin B_{12} and restorative therapy to overcome motor and sensory deficits.

Nursing Implications. The goal of nursing care is to teach the patient (1) self-care, (2) appreciation of the fact that lifelong medical supervision and parenteral vitamin B_{12} are needed, (3) restoration of function which often returns to a marked degree, and (4) maintenance of physiologic status and morale during the period when neurological symptoms tend to prevent function as a normal human being. As the physical condition improves, the older person will need encouragement to resume independent function and self-care. A special and specific objective of care should be to provide for access to the necessary vitamin B_{12} injections through home health care visits or the removal of transportation, physical, or economic barriers that prevent visits to a physician's office. This should never be left to chance. The patient with pernicious anemia usually needs help in his discharge planning.

INTRACRANIAL OR SPACE OCCUPYING LESIONS

Subdural Hematoma

Elderly people are as likely as those of any age to have tumors of the brain (the reader should consult specialized texts on this subject). The very old and the very young are the groups more likely to have subdural hematomas.

The elderly person is more likely to have a subdural hematoma than any other age group for two reasons: (1) the tendency to fall and (2) the decrease of brain substance, with a stretching of the tiny blood vessels between the cranium and the dura, which places them under tension. A fall — not necessarily a blow on the head, but a jarring of the head — will shear these small blood vessels and result in bleeding over time (Alpers and Mancall, 1971). A clot forms in several weeks to a month, and the older person begins to slowly show the signs and symptoms of a subdural hematoma.

After the fall, there is often no damage noted, but with time, there are an increase in drowsiness, a loss of interest, confusion, Jacksonian convulsions, hemiparesis, and hemiparesthesia. In diagnostic lumbar puncture, xanthochromia and excess protein are found in the cerebrospinal fluid. Computerized axial tomog-

raphy shows the mass in the skull, and electroencephalography will indicate a silent area over the hematoma. The treatment is surgical. The patient becomes a neurosurgical patient who then needs rehabilitation.

Nursing Implications. The neurosurgical patient requires highly specialized nursing, and the reader should consult a text such as Alpers and Mancall (1971) for this type of care. Nursing care is focused also on the fact that care of the elderly, while undergoing surgery of any description, is highly specialized. In addition to the care needed for neurosurgical recovery, the following nursing objectives should be followed for the elderly person with a subdural hematoma: (1) the physiology of the individual must be supported, with the need for good ventilation of the chest kept in mind; (2) activity of the body must be maintained to prevent stiffness from arthritic joints and loss of muscle strength through misuse or disuse; and in particular, (3) contact must be maintained with reality. Putting any elderly person to bed has its dangerous consequences. Assisting the patient in maintaining contact with reality may be neglected in the care which the neurological patient needs to support his physiological status. The best means of enabling the older person to maintain contact is by use of familiar faces and voices. Family members can form the bridge between life history and the present. If the family is missing, nurses should include in the nursing care plan — as a systematic and assigned task — the prevention of loss of contact with reality and restoration of links to life history. The elderly patient is a person first and a neurological patient second. The latter is a temporary state. Unfortunately, the loss of personhood often becomes permanent. Primary nursing care is the best staffing option because the same personnel should be assigned to this patient during recovery. Discharge planning should be done from the beginning to insure that recovery can continue in the posthospital period.

Cervical Spondylitis

Cervical spondylitis is quite common in the elderly and is more frequently diagnosed by x-ray than by symptoms. However, compressing lesions such as osteophytes may distort the vertebral vessels and be the cause of transient ischemic attacks (drop attacks) which are made worse by rotation and extension, particularly hyperextension of the neck (Barrowclough and Pinel, 1979). Other transvertebral barriers can interfere with circulation to the cervical cord with ischemic myelopathy (Carter, 1979).

Gait disturbances are usually the first sign noted by others, rather than the by patient. Weakness of the legs can result in a lurching gait which may be mistaken for inebriation. Sitting down may result in a "fall" into the chair instead of controlled descent. There is clumsiness and paresthesia of the hands, and the patient becomes aware of illegible writing, inability to pick up small objects, and diminishing arm strength. Frequently, these are accompanied by urinary sphincter difficulty. There is wasting of muscles and sensory loss in the peripheral nerve distribution. The picture conforms to the usual stereotype of the aged person.

Treatment is aimed at relieving cord and nerve pressure. Often a cervical collar is used to restrict neck movement. Bed rest may be required with heat and analgesics to relieve painful neck and shoulder muscle spasms. The dangers of bed rest must be offset with measures to maintain physiologic function. Occasionally, cervical laminectomy is done, but in the elderly it presents hazards (Carter, 1979).

Nursing Implications. The neurological deficits which accompany cervical spondylitis cause the older person grave distress both from a physical sense and from watching one's own strength, control, and coordination diminish. Roles change as the elderly person must accept dependence on others for the personal tasks that have been reserved for oneself. There is concern for the "drop attacks" of transient ischemia which are unpredictable, frightening, and dangerous. Safety is always a major concern (Barrowclough and Pinel, 1979). The lack of control over walking makes maintenance of balance and equilibrium precarious. Supportive aids should be available and utilized, and steps should be avoided. Chairs with high

seats and good arm supports for traction when seating or arising are important. Special tools with built-up handles should replace eating and writing instruments to make gripping easier. Clothing should be adapted with zippers with large pulls, velcro fasteners, or at least large buttons.

Independence should be fostered as long as possible. Each decrement in function and strength will be noted by the patient as a sign of his complete deterioration as a human being, although his mind is unaffected. An inventory of strengths should be made regularly to remind the older person that he is still a functioning human being. He should partake in assessing his functions. The nurse can be of great assistance here in helping the person and his family look at what is left rather than what is gone. When institutionalized, discharge planning for a thorough inventory of barriers, facilitating aids in the home, and family resources is essential to make the environment as supportive as possible.

SUMMARY

Neurological disorders of the elderly are usually coupled with other biopsychosocial limitations and motor impairments, thus compounding and exaggerating adverse effects. Vulnerability and the likelihood of immobility and dependency are increased dramatically in many neurological conditions.

The necessity for careful and detailed assessment skills cannot be overemphasized. As stated several times throughout this chapter, the older individual's condition is too easily stereotyped as inevitable deterioration. It is helpful and encouraging to remind caretakers and older individuals of the nervous system's remarkable capacity for adaptation. Because it matures late, its continuous dynamic processes and functions persist well into adult life. The nervous system has enormous reserves, and it continues to function even with the loss of considerable substance (Locke, 1971). As emphasized in Chapter 5, when working with older individuals, it is especially important to remember to assess what is left as well as what is gone.

REFERENCES

Alpers, B.J. and Mancall, E.L. *Clinical Neurology* (6th ed.). Philadelphia: F.A. Davis, 1971.

Barrowclough, F. and Pinel, C. *Geriatric Care for Nurses.* London: William Henderson Medical Books, 1979.

Bondareff, H.W. The neural basis of aging. In Birren, J.E. and Schaie, W.K. (Eds.) *Handbook of the Psychology of Aging.* New York: Van Nostrand Reinhold, 1977, pp. 157-172.

Bruno, P. Skin problems. In Patrick, M. and Carnevali, D. (Eds.) *Nursing Management of the Elderly.* Philadelphia: J.B. Lippincott, 1979.

Brumlik, J. A Question of Time: Toward Earlier Diagnosis of Parkinson's Disease, A Monograph produced by Merck and Co. Inc. Chicago 1978, pp. 9-15.

Butler, R.N. and Lewis, M.I. *Aging and Mental Health* (3rd ed.). St. Louis: C.V. Mosby, 1981, p. 303.

Carter, A.B. Neurologic aspects of aging. In Rossman, I. (Ed.) *Clinical Geriatrics* (2nd ed.). Philadelphia: J.B. Lippincott, 1979, p. 315.

Copstead, L-E. C. Effects of touch on self-appraisal and interaction appraisal for permanently institutionalized older adults. *Journal of Gerontological Nursing* 6(12):747-752 (December 1980).

Costello, M.K. Sex, intimacy, and aging. *American Journal of Nursing* 75(8):1330-1332 (1975).

Cowley, M. *The View from 80.* New York: Penguin Books, 1982, p. 2.

Duvoisin, R.C. *Parkinson's Disease, A Guide for Patient and Family.* New York: Raven Press, 1978, pp. 10-200.

Erb, E. Improving speech in Parkinson's disease. *American Journal of Nursing* 73(11):1910-1911 (1973).

Gresh, C. Parkinson's disease. *Nursing '80* 10(11):26-34 (1980).

Haber, M.E. Parkinson's disease, challenge to the health profession. *Nursing Clinics of North America.* Philadelphia: W.B. Saunders, 1969, pp. 263-273.

Hoehn, M.M. Bromocriptine and its use in Parkinsonism. *Journal of Gerontology* 251-256 (June 1981).

Holliger, L.M. Perception of touch in the elderly. *Journal of Gerontological Nursing* 6(12):741-746 (1980).

Horowitz, J. The hidden cost of mind medicines. *Human Behavior* 7(5):53-55 (1978).

Hull, J.T. The prevalence and incidence of Parkinson's disease. *Geriatrics* 25(5):128-133 (1970).

Jeste, D.V. and Wyatt, R.J. Changing epidemiology of tardive dyskinesia: an overview. *American Journal of Psychiatry* 138:297-309 (1981).

Kinney, M. Management of the person with common neurologic manifestations. In Phipps, W.J., Long, B.C., and Woods, N.F. (Eds.) *Medical-Surgical Nursing, Concepts and Clinical Practice.* St. Louis: C.V. Mosby, 1979.

Locke, S. Neurological disorders of the elderly. In *Clinical Aspects of Aging, Vol. 4:* Working with Older People. Rockville, Md.: U.S. Department of Health and Welfare, Services and Mental Health Administration, 1971, pp. 45-59.

Luckmann, J. and Sorensen, K.C. *Medical-Surgical Nursing, a Psychophysiological Approach.* Philadelphia: W.B. Saunders, 1974, pp. 499-502.

Merck, Sharp and Dohme, Company Inc. *A Clinical Notebook on Sinemet.* Chicago 1979, pp. 8-9.

Moore, G. Influenza and Parkinson's disease. *Public Health Reports* 92(1):79-80 (1977).

Parkinson's Disease Foundation. *Fact Sheet 1980.* New York: 1980.

Parkinson's Disease Foundation. *Newsletter.* New York: 1982, p. 2.

Parkinson's Disease Foundation. *Parkinson's Disease, Progress, Promise, and Hope.* New York: pp. 1-11.

Poskanzer, D.C. and Schwab, R.S. Studies in the epidemiology of Parkinson's disease predicting its disappearance as a major clinical entity by 1980. *Transactions of the American Neurological Association* 234-235 (June 1961).

Robinson, M.B. Levodopa and parkinsonism. *American Journal of Nursing* 74(4):656 (1974).

Rosal, V.L.F. The nurse's role in the management of Parkinson's disease. *Nursing Care* (February 1978).

Rossman, I. *Clinical Geriatrics* (2nd ed.). Philadelphia: J.B. Lippincott, 1979.

Wells, T. Promoting urine control in older adults. *Geriatric Nursing* 1(4):236-240 (1980).

Wolanin, M.O. and Phillips, L. *Confusion: Prevention and Care.* St. Louis: C.V. Mosby, 1981.

Yudotsky, S.C. Parkinson's disease, depression and electroconvulsive therapy: a clinical and neurologic synthesis. *Comprehensive Psychiatry* 20(6): 579-581 (1979).

Part VI
Rehabilitation in Gerontological Nursing

28
Needs and Goals in Geriatric Rehabilitation

Marilyn S. Giss

"The elements of rehabilitation nursing need to be viewed as part of basic nursing rather than as speciality."

Ruth Stryker (1972)

In some respects the term rehabilitation is a misnomer when discussing restorative treatment goals for older adults, especially the frail elderly. Complete restoration of function is more often the exception than the rule. Nevertheless, every disabled older adult should have the benefit of rehabilitation efforts for the highest possible level of wellness. Unfortunately many older individuals are not receiving adequate rehabilitation care, and there is a great need for more professionals and more professional training in the field.

It has been estimated that 40% of the elderly have some limitation of activity due to chronic conditions. This population requires advocates; it does and will need appropriate assessments, recommendations, and interventions for the patients themselves and for their families (Tager, 1979).

This chapter addresses immobility, falls, and accidents briefly, and discusses the overall needs and goals of geriatric rehabilitation. Bowel and bladder maintenance and rehabilitation, arthropathic rehabilitation, cardiorespiratory maintenance and stroke rehabilitation will be discussed in the next four chapters.

PRINCIPLES OF REHABILITATION

Generally, the concept of rehabilitation to the fullest potential means returning to home, family, community, work, and previous life-style. However, for older individuals who are disabled, this is not always realistic. Instead, for the elderly, the goal may have to be geared more toward maintaining maximum independence in the activities of daily living such as personal hygiene, grooming, dressing, eating, and hobbies. To set goals for total restoration may only invite defeat, frustration, and abandonment of the treatment plan. In other words, the focus of care should be restoring the individual to an acceptable quality of life which takes into consideration the family, community, life-style, and previous work habits (Hackler, 1976; Hunt, 1977).

Rehabilitative measures directed toward the chronically ill elderly person must involve the following factors (Boland, Murray, and Zentner, 1975; Bonner, 1974; Henriksen, 1978):

- Recognition of limitations the older person may have due to normal physiological changes as well as immediate chronic states
- Recognition of the strengths and abilities the older person brings with him
- Realization that medical and surgical interventions can facilitate well-being and foster independence
- Realization that it may take longer for the older person to learn to achieve new tasks of living
- Prevention of secondary complications that can develop from disabling chronic diseases
- Promotion of the self-worth and dignity of the older individual
- Recognition of the multiple losses (physical, psychosocial, and economic) that the older person has experienced and is experiencing
- Demonstration of a positive attitude by professional staff working with the older chronically ill patient

The importance of maximizing potential and abilities and minimizing disabilities cannot be overemphasized. It is also vitally important to establish an environment which preserves the patient's feelings of identity and self-esteem. It is imperative that the nurse be aware of the psychosocial impact of a permanent disability or chronic condition. In addition to adjusting to a new disabling condition, the older person is continually confronted with other losses to which he must adapt and adjust while expending the energy to maintain a level of independent functioning. These include loss of status and decrease in income following retirement, loss of independence, loss of spouse and significant others, decline in physical energy and well-being, and diminishing social contacts (Rees, 1979).

The impact of a disability, the length of time needed for rehabilitation, and the success of a program differ according to the stage in one's life cycle and the way in which coping skills are influenced by the disability (Steger, 1976). Brown (1978) illustrates the effect of developmental tasks for two different cohort groups of elderly on rehabilitation potential (see Table 28-1).

Note that the tasks confronting the older person affect his adjustment to the disability and his ability to actively participate in a rehabilitation program. It is essential not to give up on him and to recognize that more time may be needed to achieve an acceptable level of functioning.

The basic principles of rehabilitative nursing for working with older adults are:

- See the patient as a whole person.
- Look for and enhance the individual's abilities (i.e., maximize what is left).
- Provide an environment that promotes orientation to surroundings.
- Promote physical activity within the limitations of the patient's condition.
- Begin rehabilitative measures early, before complications and secondary disabilities develop.

IMMOBILITY

Almost 18% of the noninstitutionalized elderly report some limitation of mobility, and almost half of the population over age 65 has suffered some limitation of activity due to chronic conditions. The chronic conditions causing the greatest amount of activity limitation among the aged are heart conditions (52%), diabetes (34%), asthma (27%), and arthritis (23%). The major causes of mobility limitation among the elderly are arthritis and rheumatism, impairment of the lower extremities, heart conditions, and strokes (National Council on Aging, 1978); see Chapter 38.

Table 28-1. Developmental Tasks Affecting Rehabilitation.

THE YOUNG OLD (55–74)	THE VULNERABLE OLD (75 and Over)
Preparing for and adjusting to retirement from active involvement in the work arena with its subsequent role change (especially for men).	Learning to combine new dependence needs with the continuing need for independence.
Anticipating and adjusting to lower and fixed income after retirement.	Adapting to living alone in continued independence.
Establishing satisfactory physical living arrangements as a result of role changes.	Learning to accept and adjust to possible institutional living (nursing and/or personal care homes).
Adjusting to new relationships with one's adult children and their offspring.	Establishing an affiliation with one's age group.
Learning or continuing to develop leisure time activities to help in realignment of role losses.	Learning to adjust to heightened vulnerability to physical and emotional stress.
Anticipating and adjusting to slower physical and intellectual responses in the activities of daily living.	Adjust to loss of physical strength, illness, and the approach of one's death.
Dealing with the death of parents, spouses, and friends.	Adjusting to losses of spouse, home, and friends.

SOURCE: Brown, M. The new aged: the young old and the vulnerable old. In Brown, M. (Ed.) *Readings in Gerontology*. St. Louis: C.V. Mosby, 1978.

In our society, independence is directly related to mobility. The loss of mobility has drastic effects on all ages but the aged are most vulnerable to social, psychological, and intellectual depreciation when physically immobile (Murray Huelskoetter, and O'Driscoll, 1980; Wolff, 1979). Assessing for mobility involves more than measuring ambulation. Mobility is generally evaluated in the following terms (Wolff, 1979):

General posture	Presence and degree of kyphosis; position of head and neck; presence of contractures.
Stance	Distance between feet; position of toes.
Gait	Length of stride, shuffle, speed in walking. Is pace increased with distance; Is gait heel-toe?
Sitting	Difficulty in sitting down or coming to a standing position. Type of chair person selects in which to sit.
Balance	Use of handrails or furniture to provide support.
Devices	Use of assistive devices — canes, walkers, crutches. Is equipment used properly, fitted, and safe (e.g., rubber tip on cane)?
Stairs	Ability to climb and descend stairs.

FALLS AND ACCIDENTS

Falls

The slow, gradual process of immobility due to osteoarthritis or arthritis may not be obviously noticeable to the older person as long as he is in his familiar environment with familiar height of bed, chairs, and toilet. However, when he is forced into the unfamiliar surroundings of a hospital or a nursing home, mobility may become more of a problem. The greatest number of accidents in the hospital occur where there is the highest proportion of acutely ill old people. The aged are more accident prone, and the risk of multiple accidents increases with age (Feist, 1978; Lynn, 1980; Rogers, 1978). Decreased vision, vertigo, difficulty in regaining

balance, drop attack, and proprioceptive problems are the major physiological factors that lead to falls among the aged (Storandt, 1976). Nurses caring for the aged, whether at home or within the institutional setting, need to understand the etiology of falls and to plan care that will promote safe mobility (Witte, 1979).

Accidents

Accidents are the seventh leading cause of death in people over age 65, and a large number are due to falls. The elderly have a higher percentage of hospital falls than younger age groups, but most of their falls occur in the home (U.S. Department of Health, Education and Welfare, 1978).

For persons over age 65, the stay in the hospital due to accidents is longer than for most diseases. Although this group comprises only about 10% of the population, it accounts for 26% of accidental deaths (Lewis and Windsor, 1974). Proportionately little research has been directed toward the problem of accidents and falls of the elderly. The best approach, of course, is prevention (see Chapter 37 for hazards and risks).

MECHANICAL AIDS FOR REHABILITATION AND MOBILITY MAINTENANCE

The use of an aid to assist the elderly patients in safe ambulation is extremely important for maintaining independence. When a walking appliance is properly prescribed, it will provide the following benefits (Bonner, 1974):

- Support and redistribution of body weight
- Stability, through a wider base of support and altered center of gravity
- Relief of pain
- Decreased fear of reinjury and instability
- Early return to previous life-style
- Longer period of ambulation despite progressive disease

The elderly patient who has osteoarthritis or senile osteoporosis of the vertebral column may

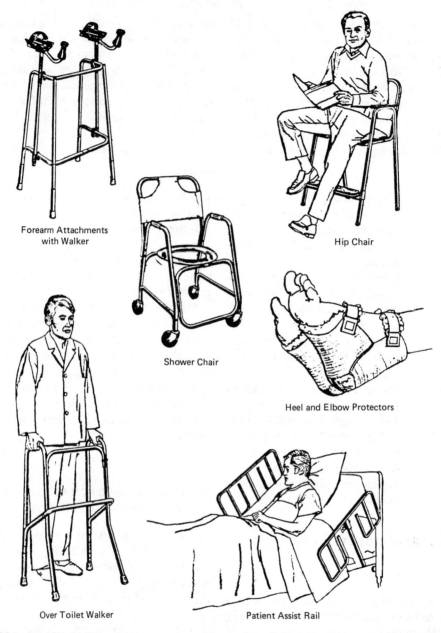

Forearm Attachments
with Walker

Hip Chair

Shower Chair

Heel and Elbow Protectors

Over Toilet Walker

Patient Assist Rail

Figure 28-1. (Reprinted with permission, courtesy of Lumex, Inc., Patient Care in the Home, Catalog of Medical Equipment. 100 Spence St., Bay Shore, N.Y. 11706.)

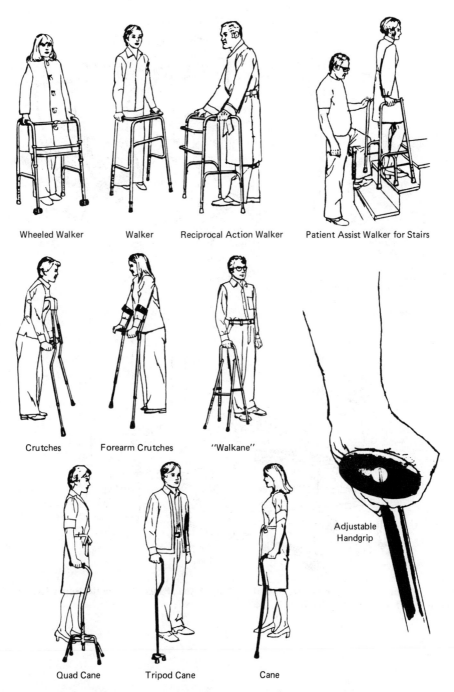

Wheeled Walker   Walker   Reciprocal Action Walker   Patient Assist Walker for Stairs

Crutches   Forearm Crutches   "Walkane"

Adjustable Handgrip

Quad Cane   Tripod Cane   Cane

Figure 28-2. (Reprinted with permission, courtesy of Lumex, Inc., Patient Care in the Home, Catalog of Medical Equipment. 100 Spence St., Bay Shore, N.Y. 11706.)

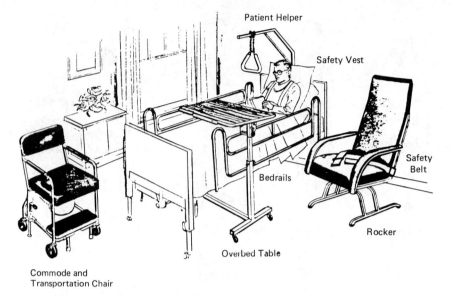

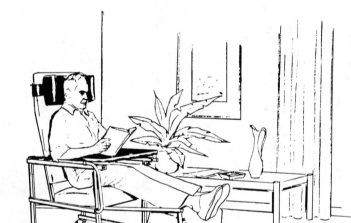

Figure 28-3. (Reprinted with permission, courtesy of Lumex, Inc., Patient Care in the Home, Catalog of Medical Equipment. 100 Spence St., Bay Shore, N.Y. 11706.)

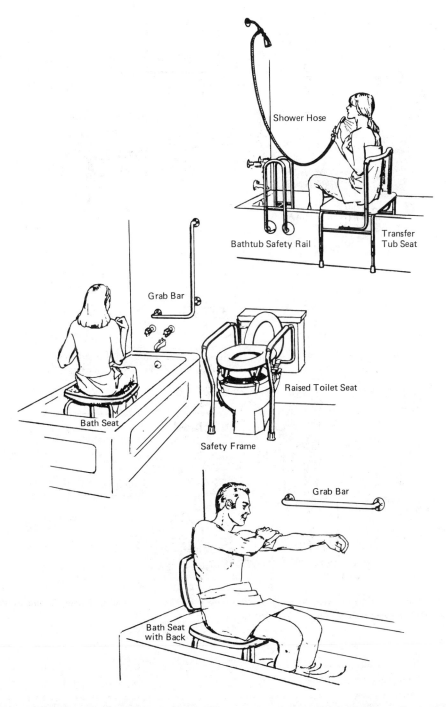

Figure 28-4. (Reprinted with permission, courtesy of Lumex, Inc., Patient Care in the Home, Catalog of Medical Equipment. 100 Spence St., Bay Shore, N.Y. 11706.)

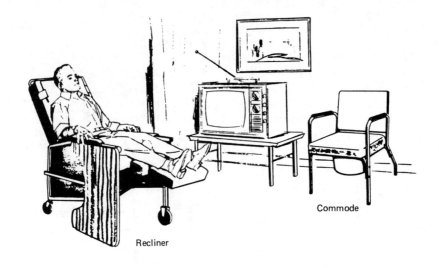

Recliner

Commode

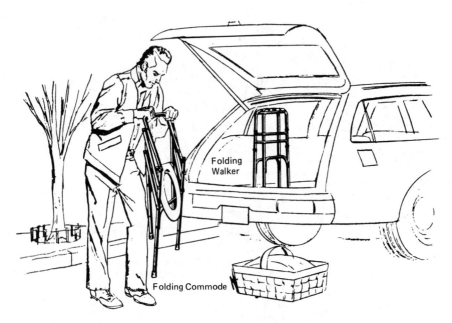

Folding Walker

Folding Commode

Figure 28-5. (Reprinted with permission, courtesy of Lumex, Inc., Patient Care in the Home, Catalog of Medical Equipment. 100 Spence St., Bay Shore, N.Y. 11706.)

particularly benefit from the use of an assistive walking appliance. Conventional walkers without wheels are the most stable of all walking appliances. There are also many varieties of axillary and forearm crutches and canes that are frequently prescribed. Figures 28-1 through 28-5 illustrate assistive and preventive devices. Nurses and families should also be aware that Sears Roebuck has a special catalogue on home health supplies. This catalogue contains and illustrates a wide variety of wheelchairs, beds, sickroom furnishings, rehabilitation devices, and clothing for individuals with physical limitations. It is available upon request from Sears.

The primary physician or physical therapist should evaluate the patient for the type of appliance and gait to use in the rehabilitation process. The nurse, however, may be the first person on the rehabilitation team to come in contact with the patient and identify the need for an appliance; she is frequently responsible for requesting the evaluation, ordering the appliance, and teaching and supervising the patient in its use.

Coordinated planning and instruction in the use of assistive devices are necessary, particularly for elderly persons who have visual and auditory loss, live alone, or take longer to learn to achieve a new and safe method of ambulation. [The reader is referred to more complete descriptions of gait training and the use of assistive devices for all activities of daily living which can be found in rehabilitation texts such as those by Bonner (1974) and Cohen (1979).] The following example illustrates coordinated preventive aspects of rehabilitation in the elderly.

Case History

Mr. Brown is 72 years old and has been admitted to the hospital with benign prostatic hypertrophy. He is to have surgery in two days. The nurse notices that he is slow getting out of bed and tends to favor his left leg. In further assessing his gait and in listening, the nurse hears Mr. Brown complain of left hip pain when walking or when having to stand for a period of time. The nurse refers him back to the physician for further evaluation. A diagnosis of osteoarthritis of the hip is made, a walker is prescribed, and Mr. Brown is taught how to use it by the physical therapist before his surgery. Information is then incorporated into the nursing care plan so that he will be able to safely and comfortably ambulate after surgery.

PSYCHOSOCIAL ASPECTS

Nurses in geriatric rehabilitation have an advocacy, assessment, and intervention role in planning, coordinating, and implementing the care of disabled elderly patients. They should be aware of family relationships, and should see that families are educated and prepared to assume responsibility to give the needed care to patients after they have been discharged from institutional care. If families are unable to care for patients at home with assistance from community services, the nurse must be supportive of their decision for placement in an appropriate facility. Too often, families are considered to be uncaring, not interested in patients' welfare, and "dumping" them in institutions. This is unjust. Nurses need to recognize the guilt, failure, and abandonment families and children often feel when they are unable to care for their aged parent or grandparent. Both the family and the patient need support and understanding in these difficult decisions. See Table 28-2 about planning for geriatric rehabilitation.

The goals in geriatric rehabilitation must be simple. They need not involve fancy or complicated equipment. They should reflect a philosophy of "caring" and, above all, should include "hope" (Patrick, 1973).

In the following chapters, rehabilitation aspects of the most common and devastating immobilizing conditions in the elderly will be discussed. Many specific disease entities are not included. However, rehabilitation measures should definitely be included in all aspects of chronic disease and long term care.

Table 28-2. Planning for Geriatric Rehabilitation.

ASSESSMENT	PLANNING AND INTERVENTION	EVALUATION
What are patient's limitations, capabilities?	Plan within patient's capabilities and limitations.	Was plan successful?
How did patient function in daily life prior to admission?	Plan consistently with what patient will be doing and where he is going when discharged.	Were goals realistic and obtainable?
What resources were used? What resources are available? What are patient's goals in relation to future life?	Plan realistic goals for patient and family.	Were new problems and needs identified? Were changes based upon patient's current status and future goals? How did patient and family cope? What would help?

REFERENCES

Boland, M., Murray, R., and Zentner, J. Assessment and health promotion for the elderly. In Murray, R. and Zentner, J. (Eds.) *Nursing Assessment and Health Promotion through the Life Span.* Englewood Cliffs, N.J.: Prentice-Hall, 1975, p. 354.

Bonner, C.D. *Homburger and Bonner's Medical Care and Rehabilitation of the Aged and Chronically Ill* (3rd ed.). Boston: Little, Brown, 1974, pp. 311.

Brown, M. The new aged: the young-old and the vulnerable old. In Brown, M. (Ed.) *Readings in Gerontology.* St. Louis: C.V. Mosby, 1978, pp. 9–19.

Cohen, S. Teaching a patient how to use crutches. *American Journal of Nursing* 79:1111–1125 (June 1979).

Feist, R.R. A survey of accidental falls in a small home for the aged. *Journal of Gerontological Nursing* 4:15–17 (November–December 1978).

Gospard, N.J. The family of the patient with long-term illness. *Nursing Clinics of North America* 5(1):77–84 (1970).

Hackler, E.S. Expanding the role of nurses in rehabilitation. *Geriatrics* 77–79 (May 1976).

Harris, C.S. *Fact Book on Aging: A Profile of America's Older Population.* Washington, D.C.: National Council on Aging, 1978.

Henriksen, J.D. Problems in rehabilitation after age sixty-five. *Journal of the American Geriatrics Society* 26(11):510–512 (1978).

Hunt, T.E. Rehabilitation of the elderly. *Hospital Practice* 89–97 (January 1977).

Lewis, D.J. and Windsor, R.J. *Handle Yourself with Care.* An instructor's guide for an accident prevention course for older Americans. Washington, D.C.: U.S. Department of Health, Education and Welfare, Office of Human Development, Administration on Aging, 1974.

Lumex Inc. Patient Care in the Home, Catalog of Medical Equipment, 100 Spence St. Bay Shore, New York 11706 pp. 4–10.

Lynn, F.H. Incidents — need they be accidents? *American Journal of Nursing* 80:1098–1100 (June 1980).

Murray, R., Huelskoetter, M., and O'Driscoll, D. *The Nursing Process in Later Maturity.* Englewood Cliffs, N.J.: Prentice Hall, 1980.

National Council on Aging. *Fact Book on Aging: A Profile of America's Older Population.* Washington, D.C.: 1978, pp. 115–116.

Patrick, M. Little things mean a lot in geriatric rehabilitation. *Nursing '73* 7–9 (August 1973).

Rees, W.L. Rehabilitation in the elderly. *Bibliotheca Psychiatrica* Vol. 59 155–162 (1979).

Rogers, P.J. The elderly: a challenge to nursing — furniture and the elderly. *Nursing Times* 32–34 (January 5, 1978).

Steger, H.G. Understanding the psychological factors in rehabilitation. *Geriatrics* 68–73 (May 1976).

Storandt, M. Psychological aspects. In Steinberg, F. (Ed.) *Cowdry's Care of the Geriatric Patient* (5th ed.). St. Louis: C.V. Mosby, 1976, pp. 321–322.

Stryker, R. *Rehabilitation Aspects of Acute and Chronic Nursing Care.* Philadelphia: W.B. Saunders, 1972, p. 236.

Tager, R.M. Gerontology: its future in the field of medical rehabilitation. *Archives of Physical Medicine and Rehabilitation* 60:537–538 (November 1979).

U.S. Department of Health, Education and Welfare. *Elementary Rehabilitation Nursing Care* (Public Health Service Publication No. 1436). Washington, D.C.: U.S. Government Printing Office, 1966 (reprinted 1970), 99 pp.

U.S. Department of Health, Education and Welfare, Public Health Service, National Center for Health Statistics. *Facts of Life and Death.* Hyattsville, Md.: 1978.

Witte, N.S. Why the elderly fall. *American Journal of Nursing* 79:1950–1952 (November 1979).

Wolff, H. Musculoskeletal problems. In Patrick, M. and Carnevali, D. (Eds.) *Nursing Management for the Elderly.* Philadelphia: J.B. Lippincott, 1979.

29
Bowel and Bladder Rehabilitation

Marilyn S. Giss
Bernita M. Steffl

Bowel and bladder incontinence is a devastating problem to the frail elderly and their families, as well as a management problem for nursing personnel. What's more, the fear of bladder incontinence and the concern about constipation are so socially crippling as to become real mental health problems. Incontinence and constipation are often taken for granted by both patients and nursing personnel because they are so prevalent. It has been estimated that from 14 to 40% of the elderly population is affected by urinary incontinence (Specht and Cordes, 1979; Wells, 1980). It might be further estimated that much of this exists among relatively well elderly women who may need counseling and evaluation for surgical repair of rectocele or cystocele.

BOWEL PROBLEMS

The idea that constipation is a normal function of aging is not valid (Bartol and Heitkemper, 1979; Brocklehurst, 1973). The term "presby-colon," when used with reference to the elderly, means constipation, complications of colon gas, and impaction. Hypertonic, hypotonic, and habit constipation are the three types of constipation commonly found in the elderly (Bartol and Heitkemper, 1979). A differentiation of the type of constipation present needs to be made for an effective treatment program to be established.

Hypotonic Constipation

In hypotonic constipation, the colon is full of feces and impactions are common. Soft putty-like stool is found in the rectum. The cause of hypotonic constipation is lack of motility, and the aim of treatment is to stimulate activity (Palmer, 1976).

Hypertonic Constipation

In hypertonic constipation, hard dry stools are present and the person may complain of lower abdominal pain. There is an increase in the contractions that mix bowel contents but not in the contractions that enhance evacuation. The result is increased reabsorption of water (Williams and Dickey, 1969).

Habit Constipation

The primary cause of habit constipation is poor eating habits, particularly a diet lacking sufficient bulk and liquids. In addition, the person either consciously or unconsciously ignores the urges to defecate (Bartol and Heitkemper, 1979). Older persons need to be educated and encouraged to drink more water.

The following factors explain the problems of constipation seen in the elderly, and must be addressed when developing and planning a rehabilitation or prevention program:

- Motility increases during and immediately following ingestion of food. Propulsiveness occurs with the physically active, not the resting person (Abbey, 1976). Therefore, it is essential that the elderly person become engaged in some form of activity.
- When the ingestion of food into the stomach causes increased colonic activity, it is referred to as the gastrocolic reflex. This activity appears to result from the effect of chyme entering the small intestine (Holdstock and Misiewicz, 1970).
- The defecation center in the medulla (diencephalon and cerebral cortex) controls and coordinates this activity (Abbey, 1976).

- When mass distension of the rectum is present, the defecation reflex is aroused. The rectum will relax if the reflex is inhibited (Abbey, 1976).
- Increased anal contractibility followed by relaxation is caused by stretching of the rectal wall.
- The length of time that the voluntary contraction of the external sphincter can be maintained is approximately one minute (Brocklehurst, 1973).
- The amount of feces decreases with age (Bertolini, 1969).
- Anatomical changes of the large bowel that occur with age are: atrophy of mucosa and muscle layers, abnormality of the intestinal glands, arteriosclerosis, and delay in peripheral nerve transmission (Abbey, 1981).

Fecal Incontinence

Fecal incontinence presents a crucial care problem of the aged person because it contributes to and compounds other problems such as the development of decubiti. It is caused by:

- Fecal impaction or gross constipation, with leakage of liquid stool around impaction
- Neurological deficits which result in increased inhibition of the rectal sphincter leading to leakage (Brocklehurst, 1973)
- Disease processes of the colon, rectum, or anus

Establishing Bowel Control

Because there is usually a lack of mobility and activity in the institutionalized or hospitalized elderly person, a bowel program should be established on admission to prevent fecal impaction, incontinence, and the use of harsh irritants and enemas.

In the process of learning the cause of constipation or fecal incontinence and the type of constipation, the nurse must assess the patient's normal bowel evacuation pattern. An initial history-assessment of the following must be documented:

- What time of day does the patient usually have bowel movement? How often?
- What is the normal consistency of the stool?
- Is a laxative taken? If so, what, when, and with what frequency? What is the normal intake of fluid and food, water, juice, other liquids, fruits, vegetables, roughage, etc.?

Once the initial history has been documented, a training program can be established. Programs vary according to individuals, but all commonly include the following activities, interventions, and goals:

- Check patient for impaction (see following section on enemas).
- Promote a daily fluid intake between 2000 and 3000 cc per day (unless the patient is on restricted fluids). Diuretic beverages such as coffee, tea, and grapefruit juice should not be given since they eliminate total body fluid as opposed to adding body fluid (Bartol and Heitkemper, 1979).
- Promote a well-balanced diet with adequate roughage (see Chapter 33) to develop a regular elimination pattern.
- Promote activities such as ambulation, sitting up in a chair, walking to the bathroom, etc., within the prescribed activities of daily living and medical orders.
- Institute a program of isometric exercises, if not contraindicated, when patient is unable to get out of bed.
- Teach patient to recognize the gastrocolic reflex and use it as a sign to defecate: distension of the stomach by food, particularly the first meal of the day, leads to contraction of the rectum and frequently to a desire to defecate (Carnevali and Patrick, 1979).
- See that patient gets laxative of choice when needed, if not contraindicated. The nurse should know the action of the laxative. Is it an emollient, a lubricant, a stimulant, bulk forming, saline, or hyperosmotic?

- Establish an evacuation time, as near as possible to patient's normal time, when personal habits and privacy can be respected.
- Strive to have patient up to bathroom, to commode, or on bedpan in sitting position or as near to that as possible.
- Have patient lie on side (if possible) when using a suppository; insert it approximately 30 minutes before defecation.
- Keep an accurate record of bowel movements (i.e., how often, time of day, consistency of stool, and problems in defecating).

Battle and Hanna (1980) found the addition of one ounce of bran cereal to the diet daily to be an economical and effective method to decrease the amount of laxatives taken by chronic laxative users.

Enemas

The use of enemas by the elderly and caretakers is hazardous. Caution is frequently ignored. Resorting to habitual enemas should be discouraged. Once a routine of taking an enema is established, it is difficult to disrupt, and normal bowel function is impaired (Mitchell, 1977; Stryker, 1972). However, the use of an enema (tap water, saline, mild soapsuds, or a commercially prepared hypertonic solution) may be needed initially to remove an impaction or when defecation has not occurred for several days before a bowel program is established (Bonner, 1974; Stryker, 1972). In some instances, it may be necessary to give an oil retention enema 2-3 hours before the cleansing enema in order to soften the stool (Mitchell, 1977). The nurse needs to remember, when giving an enema to an older person, that he may have a decrease in anal sphincter control, difficulty in taking and retaining a large amount of fluid, and difficulty in getting to the bathroom or bedside commode.

Once the bowel is free of impaction, the most vital concern is establishing a regular pattern of elimination using the steps outlined above.

BLADDER CONTROL AND URINARY INCONTINENCE

The origin of bladder control problems can be described in three broad categories: prerenal, intrarenal, and postrenal. Incontinence in the elderly is usually associated with postrenal problems (Roberts, 1981).

The most common causes of urinary incontinence in the elderly are obstruction of the bladder neck, enlarged prostate gland, fecal impaction, degenerative changes, a weakening of the muscles of the pelvic floor, atrophic senile vaginitis, atrophic urethritis, dehydration, drugs, and infections (Brink, 1980). Neurogenic disease, urgency incontinence, stress incontinence, and overflow incontinence singularly or in combination cause incontinence problems (Cape, 1978; Jaffe, 1971).

Infections

Acute and chronic infections of the lower urinary tract are some of the biggest problems affecting aged males and females. In addition to the pathological problems that lead to infection, the institutionalized aged person (hospital or nursing home) frequently has an indwelling catheter in place. When the meatus around the catheter is not properly cleansed, the area becomes a good medium for bacteria and subsequent infection. Seventy percent of persons who have an indwelling catheter can expect to have a urinary tract infection within 72 hours of insertion (Maney, 1976). The problem is, of course, compounded for the elderly person who may have a catheter in place for weeks, months, or indefinitely. Kinney, Blount, and Dowell (1980) state that the kind of catheter used makes a difference. If catheterization is necessary for longer than a week, a 100% silicone catheter should be used. The biggest problem and more important than changing the indwelling catheter is the frequent interruption of the drainage system. Some nurses recommend a side-lying position for female catheterization because it is more comfortable for the patient and technically simpler for the nurse. A detailed article on catheterization and catheter care by Kinney et al. (1980) in the *Geriatric Nursing* is highly recommended.

Types of Incontinence

Stress Incontinence. Stress incontinence can result from psychosocial pressures as well as from bladder pressures. True stress incontinence is due to an incompetent bladder outlet caused by weakness of the supporting pelvic muscles. When a person sneezes, coughs, or laughs, urine is squeezed out through the incompetent bladder outlet. This problem is particularly prevalent in the elderly female (Brocklehurst, 1973; Ebert, 1980; Field, 1979; Spiro, 1978). Because of the delicate nature of this problem, the elderly person experiencing it is often reluctant to participate in social activities and worries about accessibility of toilet facilities. Hence the person becomes increasingly isolated from friends and social activities. Surgical intervention frequently relieves this problem. At times, the problem is treated by giving 0.6 mg of atropine three times a day and by teaching the patient exercises which retrain the pelvic musculature. Depending upon the ability of the older patient to learn and follow through with exercises, the effect of the latter intervention may be minimal (Bonner, 1974).

Simple exercises (Mandelstam, 1980) to strengthen the muscles of the pelvic floor have proved helpful when the patient is given a description of the pelvic floor and its function, along with instructions in how to assess and test the functions; the aim is to increase sphincter functioning by voluntary contractions many times a day:

- The patient sits or stands and, without tensing the muscles of the legs, buttocks, or abdomen, tightens and relaxes the anal sphincter. This tightens the back part of the pelvic floor.
- The patient tries to stop the flow when passing urine, then restart it. This tightens the front muscles of the pelvic floor. Gradually, the patient learns to control the front muscles of the pelvic floor.

- The patient should practice contracting these pelvic floor muscles from back to front — counting slowly from 1 to 4 then relaxing — repeating this four times an hour (when awake) for three months (average length of time to strengthen weakened muscles).
- The patient should be told that this may take months.
- The patient may benefit from voiding "by the clock," rather than upon natural urge, and may gradually increase intervals between emptying.

Females may find a perineometer useful to monitor and register the strength of pelvic floor muscle contractions. This is an air-filled balloon which is placed in the vagina to register the strength of contractions. It is available from the Perineometer Research Institute, P.O. Box 1273, Tustin, CA 92680 (Mandelstam, 1980).

Overflow Incontinence. Retention of urine with overflow incontinence is caused by obstructive lesions or drug-induced retention. For example, diuretics increase urine volume and frequency. Bladder neck obstructions lead to retention with overflow. In these cases, eliminating or controlling the cause is as important as training or retraining.

Neurogenic Incontinence. Diseases that cause neurogenic incontinence are tabes dorsalis, diabetic neuropathy, cerebral cortex lesions, multiple sclerosis, and Parkinson's disease. They affect the sensory and motor tracts involved in bladder muscle function. Many elderly persons have these conditions.

Urgency Incontinence. Diverticulitis, pelvic tumor, vaginitis, urinary tract infection, bladder tumor, or prostatic enlargement are conditions associated with urgency incontinence.

Habit Training

Habit retraining is a tested method to regain urinary control. It is the procedure of preference and the most practical mode of management in many long term care facilities. It consists of a rather rigid scheduling of toileting. A careful nursing assessment of the type of incontinence and the individual patient's personal habits is necessary to establish a successful regime and important to maintain the human dignity of the person. A habit training chart and rigid regime protocols are the tools employed.

Research trials currently in progress in England, with patients in hospitals and at home, indicate a high degree of success for this method. In one study of a nursing team's work with 172 patients in their own homes over a period of 15 months, 150 were resocialized at home and 89 of them achieved continence by habit training (Clay, 1980).

Establishing Bladder Control

Many elderly persons are aware of their lack of bladder control and plan their lives accordingly.

They engage in social activities where they know they will have access to bathroom facilities and will see that they get up two to three times per night. For some who feel ashamed about dribbling and reluctant to discuss it, this becomes a problem by limiting and restricting socialization. However, for the elderly hospitalized patient, his pattern may be disrupted with resultant incontinence (Cape, 1978). This is most upsetting to the patient, and the nurse must work diligently to establish a program consistent with the individual patient's life-style and to assess his normal bladder elimination patterns (Brink, 1980); see Table 29-1. In addition, special questions to ascertain if the person has stress incontinence, urgency incontinence, or urinary tract infection must be included in the overall assessment to establish an effective training program (Thomas, 1980).

New products to keep patients dry and to promote their ability to remain mobile and

Table 29-1. Control of Bladder Incontinence.

BASIC ASSESSMENT	ESTABLISHING A PROGRAM
How often does patient normally void? Keep a 48-hour bedside record of input, output, color, odor, pain, or discomfort on voiding. Does patient normally experience urgency, frequency, stress incontinence? What drugs is patient taking that may induce retention or incontinence? Are there known obstructions? Is patient impacted? Can patient manage the sitting position to void (standing for male)? How much fluid does patient normally take in a 24-hour period? At what times? What kind of fluids?	Fluid intake: the amount of fluid intake may be limited due to the kidneys' inability to excrete medications patient is taking and to other pathological conditions. Whether intake is 1000 ml or 2000 ml per 24 hours, the important point is to plan how much is to be given each 8 hours. Limit fluids after 6:00 P.M. unless contraindicated. Give juices such as cranberry juice that will help to create acid urine and decrease possibility of bladder stone formation. Keep an accurate record of intake and output, making special note of times and amount of fluid given and urine voided. Teach patient/family procedure for giving perineal care to decrease the chance of infection and skin deterioration. Plan times throughout the 24 hours that patient will be offered use of bedpan, urinal, bedside commode, or bathroom. Times should be scheduled around other daily activities, such as upon arising, before and after eating, and before bedtime. A schedule may have to be based on the bladder capacity of the individual (Willington, 1975). See that patient is up in sitting position for voiding when at all possible. The bathroom or bedside commode should be close enough for the patient to reach it immediately and comfortably. See that patient is offered the urinal or bedside commode during the night. Once he has the urge to void, the elderly patient can ambulate no more than 50 feet. Be sure family/friends are aware of program!

NOTE: This table describes the steps usually taken in establishing a urine incontinence program (adapted from Kick, 1971; Field, 1979; and Willington, 1975).

active are constantly being tested. They resemble diapers and do in fact serve the same purpose. However, talking to the elderly incontinent patient about "his diapers" and referring to the "diapering" of old people is demeaning and depressing. Briefs or protective pants are better labels. No one wants to lose control, and it is physically uncomfortable. Therefore, professionals need to work at maintaining the dignity of afflicted individuals. It is most important to recognize the specific cause of urinary incontinence; it is rarely the result of one single cause, but rather of a combination of factors. Some of the factors may be irreversible, but others may be reversible, and if treated, continence may be restored (Wilson, 1976).

SUMMARY

Bowel and bladder control and rehabilitation are essential to the well-being of the elderly. They are basic to normal function in daily activities of living, maintenance of an independent life-style, and social interaction. Uncontrolled incontinence leads to devastating ostracism, isolation, and depression. With accurate assessment, professional knowledge, and skill, much can be done, such as establishing effective training programs. Above all, the patient must be given "hope," and the nurse, family, and others must exhibit a positive attitude with expectations of achievement of control.

REFERENCES

Abbey, J.C. Digestive disorders in the aged. In Burnside, I.M. (Ed.) *Nursing and the Aged*. New York: McGraw-Hill, 1981, pp. 317–345.

Bartol, M.A. and Heitkemper, M. Gastrointestinal problems. In Carnevali, D.L. and Patrick M. (Eds.) *Nursing Management for the Elderly*. Philadelphia: J.B. Lippincott, 1979, pp. 311–330.

Battle, E.H. and Hanna, C.E. Evaluation of a dietary regimen for chronic constipation. Report of a pilot study. *Journal of Gerontological Nursing* 6(9):527–532 (1980).

Bertolini, A.M. *Gerontologic Metabolism*. Springfield, Ill.: Charles C. Thomas, 1969.

Bonner, C.D. *Homburger and Bonner's Medical Care and Rehabilitation of the Aged and Chronically Ill* (3rd ed.). Boston: Little, Brown, 1974.

Brink, C. Assessing the problem. *Geriatric Nursing* 1(4):241–250 (1980).

Brocklehurst, J.C. The large bowel. In Brocklehurst, J.C. (Ed.) *Textbook of Geriatric Medicine and Gerontology*. Edinburgh: Churchill Livingstone, 1973, pp. 346–363.

Brocklehurst, J.C. Differential diagnosis of urinary incontinence. *Geriatrics* 36–39 (April 1978).

Cape, R. *Aging: Its Complex Management*. Md.: Harper & Row, 1978.

Carnevali, D.L. and Patrick, M. (Eds.). *Nursing Management for the Elderly*. Philadelphia: J.B. Lippincott, 1979, p. 325.

Clay, E. Habit training, a tested method to regain urinary control. *Geriatric Nursing* 1(4):252–254 (1980).

Dufault, Sister K. Urinary incontinence: United States and British nursing perspectives. *Journal of Gerontological Nursing* 4(2):28–33 (1978).

Ebert, N.J. Nutrition and elimination in the aged and the nursing process. In *The Aged Person and the Nursing Process*. New York: Appleton-Century-Crofts, 1980.

Field, M.A. Urinary incontinence in the elderly: an overview. *Journal of Gerontological Nursing* 5(1):12–19 (1979).

Holdstock, D.J. and Misiewicz, J.J. Factors controlling colonic motility, colonic pressures and transit after meals in patients with total gastrectomy, pernicious anemia or duodenal ulcer. *Gut* 11:100–110 (February 1970).

Jaffe, J. Common lower urinary tract problems in older people. In *Working with Older People*, Vol. 4. Washington, D.C.: U.S. Department of Health, Education and Welfare, 1971, pp. 141–147.

Kick, E.M. Rx for incontinence. *Geriatric Nursing* 7:45–49 (1971).

Kinney, A.B., Blount, M., and Dowell, M. Urethral catheterization. *Geriatric Nursing* 1(4):256–263 (1980).

Mandelstam, D. Special techniques, strengthening pelvic floor muscles. *Geriatric Nursing* 1(4):251–252 (1980).

Maney, A.Y. A behavioral therapy approach to bladder retraining. *Nursing Clinics of North America* 11(1):179–188 (1976).

Mitchell, P.H. Concepts Basic to Nursing. New York: McGraw-Hill, 1977.

Murray, R., Huelskoetter, M.M., and O'Driscoll, D. *The Nursing Process in Later Maturity*. Englewood Cliffs, N.J.: Prentice-Hall, 1980.

Palmer, E.D. Presbycolon problems in the nursing home. *Journal of the American Medical Association* 235:1150–1151 (1976).

Roberts, S.L. Renal abnormalities in aging. In Burnside, I.M. (Ed.) *Nursing and the Aged* (2nd ed.). New York: McGraw-Hill, 1981, pp. 317–345.

Specht, J. and Cordes, A. Incontinence. In Carnevali, D.L. and Patrick, M. (Eds.) *Nursing Management for the Elderly*. Philadelphia: J.B. Lippincott, 1979.

Spiro, L.A. Bladder training for the incontinent patient. *Journal of Gerontological Nursing* 4:28-35 (May–June 1978).

Stryker, R.P. *Rehabilitative Aspects of Acute and Chronic Nursing Care.* Philadelphia: W.B. Saunders, 1972.

Thomas, B. Problem solving: urinary incontinence in the elderly. *Journal of Gerontological Nursing* 6(9):533-536 (September 1980).

Vander, A., Sherman, J., and Lucian, D. *Human Physiology* (2nd ed.). New York: McGraw-Hill, 1975.

Wells, T. Promoting urine control in older adults. *Geriatric Nursing* 1(4):236-240 (1980).

Williams, R. and Dickey, J. Physiology of colon and rectum. *American Journal of Surgery* 117:849-853 (1969).

Willington, F.L. Incontinence: the nursing component in diagnosis and treatment. *Nursing Times* 71:464-467 (1975).

Wilson, T.S. A practical approach to the treatment of incontinence of urine in the elderly. In Willington, F.L. (Ed.) *Incontinence in the Elderly.* New York: Academic Press, 1976.

30
Rehabilitation in Arthropathy

Marilyn S. Giss

This chapter deals primarily with two main categories of arthropathy: rheumatoid arthritis and osteoarthritis. These two types of arthritis, which are so commonly present in the majority of older people, cause most of the joint dysfunctions and need for joint replacements. Arthropathy is an overwhelmingly disabling condition which affects about 38% of the population over age 65. More women than men are affected (National Council on Aging, 1978).

OSTEOARTHRITIS
(DEGENERATIVE JOINT DISEASE)

Osteoarthritis, a universal phenomenon of aging, is a noninflammatory disorder of the movable joints in which there is deterioration and abrasion of articular cartilage and formation of new bone at the joint edges. The joints commonly afflicted are the weight-bearing joints — the knees, hips, and lumbar and cervical spine; usually one or two joints are affected at a time (Clark, 1976; Grob, 1971; Wolff, 1979).

A typical presenting case is Mrs. Fox who is 68 years old, slightly obese, and widowed. She experiences pain in her knees when walking and has limited range of motion in knee joints with some muscle spasms. The decrease in range of motion has probably occurred gradually, due to the protective splinting that Mrs. Fox uses to prevent discomfort. Crepitation (a creaking, crackling sensation in the joint) is felt on movement. Mrs. Fox is unable to identify specifically when her problem began, but the increased pain led her to seek medical advice. If the joint becomes badly deranged, it may hurt constantly (Clark, 1976; Grob, 1971; Wolff, 1979). Although Mrs. Fox occasionally has pain upon rising, her complaints of pain center around a period of joint activity. After resting, Mrs. Fox nearly always has relief from pain. She finds she can also protect herself against pain by limiting her ambulation. The amount of pain does not indicate the extent of joint involvement. It is important to remember here that pain perception may be altered in the elderly (Clark, 1976).

Although a thorough and comprehensive history and exam should be done on Mrs. Fox, the questions listed in Table 30-1, suggested by Rogoff (1973), will help to distinguish degenerative joint disease from other diseases and will help to assess Mrs. Fox's presenting symptoms of stiff, aching joints.

An assessment must include information about the patient's home environment. This is essential to rehabilitation and health maintenance. The following should be taken into consideration by the physician and the entire health team, either upon treatment in the physician's office or upon discharge planning if the patient is hospitalized:

- The number of rooms, arrangement of rooms, and placement of furniture — are these conducive to the degree of mobility present?
- Safety measures — are there hazards present?
- How does person usually care for self?
- Who is there to assist person, at what time of day?
- What type of assistance does person presently receive to manipulate the environment?
- What else is needed?
- Is there access to household items that allow independence in activities of daily living (ADL)?
- Is there access to outside services — grocery store, doctor, church?

Table 30-1. Assessing Osteoarthritis.

Date of onset	Osteoarthritis usually occurs after age 40.
Sequence of involvement of the joints	The spine and then the knees are most commonly involved in degenerative joint disease.
Which joints are affected? Are they symmetrical?	In degenerative joint disease, the weight-bearing joints are usually affected with asymmetric involvement.
Are the symptoms migratory?	There should be a negative answer to this in degenerative joint disease.
Is there morning stiffness and for how long?	In degenerative joint disease, there may be a brief period of stiffness which disappears in about 15 minutes.
Do pain and stiffness begin after exercise?	Pain and stiffness are increased after exercise and later in the day.
What relieves the pain?	In degenerative joint disease, rest will frequently relieve the pain.
What medications are used?	The response to aspirin is not as dramatic in degenerative joint disease as in rheumatoid arthritis.
Is there limitation of movement or joint swelling?	This provides clues for thorough examination of specific joints.
Is there a family history of connective tissue disorder or gout?	There are familial tendencies for these conditions.

NOTE: Adapted from Ragoh (1973).

A thorough assessment also includes psychosocial aspects such as:

- Patient's level of motivation and ability to cooperate with a plan of treatment
- His reaction to a chronic disease that is painful and limits activity
- Family history and personal experiences with family members having osteoarthritis
- Job history for clues to course of osteoarthritis and possible need for job change
- Nearness of family or significant others

Plan of Treatment

There is no cure or complete rehabilitation for osteoarthritis. The overall goals of all treatment programs are to maximize function, prevent secondary complications, and promote comfort. Weight reduction will relieve the strain on affected weight-bearing joints in obese patients. Rest and physical therapy are of prime importance in the treatment program for all patients.

Exercise. The normal use of osteoarthritic joints for everyday activity may be overuse of joints for some osteoarthritic patients, but complete bed rest is rarely required. Rest periods of 15-30 minutes several times per day are important, and there should be a healthy relationship between exercise and rest. This must be reinforced with the elderly. An exploration with the patient about the types of activities he likes and is able to perform is necessary to determine whether these are included in his daily schedule. There should be enough exercise to maintain both joint mobility and muscle tone for joint support. Exercises are prescribed on an individual basis for specific joint involvement. The nurse should be involved in teaching and reinforcing exercises once they have been prescribed. If the patient experiences pain and stiffness after exercise, the exercise program should be reevaluated.

Conserving Energy. The patient may need nursing assistance in planning a daily schedule at home or work. For a working person, rest periods of 15-30 minutes must be provided. For the homemaker, activities should be planned so that the person is more active in the morning, with rest periods during the day. Activity is not to be discouraged, but the goal is to prevent joint overuse. Planning routine activities with a balance of rest is also important for the institutionalized elderly person. The patient must avoid carrying heavy loads. The nurse should emphasize the importance of proper body mechanics in whatever activity the patient is involved.

Avoiding Accidents and Falls

Guarding against accidents takes constant surveillance. Physical factors contributing to falls and injury are muscle rigidity and reduced range of motion, especially at the hip joints, thinning cartilage of the knee joints, and loss of strength, especially of the quadriceps muscle. These factors all contribute to instability and faulty weight bearing; thus, with these limitations, the patient may easily lose his balance when walking on uneven surfaces, going up or down curbs and steps, or hurrying across streets.

The older person who has degenerative joint disease and is also experiencing some neuromuscular incoordination finds it difficult to regain balance when changing position, adapting to change of pace, or adjusting to uneven surfaces. Therefore, an assistive device such as a cane may be indicated, at least for prolonged activity such as shopping.

As with rheumatoid arthritis, heat is often used to relieve pain. Heat should be used with caution because of the loss of pain receptors in older individuals. Aspirin, in analgesic dosages, is the primary drug used for pain control. The trial period for giving aspirin is one month, and the dosage is 8-12 300 mg tablets per day (Clark, 1976).

RHEUMATOID ARTHRITIS

The onset of rheumatoid arthritis in the elderly is usually subacute, as opposed to the acute onset in younger persons. Predominant symptoms include aching, stiffness (especially in early morning upon rising), swelling, pain on motion, tenderness, and limitation of motion. Patients also experience the more generalized symptoms of malaise, general debility, and easy fatigability. In later stages, muscle weakness is experienced. The elderly person may have involvement of joints which already have significant degenerative changes due to osteoarthritis. There is usually a greater incidence of large joint involvement, especially the shoulder joint, in elderly persons (Schissel, 1972).

Table 30-2 describes the primary objectives of the treatment program, as discussed by Bienenstock and Ferando (1976); Futrell, Brovender, McKinnon-Mullett, and Brower, (1980); and Schutt (1977). The objectives of nursing intervention should be consistent with the physical medicine treatment program.

Pain Assessment

A careful assessment of the patient's pain must be made before relief can be provided. This includes a description of location, duration, character, intensity, area of radiation, activities that induce pain, and measures that relieve pain. For the older person, joint discomfort may have developed slowly over the years, so that symptoms of joint pain and stiffness may go unnoticed and the need for medical care may not be recognized (Wolff, 1979).

In addition to assessing pain, an assessment of the patient's typical day is helpful:

- What time does the patient arise, retire?
- During what time of day is pain greatest?
- During what activities is pain greatest?
- What are peak energy levels for the patient?

Table 30-2. Treatment Goals and Nursing Intervention Objectives for Rheumatoid Arthritis.

TREATMENT GOALS	NURSING INTERVENTION OBJECTIVES
To limit disability	Determine maximum tolerance to exercise and activity
To prevent deformities	
To maintain or improve joint motion and muscle strength	Relief of pain
	Suppression of inflammation
To relieve pain and inflammation	Maintenance of function
To restore function by repairing existing deformities	Maintenance of proper body alignment

Relief of Pain and Suppression of Inflammation

The modalities available for pain relief are medication, heat, and rest. Some type of salicylate is the usual choice of medication for pain relief. The advantage of salicylates is that they decrease inflammation. Because of the high dosage that must be taken (10–15 tablets per day), some problems may be encountered (Schissel 1972):

- There is often a difficulty with compliance. Patients should not stop taking pills when they feel better. A high dose is necessary to maintain a consistent blood level of salicylates for pain relief and suppression of inflammation. It is important to remember that the elderly person may need to have a treatment plan or guide for taking pills established and written out for him. Suggestions such as setting out the amount of pills to take each day, divided into individual containers for after meals, or crossing off time and dates on a calendar as medications are taken are usually helpful.
- GI disturbances may occur so patients should be taught to take these medicines with meals. Patients should be questioned about gastrointestinal distress, bloody or tarry stools, or change in color of stools.
- Tinnitus may also occur, so hearing should be assessed periodically. Some loss of hearing is normally present in the elderly; therefore, a baseline hearing evaluation should be done prior to starting on a regime of salicylates.
- If morning stiffness is a particular problem, patients may be taught to keep the morning dose of medication at the bedside, awaken one-half hour before arising, and take their pills. This schedule is also applicable to the hospitalized patient.

Prolonged bed rest is not indicated since it leads to disuse atrophy, osteoporosis, decubitus, and thrombophlebitis (Schissel, 1972). However, bed rest may be indicated when the person is experiencing acute inflammation and when activity would cause further damage (Wolff, 1979). During these times, it may be necessary only to rest the involved joints on a daily and regular basis. The patient also needs to be instructed to place the involved joint in a position of function when resting to prevent contractures. Figure 30-1 demonstrates the use of splints in reducing and preventing contractures. In addition, a regular schedule of passive or active exercises should be followed. Active exercises should be non-weight bearing as tolerated by the patient without causing further inflammation. A balance between rest and exercise is the ultimate goal. Older persons may need additional support and encouragement to stay involved in activities. They are likely to be experiencing other losses with aging and may say, "What's the use?"

The use of heat and therapeutic massage with the guidance of a physical therapist provides relief of pain, vasodilation, and relaxation (Schutt, 1977). If the individual is using heat at home, the directions must be carefully explained and supervision in the home may be necessary. There is danger of burning oneself because of the decreased temperature perception and skin fragility of the elderly person. A hot water bottle or heating pad may be applied to painful joints but should not be left on for extended periods of time. The involved area should be checked every 10–15 minutes during application. Burns can occur when the temperature of the skin rises about 110°F. For the older individual, as for the infant, a safe temperature range when using a hot water bottle would be 105–115°F (Fuerst, Wolff, and Weitzel, 1974). A warm tub bath or shower of 102°F can help in relieving discomfort of painful joints (Schutt, 1977).

Prevention of Deformity and Maintenance of Function

The physical therapist or rehabilitation nurse needs to make an initial assessment of the range of motion of each joint and the strength of muscles adjacent to that joint to prevent deformity. Contractures may develop and muscle atrophy may occur not only from the

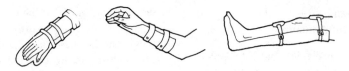

1 — Resting Splint for Hand and Wrist. Used during periods of rest and sleep, this splint is helpful in preventing hand and wrist deformities. Muscle setting exercises can be done while the splint is on.

2 — Functional Wrist Splint. This splint rests and supports an inflamed wrist and at the same time lets the fingers move so that useful routine work can be done while it is on. It is removable.

3 — Long Leg Splint. This splint rests the knee. It can be effective in preventing a knee from becoming stiff in a bend position. It is also sometimes used temporarily to support and protect the knee joint when standing or walking. Muscle setting exercises can be done while this splint is on.

Figure 30-1. Use of splints to reduce and prevent contractures. (Reproduced with permission from *Home Care Programs in Arthritis*, Arthritis Foundation, 1969.)

disease but also from maintaining joints in limited positions. Three types of exercises are used to prevent deformities or increase muscle strength: (1) range of motion, (2) strengthening, and (3) those that build endurance.

Range of motion exercise of all joints in indicated several times a day. An inflamed joint should be exercised or put through range of motion only to the point of pain tolerance. Illustrations of range of motion exercise for joints of the head, neck, and upper and lower extremities are found in Chapter 31. Increase in muscle strength can be obtained by isometric exercises. Muscles of the lower extremities, hip abductors, hip extensors, and knee extensors are the muscles in which these exercises are primarily indicated (Schissel, 1972). In isometric exercises there is no joint movement, rather tension is created and released in the muscle by the patient. Older persons learn as well as the young, but their reaction time is slower so time should be allowed for instruction and return demonstrations. Follow-up in the home is essential to see that the patient is able to do the exercises correctly and safety. Family and care givers should be involved.

Endurance exercises are best suited for upper extremity function and can be incorporated into a program through activities of daily living. They require low resistance and frequent repetition (Ditunno and Ehrlich, 1970). Examples would be brushing hair and washing and drying dishes.

The occupational therapist is the ideal member of the health team to evaluate and plan a program for retraining in the activities of daily living. However, the nurse must be aware of the program and must plan nursing care that is consistent with the training or retraining program. As previously stated, too much inactivity and rest can be disabling, especially for the older patient. Therefore, it is essential that an active life be pursued within individual limitations and pain tolerance. Practice is essential to develop and maintain muscular skills (Schwaid, 1978). In *Home Care Programs in Arthritis* (1969), specific exercises are illustrated to assist in maintaining function by working with one's hands, moving about, and maintaining good posture and breathing habits. Older patients, especially if they are "hurting," will need a great deal of education and encouragement to practice these exercises; See Figure 30-2.

JOINT REPLACEMENT

When relief of pain is not obtained through other measures and the individual's condition is progressively disabling, surgery is often indi-

Home exercises for arthritis patients

Exercise Programs Designed To Help You With 3 Functional Needs

A. The need to work with your hands

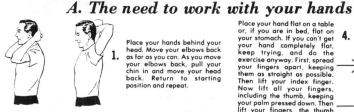

1. Place your hands behind your head. Move your elbows back as far as you can. As you move your elbows back, pull your chin in and move your head back. Return to starting position and repeat.

2. Raise your arms as high as you can over your head, keeping your elbows straight. Then swing your arms out and down to your sides. Swing your arms in as big a circle as possible. This exercise is best done when standing but it can also be performed while sitting or lying. Repeat three to six times.

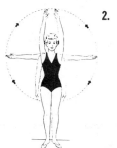

3. Grasp the handle of a medium-weight hammer firmly near its head. Keep your upper arm by your side and bend your arm at the elbow to a right angle. Turn your wrist from left to right and back so that the hammer turns out and in. Let the weight of the hammer swing your hand over as far as possible each time. Repeat with the other hand. Repeat three to six times with each hand. As you improve, shift your grip further toward the end of the handle so that the weight of the hammer makes you work harder.

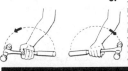

4. Place your hand flat on a table or, if you are in bed, flat on your stomach. If you can't get your hand completely flat, keep trying, and do the exercise anyway. First, spread your fingers apart, keeping them as straight as possible. Then lift your index finger. Now lift all your fingers, including the thumb, keeping your palm pressed down. Then lift your fingers, the thumb and your hand as far as possible, keeping your forearm on the table and bending your wrist up as far as you can.

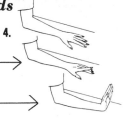

5. Open and close your hands, spreading your fingers as you open them, and making as tight a fist as possible when you close them. Repeat several times. Then touch the tip of your thumb to each finger in turn, pinching firmly each time. Try to form a letter "O" at each attempt. Do with both hands. Repeat.

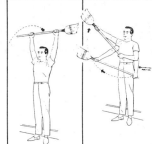

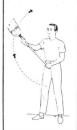

Warning to the patient

If you have arthritis—especially if you have rheumatoid arthritis— these exercises should help you to do in your home the things necessary to keep your arthritis under control and help you to get better. Discuss them with your doctor.

No two cases of arthritis are exactly the same and what may be right for one patient to do at any one time may be wrong for another patient. For this reason, always seek the advice of your doctor.

THE ARTHRITIS FOUNDATION

6a. Stand with your back against a wall with your heels, buttocks, shoulder blades and head touching it. Grasp a broomstick or cane in both hands and raise it as high above your head as possible, keeping your elbows as straight as you can. Then lower your arms. Repeat.

6b. Stand against a wall, as in 6A. With your arms straight down, move your hands two to three feet apart on the stick. Swing the stick up to the right (it helps to think of pushing with your left hand), keeping your right elbow straight and against the wall if possible. Return to the starting position and swing the stick up to the left in the same way, keeping your left elbow straight. Repeat.

6c. Grab the stick as shown and push it up as if you were shoveling snow over your right shoulder. Change your grip and repeat the motion over our left shoulder. Repeat.

Figure 30-2(A). Home exercises for arthritis patients. (Reprinted with permission from the Arthritis Foundation, National Office, 3400 Peachtree Road, NE, Suite 1101, Atlanta, GA 30326.)

cated. "Total joint replacement offers new avenues for the relief of pain and deformity and for stabilizing arthritic joints in the lower extremity" (Fitzgerald, 1977). The decision for surgery obviously involves many factors, and the risks must be carefully weighed by the physician, patient, and family (see Chapter 26).

Although there are specific exercises for the involved extremity, the maintenance and increase in muscle strength of the nonoperative extremity and both upper or lower extremities are also vitally important if the patient is to gain independence postoperatively in transfer activities and ambulation.

Exercise Programs Designed To Help You With 3 Functional Needs

B. The need to move about

Your legs must have enough strength and flexibility to get you up and carry you from place to place. Walking is good exercise, provided the joints of your knees or ankles are not swollen, painful, or stiff. If they are then limit your standing and walking but maintain strength and joint motion with Exercises 7 through 10.

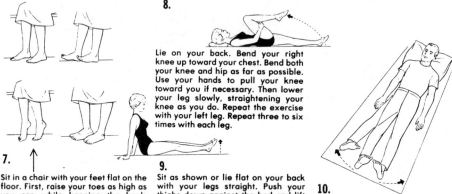

8.

Lie on your back. Bend your right knee up toward your chest. Bend both your knee and hip as far as possible. Use your hands to pull your knee toward you if necessary. Then lower your leg slowly, straightening your knee as you do. Repeat the exercise with your left leg. Repeat three to six times with each leg.

7.

Sit in a chair with your feet flat on the floor. First, raise your toes as high as you can while keeping the heels down. Then keep your toes down and lift your heels as high as possible. Next, starting with your feet flat on the floor, lift the inside of each foot and roll the weight over on the outside of the foot. Keep your toes curled down if possible. Repeat.

9.

Sit as shown or lie flat on your back with your legs straight. Push your thighs down against the bed and lift your heels up about one inch. This will tighten and straighten your knees. If you cannot straighten your knees, put a rolled towel under them, and then push your knees down against the towel and lift your heels as much as you can. Repeat.

10.

Lie flat on your back, legs straight and about six inches apart. Point the toes together. First, move the right leg out to the side and return, then the left leg out and return, still keeping your toes pointing together. Repeat.

C. The need to maintain good posture and breathing habits

Posture exercises and breathing exercises (exercises 11 through 12) go hand in hand. A series of ten very deep breaths is one of the best posture exercises you can do. One of the major reasons you need good posture is so that you can breathe properly.

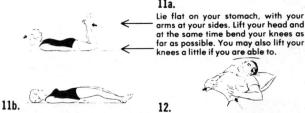

11a.

Lie flat on your stomach, with your arms at your sides. Lift your head and at the same time bend your knees as far as possible. You may also lift your knees a little if you are able to.

11b.

If you cannot lie flat on your stomach, substitute this exercise: Lie flat on your back, with your legs straight, push your heels and shoulders down against the bed and lift your buttocks off the bed. Hold the position for a few seconds. Repeat.

12.

Lie flat on your back with your hands on the sides of your chest. Now breathe in deeply and push your ribs out against your hands. Hold a moment, then breathe out. Be sure to take a breath deep enough to push the ribs outward. **Repeat.**

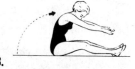

13.

Lie on your back with your knees as straight as possible. First, lift your head so that your chin is on your chest. Then come to a sitting position, reaching with your hands toward your toes. Lie back down and repeat. However, if you have low back problems, this exercise should be done with your knees bent enough so that your feet are flat on the floor (or other surface).

Figure 30-2(B). Home exercises for arthritis patients. (Reprinted with permission from the Arthritis Foundation, National Office, 3400 Peachtree Road, NE, Suite 1101, Atlanta, GA 30326.)

An experienced rehabilitation nurse emphasizes the continuous need to maintain and promote the self-worth and dignity of older individuals by recognizing their need to be active participants in their treatment. There is now increasing emphasis on involving patients in the decision-making process and in goal setting to accomplish the activities of daily living (e.g., using bathroom facilities, grooming, brushing teeth, and eating at least two meals a day out of bed). It is also important to assess the family support system. If the patient will be returning directly from the hospital to the home, there must be active involvement of family members to maintain the established goals and to assist with care that enhances independence (Tompkins, 1980).

Total Hip Replacement

Ideally, the patient prepares for surgery for several months preoperatively. During this time, rehabilitation is really begun, with emphasis placed on muscle strengthening exercises and teaching the patient crutch walking (Wolff, 1979). The surgical procedure is described briefly in Chapter 26. The importance of coughing, deep breathing, maintaining a position of abduction to prevent dislocation, and active and passive exercises is stressed during this preoperative phase (Bennage and Cummings, 1973).

Sensory losses in hearing, vision, and touch must be considered in pre- and postoperative teaching. For example, the combination of trauma, drugs, fluid imbalance, and sensory losses causes disorientation more rapidly in the elderly than in the young (see Chapter 26 regarding surgical nursing considerations for older adults).

Postoperatively the patient is assisted immediately in deep breathing and coughing, and is checked for proper body alignment. Plantar flexion and dorsiflexion exercises of the feet are initiated and continued throughout hospitalization (Bennage and Cummings, 1973).

Although there may be some variation in the postoperative rehabilitation plan, the treatment plan (Wolff, 1979) usually includes:

- Bed rest for 1-4 days
- Elevation of head of bed up to 60° for comfort
- Turning to unaffected side or back
- Use of trapeze to help lift and turn self
- Ambulation using a walker or crutches following period of bed rest
- Use of abduction splint, triangular bolster, or pillows between knees while on bed rest and at night
- Discharge in 1-3 weeks

The exercises taught preoperatively are initiated postoperatively as soon as possible (Murray, Huelskoetter, and O'Driscoll, 1980).

Discharge planning for the patient who has had a total hip replacement stresses the importance of proper hip positioning and progressively increasing activity. Specific discharge instructions for a patient with hip replacement would include the following (Wolff, 1979):

Continue with exercises as instructed.

Do not cross legs and ankles over each other until physician permits (up to three months).

Limit sitting to one hour and relieve by standing, stretching, and walking a few steps.

Avoid chairs which require bending forward to stand up.

Lie on unoperated side when in side-lying position.

When in bed use abduction splint or pillows between legs, up to 6-8 weeks after discharge.

Use crutches or walker as indicated.

Use elevated toilet seat for four weeks after discharge.

Continue to wear support hose for six weeks postoperatively.

Unless otherwise ordered, do not drive car for six weeks postoperatively.

Resume sexual activity in six weeks.

Put away scatter rugs and have clear, well-lighted path for ambulation.

The nurse should be aware that the patient and family will need individualized assistance and support to carry out these measures and to manage the activities of daily living, such as meal planning and eating, within these limitations. .

Total Knee Replacement

As with total hip replacement, ideally the patient undergoing total knee replacement should be prepared about procedures and expectations well before hospitalization. Teaching should begin as soon as the patient becomes a candidate for the procedure. Emphasis must be placed on exercises that the patient will be expected to carry out postoperatively. Usually the physical therapist instructs the patient on muscle tightening and active ankle exercises of the operative leg to maintain or rebuild muscle tone (Shoemaker, 1973). On the first day postoperatively, *gentle* flexion-extension, isometric exercises are initiated. Although the patient is free to move around in bed, ambulation may be delayed until the fifth or sixth day. At this time, the compression dressing is replaced by a plastic cylinder which provides protection for the new joint (Townley and Hill, 1974). Exercises that have been taught to the patient preoperatively are expected to be carried out by the patient postoperatively (Carpenter Conaty, Chew, and Mongon, 1976) are:

> Gluteal sets — these maintain and strengthen hip muscles.
> Calf-pumping exercises and dorsiflexion of the foot — this increases tone and strength of lower leg and foot.
> Quad sets — this strengthens the quadriceps muscle which straightens the leg.
> Straight leg raises — this also benefits the quadriceps muscle

The goals for range of motion are full knee extension with at least 60° of flexion (Shoemaker, 1973). However, the effectiveness of the replacement should be measured not only in terms of range of motion, but also in terms of the ability of the person to carry out the activities of daily living (Murray et al., 1980). By the time of discharge, the patient should be able to ambulate safely with or without assistive devices, and should have adequate knee stability and mobility.

With total joint replacement, the rehabilitation phase for the older person will most likely be longer than for a young adult. So it is important to begin rehabilitative measures early that promote dignity, well-being, and independence, and prevent secondary complications.

POSTMENOPAUSAL OSTEOPOROSIS

This disease contributes greatly to the cost of medical, nursing, and rehabilitative care of elderly women. Of prime importance is the prevention of accidents, invalidism, and deformity. Research indicates that preventive measures such as estrogen therapy, though currently controversial, have been effective. The economic, physical, and emotional consequences of deforming postmenopausal osteoporosis are enormous. Since the average age of menopause is 50 years, most symptomatic women are now 60 years of age. Medical management, rehabilitative nursing, and physical therapy are interdependent. Emphasis is placed on estrogen replacement by some. Other measures are individualized physiotherapy, orthopedic supports, optimal nutrition, safety precautions, work simplification, and occupational therapy.

Most patients with advanced osteoporosis feel more secure when they continue to wear a light corset. Braces may be helpful, but they have distinct disadvantages: (1) totally immobilizing the spine may exacerbate the osteoporosis; (2) postmenopausal women usually have thin skin and thin bones, and cannot tolerate a rigid brace. Several studies have indicated that 25% of all women with osteoporosis proceed to vertebral fracture and deformity (Vaughn, 1976). See Chapter 22 for other information on osteoporosis.

SUMMARY

When caring for the older person who is experiencing joint discomfort and limited mobility due to pathological processes, emphasis needs to be placed on the prevention of deformities, the control of pain, and the promotion of activities within one's limitations (Bienenstock and Ferando, 1976; Schutt, 1977).

Posture training and gait training are as important as the physical therapy for specific joints and muscles. The evaluation for, and instruction in, the use of assistive devices such as canes, crutches, and walkers cannot be overemphasized in the relief of weight-bearing pain. Nurses are often the first to observe the older patient's mobility; therefore, they must take the initiative in making appropriate referrals for further evaluation, as well as being knowledgeable in gait-training procedures and the use of assistive devices. Also, every nurse

should be aware of *The Arthritis Help Book* by
Friese and Loriq (1980).

Current trends in surgical procedures such as
total joint replacement are adding new dimensions to pain relief, prevention of deformities,
and stabilization of arthritic joints of the lower
extremities. Thus, many confined elderly are
now able to participate more actively in the
activities of daily living without experiencing
chronic pain.

REFERENCES

Arthritis Foundation, *Arthritis: A Manual for Patients.*
Atlanta, Georgia 1969, pp. 9–15.

Bennage, B. and Cummings, M. Nursing the patient
undergoing total hip arthroplasty. *Nursing Clinics
of North America* 8(1):107–116 (1973).

Bienenstock, H. and Ferando, R. Arthritis in the
elderly – an overview. *Medical Clinics of North
America* 60:1173–1189 (November 1976).

Carpenter, E.S., Conaty, J., Chew, V., and Mongon,
E. *Information for Our Patients about Total
Knee-Joint Replacement.* Downey, Calif.: Ranchos
Los Amigos Hospital, Arthritis Rheumatology
Service, 1976, 47 pp.

Clark, H. Osteoarthritis: an interesting case? *Nursing
Clinics of North America* 11:199–206 (March 1976).

Ditunno, J. and Ehrlich, G. Care and training of elderly
patients with rheumatoid arthritis. *Geriatrics* 25:
164–172 (March 1970).

Fitzgerald, R.H. Symposium on arthritis in older
persons. Section IV – surgery and rehabilitation.
Total joint replacement: lower extremities. *Journal of the American Geriatrics Society* 25(2):67
(1977).

Friese, J. and Loriq, K. *The Arthritis Help Book.*
Menlo Park, Calif.: Addison-Wesley, 1980.

Fuerst, E.V., Wolff, L., and Weitzel, M.W. *Fundamentals of Nursing.* Philadelphia: J.B. Lippincott,
1974.

Futrell, M., Brovender, S., McKinnon-Mullett, E., and
Brower, H.T. *Primary Health Care of the Older
Adult.* North Scituate, Mass.: Duxbury Press,
1980.

Grob, D. Prevalent joint diseases in older persons.
Working with Older People, Vol. 4. Washington,
D.C.: U.S. Department of Health, Education and
Welfare, 1971, pp. 163–171.

Murray, R., Huelskoetter, M.M., and O'Driscoll, D.
The Nursing Process in Later Maturity. Englewood
Cliffs, N.J.: Prentice-Hall, 1980.

National Council on Aging. *Fact Book on Aging: A
Profile of America's Older Population.* Washington,
D.C.: 1978, p. 110.

Rogoff, B. 20 Essentials to Differentiate Arthritis,
The Consultant, Vol. 14, September 1973, p. 119–
129.

Schissel, C.M. The elderly person with arthritis. In
Long, J. (Ed.) *Caring for and Caring about Elderly
People – A Guide to the Rehabilitative Approach.*
Rochester Regional Medical Program and the
University of Rochester School of Nursing, 1972,
pp. 49–58.

Schutt, A.H. Physical medicine and rehabilitation in
the elderly arthritic patient. *Journal of the American Geriatrics Society* 25:76–82 (February 1977).

Schwaid, M. Advice to arthritics: keep moving.
American Journal of Nursing 78:1708–1709
(October 1978).

Shoemaker, R.R. Total knee replacement. *Nursing
Clinics of North America* 8(1):117–125 (1973).

Tompkins, K. Orthopedic Nursing Coordinator, Mary-
vale Samaritan Hospital, Phoenix, Arizona. Personal communication (May 19, 1980).

Townley, C. and Hill, L. Total knee replacement.
American Journal of Nursing 74(9):1612–1617
(1974).

Vaughn, C.C. Rehabilitation in post menopausal
osteoporosis. *Israel Journal of Medical Sciences*
12(7):652–657 (1976).

Wolff, H. Musculoskeletal problems. In Carnevali, D.
and Patrick, M. (Eds) *Nursing Management for the
Elderly.* Philadelphia: J.B. Lippincott, 1979, pp.
399–425.

Yurick, A., Robb, S., Spier, B., and Ebert, N. *The
Aged Person and the Nursing Process.* New York:
Appleton-Century-Crofts, 1980.

31
Cardiac and Respiratory Rehabilitation
Marilyn S. Giss

When a new disability arrives, I look about to see if death has come and I call quietly, "Death, is that you? Are you there?" So far the disability has answered, "Don't be silly, it's me."

Florida Scott Maxwell (1968)

CARDIAC REHABILITATION

Management of hypertension includes medication, diet, follow-up care, and modification of life-style. The goal is management to maximize the state of health and functioning while treating the disease. Cardiac rehabilitation begins in the acute care setting.

Medication

The most important factor in cardiac rehabilitation is the medication regime. An assessment needs to be made of the patient's attitude toward his disease and toward taking medications, his understanding of medications, and his ability to take medications at prescribed times. Noncompliance is a major problem among the elderly. It is important to reemphasize the importance of teaching the elderly patient about his medications and their potential side effects; for example, the patient needs to know that he may develop impotence from certain drugs such as Hygroton. If patients know this, they are more apt to seek help rather than being silently fearful of what is happening to them. The development of a system for remembering to take medications is another common need. Family or significant others should be included in this teaching.

Follow-up Care. Periodic evaluation of the patient's condition is necessary to establish the effectiveness of medication, alter the dosage, and monitor compliance.

Diet

The severe adherence to a sodium-restricted diet is controversial. It might be better to restrict the use of table salt, teach the patient about avoiding salty foods, and allow for some use of salt in cooking (Jones, 1976; Roben, 1979).

Modification of Life-style

Assisting the person in gradual reduction of blood pressure is crucial. The elderly patient may feel such a sense of loss and hopelessness when confronted with a cardiac problem that extra time and effort by the nurse are essential in order for the patient to achieve a satisfactory life-style. Under the direction of the primary physician, measures should be instituted that include and emphasize the following (Roben, 1979):

- Maintenance of general healthful living
- Development of a weight-control program when appropriate
- Limitation of sodium intake (no table salt)
- Promotion of adequate rest and exercise routine
- Generation of interest in activities that increase relaxation and promote socialization

Changing human behavior is very difficult. Research and innovative intervention strategies are needed. One study reports success with a residential (live-in) therapeutic dietary and exercise program designed to change life-style through controlled and supervised activities and eating (Mannerberg, 1979). This approach might be particularly beneficial to the elderly

Table 31-1. Rehabilitative and Maintenance Measures for Heart Failure.

REDUCTION OF HEART WORK LOAD	CONTROL OF BLOOD VOLUME	IMPROVEMENT OF CARDIAC OUTPUT
Work toward balance between capacity of heart and work load of heart. Consider patient's total day and plan tolerable activities, teaching to conserve energy and avoid overexertion. Provide rest periods throughout day. Promote use of bedside commode or bathroom when prescribed. Recognize and assist with emotional stress and feelings of helplessness. Use mild sedatives when ordered to relieve insomnia and restlessness.	Recognize the normal decrease in glomerular and tubular renal function that occurs with aging. Recognize that there is decreased renal blood flow with heart disease. Monitor intake of fluids, output, salt intake, and effect of diuretics.	Use of drug therapy to increase cardiac output, particularly cardiac glycosides. Special monitoring of digitalis preparations because of increased sensitivity to drugs in older persons.

NOTE: Adapted from Atwood (1979) and Pinneo (1972).

patient who normally lives alone, may be without family or social support systems, and has to care for himself.

Cardiac rehabilitation and maintenance are directed toward teaching the individual with heart disease to restore and maintain his optimal level of physiological, psychological, vocational, and social functioning through progressive activity (Winslow and Weber, 1980). Although the elderly person may not be returning to work, the goal of restoring optimal level of functioning is critical to prevent premature institutionalization. Initially, the aim of activity is to prevent the deleterious effects of prolonged bed rest such as postural hypotension, venous thrombosis, reduced lung volume, atelectasis, reduced skeletal muscle tone, and reduced joint flexibility (Douglas, David, and Wilkes, 1975; Hoskins and Habasevich, 1978; Wenger, 1973). For the older person, this early phase is particularly crucial to prevent secondary complications. "The goal of careful mobilization is to take a patient from a position of complete dependence on admission to the CCU to full independence in activities of daily living as a comfortable convalescent by the time of discharge" (Niccoli and Brammell, 1976); see Table 31-1.

Exercises

The two basic categories of exercises are dynamic (isotonic) and static (isometric). Table 31-2 describes the results of dynamic exercises such as walking, swimming, and jogging. Lifting or pushing heavy objects and gripping a tennis racket are examples of static exercises. The results of these exercises are increased pressure load on the heart and a significant increase in myocardial oxygen consumption. Static exercises are not tolerated well by patients with coronary artery disease and limited cardiac reserve because they may develop angina, arrhythmias, or left ventricular dysfunction (Dehn, 1980).

Table 31-2. Expected Results from Dynamic Exercises. (Douglas et al., 1975).

Increased venous return to the heart
Increased heart rate
Increased cardiac output
Increased systolic arterial pressure
Moderate decrease in diastolic arterial pressure secondary to marked vasodilation in the contracting muscles
Slight increase in mean arterial pressure

Initial baseline data must be obtained about the patient's tolerance to exercise before a program is established. It is imperative that the program be individualized and supervised, with gradual increase in activity as tolerance increases and as long as contraindications do not occur (Dehn, 1980; Fardy, 1978; Hoskins and Habasevich, 1978; Williams and Fardy, 1980); see Table 31-3. In order to plan a realistic program of activity for the elderly patient, the nurse should recognize that the pattern of activity prior to cardiac insult may have been limited due to other physiological, psychological, or social problems.

Gradual progressive activity and exercise programs have been described according to phases by Cohen (1979); Comoss, Burke, and Swails (1979); Douglas et al. (1975); Fardy (1978); Hoskins and Habasevich (1978); Niccoli and Brammell (1976); and Wenger (1973). Gen-

erally phases I and II are concerned with care during the acute stage. Phase I would be in the coronary care unit (1–5 days), and phase II includes the remainder of the hospital stay (up to 21 days). Phase III is the convalescent period and is usually in the patient's home; it lasts 4–8 weeks. Phase IV is considered recovery and maintenance, and includes returning to work or to a level of activity prior to insult (Comoss et al., 1979; Wenger, 1973). Others describe essentially the same pattern in three phases (Fardy, 1978; Hoskins and Habasevich, 1978). See Table 31-4 for phases described by Wenger (1973) and Table 31-5 for a progressive activity program used at the University of Colorado Medical Center.

For safe progress in activities, the patient is taught to take the pulse before and upon completion of activity, noting change in rate and regularity. A safe limit to follow is a maximum increase of 16–20 beats per minute (Niccoli and Brammell, 1976). Douglas et al. (1975) suggest the patient take the morning resting pulse and compare it with the evening pulse.

Table 31-3. Guidelines for Dynamic Exercising. (Dehn, 1980).

Begin slowly
Avoid exercise during illness
Allow time to warm up and cool down
Dress appropriately (loose clothes, etc.)
Schedule a time for exercising at least one hour after
  a meal when environmental conditions are best
Cut back on exercise after a layoff
Avoid "all-out" efforts
Stop if chest discomfort occurs
Avoid hot showers after exercises

Patient Education

Teaching of the patient and the family is a vital component of the rehabilitation program and it begins on admission. Patients educated about their conditions are more likely to participate in their care, understand untoward signs and

Table 31-4. Phases of Cardiac Rehabilitation (Wenger, 1973).

PHASE I	PHASE II	PHASE III	PHASE IV

Begin in CCU when condition is stable:
  Self-feeding
  Shaving
  Use of bedside commode
  Passive and active movement of extremities
  Sitting on side of bed or in chair at bedside.
	Based on individual's tolerance; gradually increase activity to what would be required at home for self-care.
	Sit in chair for increased periods of time.
	Rhythmic exercises to maintain muscle tone and decrease venous stasis.
	Increase ambulation if no cardiac complications.
	Provide rest periods interspersed with activity.
		Self-care and household activities, including stair climbing, light housework (dusting, dishwashing, and desk work).
		Gradually increase the speed and distances walked to increase endurance.
			Return to work or to previous level of function, or be retrained for less demanding job.
			Pursue more active reconditioning program of exercises.
			Emphasize secondary prevention.

Table 31-5. University of Colorado Medical Center Cardiac Rehabilitation
Progressive Activity Program — Acute Myocardial Infarction.

Date of event: Name:

Type/location of event:

Acute Phase		1–4 days			Coronary Care Unit	1–2 Mets
		ACTIVITY	DATE	H.R.	COMMENTS	PLAN
		Complete bed rest until pain remits				
	1.	Orientation to rehabilitation program				
	2.	Bedside commode				
	3.	Feed self				
	4.	Active foot exercises				
1st	5.	Partial A.M. care (wash hands, face, brush				
to		teeth)				
4th	6.	May sit in chair at bedside for bed making				
day	7.	May stand to be weighed				
	8.	OT activity				
	9.	Dangle for feeding and A.M. care				
	10.	Sit in chair (15–30 min) up to 3 times daily				
Semiacute Phase		**5–10 days**			**Transfer to Ward**	**2–3 Mets**
5th	1.	Walk to bathroom				
and	2.	Up in chair 3–4 times daily as tolerated				
6th	3.	Sponge bathe self (seated)				
day	4.	Walk in room				
	5.	OT work simplification/activity				
	1.	Continue up in chair as tolerated				
7th	2.	Sponge bathe (standing)				
and	3.	Standing self-care — shaving, combing, etc.				
8th	4.	Walk 50 ft				
day	5.	Walk in room ad lib.				
	6.	OT clinic — wheelchair				
9th	1.	Bathe in tub or shower (initially trans-				
and		ported by WC)				
10th	2.	Progressive ambulation on ward				
day						
Convalescent Phase		**11–14 days**			**Ward**	**3–4 Mets**
	1.	Continue all other prior activities				
	2.	Continue walking in hall as tolerated				
	3.	Stairs before discharge as needed				

NOTES: Progressive activity will be individualized according to patient's needs and condition. *Contraindications:*
Shock, CHF, ventricular arrhythmias, angina.

symptoms, comply with drug and treatment regimes, and be able to obtain a maximum level of physiological, psychological, vocational, and social functioning (Fardy, 1978; Niccoli and Brammell, 1976). Older persons may become discouraged easily and need a great deal of support while learning about and accepting their condition.

Teaching Outline for Atherosclerotic Coronary Heart Disease (ACHD)

I. General Medical Information
The ACHD process, patient's concept and reaction, the acute clinical event

II. Definition of Terms
Myocardial infarction, angina pectoris, SVBP (saphenous vein bypass surgery)

III. Rehabilitation Overview
Goal of comfortable, independent, convalescence at time of hospital discharge and plans for care after discharge
Quality and quantity of life expected

IV. Rehabilitation Team
Who they are; what they do; expectations

V. Duration of Hospitalization
Activity progression in hospital

IV. Psychosocial Aspects
Reactions to acute event, interventions to assist with coping
Family problems, financial problems, vocational considerations, community resources

VII. Risk Factor Identification and Modification
Prevention of another clinical event and improvement of pre-event status
Identify and list patient's specific recommendations: smoking, hypertension, body fat, blood, diabetes, diet, physical inactivity, personality

VIII. Medications
List patient's medications — name, dose schedule, action, purpose, side effects
Nitroglycerin — how and when to use; action and side effects

IX. Diet
Calories, cholesterol, carbohydrates and sugar, sodium, caffeine, alcohol

X. Exercise and Exercise Prescription
Plan for return to activities
Pulse taking and heart rate response

XI. Guidelines for Patient
Warning symptoms
Work simplification
Pacing activities
Specific instructions
Driving, flying, attitude
Sex
Follow-up care

NOTE: From Niccoli and Brammell (1976).

Rehabilitation of the older cardiac patient must include planning of activities. Although the older person may not be returning to work, a careful examination of what he did prior to insult is essential. The goal is to increase independence to the greatest possible degree with conservation of energy. Specifics to remember when caring and planning rehabilitation for the older cardiac patient are:

- Length of hospitalization may be longer due to other chronic health problems.
- The patient may have an elderly spouse who also has health problems or limitations in his/her activities of daily living.
- The patient may live alone without family members nearby.
- The patient may have hearing and visual problems.
- Although new information can be learned by the older person, endurance for learning new material at any one time may be less and learning may take longer.
- An early teaching program in which new information is introduced gradually and repeated for reinforcement will be most beneficial.
- Include family members and significant others whenever possible in the teaching and rehabilitation programs.

Too often patients go home and retire to a negative state if a program is not carefully planned, reinforced, and followed up at home. Unfortunately, the result may be a nursing home placement, rather than a self-sustained individual in his home with a prescribed and supervised rehabilitation program of activity (Mock, 1977). Discharge planning should begin with admission. Every effort should be made to keep the patient in his home as long as possible. Organized discharge planning in health care facilities of all levels is just coming into practice and health delivery (Steffl and Eide, 1978).

PULMONARY REHABILITATION

Chronic obstructive pulmonary disease (COPD), chronic airway obstruction (COA), and chronic obstructive lung disease (COLD) are interchangeable terms that are used to describe a group of overlapping respiratory disorders: chronic bronchitis, reactive airway disease or asthma, and emphysema (Bither, 1979). In this chapter, the term COPD will be used, and the focus will be on maintenance rehabilitation for older individuals suffering from the two major disorders, chronic bronchitis and emphysema.

COPD represents a major health problem in the United States today. It is predicted that by 1990 there will be 27 million people over the age of 65 and that a high percentage of these people will have a chronic, and perhaps incapacitating, pulmonary condition. In 1973, Social Security disability payments reached almost 100 million dollars for such cases (Lagerson, 1974). These are strong implications that professionals and lay people should learn more about this condition — how to care for it, how to prevent complications, and how to maintain an optimal level of functioning for affected individuals.

With the normal process of aging there is diminished lung elasticity, chest wall rigidity, and respiratory muscle weakness. All of these impair pulmonary function. When this normal process is coupled with the lack of breathing reserve caused by COPD, the aged individual will have early fatigue and shortness of breath (Clark, 1972). Treatment programs are aimed at keeping patients at optimal function and preventing complications and further deterioration.

Rehabilitative and maintenance measures start with an individual assessment of the patient's home environment to ascertain if he will be able to follow a treatment program. Next the physical energy capability of the patient for performance of activities of daily living should be identified. Once the initial evaluation is made, modification of the patient's home environment and instruction in principles of work simplification, which conserve energy and promote physical activity, can be implemented. It is essential that a daily routine that is consistent with the patient's life-style, yet provides a proper balance of rest and activity, be established. (See Chapter 23 for the etiology and pathology of respiratory conditions and Chapter 19 for expected physical changes in the lungs and chest.)

It is expected that the following baseline data will always be obtained: the overall health situation at the time a program is to be initiated, the mental functioning of the older person, and the significant others available to the older person. It is imperative to elicit the patient's goals. They should involve physical activities that the patient would like to achieve, and they should be realistic, obtainable, and set down in writing. As indicated, chronic bronchitis and emphysema are the major disorders with which we will be dealing.

Chronic Bronchitis

Chronic bronchitis results from chronic inflammation and swelling of the cells lining the inside of the bronchi. With prolonged inflammation, the mucous glands lining these airways become hypertrophied and secrete excessive mucus. As mucus increases, there is increased narrowing of the airways, resulting in localized airway plugging and increased resistance to air flow in an out of the lungs (Clark, 1972; Lagerson, 1974; Modrak, Moser, Archibald, Hansen, Birgitta, Beaman, and Dunn, 1975). The signs and symptoms are similar to those found with emphysema, except that with chronic bronchitis there is a more prominent productive cough and breath sounds are usually more pronounced (Clark, 1972).

Emphysema

Emphysema results from the single-celled walls of the alveoli becoming inflamed and distended. These eventually rupture, causing damage to the surrounding capillary bed and reduced number of functioning alveoli. As this progresses, the normal lung elasticity is reduced. There is a tendency of the airways to collapse on expiration, producing expiratory obstruction. There is a decrease in alveolar ventilation, abnormal ventilation, perfusion distribution, and a reduction in gas diffusion (Clark, 1972). In both chronic bronchitis and emphysema there is severe obstruction to the flow of air, primarily during expiration.

Management of Respiratory Problems

Life-sustaining management of COPD depends on bronchial hygiene, breathing retraining, muscle relaxation, physical reconditioning, and recognition and prevention of complications.

Bronchial Hygiene. The purpose of a bronchial hygiene program is to inhibit the progression of COPD and prevent repeated infections. It should include treating bronchomucosal edema, thinning and loosening secretions, and clearing secretions from the airways (Clark, 1972; Moody, 1977).

Treating Bronchomucosal Edema. Bronchodilating agents are used to treat bronchomucosal edema. The most frequently used methods at home are the hand nebulizer and intermittent positive pressure breathing (IPPB). There is controversy as to whether or not IPPB is more effective (Brannin, 1974; Lagerson, 1974). In either case, proper instruction in use, frequency of use, type and amount of medication to be taken, and care of equipment is essential.

Thinning and Loosening Secretions. Although drugs may be employed to thin and loosen secretions, inhalation of moisture, usually in the form of hot steam, is probably the most effective means of liquefying secretions (Clark, 1972). Because of the decreased bodily sensation of the elderly person, caution should be taken when using hot moisture and the patient should be so instructed. If there are no contraindications, hydration in the form of 10–12 glasses of water daily is an excellent measure to loosen secretions. Elderly persons are frequently reluctant to increase fluid intake and need assistance in planning a schedule for taking fluids. The nurse should assess the availability of a bathroom facility and the patient's ability to use the facility.

Cleansing Secretions from the Airway. The two most effective ways of clearing secretions from the airway are postural drainage and coughing. Both are difficult and strenuous for the elderly patient. When using methods to clear secretions, steps to loosen and thin secretions must be taken first.

Postural Drainage. Although not always used with the elderly patient, postural drainage is a means by which secretions in the lungs are removed by gravity. The positions build tension which helps bring up secretions. The person slowly breathes in through the nose and out through the mouth, while he assumes various postural drainage positions. Nett and Petty (1969) have found four basic positions to be effective in helping to clear secretions. Figures 31-1 illustrates these positions. Because the elderly person may have difficulty in achieving and maintaining a particular position, this procedure should be done with a respiratory therapist, nurse, or instructed family member present to evaluate the patient's ability to tolerate the indicated position and the effectiveness of the method. Postural drainage is contraindicated for patients with increased intracranial pressure, myocardial infarction, or bleeding tendencies. The positions are also difficult and need to be carefully assessed for patients with congestive heart failure, air swallowers, obese individuals, and persons on long term steroid therapy (Bither, 1979; Brannin, 1974). To facilitate the mobilization of secretions, the person assisting the patient claps with cupped hands on the portion of the chest wall being drained. Obviously, the patient's strength and medical condition will determine his endurance of the measure and how vigorously it is carried out.

Coughing. Effective coughing also mobilizes secretion. The elderly patient must be taught how to cough, not just told to cough. For best results, the patient should be in a sitting position, leaning slightly forward, with neck flexed and feet supported. A pillow may be placed on his lap and pressure applied to assist in raising the diaphragm. The older patient may find it difficult to maintain the position, so it is best to have someone to help him do so.

Secretions are mobilized upward by repeated bending forward and sitting up. The patient drops his head, sinks his chest, and slowly bends forward while blowing out air with slightly parted or pursed lips. As he sits up, he is told to slowly breathe in through his nose. When the patient is ready to cough, he takes a deep abdominal breath, then bends

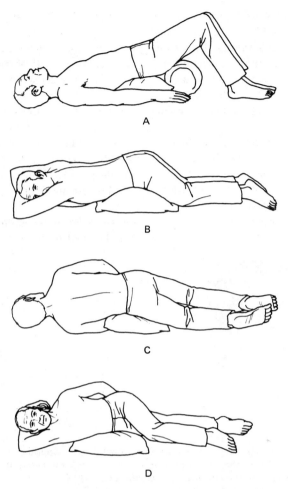

Figure 31-1. Positions for postural drainage. (a) supine position, (b) prone position, (c) right lateral position, (d) left lateral position (adapted from Nett and Petty, 1969).

forward and produces a soft, staccato cough. A slow expiratory flow should be emphasized to avoid air trapping and thus trapping of mucus. Patients, families, and caretakers need to be taught that non-productive coughing will only increase irritation and cause the bronchi to become sore and swollen. In summary, coughing measures need to be individualized, based upon age, disease state, ability to adequately generate expiratory flow, and general physical condition. (Lagerson, 1974, Modrak et al., 1975)

Breathing Retraining. The older COPD patient with dyspnea needs to be taught slowly and deliberately a pattern of slow, controlled, and relaxed abdominal-diaphragmatic breathing. It is important for him to recognize that when dyspnea is present, there is considerable muscle tension and expenditure of energy when he tries to improve the air flow by rapidly moving air in and out of his lungs. The increase in respiratory rate is wasted effort, and the patient usually does not have the necessary energy reserve. The technique of abdominal-diaphragmatic breathing will decrease respiratory effort and increase ventilation. The purpose is to reactivate and strengthen the diaphragm (Modrak et al., 1975). Have the patient relax, protrude the abdomen, and slowly draw air into his lungs through his nose. Have the patient remain relaxed, purse his lips, and let air escape through his mouth on exhalation. Have him feel how the abdomen draws in, thus putting pressure on the diaphragm. Not only does this slow the rate of breathing, but many authorities believe that by pursing the lips, pressure is exerted on the conducting airways, keeping them open and allowing more air to escape from the lungs (Clark, 1972). Pursed lip breathing is illustrated in Figure 31-2.

For abdominal-diaphragmatic breathing to be successful, there is usually the need for considerable instruction and practice of exercises which help strengthen the functional ability of the diaphragm and abdominal muscles. This is especially true for older persons. Gentle physical support, time for repetition, and evaluative feedback are needed to encourage the often weary, lonely, angry, or frightened older patient. Figures 31-3 and 31-4 illustrate exercises that aid diaphragmatic breathing.

As individual exercises are mastered, they must be combined in a pattern to be effective and must be performed every few hours. Resting after three or four deep breaths prevents light-headedness. Key points for the patient to remember are to concentrate on taking slow and deep breaths, and to use pursed lip breathing when practicing diaphragmatic breathing.

Muscle Relaxation and Physical Reconditioning. Muscle relaxation is important because of

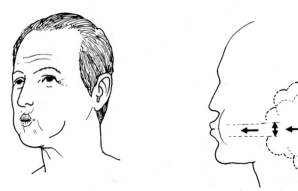

Figure 31-2. Pursed lip breathing. In pursed lip breathing, the lips are tightened as if to blow into a trumpet or other musical instrument. After inhaling, the air is forced out through the pursed lips. The patient will automatically use the diaphragm to do this (adapted from Modrak et al., 1975).

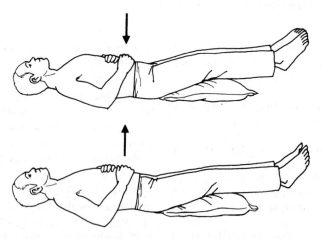

Figure 31-3. Front expansion. Place one hand in center of abdomen and other hand on upper chest. Exhale slowly, through pursed lips, pulling abdomen muscles inward and pushing gently with hand on abdomen. Inhale slowly through nose, with abdomen expanded outward. The hands help the patient know and monitor the length and depth of his respirations (adapted from Modrak et al., 1975).

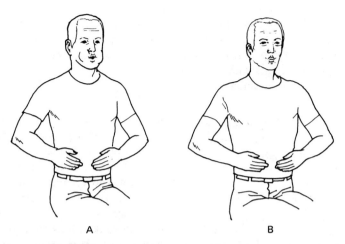

Figure 31-4. Lower side rib breathing: (a) in sitting position with good posture, place hands on sides at base of ribs and, with pursed lips, exhale slowly, (b) through nose, inhale slowly, allowing ribs to expand outward against hands (adapted from Modrak et al., 1975).

excessive oxygen consumption when a person feels tension or anxiety, and when he overworks his muscles.

Muscle Relaxation. Sitting is an excellent time to use muscle relaxation technique. The patient should sit at a desk or table, with knees under the table top and feet flat on the floor, leaning slightly forward from hips with back straight. The patient's head, shoulders, upper chest, and arms should be comfortably supported with pillows. With eyes closed, the patient then "talks" to individual muscle groups, saying, "Let go" with each sighing-type exhalation (Lagerson, 1974). Patients can also be taught to use muscle relaxation technique in bed. They should be on a comfortable surface with pillows placed under head and knees. Calm and quiet surroundings are helpful (Broussard, 1979).

Physical Reconditioning. The goals of a physical reconditioning exercise program are to prevent further muscular weakening and to increase tolerance for physical activity. A program for older individuals should consist of graded exercises, particularly walking, that are planned and individualized. The nurse can be of particular benefit to the older person by helping him to gain confidence and participate in the program (Futrell, Brovender, McKinnon-Mullett, and Brower, 1980; Murray, Huelskoetter, and O'Driscoll, 1980). The activities of

daily living are an essential part of the graded exercises for the elderly patient. As the patient participates in a graded exercise program and increases tolerance to exercises, it should become increasingly possible for him to accomplish and maintain activity of daily living tasks, expending less energy with lower oxygen consumption (Futrell et al., 1980; Murray et al., 1980; Nett and Petty, 1969); see Table 31-6.

Skeletal muscles, specialized heart muscles, and respiratory muscles are the three major groups involved in the exercises. For the patient to successfully perform all of the exercises and receive the most benefit, the airways should be cleared by methods previously described. Total body relaxation techniques should be performed if the patient is tense; if diaphragmatic and pursed lip breathing has been prescribed, this should be practiced during the exercises. Exercises that strengthen abdominal muscles and increase mobility of the rib cage are illustrated in Figure 31-5 through 31-9.

Diet

Diet is of utmost importance for older patients with COPD to enable them to meet their increased energy expenditures. A diet high in protein and low in gas-forming foods is usually recommended. Eating four to five small meals a day prevents a feeling of fullness. Keeping sputum thin by maintaining high fluid intake is important and helpful unless contraindicated (e.g., the patient with right-sided heart failure). Many elderly patients have poor nutrition, and it is not uncommon for patients with COPD to lose their appetite; therefore, assistance in meal

---

Table 31-6. Specific Breathing Rules for the Person with COPD to Maintain Activities of Daily Living (ADL).

For all activities of daily living:
Take a deep breath before performing work.
Exhale slowly while doing work.
The period of activity should not exceed the period of exhalation.
Perform all activities in rhythm with breathing.
Activities that involve any forward flex in motion such as putting on socks, tying shoes, picking things up from floor, aid exhalation.
Exhalation should be twice as long as inhalation.

To stand up from a sitting position:
Take a deep breath.
Come to a standing position while slowly exhaling through pursed lips.

To climb stairs:
Take a deep breath.
Exhale slowly while ascending stairs (pursed lips?).
Rest and repeat.

To push a broom or vacuum cleaner:
Take a deep breath.
Exhale slowly through pursed lips while pushing object.
Rest and repeat movement.

---

planning, nutrition education, socialization, and encouragement in eating are necessary (Lagerson, 1974; Modrak et al., 1975).

Education

Since the majority of elderly pulmonary patients are being cared for in home settings, the education of patients and those caring for them is critical to the success of the treatment program. The teaching-learning process includes: description of the disease, understanding and acceptance of the disease, knowledge of the limitations the disease imposes, and the role of patient and care givers in the treatment program (Clark, 1972). Chronic obstructive pulmonary disease is frightening and life threatening, and it restricts mobility. This is most significant for older patients. Therefore, enough time should be planned to provide for teaching and reinforcement of material, while keeping in mind that the hearing and vision of the older person may also be affected.

Psychosocial Aspects

The psychosocial aspects of aging are discussed in detail elsewhere in this book, but it must be emphasized again that they have crucial significance for older patients with COPD. The patient with COPD is faced with living with a chronic,

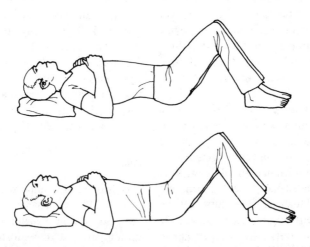

Figure 31-5. Contraction of abdominal muscles with pelvic tilt: lie on back, knees flexed, feet flat on floor; exhale, contracting abdominal muscles and rolling hips under, so back is flat on floor; relax, rest, then repeat (adapted from Modrak et al., 1975).

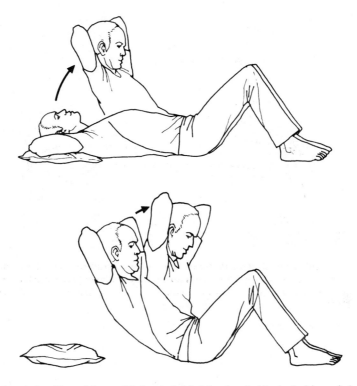

Figure 31-6. Head and shoulder raising: with hands behind head and chin tucked in, exhale slowly and raise head and shoulders as far as possible; return to starting position, rest, and repeat (adapted from Modrak et al., 1975).

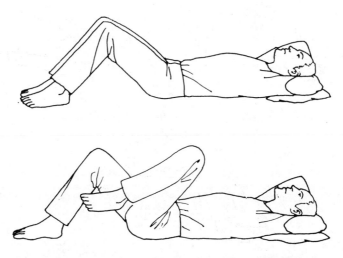

Figure 31-7. Knee bending: Lie on back, knees flexed, feet flat on floor; bring left knee toward left shoulder while exhaling, pressing small of back against floor; return to original position, relax, repeat on right side (adapted from Modrak et al., 1975).

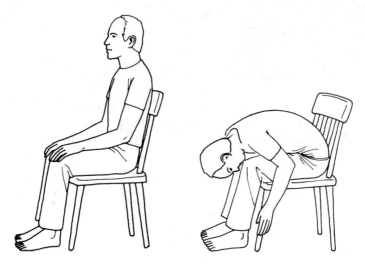

Figure 31-8. Forward bending: sit in straight-backed chair — feet slightly apart and flat on floor, shoulders and arms relaxed; drop head to chest, slowly rolling body forward toward knees while exhaling; return slowly to upright position — pushing lower, then middle, then upper back against the chair; relax, inhale, and repeat (adapted from Modrak et al., 1975).

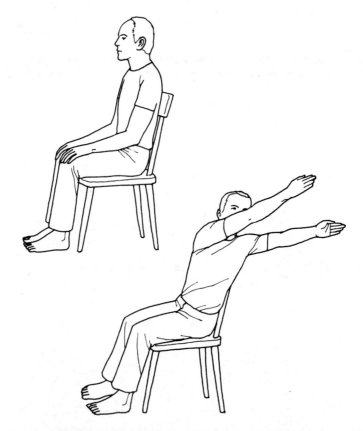

Figure 31-9. Trunk turning with shoulder loosening: sit in straight-backed chair; turn trunk to left, swinging outstretched arms over left shoulder (head should follow movement of hands); bounce arms a few times; return to starting position, rest, and repeat on other side (adapted from Modrak et al., 1975).

sometimes disabling, progressive, and irreversible condition that affects major organ systems and is threatening to life. There is usually a response of apprehension, anxiety, and fear of the unknown, as well as a fear of death. This fear is often expressed in anger, denial, depression, dependency, or demanding behavior (Clark, 1972). The most common response is depression. The elderly person may already be experiencing a number of losses — physical, personal, and social. It is essential that the nurse empathize and view these elderly patients as unique individuals coping with devastating conditions that have little promise of reversal (see Chapter 5 for basic human needs).

REFERENCES

Atwood, J. Cardiovascular problems. In Carnevali, D.L. and Patrick, M. (Eds.) *Nursing Management for the Elderly*. Philadelphia: J.B. Lippincott, 1979, pp. 247–273.

Bither, S. Respiratory Problems. In Carnevali, D.L., and Patrick, M. (Eds.) *Nursing Management for the Elderly*. Philadelphia: J.B. Lippincott, 1979. pp. 427–456.

Brannin, P.K. Oxygen therapy and measures of bronchial hygiene. *Nursing Clinics of North America* 9(1):111–121 (1974).

Broussard, R. Using relaxation for COPD. *American Journal of Nursing* 79:1962–1963 (November 1979).

Clark, N. The elderly person with chronic obstructive pulmonary disease. In Long, J.M. (Ed.) *Caring for and Caring about Elderly People*. Rochester Regional Medical Program and the University of Rochester School of Nursing, 1972.

Cohen, J.D. Cardiac rehabilitation: a multidisciplinary team approach. *Journal of Cardiovascular and Pulmonary Technology* 7:45–46 (October-November 1979).

Comoss, P.M., Burke, E.A., and Swails, S.H. *Cardiac Rehabilitation: A Comprehensive Nursing Approach*. Philadelphia: J.B. Lippincott, 1979, p. 334.

Dehn, M.M. The effects of exercise. *American Journal of Nursing* 80(3):435–440 (1980).

Douglas, J.E., David, T., and Wilkes, I. Reconditioning cardiac patients. *American Family Physician* 2(1):123–129 (1975).

Fardy, P.S. Cardiac rehabilitation program focuses on total patients. *Hospitals, Journal of the American Hospital Association* 52:101–108 (November 1978).

Futrell, M., Brovender, S., McKinnon-Mullett, E., and Brower, H.F. *Primary Health Care of the Older Adult*. Mass.: Duxbury Press, 1980.

Harris, R. Special features of heart disease in the elderly patient. *Working with Older People*, Vol. 4. Washington, D.C.: U.S. Department of Health, Education and Welfare, 1971, pp. 81–102.

Hoskins, T.A. and Habasevich, R. Cardiac rehabilitation – an overview. *Physical Therapy* 58(10):1183–1190 (1978).

Jones, L.N. Hypertension: medical and nursing implications. *Nursing Clinics of North America* 2(2):283–295 (1976).

Lagerson, J. Nursing care of patients with pulmonary insufficiency. *Nursing Clinics of North America* 9(1):165–179 (1974).

Mannerberg, D. Rehabilitation of cardiovascular diseases in a USA centre. *Chest Heart Stroke Journal* 3:62–65 (May 1979).

Maxwell, F.S. *The Measure of My Days*. New York: Penguin Books, 1968.

Mock, M.B. Rehabilitation of the elderly cardiac patient hampered by bias. *Geriatrics* 22–23 (December 1977).

Modrak, M., Moser, K., Archibald, C., Hansen, P., Birgitta, E., Beaman, A., and Dunn, D. *Better Living and Breathing: A Manual for Patients*. St. Louis: C.V. Mosby, 1975.

Moody, L. Primer for pulmonary hygiene. *American Journal of Nursing* 77:104–106 (1977).

Murray, R., Huelskoetter, M.M., and O'Driscoll, D. *The Nursing Process in Later Maturity*. Englewood Cliffs, N.J.: Prentice-Hall, 1980.

Nett, L. and Petty, T. Patient education and emphysema care. *Medical Times* 97:117–130 (1969).

Niccoli, A. and Brammell, H.L. A program for rehabilitation in coronary heart disease. *Nursing Clinics of North America* 2(2):237–250 (1976).

Ogden, L.D. Activity guidelines for early subacute and high-risk cardiac patients. *American Journal of Occupational Therapy* 33(5):291–298 (1979).

Pathy, M.S. Clinical presentation of myocardial infarction in the elderly. *British Heart Journal* 29:190 (1967).

Pinneo, R. The elderly person with congestive heart failure. In Long, J.M. (Ed.) *Caring for and Caring about Elderly People – A Guide to the Rehabilitative Approach*. Philadelphia: J.B. Lippincott, 1972, pp. 59–68.

Roben, N.L. Hypertension. In Carnevali, D.L. and Patrick, M. (Eds.) *Nursing Management for the Elderly*. Philadelphia: J.B. Lippincott, 1979, pp. 371–385.

Roberts, S. Cardiopulmonary abnormalities in aging. In Burnside, I.M. (Ed.) *Nursing and the Aged*. 2nd Ed. New York: McGraw-Hill, 1981, pp. 286–316.

Steffl, B. and Eide, I. *Handbook on Discharge Planning*. Thorofare, N.J.: C.B. Slack, 1978.

Timiras, P.S. Disease of aging. In Timiras, P.S. (Ed.) *Developmental Physiology and Aging*. New York: Macmillan, 1972, p. 474.

Waxler, R. The patient with congestive heart failure – teaching implications. *Nursing Clinics of North*

America 2(2):297–307 (1976).

Wenger, N.K. Benefits of a rehabilitation program following myocardial infarction. *Geriatrics* 64–67 (July 1973).

Williams, M. and Fardy, P.S. Limitations in prescribing exercise. *Journal of Cardiovascular and Pulmonary Technology* 8:33–36 (December-January 1980).

Winslow, E.H. and Weber, T.M. Progressive exercise to combat the hazards of bedrest. *American Journal of Nursing* 80(3):440–445 (1980).

32
Stroke Rehabilitation

Marilyn S. Giss

All human capabilities must be used regularly if they are to be kept at the highest peak of efficiency.

U.S. Department of Health, Education and Welfare and U.S. Public Health Service (1969)

Of the two million Americans who survive a stroke every year, most are elderly and will be hemiplegic (Hirschberg, 1976). Stroke is the third leading cause of death and the main cause of locomotor defects (Murray, Huelskoetter, and O'Driscoll, 1980). Although there will be differences in the amount and kind of rehabilitation needed for these persons, the overall goal for anyone with a stroke should be to prevent complications and resulting secondary disabilities, and to promote activity within the patient's current limitations to enhance his quality of life.

It has been estimated that approximately 90% of elderly hemiplegics have positive rehabilitation potential soon after a stroke, but if prolonged bed rest and an effective rehabilitation program are not implemented, this potential is diminished (Hirschberg, 1976). Strength and endurance are lost for every day of immobility, and three days of activity are required to regain the loss of each day (Kottke, 1966). Eric Muller (1970) reports that strength is lost at a rate of 5% a day. With elderly persons, there is frequently a loss of strength that was present prior to the stroke, and if the patient is kept inactive for two or more weeks after the stroke, disuse atrophy further weakens muscles. All too often there is the misperception that little or nothing can be done for the patient suffering from a stroke (Anderson and Kottke, 1978).

The objectives of stroke rehabilitation are to maintain medical stability, improve functional status, and assist family and patient in adjusting to any residual long term disability (Granger, Dewis, Peters, Sherwood, and Barrett, 1979). Therefore, it is essential that early rehabilitation measures be instituted at the time of the stroke, whether or not the patient is admitted to the hospital. In addition to seeing that major physical needs are met, such as maintenance of a patent airway and adequate nutrition, two other primary aspects of physical care must be provided during this acute or bed phase: proper positioning and passive range of motion exercises.

POSITIONING

Positioning is vital during this acute stage. When an extremity is paralyzed, muscle action that would normally assist venous return to the heart and lymphatic drainage of tissue fluids is not present, and there is accumulation of fluid in the tissues. As a result, there is inadequate nutrition to cells which leads to tissue breakdown. The arm, hand, leg, and foot need to be supported to prevent secondary disabilities, e.g., contractures, decubiti, pain (Kavchak-Keyes, 1979). Figures 32-1, 32-2, and 32-3 demonstrate the correct alignment for the person in the supine, lateral, and prone positions.

The prone position, although not frequently used, is an excellent position to maintain good body alignment. If a patient is not used to sleeping on his abdomen and/or is fearful of this, the amount of time that he will be able to maintain this position may be very limited at first. In working with older patients, the writer has found that with careful explanation this position can be tolerated initially for 5–10 minutes, as long as the patient is not having respiratory complications. If someone stays with the patient during this time, there is less resistance to being in the prone position and

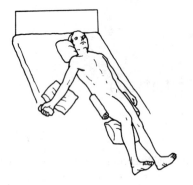

Figure 32-1. Supine position.

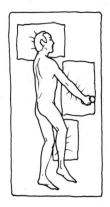

Figure 32-2. Lateral position.

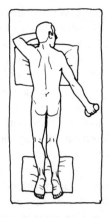

Figure 32-3. Prone position.

the amount of time can be increased gradually. Proper positioning of all extremities, head, neck, and torso is extremely important, and with the use of pillows this can be done so that complications do not develop.

The routine time established for turning a patient is every two hours. This is too long for the stroke patient to lie on the affected side because of the accumulation of fluid which can result in edema. A more appropriate and effective method is to position the patient on his unaffected side for two hours at a time and on the affected side for no more than 20 minutes, four times a day (Large et al., 1969).

EXERCISES

Passive Range of Motion Exercises

The purpose of passive range of motion (ROM) exercises is to aid in lessening edema and preventing contractures. They are not used to strengthen muscles and should be done within the framework of the patient's activity orders. Although a physical therapist may be involved in prescribing exercises, every nurse caring for the stroke patient should be able to perform the exercises competently. Equally important as exercise is establishing a schedule for doing them (a minimum of three times a day) and deciding the number of times each exercise should be repeated. All should be individualized for the patient. The numbers should be gradually increased to the patient's tolerance. Each exercise is only carried out to the point of pain or resistance. Exercises for the uninvolved side are also needed. Range of motion movements for the head and neck and for the upper and lower extremities, although not all inclusive, are diagrammed in Figures 32-1 through 32-9. As the medical condition stabilizes and activity is increased, these exercises should be incorporated into daily activities during bathing, eating, turning in bed, standing, etc. Encourage the patient to do as much for himself as possible.

Isometric and Isotonic Exercises

Isometric exercises are those in which muscles are alternately tightened and relaxed without moving joints, and isotonic exercises are those in which muscles shorten under a constant load in the process of doing work (Brower and Hicks, 1972). A physical therapist usually sees

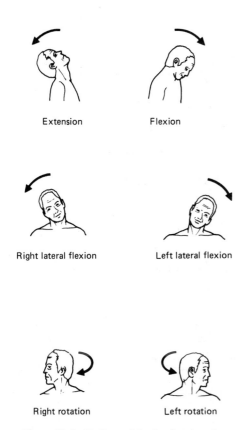

Extension   Flexion

Right lateral flexion   Left lateral flexion

Right rotation   Left rotation

Figure 32-4. Motions of the head and neck.

patients for progressive resistive exercises (isotonic).

Kelly (1966) found that isometric exercises "are of value and particularly useful for maintaining the tone of the postural muscles of the buttocks, abdomen, and thighs. The patient can set the quadriceps, gluteal and abdominal muscles separately, or he may set all of them simultaneously by lying supine with legs extended and hands at his sides, then lifting his buttocks off the bed, bearing his weight on shoulders and heels." The hemiplegic patient is not likely to be able to set the muscles simultaneously, but he may be able to set each muscle group individually as return in muscle function increases. The patient's ability to follow through with exercises will also depend upon his ability to understand and comprehend tasks and to retain information for repeating the exercise program at a later interval. Remember that in teaching any new task, it normally takes the older person longer to learn, and there

always needs to be reinforcement of information. Consistency in approach and having the same nurse care for the patient on a daily basis are ideal ways to achieve this.

Exercises that are incorporated into a program for the patient should be written out as to kind, amount, and frequency. Exercises are then increased as the patient's condition and activity level dictate, and progress is recorded for long range evaluation.

It is important to remember that ROM exercises are intended to maintain normal range of motion of joints and prevent contractures; they do not strengthen the muscles. However, by starting immediately with a series of sit-up or stand-up exercises, mobility is initiated and strengthening of muscles is begun (Cummins, Harris, Materson, Sarno, and Shahani, 1979; Hirschberg, 1976). Cummins et al. (1979) identify a "sit-up" phase in which the patient practices sitting at the edge of the bed in order to regain his balance.

Guidelines for Sit-up Phase.

- Slightly elevate head of bed initially. This will make it easier and less discouraging for the patient.
- Have half of side rail in up position. Patient should be close to side of bed from which he is getting up, but safe so that he will not roll off edge when he turns on side.
- Patient, using uninvolved hand, grabs hold of side rail and turn toward uninvolved side.
- Patient pulls self to sitting position, lowering legs off bed by putting uninvolved leg under involved ankle. This latter step may not be feasible initially so assistance should be given when needed. Protection of the involved arm is also important to avoid subluxation of the shoulder.
- Patient sits on side of bed to regain balance.

This procedure should be done 3–6 times per day. The older person can easily become discouraged, particularly if other losses have

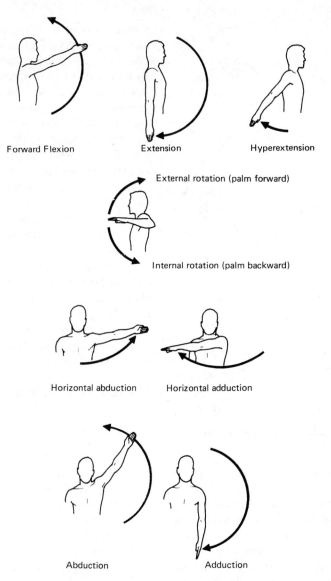

Figure 32-5. Motions of the upper extremities.

recently occurred and he feels that there is nothing worth living for. Therefore, it is imperative that the nurse encourage the patient and explain the steps to be followed throughout the procedure. As stated in earlier chapters, it is important to instill and restore "hope."

Guidelines and Steps for Stand-up Exercise.

- Have patient sitting in stable chair with armrests. If using wheelchair, brakes should be locked. The seat of the chair should be high enough so that patient can move forward and stand up unassisted. As patient's strength increases, the seat is lowered.
- Patient should sit toward edge of chair so that he is able to rise nearly straight up, rather than having to lean forward and stand.
- Both feet should be flat on the floor, approximately shoulder width apart and perpendicular to the knees.

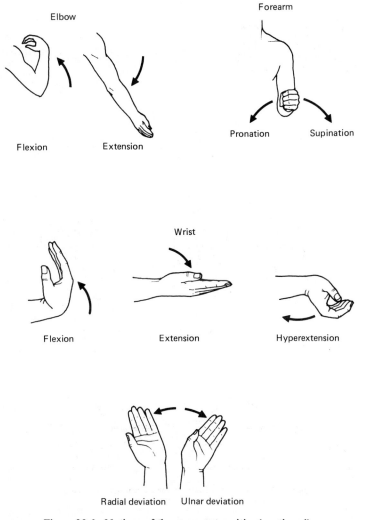

Figure 32-6. Motions of the upper extremities (continued).

- Explain the procedure slowly, looking directly at patient while demonstrating. Have patient push with uninvolved hand on armrest, while bringing self to standing position.
- Plan exercise period around other activities and when patient's energy level is high.
- The number of times the patient stands up in one exercise period and the number of exercise periods should be individualized and reassessed regularly. One may start by doing 2–5 stand-up exercises 3–4 times per day. Whatever is initiated has to be recorded as to time, amount, and patient's ability and tolerance. The number of exercises in each period and the number of exercise periods can then gradually be increased according to patient's strength and endurance.
- The nurse needs to know patient's overall general medical condition, as well as the amount of exercise and activity patient had prior to stroke, in order to set realistic goals (Hirschberg, 1976).

The advantages of a stand-up exercise program (Hirschberg, 1976) are:

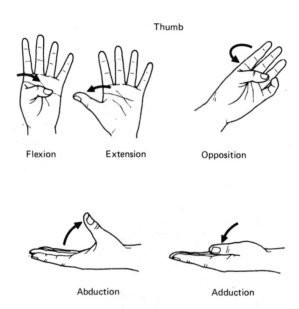

Figure 32-7. Motions of the upper extremities (continued).

- It can be started immediately after a Cerebrovascular Accident (CVA).
- It can be used with aphasic (and slightly obtunded) patients.
- Patient's strength is improved.
- Patient's self-confidence is enhanced.
- Secondary disabilities are prevented.

After several weeks, when the patient is able to support his body with the uninvolved leg, a two-legged exercise program, such as stair climbing, should be initiated. "Stair climbing arouses less fear in the patient if he can begin by coming down the stairs backward" (Hirschberg, 1976). This continues to strengthen the leg; in addition, the patient learns to raise the uninvolved leg and take even, measured steps. During this time, the patient should be wearing a short leg brace.

ACTIVITIES OF DAILY LIVING (ADL)

The evaluation, treatment plan, and ongoing therapy provided by occupational therapy are invaluable for the patient who has had a stroke. Unfortunately, these are often neglected simply because the person is old! Whenever this modality of care can be provided, the referral for an evaluation and plan of therapy should be initiated early. Although there is some overlap in the therapy provided by the occupational therapist and the physical therapist, the goals of each are specific. An evaluation by the occupational therapist (Wingerson, 1976) includes:

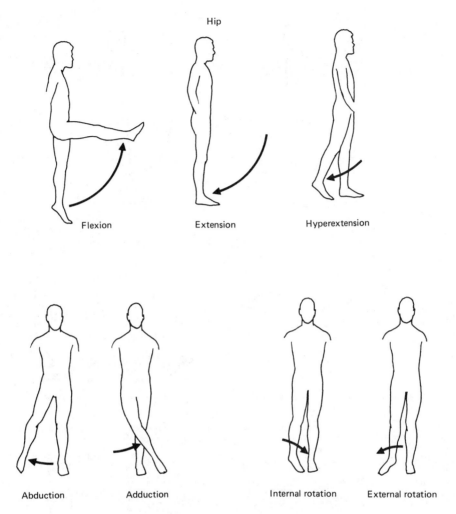

Figure 32-8. Motions of the lower extremities.

- Objective measurements of joint range of motion.
- Measurement of muscle strength.
- An assessment as to the presence or absence of increased muscle tone. With severe spasticity, deformities may result unless preventive measures are instituted.
- Testing for proprioception and sensation. When there are deficits in this area, the patient may not be using his extremity in a functional manner even though range of motion and strength are sufficient.
- Evaluation of how patient uses or attempts to use an affected extremity.
- Evaluation of self-care level:

a) How much assistance does person need from someone else, and what equipment is necessary?
b) How safe and efficient is person in performing tasks such as feeding, dressing, personal hygiene?
- Evaluation of sensorimotor skills.
- Evaluation of short term and long term memory. It will be important to know a patient's ability to register and retrieve information in teaching relearning of tasks or new ways to do tasks.

In promoting the ADL of an individual, the nurse may be the first one to assess the individual

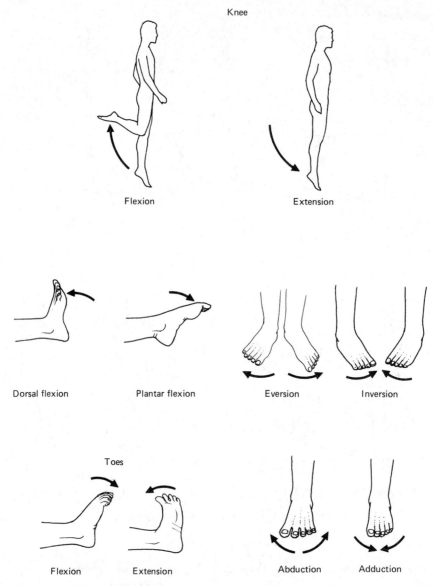

Figure 32-9. Mobility of the lower extremities (continued).

and, in certain instances, may not have the resources of an occupational therapist. The following guidelines are offered to assist the nurse in planning care to increase the functional ability of the older person when occupational and physical therapists are not available.

- Establish a baseline as to what the patient can do, either on his own initiative or with instruction. Feeding, dressing, and bathing are examples of ADL to be assessed.

- Assess amount of assistance that is needed.
- Assess whether person is neglecting one side of his body or one side of object on which he is working.
- Assess the amount of difficulty the person has in relating objects to other things in space, e.g., putting a glass on a table, an arm in a sleeve, a washcloth in a pan of water.
- Assess ability to follow directions.
- Assess safety measures that patient takes in performing tasks.

After the initial baseline data are obtained, the information should be available to all who will be caring for the patient, as well as to the patient and significant others. Some type of chart kept in the patient's room is helpful. The following ongoing assistance should be included in the patient's plan of care:

- Continue to have patient do those things he is capable of doing.
- Introduce new tasks one at a time, using simple directions, given one at a time, by the same person over a period of time.
- Update chart as to what patient can do.
- Encourage patient in what he is doing. Set realistic goals consistent with life-style.
- Have family members or a significant other observe what patient can do. Encourage them to participate in his care as indicated and needed.

COMMUNICATION

Following a CVA, the patient is frequently not able to express his needs. This may be due to coma, confusion, disorientation, or aphasia. The patient with aphasia will be apprehensive and frustrated. Family members and those caring for him will also find this a frightening and frustrating problem. Aphasia in its broadest sense means loss of language. Generally, *expressive aphasia* is the inability of a person to communicate verbally or in writing. *Receptive aphasia* is the inability to understand verbal or written communication. Most often the person with aphasia has a mixture of both expressive and receptive aphasia. In order to establish effective communication and help the patient, family members, and staff to understand the specific problem, a speech evaluation followed with a specific treatment program by a speech pathologist is crucial. Nurses should be aware of this, facilitate referral to the speech pathologist, and incorporate the approach or plan into the nursing care plans. All personnel and family members must be consistent in the approach that is established. Whether or not a speech evaluation has been initiated, the following are some general rules to follow when caring for the patient who has aphasia.

- Speak slowly; do not shout.
- When talking to patient, give simple directions — *one at a time*. Let patient attempt to perform action; then continue with another step in the procedure.
- When communicating with patient, limit other distractions such as TV, radio, or other conversation in the room.
- Associate words with objects either by using pictures or by pointing to objects.
- Do not assume that the patient who answers yes and no comprehends what you are saying or asking.
- Use repetition and redundancy in explaining procedures to be done. Orient person frequently to who he is, where he is, day, time, and who you are.
- Even if patients do not respond verbally, do not stop talking to them throughout the day.
- Encourage family members to talk to afflicted person.
- Encourage family members to bring in small, familiar objects and to name them.

See Table 32-1 for a list of the types of aphasia.

The nurse must assess the patient's level of orientation and communication patterns prior to the CVA and whether there was a visual or hearing problem. Usually this is done by talking with the family and or significant others and asking questions such as, Was the patient oriented to date, time, place, and name? Does the patient normally use a hearing aid?

PSYCHOLOGICAL SUPPORT

Physical changes in the body that normally occur with aging often represent a loss to the older person, such as loss of function and loss of energy. When a catastrophic condition such as a stroke occurs in addition to normal changes and losses, this represents devastating changes in one's body image.

The patient with a stroke generally finds himself with a sudden disabling condition; he is confronted with the necessity of adjustment to a far more disabling problem than existed in his residual condition. He finds himself uncertain

Table 32-1. Types of Aphasia.

Expressive aphasia (apraxia)	Also called Broca's aphasia. Inability to produce desired language. Loss of facility of using or understanding spoken and written language.
Receptive aphasia (agnosia)	Also called Wernicke's aphasia. Inability to comprehend language. Partial or total inability to recognize objects by use of senses.
Global aphasia (mixed)	Combines all of the above. No communication is retained.
Dysphasia	Partial impairment.
Dysarthria	Articulatory dysfunction.

in his ability to cope with physical surroundings, to participate in his social world, and to see himself as a valued person (Elwood, 1970). The impact of a stroke in a loved one, its residual effects, and long term rehabilitation measures also present tremendous problems for spouse and family (McCormick and Williams, 1979).

The importance of ascertaining information about the person's previous life-style, habits, activities, and work cannot be overemphasized. Realistic goals can be established from this, and potential problems and needs can be identified. Setting goals that are unrealistic, unobtainable, and incompatible with the patient's expectations will only promote an environment that is frustrating for the patient, family, and staff. From the onset and throughout the rehabilitation process, it is necessary that the patient and family be included in planning his care and in setting goals and that you let the patient know what you want him to do. Make sure that the patient is given an opportunity to make choices that affect his welfare. For example, if you plan to see that a patient is up in a wheelchair four times a day, you need to share this with him at the beginning of the day and reinforce it as the day progresses. He may indicate that he does not want to get up, but you can let him make choices by asking, for example, "Do you want to get up now for 15 minutes or in an hour for 15 minutes?" "Do you want to sit at the nurses' station or here by the window?"

Although depression is common among patients who have a chronic and often irreversible condition, it can be a favorable sign that the patient is facing reality, which is essential if he is to participate successfully in the rehabilitation process. To help regain a feeling of self-worth, he needs to succeed in tasks that increase his independence. In summary, some important points in the care of an elderly stroke victim are:

- Give him time to complete a task.
- Set goals that are realistic, recognizing that the patient's disability is as he perceives it. Asking him to reach goals of others leads to frustration and failure.
- Emphasize his strengths and abilities rather than his disabilities.
- Obtain accurate data as to how he functioned physically, socially, psychologically, and intellectually prior to the insult of stroke.

REFERENCES

Anderson, T.P. and Kottke, F.J. Stroke rehabilitation: a reconsideration of some common attitudes. *Archives of Physical Medicine and Rehabilitation* **59**: 175–180 (April 1978).

Bonner, C.D. *Homburger and Bonner's Medical Care and Rehabilitation of the Aged and Chronically Ill* (3rd ed.). Boston: Little, Brown, 1974.

Brower, P. and Hicks, D. Maintaining muscle function in patients on bedrest. *American Journal of Nursing* **72**(7):1250–1253 (1972).

Cummins, B.J., Harris, T.R., Materson, R.S., Sarno, J.E., and Shahani, B. Stroke: mobilizing and planning therapy. *Patient Care* **13**:50–52 (January 1979). (a)

Cummins, B.J., Harris, T.R., Materson, R.S., Sarno, J.E., and Shahani, B. Stroke: post hospital care and follow-up. *Patient Care* **13**:94–95 (January 1979). (b)

Elwood, E. Nursing the patient with a cerebral vascular accident. *Nursing Clinics of North America* **5**(1):47–53 (1970).

Granger, C.V., Dewis, L.S., Peters, N.C., Sherwood, C.C., and Barrett, J.E. Stroke rehabilitation: analysis of repeated barthel index measures. *Archives of Physical Medicine and Rehabilitation* **60**:14–17 (January 1979).

Hirschberg, G.G. Ambulation and self-care are goals of rehabilitation after stroke. *Geriatrics* 61–65 (May 1976).

Hirschberg, G.G., Lewis, L., and Vaughn, P. *Rehabilitation, A Manual for the Care of the Disabled and Elderly* (2nd ed.). Philadelphia: J.B. Lippincott, 1976.

Kavchak-Keyes, M.A. Come back from disaster: helping the stroke patient to learn to help himself. *Nursing '79* 9:32–35 (January 1979).

Kelly, M.M. Exercises for bedfast patients. *American Journal of Nursing* 66(10):2209–2213 (1966).

Kottke, F.J. The effects of limitation of activity upon the human body. *Journal of the American Medical Association* 196: 826 (June 1966).

Large, H., Tuthill, F., Bryan, K., and Dogen, T.J. In the first stroke Intensive Care Unit. *American Journal of Nursing*, Vol. 69, January 1969, pp. 76–80.

Linde, M. Cerebrovascular accidents. In Carnevali, D.L. and Patrick, M. (Eds) *Nursing Management of the elderly*. Philadelphia: J.B. Lippincott, 1979.

McCormick, G.P. and Williams, M. Stroke: the double crisis. *American Journal of Nursing* 79:1410–1411 (August 1979).

Muller, E.A. Influence of training and of inactivity on muscle strength. *Archives of Physical Medicine and Rehabilitation* 51:449 (August 1970).

Murray, R., Huelskoetter, M.M., and O'Driscoll, D. *The Nursing Process in Later Maturity*. Englewood Cliffs, N.J.: Prentice-Hall, 1980.

Stryker, R.P. *Rehabilitative Aspects of Acute and Chronic Nursing Care*. Philadelphia: W.B. Saunders, 1972.

U.S. Department of Health, Education and Welfare and U.S. Public Health Service. *Working with Older People* (Publication No. 1459), Vol. 1. Revised March 1969.

U.S. Government Printing Office. *Elementary Rehabilitation in Nursing Care* (Publication No. 1436). Washington, D.C.: U.S. Department of Health, Education and Welfare Division of Nursing, 1966 (reprinted 1970), 99 pp.

Wingerson, E. The value of occupational therapy in rehabilitation. *Geriatrics* 99–101 (May 1976).

Part VII
Special Concerns in
Gerontological Nursing

33
Nutrition and the Elderly

Marianna Cadigan

Let food be thy medicine.

Hippocrates

Nutrition is one of the basic elements of health and health maintenance in all age groups; it becomes even more crucial as we age. There is ample evidence in medical and research literature to indicate that the nutritional status and nutrition behavior of an individual are directly related to health and longevity.

Some obstacles to the maintenance of adequate nutrition in the older population are:

Limited income
Inadequate dentition
Reduced activity leading to poor appetite
Reduced caloric requirements
Sensory alterations leading to fewer taste buds, decreased smell, and lessened sight
Magnitude of medication (drug and alcohol) use
Loneliness, anxiety, fear, and depression

Professionals often fail to realize that older persons are individualistic and become more so with age. Furthermore, in no aspect of their lives is this more formidable than in what they eat and what they believe about food. Actually, the belief in the special magic of foods goes back to the ancient Greeks and Egyptians and, indeed, to the days when Eve convinced Adam to bite the apple and to know good and evil.

Instructions in diet and nutrition practices can help prevent the late life development and progression of disease. Even in disorders of structure or function, not necessarily nutritional in origin, dietary management can improve the results. Good nutritional status of the elderly patient is known to promote the successful outcome of medical treatment.

In addition to promoting the physical health of the elderly, nutrition also contributes to mental and emotional health. The elderly patient's desire to eat is a well-recognized sign of improved physical and mental well-being. The social value of eating meals with others cannot be overemphasized and is needed by so many older adults.

Older individuals are at increasingly high risk for malnutrition as they age. This chapter discusses preventive and therapeutic aspects of nutrition information for professionals, with implications for the counseling and guidance of older people.

NUTRIENT REQUIREMENTS FOR THE ELDERLY

Nutrient requirements remain the same throughout life, but calorie requirements change. The energy and calorie needs are generally reduced as aging progresses, which means calories should be given special consideration. A gradual reduction of caloric needs begins during the young adult years and continues until there is a reduction of approximately 10% in the intake of the adult from 69 years on. A woman's caloric allowance from 51 to 75 years of age is 1800 calories; this decreases to 1600 calories after 76 years of age. The daily caloric allowance for a man from 51 to 75 years of age is 2400 calories; this decreases to 2050 calories after 76 years of age. The decline in energy needs is due to the change in body mass, resting metabolic rate, and reduced physical activity which occur in the aging process. Food intake is often reduced in people entering the late middle years, which helps to meet the reduced energy needs. If this does not occur, there is apt to be a buildup of fat tissue which contributes to the incidence of obesity in the elderly.

Physical activity varies among the elderly, and those who remain active or participate in new physical activities may not need to reduce caloric intake. The best guideline for an individual is to adjust consumption of food to prevent overweight or underweight (Harper, 1978).

Proteins

The protein allowance for the adult over 50 years of age is the same as for the younger adult, .8 gram per kilogram of body weight. The recommended daily allowance of protein for adults is 56 grams for men and 44 grams for women. Since many foods high in protein are also good sources of iron, thiamine, riboflavin, and niacin, they are considered important food sources when caloric intake must be reduced. Because renal function tends to deteriorate with age and the work of the kidney is increased when protein intake is high, the protein content of the diet should be kept close to 12% of the caloric total (Harper, 1978). A low protein intake usually accompanies a low caloric intake.

Fats

Most sources recommend that the elderly should restrict fat intake to no more than 30-35% of the caloric value of their daily food intake. The controversy over the relationship between fat intake and atherosclerosis and heart disease continues, and little seems to have been done to support the need for a fat-modified or cholesterol-lowering diet for the elderly (Goodhart and Shils, 1975).

Fats and oils are concentrated sources of energy and contribute to caloric intake. Fats are good sources of fat-soluble vitamins A,D,E, and K, and contain essential fatty acids. In general, there is reduced tolerance for fat in later adult years due to slower digestion and metabolism.

Carbohydrates

Adequate carbohydrates are used in the diet as an immediate source of energy to meet the needs of tissue cells, thus sparing protein for tissue building. If the energy needs of the body are not met with carbohydrate, adipose and protein tissue will be used. One gram of carbohydrate provides 4 calories of energy. A diet high in carbohydrate may contribute to overweight in the elderly, since excessive amounts are converted to fat for an energy reserve. See Table 33-1.

Vitamins and Minerals

The need for vitamins and minerals in the elderly differs little from that of younger adults; however, concern for adequate intake may have to be stressed with individuals whose food intake is reduced. Food choices of the elderly may also be limited to foods easy to chew and to likes versus dislikes, thereby reducing adequate nutrient intake. Emphasis should be placed on a diet which includes a variety of foods with the necessary vitamins and minerals.

Since older adults are inclined to preserve, maintain, or improve their health (sometimes in

Table 33-1. Energy/Calorie Sources and Recommendations (Cadigan, 1980).

| SOURCE | PERCENT OF DAILY INTAKE | CALORIC VALUES | | | |
| | | WOMEN | | MEN | |
		51-75 YEARS	76+ YEARS	51-75 YEARS	76+ YEARS
Carbohydrate	50-58	900-1044	800-928	1200-1392	1025-1189
Fat	30-35	540-630	480-560	720-840	615-717
Protein	10-12	180-216	160-192	240-288	205-246
Total caloric intake		1800	1600	2400	2050

NOTE: Based on *Recommended Daily Dietary Allowances* as revised in 1980, Food and Nutrition Board, National Academy of Sciences – National Research Council.

Table 33-2. Essential Nutrients for Older Adults.

NUTRIENT	FOOD SOURCES	FUNCTIONS
Protein	Meat, poultry, and fish Eggs Milk and dairy products Soybeans, dried beans, and peas Nuts Peanut butter	Maintenance of cells and tissues Essential part of body cells, blood enzymes, hormones, and body secretions Synthesis of enzymes needed for digestion and cellular metabolism Formation of antibodies as defense against disease May be used to supply energy
Fat	Vegetable oils Animal fats Butter, margarine Egg yolk Salad dressings Bacon and fatty meats	Supplies essential fatty acids which help maintain normal membranes and skin structure Provides concentrated source of energy Carries fat-soluble vitamins A, D, E, and K
Carbohydrate	Breads and cereals Potatoes, corn, and dry beans Pastas Fruits Sugar, syrup, jam, jelly, honey	Supplies energy Spares protein for tissue building and repair Aids the body in using fat efficiently
Calcium	Milk Cheese and ice cream Canned salmon, sardines (with bones) Dark green leafy vegetables	Helps in building and repairing bones Maintains calcium balance to help prevent bone loss Helps blood clot normally Helps in normal functioning of muscles and heart Aids in transmitting nerve impulses
Phosphorus	Milk, cheese Meat, fish, poultry Egg yolk Whole grain ceral products	Promotes bone formation Helps regulate acid-base balance in body fluids Helps body utilize carbohydrate and fat
Potassium	Banana, avocado, citrus fruit juice, tomato, and apple Meat, poultry Potato, tomato, broccoli	Helps maintain osmotic pressure of the cell and acid-base balance Helps in transmission of nerve impulses and muscle contraction
Iron	Liver, other organ meats Meat and poultry Egg yolk Dried beans and peas Enriched or whole grain cereals Dried fruit, prune juice Dark green leafy vegetables	Combines with protein to make blood hemoglobin which carries oxygen to the cells and tissues Helps cells use oxygen
Zinc	Seafood and meat Whole grain cereals Legumes Nuts Egg yolk	Constituent of enzymes involved in digestion Helps in healing wounds Helps regain appetite, taste, and smell if zinc loss occurred during illness
Fluorine	Water, tea Seafood	May be helpful in maintaining bone structure
Vitamins: A	Liver Yellow and dark green vegetables Yellow fruits Egg yolk Milk and cheese Butter and fortified margarine	Needed in formation of visual purple which helps the eye to adapt to dim light Helps preserve health of epithelial cells Helps keep mucous membranes firm and resistant to infections
D	Fish liver oil Milk (vitamin fortified) Butter and fortified margarine Sunshine (not a food) produces vitamin D from a form of cholesterol in the skin	Enhances absorption of calcium and phosphorus from digestive tract Promotes mineralization of the bones

Table 33-2. Essential Nutrients for Older Adults. (continued)

NUTRIENT	FOOD SOURCES	FUNCTIONS
Vitamins (continued):		
E	Wheat germ oil, vegetable oils Margarine Shortening Wheat germ and cereal products Fruits and vegetables Nuts	Acts as an antioxidant Apparent role in maintaining stability and strength of cell membrane
K	Green leafy vegetables Egg yolk Soybean oil	Appears to be necessary for synthesis of pro-thrombin needed for normal blood clotting Believed to help arrest bone degeneration
C	Citrus fruits and juices Broccoli, cabbage Tomatoes Green peppers Leafy green vegetables White and sweet potatoes Strawberries, cantaloupe	Contributes to the normal functioning of cells Essential in the formation of collagen and to strengthen walls of blood vessels Converts the inactive form of folic acid to the active form Helps in the metabolism of some proteins Enhances the absorption of iron and calcium Helps resist infections and aids in healing wounds
B_1 (thiamine)	Lean pork, organ meats Eggs Whole grain and enriched breads and cereals Green leafy vegetables Nuts and legumes	Aids in the utilization of carbohydrate as a source of energy Appears to be related to functioning of the nervous system Promotes normal appetite and digestion
B_2 (riboflavin)	Milk and cheese Organ meats Eggs Lean meat Leafy green vegetables Whole grain and enriched breads and cereals	Aids in the metabolism of protein, fat, and carbohydrate Necessary for release of energy in the cell Helps keep skin healthy, especially around the mouth, nose, and eyes
Niacin	Liver, lean meat, fish, and poultry Peanuts and peanut butter Beans, peas, other legumes Whole grain or enriched cereals and breads	Aids in the release of energy from carbohydrate, fat, and protein Helps maintain healthy nervous system, healthy skin, and normal digestive system
B_6 (pyridoxine)	Liver, meat, kidney, other meats Dried beans, peanuts, and nuts Whole grain and enriched cereals Egg yolks Bananas, avocados, and corn	Aids in metabolism of protein Helps maintain healthy skin, normal digestion, and healthy nervous system
Folic acid	Green leafy vegetables Liver and kidney Asparagus, lima and kidney beans Whole grain cereals	Helps prevent macrocytic anemia; stimulates the regeneration of red blood cells and hemoglobin Involved in the synthesis of protein
B_{12}	Liver, kidney, and lean meats Milk and cheese Fish Eggs	Aids in normal functioning of nervous tissue Needed for formation of red blood cells Aids in protein synthesis
Water	Drinking water Beverages: coffee, tea, fruit juice, and fruit drinks Soup Milk	Constituent of all body cells Constituent of all body fluids Aids in mastication and softening of food Aids in elimination of waste Helps in moving material through the digestive tract Helps regulate body temperature

desperation), they find dietary supplements such as multivitamin and mineral preparations very appealing. Millions of dollars are spent for these supplements each year — a good percentage of that amount by older adults. The money would be better spent on nutritious foods containing essential requirements. See Table 33-2 for essential nutrients and Table 33-3 for recommended dietary allowances for older age.

The recommended dietary allowances (RDA) were developed to serve as goals for food planning and to act as guides for the interpretation of food intake. The Food and Nutrition Board (1980) designed these guides to be adequate for practically all age populations of the United States; an allowance for a margin of safety for individual variations is included. The RDA are used only as a reference; individuals whose diets do not meet the guidelines are not necessarily suffering from malnutrition. Though the RDA should not be used for absolute judging of the adequacy of the diet of an elderly person, they may serve as a means for comparison of daily dietary intakes from which individual nutritional status can be estimated, and dietary recommendations and counseling can be planned and provided.

Fiber

Recent interest has been directed to fiber, the nondigestible portion of the diet. Lack of fiber in the diet has been implicated in the incidence of certain diseases common to the aged population such as diverticulitis, gallstones, bowel cancer, constipation, hemorrhoids, atherosclerosis, diabetes mellitus, and obesity.

Fiber in the diet increases bulk and moisture content of the stool, thus aiding in the prevention

Table 33-3. Recommended Daily Dietary Allowances for Adults 51 Years of Age and Older as Revised in 1980.* Designed for the Maintenance of Good Nutrition of Practically All Healthy People in the United States.

	MEN		WOMEN	
	51–75 YEARS	76+ YEARS	51–75 YEARS	76+ YEARS
ENERGY (kcal)	2400 (RANGE = 2000–2800)	2050 (RANGE = 1650–2450)	1800 (RANGE = 1400–2200)	1600 (RANGE = 1200–2000)
Protein, g	56	56	44	44
Vitamin A, µg RE†	1000	1000	800	800
Vitamin D, µg	5	5	5	5
Vitamin E, mg α-TE‡	10	10	8	8
Vitamin C, mg	60	60	60	60
Thiamine, mg	1.2	1.2	1.0	1.0
Riboflavin	1.4	1.4	1.2	1.2
Niacin, mg NE §	16	16	13	13
Vitamin B$_6$, mg	2.2	2.2	2.0	2.0
Folacin, µg	400	400	400	400
Vitamin B$_{12}$, mg	3.0	3.0	3.0	3.0
Calcium, mg	800	800	800	800
Phosphorus, mg	800	800	800	800
Magnesium, mg	350	350	300	300
Iron, mg	10	10	10	10
Zinc, mg	15	15	15	15
Iodine, µg	150	150	150	150

SOURCE: *Recommended Daily Dietary Allowances,* Ninth Revised Edition (1980), the National Academy of Sciences, Washington, D.C.
*For men, the average height was 70 inches and the average weight 154 pounds (70 kg). For women, the average height was 64 inches and the average weight was 120 pounds (55 kg).
†Retinol equivalents.
‡Alpha-Tocopherol equivalents.
§Niacin equivalent = 1 mg niacin or 60 mg dietary tryptophan.

and treatment of constipation. Since the correction of fiber deficiency is one of the more manageable aspects of the diet which will help relieve constipation, it is advisable to encourage foods that provide a moderate, not excessive, amount of fiber in the diet. Good sources of foods with fiber are whole grain bread and cereals (especially bran), legumes, fresh cooked vegetables, and fruits. At least eight glasses of water a day should be included for adequate hydration.

Researchers and clinicians support the hypothesis that diverticulosis may be caused by a deficiency of vegetable fiber in the diet. Nutrition is, therefore, a major consideration in its prevention and treatment (Weg, 1978). Although claims are high for the benefits of fiber to alleviate other conditions, further research is needed before specific recommendations can be made (Almy, 1976).

COMMON NUTRITION-RELATED PROBLEMS

There are a number of degenerative diseases and conditions associated with aging that are directly related to nutrition and require dietary modification for their treatment.

"We are what we eat and what we have eaten all our lives" is an old adage containing more truth than fiction. Unfortunately, many older adults ignore nutrition till they are confronted with a problem related to nutritional neglect or ignorance; then, they engage in a frantic, sometimes fanatic, effort to reverse the results of a lifetime of unhealthy eating. The following sections contain a brief description of the most common nutrition-related problems of older adults.

Drugs and Alcohol

Older people use more drugs than any other age group. In 1971, it was estimated that 50% of older Americans drank alcohol, and it has been well documented that the elderly self-administer excessive quantities of nonprescription drugs. This figure emphasizes the fact that as the individual ages, greater use is made of many different types of chemicals (Eckhardt, 1978).

It has been estimated that the expenditure for prescription drugs for people over 65 years of age is four times more than that for people under 65. This greater use of drugs in the older population seems to have a physiological and psychological basis. As the individual grows older, there is an increased incidence of physical illness accompanied by more frequent intervention with medicine. The body's ability to remove toxic substances is reduced, the effective use of energy reserves is limited, and the body becomes more susceptible to illness and other debilitating conditions. The psychological stresses which accompany forced retirement, the loss of family and friends, economic insecurity, isolation, a decrease in feelings of self-worth, and poor physical health cause depression and anxiety. Medication has been used by the aged, by the family, and by physicians as a way of helping to relieve these pressures on the elderly. Unfortunately, the aged may rely on the medication as a means of coping, and psychological or physical addiction may result. In addition, the elderly may be lured, by advertising directed at them, to the use of nonprescription-type drugs and medications to alleviate signs of impaired physical health and mental stress.

Increased drug use in the elderly may cause adverse side effects and can have significant influence on dietary and nutritional status. Since the range of drugs and their effects on diet and food are so extensive, only a few will be included in this discussion. Detailed references are available on diet implications caused by interactions of foods and specific medications.

Diuretics. Most diuretics are capable of precipitating severe hypokalemia through excessive loss of potassium (Lambert, 1975). The individual on thiazide therapy should consume foods which are high in potassium, such as bananas, citrus fruits and juices, and dried fruit, to help maintain the potassium level in the body. Potassium drug supplementation may be advisable, but the use of potassium-containing foods is still helpful and usually more acceptable since this substance is found in commonly liked foods.

Cardiovascular Medications. Various antihypertensive medications may increase gastrointestinal motility and secretion, anorexia, and diarrhea. Other possible problems relating to food and diet include nausea, dry mouth, vomiting, and abdominal cramping. Since digoxin and digitoxin (drugs in the digitalis family) may increase the excretion of calcium and magnesium, it is especially important to include an adequate amount of these minerals in the diet.

Antibiotics. Nutrient absorption is affected by commonly used anti-infective medications such as sulfa drugs, tetracycline, and penicillin. Antibiotics, in general, are found to alter the bacterial flora or influence enzymic systems responsible for the digestion or absorption of foods and nutrients.

Gastrointestinal Medications. Mineral oil which has been a popular laxative among the elderly for years is known to interfere with the absorption of fat-soluble vitamins A, D, E, and K in the gastrointestinal tract. The vitamins are soluble in mineral oil and are excreted instead of being absorbed.

Antacids. Antacids commonly taken by the elderly may interfere with mineral absorption and cause thiamine destruction (Christalkis and Mardianian, 1968). Abuse can lead to phosphate depletion and, in some patients, to the development of osteomalacia (vitamin D deficiency; Roe, 1978).

Alcohol. Alcohol is one of the most commonly used nonprescription drugs. The effects of alcohol consumption will depend upon the amount consumed. The older person who consumes a moderate amount of alcohol on a regular basis may show adverse effects, disease complications, or altered therapeutic effects of other drugs. In addition, the person who consumes alcohol regularly is quite apt to be substituting this product for the regular consumption of food, thereby depleting the body's store of some nutrients.

The effects of a diet containing excessive amounts of alcohol include malabsorptive problems and alterations in liver and pancreatic functions. Damage to the mucosal lining of the gastrointestinal tract alters the absorption of many nutrients, thereby reducing the availability of these nutrients for metabolic function. Alcohol also has a direct toxic effect on the liver and pancreas, producing alcoholic cirrhosis and pancreatitis (Moore and Powers, 1981).

Deficiency diseases to which alcoholics are prone are those of proteins; water-soluble vitamins, particularly the B complex — thiamine, niacin, riboflavin, pyridoxine, and folic acid; and the minerals magnesium, potassium, and zinc. Deficiencies occur for multiple reasons, such as impaired appetite and reduced intake, poor absorption, reduced storage, and the need for increased requirements (Stone, 1978). The degree of deficiency depends on the length of time the person has been drinking and the quality of the diet during this time (Moore and Powers, 1981).

Obesity

Obesity, a common disorder of the elderly, is associated with other degenerative diseases. A body weight 15% above the ideal or desirable weight usually indicates obesity. A weight increase to this amount indicates that the fat content of body cells has increased because of excessive intake and that adipose tissue has been formed to store energy.

In aging, there is an increased proportion of adipose tissue at the expense of lean body mass. In addition, bone and muscle mass are reduced. This overall reduction of lean body mass lowers caloric requirements with age (Bierman, 1976). Calorie needs for energy expenditures are reduced because physical activities are usually limited in the elderly. These two factors are the main indicators for a reduced caloric intake. However, complying with these changes is difficult for the aging who have long-standing eating habits that were built on the physiological, sociocultural, and environmental influences of earlier years. Ideally, a gradual reduction in caloric intake throughout the adult years will result in maintaining the normal or desirable weight of the individual.

It is well established that chronic illness is more prevalent among the obese than the nonobese and that even for people 10-15% overweight, mortality rates are higher. The risk of coronary artery disease, diabetes mellitus, and nephritis is higher among obese than non-obese persons (Guthrie, 1975). Other chronic ailments common to the elderly are worsened by an obese condition. The work of breathing is made more difficult if weight is added to the chest wall of the individual who has a respiratory infection or suffers from a chronic pulmonary disease. Congestive heart failure may also result from pulmonary difficulties due to obesity. Hypertension is generally more prevalent among obese than nonobese persons. Obesity also causes greater discomfort to those who suffer from bone and joint diseases.

Weight reduction is best accomplished in the elderly by a slow, gradual decrease in caloric intake. Since it is difficult to change long established habits, careful consideration of the individual is needed in working out a weight-reduction plan which encourages only small changes. The reduced caloric intake of the elderly person makes it essential to choose foods with high nutrient content. The diet should include lean meats, eggs, milk, enriched or whole grain cereals and breads, fruits, and vegetables. Food that should be restricted are those high in calories and low in nutritional value.

Modifications which will lower the caloric intake include decreasing the intake of fats and oils, rich pastries, and sweetened carbonated beverages. These should be replaced by foods low in calories and high in nutrition such as fresh or canned fruits and raw or cooked vegetables. Meals should be eaten regularly, and serving sizes should be controlled.

Not only is regular exercise an important means of reducing or maintaining body weight, but it also helps improve muscle tonus, stimulates circulation, and promotes a sense of well-being.

Cardiovascular Problems

Epidemiological studies have shown that cardiovascular disease occurs more frequently in groups with certain characteristics. Although close to 40 different factors have been implicated, three of the major contributors are elevated serum lipid levels (particularly of cholesterol), hypertension, and cigarette smoking. Additional risk factors indicated are obesity, diabetes mellitus, personality factors, and a family history of atherosclerosis.

Dietary factors continue to be strongly implicated in cardiovascular disease; however, there are still conflicting data regarding the proper dietary regimen to reduce the incidence of heart disease and hypercholesterolemia. As the controversy regarding the effects of diet cholesterol on human blood levels continues, it is evident that further work on a long term basis is required to determine how diet interacts with other variables in the development and treatment of atherosclerosis.

A diet restricted in sodium has been used in the treatment of hypertension for many years. When diuretics are used in the treatment of hypertension, consideration must be given to the possibility of hypokalemia due to a loss of potassium from the body. Consumption of foods high in potassium on a daily basis will help to alleviate this condition. (These include foods such as bananas, citrus fruit or juice, prune juice, spinach, dried beans, potatoes, etc.)

Anemia

Iron deficiency anemia is a common problem among the elderly. Dietary iron deficiency usually results from an inadequate diet, impaired absorption of iron, or blood loss. The diet of the older person may be low in the protein foods which are high in iron because of poor selection, low income, or inability to chew certain foods. Malabsorption frequently results from a partial or total gastrectomy. Problems not uncommon to the elderly which may result in blood loss are peptic ulcers, excessive salicylate ingestion, diverticulitis, gastrointestinal tumors, ulcerative colitis, and hemorrhoids.

A combination of a diet high in iron-containing foods and oral iron medication is often the treatment used for nutritional anemia. Iron-containing foods include liver and other meats, poultry, fish, eggs, green leafy vegetables, and enriched or whole grain breads and cereals. Alterations in the form of meats eaten may have to be made to accommodate the chewing ability of the individual.

Ascorbic acid (vitamin C), a nutrient frequently found to be limited in the diet of the elderly, is helpful in promoting the absorption of iron. At least one serving of a food high in vitamin C should be included in the daily diet. These foods include citrus fruits or juices, broccoli, greens, green or chili peppers, cabbage, cauliflower, strawberries, and tomatoes.

Diabetes

Controversy has persisted as to whether changes in insulin secretion in man are characteristic of aging. We do have well-substantiated data drawn from nonobese subjects indicating that advancing age is characterized by decreased insulin release (Davis, 1978). This may account for the gradual increase of blood glucose levels after meals in both men and women as aging occurs. Elderly individuals may be diagnosed as diabetics even though true diabetes mellitus may not be present. However, these are included in the general definition of diabetes as a disorder in blood sugar regulation.

Dietary treatment for the individual with diabetes acquired during the later years (maturity onset) is essential and will often be effective in controlling diabetes without the use of insulin or oral drugs. The most important objective of dietary treatment of diabetic patients is control of total caloric intake to attain and maintain desirable body weight, since the majority of diabetics are obese (Goodhart and Shils, 1975). Obesity is associated with diabetes and tends to complicate the condition.

Revisions for diabetic meal planning by the American Diabetes Association and the American Dietetic Association (Guide for Professionals, 1977) reaffirmed the importance of the reduction of total caloric consumption and the restriction of foods high in fat. Caloric intake should be adjusted according to standard height and weight scales, with consideration of physical activity, sex, and age. The recommended dietary allowances, as revised in 1980, are 2400 calories for men 51-75 years of age and 2050 calories of those over 75. For women, the recommended dietary allowances are 1800 calories for those 51-75 years old and 1600 calories for those over 75. The recommended dietary allowance is indicated for healthy, moderately active adults.

The lower calorie needs of the older individual make it especially important that foods be chosen for nutritive value. Therefore, in the diabetic diet, foods must include lean meats, eggs, milk, fruits and vegetables, legumes, and whole grain and enriched breads and cereals.

Osteoporosis and Periodontal Disease

Osteoporosis is a skeletal disease characterized by decreases in the amount and strength of bone tissue. Bones are reduced in size and density, which makes them weak and susceptible to fracture that may occur from physical stress or even spontaneously under normal mechanical stress. Surveys indicate that approximately 25-30% of women and 15-20% of men over the age of 50 have osteoporosis severe enough to involve vertebral compression (Nutrition and Aging, 1979).

The decrease in bone density appears to be due primarily to resorption of bone which occurs to maintain blood levels of calcium. Absorption of calcium by the body decreases with age, and bone calcium is expended if calcium intake is low and absorption is poor.

Jowsey (1976) states that the most important etiologic factor in osteoporosis appears to be nutrition. Most people have greater calcium excretion than dietary intake during their adult years, which causes the necessary calcium supply to come from the skeletal structure. Additional factors considered to contribute to reduced bone mass include poor utilization of calcium, reduced action of the parathyroid, lack of exercise, and loss of stimulus to bone formation which is provided by estrogen.

Periodontal disease is a disorder affecting the structures that surround and support the teeth. The deterioration of these structures affects the supporting alveolar bone and may result in detachment of the teeth. Some studies indicate that the alveolar bone loss bears a relationship to bone changes and may precede bone deterioriation elsewhere in the body; thus it may be an indicator of osteoporosis. Lowered calcium intake may contribute to the loss of alveolar bone in some patients (Albanese et al., 1978). Although the dentin and enamel of the teeth do not readily release calcium to meet the body's needs, the periodontal tissues experience active exchange with the vascular nutrient supply as do bone and soft tissues.

Since osteoporosis and periodontal disease involve the loss of minerals and bone matrix, other nutrients in addition to calcium are considered in their treatment. A diet generous in protein, calcium, phosphorus, and vitamin D is recommended. The 1980 recommended dietary allowance for calcium and phosphorus was established at 800 mg per day for an adult. Two cups of milk, the usual recommendation for an adult, contributes only about three-fourths of this amount.

Cancer

The great majority of cancer cases occur in the older adult population, and diet and nutrition are of special concern. Research studies indicate that the well-nourished body is better able to tolerate and benefit from chemotherapy and other kinds of therapy, including surgery. (JAMA, 1977).

Cancer and chemotherapy or radiation therapy are frequently associated with anorexia and weight loss. Malnutrition may result because food intake does not meet the body's need for calories and nutrients. Patients undergoing therapy may complain of nausea, changes in taste and smell, and feeling full quickly. Taste changes cause some individuals to refuse to eat meat, fish, poultry, eggs, and fried foods. Foods not tolerated are often reported as tasting bitter, sour, salty, or spoiled. Extremes in the temperature of food may cause or intensify mouth discomfort.

Nutritional treatment of the elderly person with cancer is best determined on an individual basis. Concern should center on an adequate caloric and protein intake. It is necessary to explore with the patient and caretaker what are acceptable foods for the patient. In general, tolerated foods include milk, skim milk powder, and cottage cheese; other cheese and dairy products served in meat, fish, egg, and protein combination dishes help meet the protein and caloric needs. Between-meal feedings of eggnog, custards, puddings, ice cream, milk shakes, and commercial liquid supplements seem to be well tolerated.

Vegetables and fruits contribute mainly to the mineral and vitamin content of the diet, and vary in their acceptability to patients with cancer. It may be advisable to add vitamin and mineral supplements to the diet for adequate intake of these nutrients.

As therapy progresses, changes in texture and consistency of food make chewing and swallowing easier. Regular encouragement and support are necessary through all stages of the disease and treatment for good nutritional intake.

NUTRITION ASSESSMENT

Ideally a nutrition assessment should include a medical history, a clinical examination, indicated laboratory data, and a dietary history. Whether or not all of these are available, a nutrition data base is essential and should be obtained during initial counseling. The data base should include information about eating habits, attitudes toward food, and food resources. Information about socioeconomic status, living conditions, availability of food, and food assistance programs will be especially helpful in working with older individuals. See Figures 33-1 and 33-2 for nutrition data base formats which may be useful to all professionals working with older individuals. The following sections deal with methods commonly used to gather food intake information and dietary history.

Dietary Intake. Dietary intakes may be done by the nurse, nutritionist, or a trained paraprofessional. Questions are asked about the frequency and types of foods eaten during a specified period of time, usually a day or a week. A dietary intake is shown in Figure 33-1 as part of the nutrition data base. This method is helpful in identifying the individual who limits variety in the diet or who regularly uses excessive amounts of some foods. It is also a good indicator of the regular consumption of foods with little nutritive value, such as the "tea and toast syndrome."

MARICOPA COUNTY DEPARTMENT OF HEALTH SERVICES
BUREAU OF NUTRITION
NUTRITION DATA BASE I

PID NO.:

SUBJECTIVE: _____

PT.S NAME
(LAST, FIRST):

PATIENT TYPE
☐ MATERNITY   ☐ BREAST FEEDING   ☐ FAMILY PLANNING

BIRTHDATE:

☐ OTHER:
(SPECIFY):

AGE:

NO. PERSONS _____ WHO _____ WHO _____
IN HOME   SHOPS? _____ COOKS? _____

SEX: ☐ M   ☐ F   ETHNICITY: W B M I O

MEALS/DAY ☐ B ☐ L ☐ D ☐ EXTRA   NO. OF MEALS EATEN
NO. OF SNACKS/DAY: _____   AWAY FROM HOME/WK? _____ WHERE? _____

FACILITIES: ☐ REFRIGERATOR ☐ STOVE ☐ OTHER: _____

ASSISTANCE: ☐ FOOD STAMPS ☐ WIC   ☐ OTHER: _____

Rx/OTC: _____ VIT./MIN. _____

DIET: _____ SUPPLEMENTS: _____

DIETARY INTAKE	NO. SERVINGS		DIS-LIKES	CANT AFFORD		NO. SERVINGS		DIS-LIKES	CANT AFFORD
ITEM	DAY	WK			ITEM	DAY	WK		
EGGS					TORTILLAS F C				
BEANS, DRIED					CRACKERS				
LUNCH MEAT/HOT DOGS					BISCUITS/CORN BREAD				
FISH, TUNA					CEREAL				
MEAT/CHICKEN/PORK					PANCAKES/FR. TOAST				
P. BUTTER/NUTS/SEEDS					MARGARINE/BUTTER				
MILK/H. CHOCOLATE					FATS/OIL/LARD				
CHEESE/COTT. CHEESE					SWEETS/DESSERT				
ICE CREAM/YOGURT					HONEY/SYRUP/JELLY				
GREEN LEAFY VEG.					CHIPS/POPCORN				
OTHER VEGETABLES					SODA POP				
CITRUS FRUIT/JUICE					KOOL-AID/OTHER				
OTHER FRUIT/JUICE					COFFEE/TEA				
SOUP					NON-FOOD (PICA)				
POTATOES					WATER				
PASTAS/SOPAS/RICE									
BREAD/ROLLS									

PRIOR   PRESENT

SMOKE: _____

ALCOHOL: _____

KEY NUTRIENT SUMMARY

PROTEIN	HIGH	ADEQ	LOW
IRON	HIGH	ADEQ	LOW
CALCIUM	HIGH	ADEQ	LOW
VIT. A	HIGH	ADEQ	LOW
VIT. C	HIGH	ADEQ	LOW
FAT	HIGH	MOD	LOW
STARCH	HIGH	MOD	LOW
SUGAR	HIGH	MOD	LOW
SODIUM	HIGH	MOD	LOW
_____	HIGH	MOD	LOW
_____	HIGH	MOD	LOW
CALORIES	HIGH	MOD	LOW

DIET SUMMARY
GOOD   FAIR   POOR

OBJECTIVE:

Hgb/Hct	WT.	HT.	GRAVIDA:	PARA:	DATE LAST PG ENDED:	OTHER:

ASSESSMENT:

PLAN:

Figure 33-1. Nutrition data base I. Reprinted with permission of Bureau of Nutrition Services, Maricopa County Department of Health Services, Phoenix, Arizona.

Food Intake/Meal Pattern. Figure 33-2 provides an example of a nutrition data base form which is useful in obtaining food intake information through a discussion of daily food patterns. This method involves inquiring about foods and the quantities of these foods which are usually consumed at meals or at certain times of the day. Family members or caretakers may find providing information through this system more acceptable than attempting to recall specific foods that the patient consumes. The key nutrient summary provides an assessment

```
MARICOPA COUNTY DEPARTMENT OF HEALTH SERVICES      PID NO.:
              BUREAU OF NUTRITION
           NUTRITION DATA BASE II                  PT.S NAME
                                                   (LAST, FIRST)
        SERVICE:  □ PCC/CLINIC   □ HHC

TYPE    □ INFANT  □ CHILD  □ TEEN  □ ADULT   BIRTHDATE:
OF      □ OTHER
PATIENT   (SPECIFY)                          AGE:

    THERAPEUTIC
       DIET:                                 SEX: □ M  □ F   ETHNICITY: W  B  M  I  O

SUBJECTIVE:
NO. PERSONS      WHO            WHO            NO. OF MEALS EATEN
IN HOME          SHOPS?         COOKS?         AWAY FROM HOME/WK. ____ WHERE? _____
MEALS/DAY □B □L □D □EXTRA       OCCUPATIONAL
NO. OF SNACKS DAY ____                SKILLS: _____  SMOKE: _____  ALCOHOL: _____
                          □ OTHER
FACILITIES: □ REFRIGERATOR □ STOVE   (SPECIFY): _____

ASSISTANCE: □ FOOD STAMPS  □ WIC  □ SSI  □ AFDC  □ SS  □ DISABILITY  □ OTHER: _____

Rx/OTC _____          VIT./MIN.: _____

         FOOD INTAKE/MEAL PATTERN            SUPPLEMENTS: _____

 BREAKFAST     LUNCH      SUPPER     SNACKS       KEY NUTRIENT SUMMARY
                                          PROTEIN  HIGH  ADEQ  LOW
                                          IRON     HIGH  ADEQ  LOW
                                          CALCIUM  HIGH  ADEQ  LOW
                                          VIT. A   HIGH  ADEQ  LOW
                                          VIT. C   HIGH  ADEQ  LOW
                                          FAT      HIGH  MOD   LOW
                                          STARCH   HIGH  MOD   LOW
      LIKES/DISLIKES      FOOD ALLERGIES   SUGAR    HIGH  MOD   LOW
                                          SODIUM   HIGH  MOD   LOW
                                                   HIGH  MOD   LOW
                                                   HIGH  MOD   LOW
                                          CALORIES HIGH  MOD   LOW

  COMMENTS:                                     DIET SUMMARY
                                          GOOD    FAIR    POOR
  OBJECTIVE:                               OTHER
Hgb/Hct. ____ HT. ____ WT. ____ B.P. ____  LAB: _____
DIETARY RELATED
MEDICAL PROBLEMS _____
LAB., X-RAY
OTHER (SPECIFY) _____

  ASSESSMENT:


  PLAN:


081-1590-8-82       (DATE)        (INTERVIEWER'S SIGNATURE)
```

Figure 33-2. Nutrition data base II. Reprinted with permission of Bureau of Nutrition Services, Maricopa County Department of Health Services, Phoenix, Arizona.

tool for determining the adequacy of the food intake of the basic food groups.

The 24-hour Recall. The 24-hour recall method for acquiring food intake information requires the individual to remember everything consumed in the past 24-hour period. This method may be somewhat time consuming and trying to the patience of the interviewer since the subject must rely on memory. Also, it is important that the past 24-hour period be typical of the subject's regular food intake and eating pattern. If done in a relaxed atmosphere, this method may give the interviewer an opportunity to become acquainted with the individual and to establish a good teaching environment through the common topic of food.

Food Records and Comparisons. Food records which indicate the specific food and the amount eaten within a time period may be kept by the individual. This method requires a person who is motivated to keep careful records of foods consumed. The elderly patient may find this difficult.

Comparison with the basic food groups is a simple means of determining areas of strengths and weaknesses in the daily diet. When this means is used, careful consideration must be applied to the great variety of foods consumed by the elderly who represent many cultural and ethnic groups and reflect a lifetime of environmental, economic, and social influences.

Taste and Smell

Taste and smell decline with age and are important because they have a direct effect on appetite and on the consumption of salt, sugar, and condiments. We now have scientific data indicating that the olfactory bulb, which is the crucial organ controlling smell, atrophies with age (Schiffman and Pasternak, 1979). We have known for a longer time that taste buds atrophy with age and that this may affect nutrition behavior. Older people do seem able to detect "sourness" and "bitterness" well into old age. This is thought to be due to the slower atrophy of the large taste buds at the back of the tongue which seem to be the most sensitive to sour and bitter flavors (Schiffman, 1977). Since taste and smell are crucial in many of the daily functions of older people such as detecting smoke, information about them is essential in a basic nutrition assessment.

NUTRITION EDUCATION AND COUNSELING

Most of the elderly population is at nutritional risk. Nutritional guidance to maintain and promote better health in the elderly individual can be effective only if the care provider is knowledgeable about nutrition requirements and understands the psychological, sociological, cultural, and economic factors that influence the eating behavior of the individual. This understanding must be accompanied by the ability to use the information in counseling, motivating, and guiding individuals to improve their food and nutrition practices.

This is not easy; true health education does not take place unless there is a positive change in behavior. Although many have heard or know quite a bit about nutrition and diet, they will try current fads rather than struggle with self-discipline or restrictions on what they eat.

Sociocultural Aspects and Diet Modifications

No other group includes as many individuals with diversified eating habits and patterns as the aging population. The elderly have arrived at this stage in life with dietary practices of many years which were influenced by varied cultural, socioeconomic, religious, health, and family backgrounds. A change in life-style and adjustments to the daily needs of the later years contribute further to their eating patterns and the nutritional content of their diets. Limited socialization and companionship may affect what the person eats and the quantity consumed. Lack of transportation or a change in the type of transportation available will influence the eating pattern of the individual. Limited financial resources for food restrict the variety of foods, especially fruits, vegetables, protein foods, and dairy products. Even in this modern age, ethnic patterns remain very influential in health and illness. Food and language remain most important (Hall, 1979).

The older person who has looked forward to this period in life as a time for reward or doing as one chooses may relax to an eating style that reduces nutrient quality or increases caloric intake from less nutritious foods. Instead, this is a time in life when the individual needs to pay special attention to the nutrient density of food intake by consuming foods high in nutritional content and maintaining or reducing caloric levels.

General Guidelines for Nutrition Counseling

Changing food and nutrition ideas or practices is not a single event but requires a multiplicity of steps. The health professional can best help the elderly patient by following these general guidelines:

- Clearly explain the reason for nutritional needs or dietary modification (see Figure 33-3).

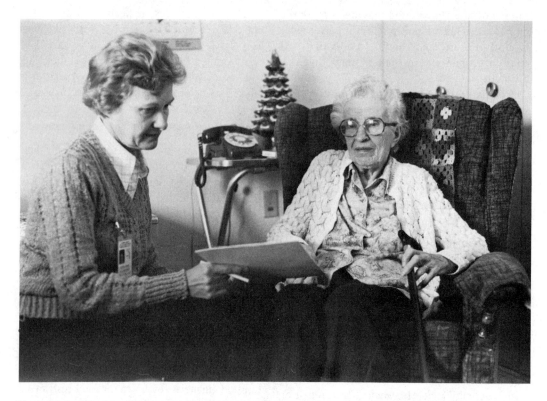

Figure 33-3. Older clients respond well when counseling is geared to their individual needs, when the setting is free of excessive noise, and when their sensory losses (hearing and vision) are considered. (Photo courtesy of M. Cadigan.)

- Indicate the results one can expect from making the changes or, in some cases, reflect upon the consequences if the changes are not made.
- Emphasize the positive results of change, since nutritional concerns for health maintenance have been demonstrated in the elderly (Elwood, 1975).
- Provide information in two or more sessions when counseling older adults. The intervals between sessions provide an opportunity to explain and question what was taught. Counseling or education sessions may be presented by different providers as long as they are reinforcing the teaching.
- Include the caretaker during counseling on food needs. This is vital since the caretaker may be the key person in a successful nutritional outcome for the patient, through motivation and fulfillment of dietary plans.

- Individualize the diet plan according to the patient's specific needs, resources, and capabilities. This will encourage patient compliance.
- Prescribe foods which are within the patient's economic means, are adapted to his established food likes and dislikes, as well as to his ethnic and cultural food habits, and are available whether dining out or at home.
- Clearly state the number of meals to be consumed daily and the distribution of foods between meals. Ways of improving attractiveness and palatability of food should also be included (Todhunter and Darby, 1978).

Specific Nutrition Guidelines

- Foods in the diet should be high in essential nutrients because of gradually decreasing caloric requirements and decrease in appetite.

- Frequent small feedings during the day are often more acceptable and appealing to the older individual with a lessened appetite than three full meals. The daily food plan may be in the form of four to six small meals or three small meals with two or three nutritious snacks in between.
- Fruit, fruit juices, milk or milk-based beverages, yogurt, puddings, soups, and cereals are the best between-meal feedings. Eating slowly and chewing food thoroughly will help digestive processes and reduce the swallowing of air which often causes discomfort for older adults.
- A moderate amount of fiber should be included in the daily diet. Moderately high fiber foods which are generally acceptable to the elderly are whole grain breads and cereals, cooked vegetables, some raw vegetables such as lettuce and shredded salad vegetables, and cooked or raw fruit.
- Fried foods contribute additional calories and are often difficult to digest.
  When chewing is difficult, protein foods such as fish, ground meats, poultry, dried beans, peanut butter, and eggs are usually acceptable. Milk, milk products, yogurt, cheese, and cottage cheese are good sources of calcium and protein which are usually tolerated by the individual with chewing concerns.
- If milk intolerance is a problem, small amounts of milk or milk products added gradually to the daily food intake may help to increase the ability to consume milk. Some people are able to consume yogurt, cheese, buttermilk, or acidophilus milk as a replacement for other milk products.
- A low to moderate intake of salt is usually advisable. The use of canned foods, convenience foods, and salted snack foods contributes greatly to the salt intake of the daily diet and should be avoided.
- Water and other fluids should be consumed throughout the day. Reminders for fluid consumption may be necessary and/or helpful.

- Sugar and concentrated sweets should be limited. Fruit, desserts containing fruit, puddings, custards, and ice cream, rather than rich cakes and pastries, are recommended for those who enjoy sweets and desserts.

COMMUNITY NUTRITION PROGRAMS

Concern for the dietary adequacy of the elderly has resulted in local, state, and federal intervention programs to help meet food and nutrition needs. In addition, some programs contribute to the maintenance of a social life or to the resocialization of the widowed and isolated.

CONGREGATE MEALS

Feeding programs administered under Title III of the Older American's Act are designed to provide the older population, particularly those with low incomes, with meals that supply one-third of the recommended daily allowances. Regulations of this federally funded program allow individuals aged 60 and over and their spouses of any age to receive meals if the following conditions exist:

- They cannot afford to eat adequately.
- They lack the skills and knowledge to select and prepare nourishing and well-balanced meals.
- They have limited mobility which may impair their capacity to shop and cook for themselves.
- They have feelings of rejection and loneliness which obliterate the incentive necessary to prepare and eat a meal alone.

Emphasis is given to providing meals in group settings such as community centers, churches, schools, senior centers, public housing, and other public and private facilities where other social and rehabilitation services may also be delivered. Thus, in addition to promoting better health among the older segment of the population through improved nutrition, the program can help reduce the isolation of the aged by offering older Americans an opportunity to participate in community activities. Meals are served at least five days a week, usually at noon, with some centers serving morning or evening meals. Participants are encouraged to make voluntary contributions, but payment is not required.

The nutrition programs include plans for outreach to search out those in need of services, transportation, information and referral to supporting services, health and welfare counseling, nutrition education, shopping assistance, and physical and recreational activities.

Home-delivered Meals

A limited number of meals are delivered from congregate sites. In addition, volunteer or community agencies such as "Meals on Wheels" supply home delivered meals to elderly homebound individuals. These programs usually provide one hot meal and a cold meal which are delivered five days a week for a low cost. Special diets are available through this program.

The Food Stamp Program. Food stamps are available to the low income elderly through local welfare offices. Many older Americans are not aware that their limited incomes allow them to participate in the Food Stamp Program. Others choose not to participate because of pride and the determination that they will not accept "welfare" during their lifetimes. Recent legislation has eliminated the requirement of paying for a portion of the cost of the stamps. In some areas, the elderly may use food stamps to purchase meals at specified restaurants.

CONCLUSION

Nutrition is an environmental factor which is often directly under man's control; it contributes directly to the prevention of disease and disability, and assists in recuperation from illness and accident. The beneficial results of good nutrition often manifest themselves slowly. The elderly cannot expect immediate miracles from improved nutrition alone, but they can receive substantial benefits from a well-planned health care program with a focus on nutrition.

Proper nutrition throughout life has been suggested as one of the best means of minimizing

degenerative changes as well as increasing life span. Most references and sources of information on nutrition and the elderly indicate that more research, especially longitudinal studies, is needed to add to the increasing knowledge of the role of nutrition in the aging process.

The following current, reliable materials may be helpful in counseling and teaching elderly patients:

- *Help Yourself to Better Health* (16-mm film)
- *Journal of Nutrition Education* (Society for Nutrition Education)
- *Journal of the American Dietetic Association*
- *Journal of Nutrition for the Elderly*
- *Nutrition Today* (Nutrition Today Society)
- *Nutrition and the M.D.* (monthly publication)
- *Advisory Dietary Guidlines* (pamphlet available from the Office of Governmental Public Affairs, U.S. Department of Agriculture, Washington, DC 20250)

REFERENCES

Albanese, A.A. et al. *Calcium throughout the Life Cycle.* National Dairy Council, 1978, p. 21.

Almy, T.P. The role of fiber in the diet. In Winick, M. (Ed.) *Nutrition and Aging.* New York: Wiley, 1976, pp. 155-170.

Bierman, E.L. Obesity, carbohydrate and lipid interaction in the elderly. In Winick, M. (Ed.) *Nutrition and Aging.* New York: Wiley, 1976, p. 171.

Christalkis, G. and Mardianian, A. Diet, drugs and their interrelationships. *Journal of the American Dietetic Association* 52:21-24 (1968).

Davis, P.J. Endocrinology and aging. In Behneke, J.A., Finch, C.E., and Moment, G.B. (Eds.) *The Biology of Aging.* New York: Plenum Press, 1978.

Eckhardt, M.J. Consequences of alcohol and other drug use in the aged. In Behnke, J.A., Finch, C.E., and Moment, G.B. (Eds.) *The Biology of Aging.* New York: Plenum Press, 1978, pp. 191-203.

Elwood, T.W. Nutritional concerns of the elderly. *Journal of Nutrition Education* 7:50-52 (April-June 1975).

Fleck, H. *Introduction to Nutrition.* New York: Macmillan, 1976.

Food and Nutrition Board, National Academy of Sciences–National Research Council. *Recommended Daily Dietary Allowances.* Washington, D.C.: 1980.

Friedman, G.J. Diet in treatment of diabetes mellitus. In Goodhart, R.S. and Shils, M.E. (Eds.) *Modern Nutrition and Disease.* Philadelphia: Lea and Febiger, 1975, p. 844.

Goodhart, R.S. and Shils, M.E. *Modern Nutrition and Disease.* Philadelphia: Lea and Febiger, 1975.

Guide for Professionals: The Effective Application of Exchange List for Meal Planning. American Diabetic Association, Inc., New York, and The American Dietetic Association, Chicago, 1977.

Guthrie, H.A. *Introductory Nutrition.* St. Louis: C.V. Mosby, 1975.

Hall, G. Lecture at Arizona State University College of Nursing, November, 1979.

Harper, A.E. Recommended dietary allowances for the elderly. *Geriatrics* 33:75 (1978).

Harper, A.E. Nutrition, aging and longevity. *American Journal of Clinical Nutrition* 36:737-749 (1982).

JAMA. Well-fed patients are more likely to benefit from their therapy. *Journal of the American Medical Association* 237:1303-1305 (1977).

Jowsey, J. Prevention and treatment of osteoporosis. In Winick, M. (Ed.) *Nutrition and Aging.* New York: Wiley, 1976, p. 136.

Jowsey, J. Why is mineral nutrition important in osteoporosis? *Geriatrics* 33:39-49 (1978).

Lambert, M.L. Drug and diet interactions. *American Journal of Nursing* 75:402-408 (1975).

Moore, A.O. and Powers, D.E. *Food-Medication Interactions.* Tempe, Arizona: 1981.

Natow, A.B. and Heslin, J. *Geriatric Nutrition.* Boston: CBI Publishing Company, 1980.

Nutrition and Aging. Washington, D.C.: U.S. Department of Health, Education and Welfare, Public Health Service, National Institutes of Health, 1979, p. 12.

Recker, R.R. Diet, osteoporosis and health. *ADA Abstracts,* 65th Annual Meeting of the American Dietetic Association (October 18-22, 1982).

Roe, D.A. Drugs, diet and nutrition. *Contemporary Nutrition* 3:6 (1978).

Rose, J.C. Nutritional problems in radiotherapy patients. *American Journal of Nursing* 78:1194-1196 (1978).

Schiffman, S. Food recognition by the elderly. *Journal of Gerontology* 32:586-592 (1977).

Schiffman, S. and Pasternak, M. Decreased discrimination of food odors in the elderly. *Journal of Gerontology* 34:73-79 (1979).

Shannon, B. and Smiciklas-Wright, H. Nutrition education in relation to the needs of the elderly. *Journal of Nutrition Education* 11:86 (April-June 1979).

Stone, O.J. Alcoholic malnutrition and skin infections. *Nutrition Today* 6-10 (November-December 1978).

Todhunter, E.N. and Darby, W. Guidelines for maintaining adequate nutrition in old age. *Geriatrics* 33:49-56 (1978).

Weg, R.B. *Nutrition and the Later Years.* Los Angeles: University of Southern California Press, 1978, p. 89.

Williams, S.R. *Nutrition and Diet Therapy.* St. Louis: C.V. Mosby, 1973.

Wilson, E.D., Fisher, K.H., and Fugua, M.E. *Principles of Nutrition.* New York: Wiley, 1975.

Winick, M. (Ed.). *Nutrition and Aging.* New York: Wiley, 1976.

34
Drugs and the Elderly

Eleanor Sidor Sheridan

Our body is a well-set clock, which keeps good time, but if it be too much or indiscreetly tampered with, the alarm runs out before the hour.

Joseph Hall (1981)

From the beginning of time, man has searched for a drug to cure his ills, provide pleasure, decrease anxiety, and prolong life. He has made great strides in developing drugs, curing certain illnesses, easing some discomforts, and prolonging life. However, the advantages of modern drugs have been clouded by adverse side effects, misuse, and abuse. The lesson learned is that the use of drugs should proceed with caution.

THE ELDERLY AS CONSUMERS OF DRUGS

Extent of Drug Use

Drug use in the elderly must be viewed from three perspectives: prescribed drugs administered by health professionals, prescribed and self-administered drugs, and self-prescribed and self-administered drugs.

In the study *Out of Pocket Cost and Acquisition of Prescribed Medications,* (U.S. Department of Health, Education and Welfare, 1977), there was found to be an average of 5.8 acquisitions per person per year at an average cost of $4.80 per purchase. This money was paid directly by the individual, exclusive of any payment by insurance companies or other agencies. With age, the number of acquisitions rose sharply. The annual out-of-pocket expense per person for individuals aged 65 years and older was $61.40. There was a greater expense for females than for males. Individuals having chronic illnesses with associated limitation of

activity had a greater expenditure for medicines, averaging 23.5 acquisitions per year. To translate this study to the present, one must consider the introduction of new drugs on the market, which increases the number of prescribed drugs, and the influence of inflation on drug costs.

Whittington and Petersen (1979) cite the frequently used statistic that the elderly constitute only 10% of the population and receive roughly 25% of all prescriptions; they further state that it is probably safe to assume that the elderly share of the over-the-counter (OTC) drug market is at least as large. The self-prescribed use of OTC drugs and home remedies provides advantages as well as disadvantages; e.g., OTC drugs, when properly used, can provide economic and time savings. Warren (1979) sees OTC drug use as safe if the symptom being treated is minor, short term, and simply relieved, and if the individual is able to recognize when self-treatment has failed and is willing to seek medical care. The challenge is proper education.

A national survey of skilled nursing facilities (U.S. Public Health Service, 1976) revealed that the average number of prescriptions per patient was 6, with a range from 2 to 23. Prescribed drugs were classified in 30 categories. Cathartics were the single largest class of drugs prescribed. Other frequently ordered categories included analgesics, tranquilizers, vitamins, sedative/hypnotics, and cardiac drugs, in decreasing order of frequency. The majority of patients had only one prescription in any one drug category.

Drug Misuse

Drug misuse refers to the use of drugs (prescribed and OTC) either for purposes that are appropriate but in improper in dosage or for inappropriate purposes. Drug misuse is varied and depends on the view of the patient, the physician, and other health professionals caring for the patient. A patient's misuse of drugs usually includes mistakes made in following the physician's prescription, the misuse of OTC drugs in self-treatment, and the illegal acquisition of prescription drugs. Drug misuse of this latter type is subtle, and few studies explore all of its aspects.

The majority of studies on drug misuse deal with patient compliance with medical regimens (Barofsky, 1977; Hulka, 1976; Komaroff, 1976; Schwartz, 1975). It has been reported that 25-50% of outpatients fail to take their medications. Hulka et al. (1976), in their study of medication compliance of 357 outpatients aged 50-75 years, identified an average of 58% error in taking medication prescribed for hypertension and congestive heart failure. Four types of medication errors were identified: (1) errors of omission constituted 18-20%; (2) errors of commission (i.e., the proportion of drugs taken which the physician had not prescribed) constituted 19-20%; (3) scheduling misconceptions constituted 17%; and (4) scheduling noncompliance constituted 3% of the errors identified. Neither patient characteristics nor the severity of the disease was influential in determining the extent of medication errors. Specific aspects of the medication regimen associated with increased errors included the following facts:

- The more drugs involved in the regimen, the greater was the number of errors of omission and commission.
- The greater the complexity of the scheduling, the greater were the errors of commission and scheduling.
- When patients did not know the function of the drug, errors of commission and scheduling misconception increased.

The authors concluded, "Good communication of instructions and information to the patient was associated with a lower level of all types of errors" (Hulka, 1976).

Drug misuse of nonprescription drugs is not as well documented, yet the problem exists and may be evidenced only if health professionals ask the patient about his use of OTC drugs, home remedies, herbs, and illegally prescribed drugs.

Misuse of Prescribed Drugs by Health Professionals. Health professionals may prescribe/administer drugs that are appropriate but in improper dosage or for inappropriate purposes. Misuse in this sense is viewed by Stimmel (1978) "not as intentional inappropriate prescribing, but as deficiencies in monitoring and tailoring of drugs to the individual patients." The goals of drug therapy are to maximize the therapeutic benefit to the patient, to minimize adverse effects, and to avoid drug duplication, interactions, and toxicity.

Weg (1978) and Butler (1976) identify a lack of geriatric pharmacology content in medical school curricula (however, the situation does appear to be improving). The lack of geriatric knowledge is compounded by the explosion of knowledge in the field of pharmacology. The "life" of a new drug in the current drug market is about five years. Seventy percent of all drugs now available were either unknown or unavailable 15 years ago. The need for continuing education in the proper therapeutic use of drugs is most apparent. Weg (1978) concluded:

While aging is not a disease, greater susceptibility to disease is a fact and proportionately there is a greater incidence of multiple disease in those over 65. Many of the very new, potent drugs being used to treat morbid conditions of the elderly often are in the hands of people who understand little about the changing physiology of the aging human being.

To summarize, drug misuse is far more subtle than drug abuse, far less documented, and far more prevalent in our society. Four actions of health professionals which contribute to the problem include: (1) inaccurate diagnosis; (2) inaccuracies in drug treatment; (3) polypharmacy, including failure to consider drug interactions; (4) deliberate overmedication or arbitrary medication (especially in the institutionalized psychiatric elderly patient; Gollub, 1978).

Drug Abuse

Whittington and Petersen (1979) state that individuals over age 50, involved in federally reported drug abuse incidents, constituted 6% of the total. Drugs involved in these incidents included barbiturate sedatives, tranquilizers, and other drug interactions with alcohol. In a study of hospital emergency room admissions for acute drug reactions (overdosages), only 5% of those treated were over 50 years (Petersen and Thomas, 1979). All admissions for the older age group resulted from an acute reaction to a legally available drug. (This was not the finding with the younger age groups.) Over 80% of the older admissions involved misuse of a sedative or a tranquilizer. An additional 10% resulted from the misuse of the nonnarcotic analgesic Darvon. The study concluded that the older person is underrepresented among those who come to the attention of the public; it is speculated that the problem of the elderly may be unmanaged or unreported.

Drug misuse and abuse in the elderly seem to result from those drugs most often prescribed for them (Whittington and Petersen, 1979). This is seen in both the ambulatory and the institutionalized elderly. In many institutions, the practice of continuing a physician's prescription for drugs having no therapeutic function other than to aid in the management of difficult patients has been cited (Gollub, 1978).

Suicide may be viewed as a problem of drug abuse. It is one of the ten leading causes of death in the United States for persons 45 years of age and older. Payne (1979) estimated that one in three suicides is accomplished by a drug prescribed by a physician. Major factors implicated in the suicide attempts of older persons include chronic illness, social losses, insomnia, and depression, all of which can be alleviated by prescription drugs. At times, the drugs may intensify preexisting depression and suicidal tendencies. Ingestion of alcohol or another easily available depressant drug potentiates the action of the hypnotic or tranquilizer. This combination of drugs can be fatal, even when suicide is not intended.

Alcohol Abuse

The true prevalence of alcohol abuse among the elderly has not been documented. Yet alcohol is man's most ancient and widely used beverage. Zimberg (1979) states that with current consumption rates rising rapidly in the United States, we can expect more alcoholism. The Arizona Community Advisory Committee on Aging and Addiction (1979) estimates that 10–12% of the elderly have a problem related to alcohol abuse themselves or in their family.

Studies indicate that there are two types of elderly alcoholics (Zimberg, 1979). Two-thirds of those studied had a long-standing drinking problem which persisted as they grew older. This group shared personality factors similar to young alcoholics. Apparently the stresses of aging perpetuate the drinking problem. One-third of the alcoholics studied developed drinking problems later in life, associated with bereavement, loneliness, depression, marital stress, and physical illness. There are more women than men in this group, in contrast to a prevalence of men in the younger alcoholic group.

Treatment and prevention of alcoholism in the elderly will differ somewhat physically and psychosocially from that of youth. Therefore, knowledge of the aging process is required.

Narcotic Abuse

Little research has been reported on the older narcotic abuser and addict. One reason given is the high visibility of adolescents and young adults who abuse drugs. Secondly, researchers have long believed that the narcotic abuser either dies an early death or "matures out" of his addiction in later years. Professionals, researchers, and clinicians also often overlook and discount the importance of drug abuse among the elderly (Whittington and Petersen, 1979). Studies are further plagued by the lack of standard definitions of drug abuse.

Using admissions to the United States Public Health Service Hospital in Lexington, Kentucky, Whittington and Peterson (1979) note that only 10% of those admitted were over age 50 and that persons 60 years of age comprised less than 4% of the total. The "maturing out" and "burning out" hypothesis has been used to explain these low admissions. Others believe that sufficient evidence is lacking and that older addicts do exist whether they come to the attention of health professionals or not.

Two special groups of addicts tend to be older than the overall population. One consists of Chinese-American opium addicts, most of whom became addicted early in this century; this group is gradually disappearing. The other consists of addicted physicians. This group has an established addiction rate of 1% or 30 times that of the general population. The mean age for the group, established by studies, is 44–52 years (Whittington and Petersen, 1979).

THE ELDERLY AS RESPONDERS TO DRUGS

It is a well-known fact that individuals respond differently to drugs; old people are very individualistic and become more so as they age. Individual variations influence absorption, distribution, metabolism, and elimination of drugs. Other factors influencing these variables are age, body mass, developmental state, physiological and psychological state, and drug history. Drug history includes genetic factors, allergies, and present and past drug usage.

Individual variation in drug response increases with age. The threshold for side effects is often lowered in the elderly, which necessitates a comparable lowering of drug dose to produce

therapeutic effects. They also show altered and unexpected response to medication as a result of the interaction of several drugs being taken for other acute and chronic disease states. Another problem experienced by the elderly is that of adverse drug reactions. Three to five percent of all hospital admissions are the consequence of adverse drug reactions. There are proportionately more drug-induced illnesses leading to hospitalization in patients over 61 years of age than for those younger (Caranasos, Steward, and Cluff, 1974). It is estimated that one-seventh of all hospital days are devoted to the care of patients with drug reactions (Kayne, 1976). To avoid such iatrogenic problems, it is important that health professionals understand the variables that influence a drug's mechanisms of action and the patient's response.

Pharmacokinetics

Pharmacokinetics — the study of the fate of drugs in the body — has provided some insights into the action of drugs in the elderly. A brief review follows.

Absorption. The majority of drugs are absorbed by passive diffusion through the intestinal mucosa; a few are absorbed through the stomach. In any age group, factors interfering with absorption of drugs include the presence of food, low gastric pH, nausea, and pain. With the elderly producing less gastric acid than the young, one can anticipate slower absorption. The presence of certain drugs that delay gastric emptying will also influence the absorption of other drugs when given concurrently. Drugs which delay gastric emptying include the anticholinergic drugs, tricyclic antidepressants, and phenothiazines. Another important factor is that old people have fewer secreting cells in the mucous membrane. As a result, the absorption of certain foods or drugs such as fat, glucose, thiamine, iron, and xylose may be reduced (Cape, 1978).

Studies do show that absorption in the duodenum and jejunum (where the majority of drugs are absorbed) is as efficient in the elderly as in the young (Cape, 1978). However, mesenteric blood flow in the elderly may be reduced secondary to cardiovascular changes, and these changes can affect absorption (Vancura, 1979). Another important factor that must be considered in absorption is the rate of passage of the drug through the intestine. Conditions which increase or decrease motility of the intestine influence the amount of time available for the drug to be absorbed through the intestinal mucosa. Gastrointestinal motility can be increased with the use of certain laxatives, thus causing more rapid drug elimination than usual (Vancura, 1979). Malabsorption conditions also increase the rate of passage of intestinal contents, including drugs. Diverticuli in the small bowel may create areas of stagnation, altering intestinal flora and in turn affecting absorption. No studies of this aspect have been carried out, yet diverticuli are a frequent problem associated with age (Cape, 1978).

Distribution. Once absorbed, a drug must be distributed to its sites of action in order to bring about its effect. Drugs exert systemic effects at the cellular level where cellular receptors are thought to bind chemically with the active chemical compound. To achieve this action, an adequate amount of "free" drug must be delivered from the blood to the tissue. Some drugs are present in the bloodstream in simple solutions; however, the majority of drugs are bound or attached to other constituents of the blood. Some drugs may be bound or stored in other body tissues such as fat or muscle. These bound drugs affect serum levels of the substance but exert no pharmacological action. They act as "reservoirs," releasing drug as "free" drug is metabolized or eliminated. Alteration in the extent of binding/storage will have considerable therapeutic importance.

The distribution of drugs is also influenced by body composition (body fluid and mass), plasma protein concentration, cardiac output, and organ blood flow. With age, there is a decrease in total body water and total muscle mass. In addition, there is an increase in total body fat compared to total body mass. If a drug is highly bound to protein tissues, its tissue distribution will be affected by the decrease in muscle mass. If a drug such as a barbiturate, diazepam, or chlorpromazine is bound to fat tissues, one can anticipate prolonged and possibly decreased effects.

Other changes noted in the elderly include decreases in protein binding, regional blood flow, red cell binding, and tissue permeability. There is an increase in gamma globulin and a decrease in total serum protein. These changes increase the free drug concentration, potentiating the response to drugs and accounting for increased drug sensitivity (Exton-Smith and Windsor, 1979; Vancura, 1979). Drugs strongly bound to protein which reflect such a response include the salicylates, sulfadiazine, and phenylbutazone. It has also been said that side effects of steroid therapy are frequent in patients with low serum albumin levels (Exton-Smith and Windsor, 1979). To further complicate the matter, given two drugs which form complexes with protein, one may expect competition for binding sites. If one drug displaces the other, the freed molecules then diffuse into the tissues at an abnormally rapid rate and may thus tend to reach toxic concentrations. This is of particular significance with potent drugs; reactions of this kind include the coumarin-type anticoagulants and anti-inflammatory agents such as phenylbutazone. Drug interactions of this sort must be carefully evaluated before therapy is initiated.

Decreased regional blood flow and tissue permeability influence the amount of drug carried to the receptor sites. It is important to note that cardiac output decreases approximately 1% per year from ages 19 to 86 years. In the elderly, cardiac output may be further decreased secondary to pathological conditions.

Alterations in the distribution of drugs, in addition to cellular changes in aging which alter drug receptors, make it difficult to predict effects of drugs on the elderly. Individual variation in the elderly compounds the problem, so careful monitoring of drug therapy and response is a must.

Metabolism. Drug concentration in the body is influenced by the rate at which the drug is metabolized into less active or inert compounds, as well as by elimination of the drug from the body. The liver and kidneys are the key sites for these processes. Age-related changes in these organs are of profound pharmacological importance. Reduction in metabolic activity would reduce drug elimination and may lead to toxicity.

Two metabolic routes are involved: oxidation and acetylation. Individual variations in these processes are as important as age. Genetic differences in the rate and manner in which drugs are oxidized have been identified. It is also known that certain drugs stimulate the production of enzymes and thus increase the rate of oxidation of other drugs given concurrently. Phenobarbital is known to stimulate this process. At other times, oxidation of drugs may be inhibited by other drugs.

Genetic differences also account for individuals in whom drugs are acetylated rapidly or slowly. Individuals who metabolize drugs more slowly will have prolonged and higher plasma drug levels, leading to adverse effects. Genetic differences in acetylation of drugs further reflect individual variations in metabolism that are unrelated to aging.

There is evidence that the production of liver enzymes for oxidation of drugs is reduced in old age. This reduction in enzymes may delay or slow the metabolism of drugs, leading to increased drug plasma levels and contributing to the known high incidence of adverse reactions in the elderly. Drugs that have been identified to be more slowly metabolized in the elderly include phenylbutazone, antipyrine, propranolol, and diazepam (Cape, 1978; Vancura, 1979).

An individual's past response to drugs gives an indication of his genetic variations in drug metabolism. Age-related changes in drug metabolism may not be as evident as genetic differences. Liver function studies may not indicate diminution in drug metabolism activity. In an attempt to identify delays and increases in drug metabolism, it is important to observe whether the patient responds to the drug as anticipated.

Elimination. Even though all excretory organs participate in the elimination of drugs, the majority of drugs are ultimately excreted by the kidneys. With advancing age, there is a cumulative loss of functioning nephrons as well as decreases in renal blood flow, glomerular filtration rate, and tubular function. Such age-associated changes have important pharmacokinetic implications for many drugs.

Studies have indicated that drugs which are mainly eliminated by the kidneys have a longer half-life in old people. This factor can lead to drug accumulation and possible toxicity. Drugs identified in these studies include digoxin, penicillin, sulfamethizole, methotrexate, and practolol (Cape, 1978). Even though some of these drugs are excreted partly by filtration through glomeruli and partly by active secretion by the tubules, Cape (1978) and Davison (1978) state that it is seldom possible to correlate creatinine clearance levels with the possible excretion rates of these drugs. Others however, disagree with them (Lamy and Vestal, 1978; Thompson and Floyd, 1978). All authors agree that measurement of drug serum levels should be used to establish proper regimens for many potent drugs.

It has also been found that deteriorating glomeruli filtration rate in the elderly results in a very slow elimination of protein-bound drugs, increasing their half-life appreciably. Diazoxide is an example of such a drug. With a reduction in renal filtration by 50%, elimination becomes extremely slow, with an obvious effect on increased plasma level (Cape, 1978). Other drugs eliminated unchanged by glomerular filtration include the cardiac glycosides (e.g., digitalis preparations) and aminoglycoside antibiotics.

Drugs eliminated by the renal tubules are not affected in the same way. Active tubular secretion decreases the serum concentration of a free drug, which is quickly replaced since there is a constant equilibrium between bound and free drug. Certain penicillins are 90% bound to serum albumin but are excreted through the renal tubules.

Thus, normal changes in renal function can cause inefficient and slowed drug excretion in the elderly. In addition, many elderly show a further decrement in renal function due to dehydration, congestive heart failure, pneumonia, urinary tract infections, and renal disease (Cape, 1978; Exton-Smith and Windsor, 1979). Close observation and monitoring of drug response, plus precise modification of the dosage regimen, can minimize drug problems (Vancura, 1979).

Adverse Reactions

Ronald Cape (1978) has summarized a number of reports on problems of drug utilization and drug induced illnesses in the United States and Canada and Australia. Findings indicate (1) a peak incidence of adverse reactions in the age group 66 to 75 years, (2) almost one third of this age group suffer reactions, (3) about 10% have severe problems, (4) those receiving 6 or more drugs had a greater chance of developing adverse reactions and (5) the majority of reactions from studies received were related to the gastrointestinal tract and neuromuscular disturbances.

The Caranasos et al. (1974) study of 6063 patients admitted to the medical services at the University of Florida Teaching Hospital over a three-year period identified adverse drug reactions as a reason for 2.9% of all admissions. Of these patients, 41.7% were in the 61–90 age group. The severity of the adverse drug reactions was identified as 28.8% moderate, 65.0% severe, and 6.2% lethal. These figures vary some from the Boston study.

In the Florida study, hemorrhagic effects occurred frequently. Organ systems implicated most frequently in adverse reactions included the cardiovascular (22.2%), gastrointestinal (18.5%), and hematologic (13.2%). Drug allergy was cited in 17.6% of all cases, whereas the remainder were

due to pharmacologic mechanisms. Eight drugs produced one-third of the drug-induced illnesses; these included aspirin, digoxin, sodium warfarin, hydrochlorothiazide, prednisone, vincristine sulfate, norethindrone, and furosemide.

The Florida researchers added that 60% of patients cannot correctly identify their medications. Forty percent receive drugs prescribed by two or more physicians. Twelve percent take drugs prescribed for someone else. Sixty percent consider their drugs completely safe.

Davison (1978) identifies a profile of the individual apt to develop an adverse reaction as a small elderly female, with a history of allergic illness, previous adverse reactions, multiple chronic illnesses, and renal and mental failure. Because of the erosion of reserve capacity in the elderly, the safety margin between the therapeutic and the toxic dose of many drugs is narrowed.

Although there are some variations in these studies, the message is clear. The incidence of adverse drug reactions is greater in the elderly. With the 1–6% incidence of adverse reactions leading to death, it becomes most clear that "therapeutic enthusiasm must clearly be tempered with caution" (Cape, 1978).

DRUG SIDE EFFECTS IN THE ELDERLY

The following pages list drugs most commonly prescribed for the elderly, their characteristics, side effects, and nursing implications. This is by no means a complete discussion of drug actions and precautions. For further information, refer to the pharmacology texts listed in the references.

SUMMARY

This discussion of drugs has demonstrated that the elderly frequently take a large number of drugs over long periods of time, have decreased reserves, and are prone to increased hazards as a result of drug action and side effects. All health care providers need to work as a team to provide for patients' safety and to promote the therapeutic effectiveness of drug therapy for

DRUG (Trade Name)	CHARACTERISTICS	ADVERSE EFFECTS/TOXICITY	NURSING IMPLICATIONS
CARDIOVASCULAR DRUGS			
Digitalis preparations Digitoxin (Crystodigin, Purodigin, etc.) Oral maintenance dose: 0.05–0.2 mg Onset of action: 3–4 hr Duration of action: 14–21 days Digoxin (Lanoxin, Natigoxin, etc.) Oral maintenance dose: 0.25–0.75 mg Onset of action: 1 hr Duration of action: 3 days Usually administered with meals	A variety of preparations with varying potency and pharmacokinetics. All preparations increase the force of myocardial contractions; these are the mainstay in the treatment of congestive heart failure. Digitoxin has the lowest margin of safety, i.e., the therapeutic dose is very nearly the toxic dose. A leading drug implicated in drug-induced illnesses requiring hospitalization (Ziance, 1979). Elderly more apt to develop toxicity since the drugs are eliminated more slowly than in younger persons (Cape, 1978; Davison, 1978).	Toxicity associated with hypokalemia, hypocalcemia, hypomagnesemia, hypothyroidism, ischemic heart disease, and those "susceptible to toxic effects of digitalis." Serum potassium levels are decreased through the concurrent use of diuretics and laxatives, and from poor dietary intake, vomiting, diarrhea, or continuous nasogastric suctioning. Hypomagnesemia may be seen with chronic alcoholism. Symptoms of toxicity vary with the elderly. Classical symptoms of nausea and vomiting with marked slowing of heart rate are seen less frequently. Elderly may first experience anorexia and/or cardiac arrhythmias in absence of other signs. Color vision can be disturbed; a brown or yellowish hazy vision is reported in 25% of patients. Neurological effects are seen more in the elderly, including extreme weakness, lethargy, mental confusion, depression, and toxic psychosis. Dizziness due to cardiac arrhythmias may be seen with toxicity. Nausea, vomiting, and diarrhea may be seen. Abdominal pain due to mesenteric ischemia is fairly common in elderly (Davison, 1978).	Note differences in preparations, dosages, and elimination patterns. Therapeutic doses are determined by individual response. Patient must be monitored closely during initial treatment as well as during maintenance. Note pulse rate and rhythm, EKG patterns. Report alterations indicative of toxicity. Observe patient for improvement of condition. Note intake and output, weight, presence/absence of edema, and/or rales. Monitor laboratory reports for potassium and magnesium, especially in those having losses of these ions. Serum drug levels may be used to monitor patient therapy.

DRUG (Trade Name)	CHARACTERISTICS	ADVERSE EFFECTS/TOXICITY	NURSING IMPLICATIONS
DIURETICS			
Thiazides Bendroflumethiazide (Naturetin) Usual oral dose: 5–20 mg qd or bid Duration of action: 18–24 hr Chlorothiazide (Diuril) Usual oral dose: 500 mg–1 g qd Duration of action: 6–12 hr Hydrochlorothiazide (Esidrix, Hydro-Diuril, Oretic) Usual oral dose: 25–100 mg qd Duration of action: 6–12 hr *Thiazide-like drugs* Chlorthalidone (Hygroton) Usual oral dose: 50–100 mg qd Duration of action: 24–72 hr Metolazone (Zaroxolyn) Usual oral dose: 5–20 mg qd Duration of action: 12–24 hr Quinethazone (Hydromox) Usual oral dose: 50–100 mg qd Duration of action: 18–24 hr	Diuretics are frequently used in the treatment of acute and chronic cardiovascular disease. They are the cornerstone of hypertensive therapy, used alone or in combination with other drugs. Thiazides reduce extracellular fluid volume by increasing output of water and electrolytes, mainly sodium, but also chloride and potassium. To avoid hazards of hypokalemia, potassium and chloride supplements are frequently ordered with the thiazides.	The possibility of adverse side effects increases with age (Gotz and Gotz, 1978; Ziance, 1979). With prolonged and poorly monitored therapy, serious fluid and electrolyte disturbances can occur, symptoms of which are easily missed. Mild dehydration, hyponatremia, hypokalemia, and hypochloremia may occur. Thiazides can also induce hyperglycemia and aggravate preexisting diabetes mellitus; they can cause uric acid retention and precipitate an attack of gout in susceptible persons. With concomitant digitalis therapy, lowered levels of serum potassium can lead to digitalis toxicity. With concomitant antihypertensive therapy, thiazides can cause orthostatic hypotension.	Schedule dose in the A.M. to minimize nocturia. Patient should be taught how to monitor edema. Note weight, tightness of shoes, etc. Instruct patient to avoid excessive ingestion of water which can lead to hyponatremia when taking thiazides or potassium-sparing diuretics. Observe for side effects of fluid and electrolyte imbalance, specifically that of hypokalemia (i.e., muscle weakness, lethargy, changes in mental status and behaviors, and vague gastrointestinal complaints). Observe for hypokalemia when conditions contributing to potassium loss are present, i.e., inadequate dietary intake or excessive gastrointestinal losses (e.g., due to protracted vomiting, diarrhea, nasogastric suction, and excessive use of laxatives and enemas).

Drug	Action/Use	Adverse Effects	Implications
Loop diuretics (kidney loop) Furosemide (Lasix) Ethacrynic acid (Edecrin) Dosage varies with situation. Both administered orally or parenterally Duration of action: 6–8 hr	Short acting, more potent, more expensive diuretics than the thiazides. Used to treat refractory edema.	Greater potential for adverse effects of fluid and electrolyte imbalance as well as hypotension. Other adverse effects such as gastrointestinal disturbances and hyperuricemia occur less frequently.	Can produce large quantities of urine quickly and cause urinary incontinence in the elderly (Davison, 1978). (See thiazides for additional implications.)
Potassium-sparing diuretics Spironolactone (Aldactone) Triamterene (Dyrenium) Amiloride (Midamor) Dosage varies	Diuretics which spare the loss of potassium in their action. Used for intermittent treatment or for limited periods of time; can be used concurrently with the thiazides. Peak effect occurs in 4–8 hr.	These drugs do not seem to disturb glucose and purine metabolism like the thiazides but may cause potassium retention, especially with spironolactone.	Review the patient's dietary habits and caution against excessive intake of potassium. Note that salt substitutes contain large amounts of potassium. (See thiazides for additional implications.)

ANTIHYPERTENSIVE DRUGS

Although hypertension is common in the elderly, it is not necessarily an indication for drug therapy. When therapy is indicated, diuretics may be all that is necessary. Only when there is an inadequate response to diuretics, are antihypertensive drugs added. A minimal number of drugs should be used in the lowest possible dosage (Colman, 1979; Moser, 1979). The goal of hypertensive therapy is a gradual reduction in blood pressure to prevent coronary and cerebral insufficiency.

Drug	Action/Use	Adverse Effects	Implications
Methyldopa (Aldomet) 500 mg–2 gm Given orally in divided doses	Thought to bring about its effect by reducing serotonin and norepinephrine in the brain and peripheral tissues.	Regularly occurring side effects are sedation (which may decrease with continued therapy), weakness, drowsiness, headaches, vertigo, and nasal congestion. Postural hypotension develops infrequently. Alcohol, taken with methyldopa, has an addictive effect. Adverse reactions of hemolytic anemia and reversible liver damage have occurred (Blaschke and Melman, 1980; Caird and Dall, 1978).	All effective antihypertensive drugs produce significant adverse effects, some of which may interfere with patient compliance with the therapeutic regimen. The patient needs help to understand the reasons for therapy and measures to minimize side effects. Drug treatment is a long term matter; careful monitoring of response becomes important in determining treatment effectiveness and adverse effects.

DRUG (Trade Name)	CHARACTERISTICS	ADVERSE EFFECTS/TOXICITY	NURSING IMPLICATIONS
Hydralazine (Apresoline) Dosage individualized Administered orally (40–300 mg in divided doses) or parenterally (20 mg)	Lowers blood pressure through direct relaxation of vascular smooth muscle with a greater effect on arterioles than on veins. This decrease in pressure is thought to cause a reflex tachycardia that precipitates chest pains in patients with a history of angina. This effect can be prevented by adding a ganglionic or beta-adrenergic blocking agent such as propranolol (Inderal) to the therapeutic regimen. Reflex tachycardia contraindicates the use of this drug in patients with coronary artery disease and mitral valvular rheumatic heart disease. Elderly may not experience as great tachycardia as younger persons.	Incidence of untoward effects is high. Anorexia, nausea, headache, palpitation, dizziness, and sweating are common. Nasal congestion, flushing, lacrimation, conjunctivitis, paresthesias, edema, tremors, and muscle cramps occur less frequently (Blashke and Melman, 1980). When taken with alcohol, drug hypotensive effects are increased. Drug fever, polyneuritis, gastrointestinal bleeding, and pancytopenia occur rarely but require termination of therapy.	Most antihypertensive drugs are given orally with meals. Patients should be advised of possible postural hypotension which is a frequent side effect of antihypertensive drugs. Instruct patients to rise slowly from a recumbent position and to lie down at the first feeling of dizziness. Patient should avoid prolonged standing and should not attempt strenuous exercise until adjusted to new blood pressure levels because of danger of syncope. Advise patients of adverse symptoms which may occur and should be reported to physician.
Prazosin hydrochloride (Minipress) Dosage adjusted to response (1–20 mg in divided doses)	Blocks alpha-adrenergic responses, thus lowering vascular resistance and decreasing blood pressure.	Marked orthostatic hypotension and syncope may occur with the first dose but disappear with continued therapy. Most common side effects of dizziness, drowsiness, lack of energy, weakness, palpitation, and nausea appear in 5–10% of patients and diminish with continued use.	Dizziness and resultant falling may be the greatest threat to the elderly. Experience with this drug in the elderly is limited; thus the values and risks are not clear at this time (Caird and Dall, 1978).
Beta-adrenergic blocking agents Propranolol hydrochloride (Inderal) Given orally Dosage individualized (160–180 mg in divided doses) Nadolol (Corgard) Dosage individualized Oral dosage: 40–320 mg in divided doses	Propranolol and nadolol are used in the treatment of hypertension as well as cardiac arrhythmias. These drugs block both the cardiac and smooth muscle receptors from responding to sympathetic nerve impulses or to the circulating catecholamines and adrenergic drugs.	Side effects are slight and include fatigue, light-headedness, and gastrointestinal discomforts. Drugs are contraindicated in patients with chronic obstructive lung disease since airway resistance can be increased with the drugs and the condition worsened. Drug is contraindicated in most patients with congestive heart failure, bradycardia, and second or third degree heart block. Propranolol masks early signs of hypoglycemia, and caution is advised when it is administered to insulin-dependent diabetics.	See implications discussed with antihypertensive drugs (p. 403). The primary advantages of propranolol use in the elderly are the minimal/slight side effects; the number of older patients who respond to beta blockers is considerably fewer than younger patients (Moser, 1979). There should be routine monitoring as for other antihypertensive drugs.

Metoprolol tartrate (Lopressor) Oral dosage: 50 mg bid but may be individualized higher	Metoprolol selectively blocks β_1-adrenergic receptors and blocks β_2-adrenergic receptors only in high doses. It is used basically in the treatment of hypertension.	Metoprolol is thought to cause less adverse effects than propranolol.
Other agents Reserpine (Serpasil) Oral or parenteral 0.25–1 mg bid to qid	This drug gradually drops the blood pressure by partially blocking transmission of tonic vasomotor and cardioaccelerating impulses from the sympathetic nerves. Its effects are believed to result from the release and depletion of the neurotransmitter norepinephrine in the adrenergic nerve endings.	Reserpine side effects present serious deterrents to its use in geriatric patients. Mental depression, estimated to occur in 18% of all patients, is the chief deterrent. This depression can be subtle and insidious but may also be of the magnitude to demand hospitalization. Effects may continue for several weeks after treatment is discontinued. Other effects include nasal congestion, drowsiness with feelings of weakness and fatigue, gastric distress, decreased libido, impotence, increased appetite, and weight gain (Caird and Dall, 1978).
Clonidine hydrochloride (Catapres) 0.1–0.8 mg orally	Clonidine acts as an agonist at central alpha-adrenergic receptors, reducing the outflow of sympathetic nerve impulses. The hypotensive effect is associated with a decreased heart rate and fall in cardiac output.	Common side effects are a persistent drowsiness and dryness of mouth. Impotence, constipation, postural hypotension, and depression occur less commonly. Abrupt withdrawal may lead to hyperirritability and marked rebound in blood pressure. The rapid rise in blood pressure may cause central nervous system complications but can be controlled by intravenous administration of an alpha-adrenergic blocking agent such as phentolamine (Regitine).
		Because of disturbing adverse effects, clonidine therapy is reserved for those patients whose blood pressure cannot be adequately controlled by other drugs (Blaschke and Melman, 1980).
Guanethidine sulfate (Ismelin) Dosage individualized Administered orally: 10–50 mg	Guanethidine is used only in selected cases (Blaschke and Melman, 1980). This drug is a postganglionic sympathetic blocking agent which reduces venous return and cardiac output. This is not always a desirable effect in the elderly.	A dramatic postural hypotension, relatively rare in younger patients, presents itself as a common side effect in the elderly. This hypotension is potentiated by other drugs such as alcohol, and is accentuated by high temperatures and exercise. The postural hypotension is quite hazardous in the elderly. Other disquieting side effects include diarrhea and interference with normal ejaculation in sexually active men.
		See p. 399 for nursing implications.
		See p. 404 for implications. Note those dealing with postural hypotension.

DRUG (Trade Name)	CHARACTERISTICS	ADVERSE EFFECTS/TOXICITY	NURSING IMPLICATIONS
NITRATES Amyl nitrite (Aspirols, Vaporole) Inhalation route: 0.2 ml Erythrityl tetranitrate (Cardilate) Dosage: 5–30 mg orally prn; 5–15 mg sublingually Isosorbide dinitrate (Isordil, Sorbitrate) Sublingual and oral: 2.5–20 mg prn Mannitol hexanitrate (Maxitate, Nitranitol) Oral route: 15–60 mg q 4–6 hr Nitroglycerin (Nitrol, Nitrostat, Glyceral trinitrate, Nitro-Bid, etc.) Sublingual, oral, and topical routes Oral: 0.1–0.6 mg prn; sublingual: 2.6–6.5 mg bid Pentaerythritol tetranitrate (Peritrate) Oral route: 5–20 mg Trolnitrate phosphate (Metamine, Nitretamin) Oral route: 2–4 mg tid pc and hs	The nitrates relax vascular smooth muscle and are used mainly in the management of angina pectoris. It is through the resultant vasodilation that nitrates increase circulation to ischemic areas of myocardium, decreasing anginal pain. Indirectly, the nitrates decrease myocardial oxygen requirements by decreasing peripheral resistance and reducing the work load on the heart. Preparations vary in route of administrations, onset, and duration of action. Rapidly acting preparations are used to abort an acute anginal attack. Slower acting drugs like isosorbide dinitrate and erythrityl tetranitrate may be used to prevent an anginal attack from occurring. These two drugs produce a vasodilation effect in about 5 min, reach a peak in 30–45 min, and lasting 2 hr or more. Slower acting nitrates may be used for the long term management of angina. Pentaerythritol and a 2% nitroglycerin ointment may be used for this purpose. In theory, these nitrates are supposed to help stimulate the development of collateral coronary circulation. Long term therapy should reduce the number, duration, and intensity of attacks.	The vasodilation caused by nitrates produces a fall in blood pressure, and the patient may feel weak, dizzy, and faint. If the blood pressure drops too low, a reflex tachycardia may be precipitated. The concurrent use of alcohol and nitroglycerin can intensify the drop in blood pressure, producing a severe shock-like state called "nitrite syncope." A throbbing headache is generally seen with high doses and can be controlled with a dose reduction. The longer acting nitrates are more apt to cause severe headaches. Tolerance and cross-tolerance also occurs with long term use of nitrates. Therefore, the lowest possible effective dosage is recommended. There are arguments against the use of nitrates for sustained prophylactic therapy. One argument is that around-the-clock nitrate blood levels favor the development of cross-tolerance to all nitrates. This tolerance would limit the effectiveness of nitroglycerin in alleviating acute anginal attacks.	The rapidly acting nitrates, such as nitroglycerin, are used to abort an acute anginal attack. The patient needs to know that the nitroglycerin is placed under the tongue at the first sign of pain, allowing the tablet to dissolve completely in the mouth. Full effects of the drug are reached in 2–3 min. After taking nitroglycerin, the patient should rest in a sitting or lying position to minimize hypotensive effects. If the drug is not effective, a second or third tablet may be taken at 5-min intervals. If pain is not relieved in this time period, the physician should be notified (Sheridan, 1982). To prevent deterioration of nitroglycerin, tablets should be stored in a dark glass bottle, tightly capped, and kept in a cool area. The tablet causes an initial burning sensation under the tongue; lack of this sensation may indicate deterioration of the medication.

CALCIUM BLOCKERS			
Nifedipine (Procardia) Dosage individualized Oral: start with 10 mg tid Verapamil (Calan, Isoptin) Dosage individualized Oral: start with 80 mg tid or qid Available parenterally as Calan	Calcium blockers are newly approved drugs used in the management of angina pectoris. They inhibit the influx of extracellular calcium into cardiac and vascular smooth muscle. This causes vasodilation with a reduction of peripheral vascular resistance, lowering of blood pressure, and reversal of coronary spasm. The cardiac effects are less prominent; they include negative inotropic effects and depressed sinoatrial (SA) and atrioventricular (AV) node function (FDA, 1982).	Side effects of these drugs are similar but not identical. Nifedipine has a greater tendency to lower blood pressure and cause slight increases in pulse, dizziness, palpitation, flushing, numbness, and tingling of extremities. Excessive hypotension is most probable during initial treatment. Concomitant use with beta blockers and nitrates is possible but not without problems. Further study is needed. Verapamil has a greater tendency to inhibit SA and AV nodal conduction, and may cause sinus bradycardia and AV block. Marked decreases in blood pressure are usual. Contraindicated in patients with heart failure and liver failure. Both drugs may increase serum digoxin levels in chronic digoxin therapy.	Use of these new drugs has not generated sufficient data as to their specific effects on the elderly. Patients should be advised of possible adverse effects, how they can be controlled, and when medical attention is indicated. With verapamil, monitoring of the pulse is important.

CENTRAL NERVOUS SYSTEM DRUGS SEDATIVE/HYPNOTICS

Principle use of the sedative/hypnotics is to produce drowsiness and sleep. Most drugs in this classification bring about effects by depressing a wide range of cellular function in many vital organ systems. The proper use of sedative/hypnotics is for temporary induction of sleep over short periods of time, no longer than a matter of days (Pfeiffer, 1978).

Barbiturates Wide variety of dosages (consult PDR and drug references)	Barbiturates suppress rapid eye movement (REM) sleep.	Barbiturates should be avoided in the elderly. They frequently produce a "hangover" effect, impairing judgment and motor coordination. With long term use in the elderly, barbiturates accumulate and cause a syndrome suggestive of arteriosclerotic dementia. This syndrome is manifested by intellectual impairment, slurred speech, and an unsteady gait (Cape, 1978; Davison, 1978). Upon cessation of therapy, the patient may be temporarily worse, suffering nightmares and delirium.	Insomnia is a subjective symptom, and a careful history of the patient's sleep habits is a necessary part of assessment and treatment. Attempt nondrug methods to deal with insomnia: daytime exercise, bedtime relaxation techniques, pain relief, scheduling of sleep-related activities, warm milk, control of the environment. These activities should also be included when hypnotics is taken.

DRUG (Trade Name)	CHARACTERISTICS	ADVERSE EFFECTS/TOXICITY	NURSING IMPLICATIONS
Barbiturates (continued)		Tolerance and dependence are problems with long term use of barbiturates. Long term use also allows the use of the drugs as a "magnificent suicidal tool" (Pfeiffer, 1978). Concurrent use of barbiturates and alcohol is dangerous because of synergistic effects. The lethal dose for barbiturates is nearly 50% lower in the presence of alcohol than when used alone. Death can occur as a result of respiratory depression. Alcohol abusers who have developed tolerance to alcohol exhibit cross-tolerance to the barbiturates (FDA, 1979a).	Elderly patients awakened from a drug-induced sleep may experience dizziness and need assistance getting out of bed. Hypnotics are used in suicide attempts (Sheridan, 1982).
Chloral hydrate 250–600 mg Administered orally and rectally	One of the oldest and perhaps most effective hypnotic drugs for the elderly. The drug does not appear to modify REM sleep and is fairly quickly removed from the body.	The chief side effect may be gastric distress. Hangover may occur but not as frequently as from barbiturates. Should not be given with alcohol because central nervous system effects will be potentiated. The drug may also affect the metabolism of oral anticoagulants, causing unexpected bleeding. As with barbiturates, tolerance and dependence are possible (Cape, 1978; Davison, 1978; Harvey, 1980b).	See barbiturate implications.
Ethchlorvynol (Placidyl) Administered with food 500–700 mg orally hs for hypnosis; 100–500 mg for sedation	Ethchlorvynol is another nonbarbiturate hypnotic recommended for use in the elderly.	May cause mild gastrointestinal effects. Mild hangover is common despite the short half-life of the drug. Tolerance and dependence can occur with long term use. Reduces the effectiveness of oral anticoagulants.	See barbiturate implications.

Drug/Dosage	Action	Implications
Flurazepam (Dalmane) 15–30 mg hs orally	Flurazepam is a benzodiazepine that is frequently used as a hypnotic. Although the drug does not supress REM sleep, it does suppress stage 3 and 4 sleep. This may be a disadvantage in the treatment of insomnia (FDA, 1979b).	
	Metabolites of flurazepam have a half-life of 50–100 hr, compared to the half-life of 14–42 hr for amobarbital, pentobarbital, and secobarbital. There are potential risks with the buildup of flurazepam in the body. Unwanted daytime carry-over effects of drowsiness and poor coordination may occur. These effects are more profound in the elderly, with symptoms similar to organic brain syndrome occurring at times (Ivey, 1979).

Unexpected toxic reactions with alcohol can also occur with these prolonged drug serum levels (FDA, 1979a). | See barbiturate implications.

Short term therapy with instructions to the patient can prevent some of the adverse reactions. |
| PSYCHOTROPICS PHENOTHIAZINES

Aliphatic subgroups
Chlorpromazine hydrochloride (Thorazine)
10–200 mg tid orally
Promazine hydrochloride (Sparine)
10–50 mg tid orally
Triflupromazine hydrochloride (Vesprin)
10–50 mg orally
Piperazine subgroups
Acetophenazine dimaleate (Tindal)
20–40 mg tid
Butaperazine maleate (Repoise)
Up to 100 mg qd
Carphenazine maleate (Proketazine)
12.5–50 mg daily | When administered to mentally disturbed patients, phenothiazines are tranquilizing and antipsychotic in action. In addition, these drugs have autonomic blocking action and antiemetic effects. They also potentiate the action of other depressant drugs and decrease the seizure threshold.

Phenothiazines are classified into three groups, all essentially similar in action, differing however in potency and side effects.

The aliphatic group is more likely to produce sedation and blockade of peripheral sites innervated by the autonomic nervous system.

The piperazine subgroup is more likely to cause extrapyramidal motor side effects; it has more antiemetic effects. Haloperidol resembles this group of drugs. | Used faily commonly with the elderly, these drugs provide great therapeutic benefits, but not without some problems. There is a wide margin of safety, but phenothiazines are capable of causing many different types of adverse effects. Many side effects are dose related. Massive doses used in psychotic disorders of younger patients have been most beneficial; however, this is not so with the elderly (Ziance, 1979). Adverse effects may deter compliance and present hazards for the elderly.

Autonomic effects include drug-induced postural hypotension with a reflex tachycardia, a common and dangerous effect in the elderly. These effects lead to dizziness, weakness, fainting, and heart palpitation. Individuals may fall and sustain bodily injury.

Direct cardiac depressant effects with conduction defects, arrhythmias, and cardiac | Postural hypotension causes a reduced cerebral oxygenation in the elderly, worsening agitated states. To minimize this hypotension, elastic hose are recommended. Caution patients to change from recumbent to sitting position slowly and to avoid standing for prolonged periods.

Ziance (1979) recommends initiation of drug therapy at low dosages and increasing very slowly as needed in the elderly.

Baseline data on physiological and psychological status before therapy is initiated are necessary in determining patient progress.

Dryness of mouth can be diminished with sugar-free gum or candies and frequent sips of water. |

DRUG (Trade Name)	CHARACTERISTICS	ADVERSE EFFECTS/TOXICITY	NURSING IMPLICATIONS
Piperazine subgroups (continued) Fluphenazine hydrochloride (Permitil, Prolixin) Perphenazine (Trilafon) 2–16 mg tid orally; 5 mg IM q 6 hr Prochlorperazine dimaleate (Compazine) Thiopropazate hydrochloride (Dartal) Trifluoperazine hydrochloride (Stelazine) *Piperidyl subgroup* Mesoridazine besylate (Serentil) 10–400 mg orally or IM daily Piperacetazine (Quide) 10–160 mg orally daily Thioridazine hydrochloride (Mellaril) 10–200 mg tid or qid orally *Other* Haloperidol (Haldol) 1–5 mg bid orally or IM	The piperidyl subgroup has effects more like those of the aliphatic group. Starting dose should not exceed 40 mg daily.	arrest may occur; these are more prominent with parenteral administration of the aliphatic subgroup and have been reported in the elderly. Cholinergic blockage action causes dryness of the mouth, blurring of vision, constipation with possible obstipation and paralytic ileus, urinary retention, failure to sweat, nasal stuffiness, and inhibition of ejaculation. These effects can be disturbing to the elderly. Central nervous system effects may be the result of either excessive depression or excessive stimulation. Depressive effects of drowsiness, lethargy, weakness, and fatigue are more common in the elderly (Cape, 1978; Ziance, 1979). Mood depression and toxic confusion reactions also occur in the elderly. Adverse effects due to stimulation of the extrapyramidal motor system are classified into four categories: 1. Parkinsonism — a lack of activity, or akinesia; tremor, mask-like facies, and shuffling gait. 2. Acute dyskineasia or dystonias — an acute reaction of sudden contractions of muscle groups in spasms resembling convulsive seizures. 3. Akathisia — extreme mental and motor restlessness; the patient finds it impossible to sit still or to sleep. 4. Persistent tardive dyskinesia — characterized by abnormal, repetitive, involuntary movements which are not present during sleep. Lips, tongue, and jaw involvement make	With the elderly, monitor urinary and bowel output. Constipation can become quite a problem. With decreased sweating, caution the elderly to avoid excessive heat in hot weather to prevent heat stroke. Monitor the patient closely for signs of extrapyramidal motor system stimulation (dyskinesia). Observe and document involuntary movements, body part involved, intensity, and duration (Rosal-Grief, 1982). Observe for hypersensitivity reactions. Provide protection from sunlight. Extrapyramidal adverse reactions occur more frequently in the elderly. It has been estimated that 50% of geriatric patients receiving chlorpromazine will develop parkinsonism and dyskinesias. Elderly women are particularly prone to develop akathisias (Ziance, 1979). These reactions are best controlled by reduction of dosage or cessation of therapy. Many times these symptoms are misinterpreted as increased agitation, with a resultant increase in dosage and subsequent exacerbation of symptoms. Antiparkinsonism drugs may also be given, but these drugs have similar side effects which only produce more patient discomfort. One method to prevent persistent tardive dyskinesia is to give the patient annual drug holidays of 6–12 weeks. The holidays decrease the total cumulative drug dosage, as well as allowing time

Other (continued)	speech and swallowing difficult. Muscles of the extremities may twitch and jerk uncontrollably (Figure 34-1). This reaction differs from the others in that it develops gradually in patients on long term antipsychotic therapy, is persistent, and can be irreversible. At present there is no known treatment except prevention and the use of lower drug dosages. Hypersensitivity reactions occur, including hematologic, hepatic, and dermatologic types. Chlorpromazine-induced jaundice is common in the elderly. Many elderly also develop scaling of the skin upon exposure to sunlight (Ziance, 1979). Other skin reactions such as diffuse melanosis are also seen frequently in the elderly (Davison, 1978). Ocular changes do occur, and manifest as cataracts and corneal opacities. Hypothermia is another possible hazard of phenothiazine therapy (Ivey, 1979).	to uncover "masked" dyskinesias (DeVeaugh-Geiss, 1979).
ANTIANXIETY AGENTS *Benzodiazepines* Chlordiazepoxide hydro- chloride (Librium) 5–10–25 mg tid or qid orally; 100 mg IM or IV q 4–6 hr Clorazepate mono- or dipotassium (Azene, Tranxene) Diazepam (Valium) 15–30 mg daily in divided doses Flurazepam hydrochloride (Dalmane) – a hypnotic 15–30 mg hs orally	The benzodiazepines are used in the elderly to alleviate anxiety, calm agitation, and treat withdrawal from alcohol. Some drugs in this group have skeletal muscle-relaxant properties. This group probably constitutes the most commonly used drugs in the Western world. Tolerance and dependence occur with prolonged therapy. The benzodiazepines are frequently misused and abused.	Common side effects in the elderly are excessive sedation, dizziness, weakness, unsteadiness, and confusion. The frequency of drowsiness is almost twice as high in people over 70 years receiving chlordiazepoxide as in those under 40. Increased lethargy is seen. Most geriatricians recommend cautious use of these drugs, especially with the elderly who become confused. The biological half-life of most drugs is increased in the elderly, causing the potential for accumulation and toxicity. Clinical effects of these drugs may not be evident for several	These drugs are not substitutes for helping patients deal with anxiety. Patients should understand the need for other therapies that may be used. Remember that the elderly and debilitated are more prone to drowsiness. Patients should be monitored and cautioned about avoiding activities requiring mental alertness so that their safety is not jeopardized. The commonly seen side effects in the elderly are also prominent symptoms of illness; this makes diagnostic decisions more difficult (Cape, 1978; Ziance, 1979).

DRUG (Trade Name)	CHARACTERISTICS	ADVERSE EFFECTS/TOXICITY	NURSING IMPLICATIONS
Benzodiazepines (continued) Lorazepam (Ativan) 1–10 mg orally in divided doses Oxazepam (Serax) Prazepam (Verstran) 10–30 mg tid or qid orally		days, and effects will persist after the drugs are discontinued.	Cape (1978) states that benzodiazepines should seldom be used for the elderly because of debilitating effects. If necessary, he recommends oxazepam because of its shorter half-life. Caution patients against drinking alcohol without permission of physician.
ANTIDEPRESSANTS *Tricyclic preparations* Amitriptyline hydrochloride (Elavil) 10–50 mg tid orally; 20–50 mg qid IM; 100–200 mg hs Desipramine hydrochloride (Norpramin, Pertofrane) 20–50 mg tid orally Doxepin hydrochloride (Adapin, Sinequan) 75–300 mg daily orally Imipramine hydrochloride (Tofranil, Presamine) Dosage is individually determined Nortriptyline hydrochloride (Aventyl) 25 mg tid orally Adjust dose to patient Protriptyline hydrochloride (Vivactil) 15–40 mg orally in divided doses	Tricyclic antidepressants are drugs of choice in treatment of depression in the elderly. These drugs are similar in chemical structure to the phenothiazines. They exert a sedative effect during the first days of therapy, with mood elevation not evident for 2–3 weeks. This necessitates initiation of other supportive therapies to assist the patient during this time.	Low dosages are recommended for the elderly because of their lower threshold for toxic side effects (Ziance, 1979). The most common adverse effects are related to the anticholinergic activity of these drugs. Symptoms most uncomfortable to the elderly are dry mouth, constipation, blurred vision, postural hypotension, dizziness, tachycardia, and urinary retention. Cardiac rhythm changes are possible, and care must be exercised in administering these drugs to the elderly with known cardiac rhythm problems. These drugs are also used cautiously in the elderly who have glaucoma or prostate enlargement. With higher doses, extrapyramidal effects are possible. These drugs can produce synergistic or antagonistic interactions with alcohol, depending on the drug. Desipramine has a tendency to antagonize depressant effects of alcohol, whereas amitriptyline can potentiate alcohol's sedative effect (FDA, 1979).	Tricyclic antidepressants have a 24-hr half-life, allowing for a single bedtime dosage. This allows inconvenient side effects to occur while sleeping but can be hazardous to those who get up during the night. Single dosage assists in promoting compliance. Antidepressant drugs have side effects similar to those experienced with the phenothiazines (postural hypotension, cardiovascular effects, gastrointestinal and urinary effects, extrapyramidal effects, and hypersensitivity reactions). (See p. 000 for a discussion of implications.)

ANTIPARKINSONISM DRUGS

Parkinson's disease is one of the most common degenerative diseases of the nervous system, affecting at least 1% of those over age 50 (Gresh, 1980). The classical symptoms of bradykinesia, loss of postural reflexes, rigidity, and tremor at rest are easily envisioned.

In Parkinson's disease, the normally high level of dopamine (a neurotransmitter) in the corpus striatum is severely reduced. The cause of this reduction is unknown. It is known that some drugs reduce dopamine stores in the nerve endings, and the pheno-thiazines block dopamine receptors in the striatum. A variety of parkinsonian syndromes (idiopathic, postencephalitic, arteriosclerotic, etc.) have also been associated with striatal dopamine deficiency. Lack of the inhibitory dopamine activity leads to unbridled excitatory acetylcholine activity, resulting in the extrapyramidal disorder of parkinsonism. Thus the treatment of parkinsonism is designed to reduce cholinergic activity and/or increase dopaminergic activity in an attempt to restore striatal neurotransmitter balance (Davison, 1979).

Levodopa and combinations

Levodopa (Dopar, Larodopa)
Dose is individually adjusted

Carbidopa and levodopa (Sinemet)

Maximum daily dose:
200 mg of carbidopa and 2000 mg of levodopa

The administration of dopamine itself is ineffective in treating parkinsonism since dopamine does not cross the blood-brain barrier. Therefore, the biologic precursor of dopamine, levodopa, and its combinations are used rather successfully in the treatment of moderate to severe parkinsonism. Levodopa allows the patient more optimal function but does not prevent progressive deterioration due to the underlying disease.

With chronic levodopa therapy, rapid swings in intensity of patient symptoms have been noted. Such variation in intensity of signs and symptoms may be related to the chronic use of levodopa. These dramatic and rapid changes in mobility (called the "yo-yo" and "on-off" effects) are seen after 2–3 years of therapy. It is believed that these effects may be related to dosage and readjustments should be made. If these effects are accompanied by postural hypotension and mental deterioration, this is thought to represent a more advanced stage of the disease and readjustments in drug therapy will not be effective (Davison, 1978).

Side effects of levodopa therapy may limit its usefulness. Common side effects include gastrointestinal disturbances, postural hypotension, urinary retention, cardiac arrhythmias, involuntary movements, and gross mental changes.

If cardiac irregularities occur, the physician may prescribe a beta-adrenergic blocker such as propranolol. The patient will need continued monitoring of drug therapy to assure continued adequate cardiac functioning.

Involuntary movements (choreoathetosis and dyskinesias) occur at dose levels that are necessary to produce maximum benefits for rigidity and bradykinesia, but dosages must be reduced or readjusted to avoid the involuntary movements.

Mood swings are also seen with levodopa therapy. Generally, elevation of mood is experienced, leading to overstimulation with resultant agitation, mental confusion, delirium, hallucinations, and psychosis. Depression of mood is also seen and may necessitate addition of other therapies (Davison, 1979).

It has been reported that levodopa may enhance libido and activate sexual behavior in a small number of patients.

Presently most patients starting therapy are given levodopa concurrently with a decarboxylase inhibitor which blocks the peripheral metabolism of levodopa, thus enhancing its therapeutic effectiveness in the brain. This drug combination minimizes the gastrointestinal disturbances, postural hypotension, and cardiac arrhythmias. The main adverse effects of the combination therapy are involuntary movements and mental disturbances (Davison, 1979).

The gastrointestinal side effects may be minimized by administering the drug after meals or with an antacid or milk.

Postural hypotension may be minimized by advising the patient to change positions slowly and to wear elastic hose.

Patients need to know that therapeutic effects may not be evident for at least 2–3 weeks after treatment is started. Once drug effects have occurred the patient should increase activity gradually, within limits of his cardiovascular system.

In patients experiencing increased libido, the nurse should be aware of opportunities to counsel and assist these patients and their spouses regarding needs for

DRUG (Trade Name)	CHARACTERISTICS	ADVERSE EFFECTS/TOXICITY	NURSING IMPLICATIONS
Levodopa and combinations (continued)		Levodopa should not be given concurrently with monoamine oxidase inhibitors or with pyridoxin. Patients receiving monoamine oxidase inhibitors must have these drugs discontinued at least two weeks prior to levodopa therapy to avoid possible hypertensive crisis. Pyridoxine interferes with the amount of levodopa that can reach its central site of action. Multivitamin preparation containing pyridoxine must be avoided.	sexual intimacy and, if necessary, to prevent punitive reactions to a "sexy" old man or lady. Gather baseline physiological and psychological data so that patient progress can be monitored.
Ergolines Bromocriptine 20–150 mg daily	Newest drug for treatment of Parkinson's disease, approved by the FDA in November 1981. Has had extensive testing in past 5 years. Usually given in combination with levodopa or Sinemet. This allows dose of standard drug to be reduced and to be longer acting. Fifty to seventy percent of patients respond. Greatest improvement in early stages. Still very expensive (Hoehn, 1981; Parkinson's Disease Foundation, 1982).	Ten percent of patients do not respond. A considerable number have serious side effects of nausea, vomiting, or visual, auditory, and mental disturbances. Bromocriptine induces less dyskinesia than levodopa.	Patient and family need to be educated about idiosyncrasies of parkinsonism drugs. Watch for dyskinesia and monitor dosages carefully. The medication controls rather than cures. Patient may have problems swallowing. Monitor for adequate fluid and nutrition.
Lergotrile (experimental at this time)			
Anticholinergic drugs Benztropine mesylate (Cogentin) Biperiden hydrochloride (Akineton) Cycrimine hydrochloride (Pagitane) Procyclidine hydrochloride (Kemadrin) Trihexyphenidyl hydrochloride (Artane, Pipanol, Tremin)	The anticholinergic drugs are used in all forms of parkinsonism, for those patients with minimal symptoms or for those unable to tolerate levodopa. The drugs may be used as adjuncts to levodopa therapy. These drugs are all given in small doses individually adjusted.	The side effects of these drugs may limit their use. Common atropine-like effects are seen: dry mouth, blurred vision, constipation, and urinary retention. Large doses lead to central symptoms of mental confusion, delirium, ataxia, hallucinations, somnolence, and rarely, coma.	Drug administration depends on the patient's symptoms: if excessive salivation, administer after meals; if excessive dryness, administer with meals unless nausea occurs. Patients need to know that they will experience some side effects to gain relief from the disease.

Drug	Comments	Nursing Interventions
Antihistamine drugs Chlorphenoxamine hydrochloride (Phenoxene) 50–100 mg qid orally; 10 mg IM or IV Diphenhydramine hydrochloride (Benadryl) Orphenadrine hydrochloride (Disipal) 50 mg tid orally	Antihistamines possess some central anticholinergic properties and may be better tolerated by the elderly than other antiparkinsonism drugs.	Mouth care is important. Alleviate dryness of mouth with sugar-free gum or candies and frequent sips of water. Constipation should be avoided by adequate fluid intake, dietary planning, and establishment of regular habits.
Phenothiazines Ethopropazine hydrochloride (Parsidol)	Antihistamines produce fewer side effects but do not benefit the tremor and sialorrhea as well as anticholinergic agents. They are helpful in some patients because of their sedative effect, and their tendency to improve mood and muscle strength. This phenothiazine has properties similar to that of diphenhydramine and trihexyphenidyl.	Activities that require alertness and skill should be planned when blurred vision and sedation are at a minimum.
ANALGESICS AND ANTIRHEUMATICS *Narcotics* Morphine Usually ordered and given in traditionally established doses Meperidine hydrochloride (Demerol) 20–100 mg q 3–4 hr prn orally	With morphine, the elderly appear more sensitive to side effects of respiratory depression, urinary retention, and constipation. However, tolerance to respiratory depression occurs over time. Morphine produces a "detached" feeling creating problems for some elderly (Davison, 1978). Hypotension, confusion, and nausea are seen in the elderly receiving meperidine (Cape, 1978). This may be due to increased quantities of free drug circulating because of meperidine's inability to bind to the red blood cells of the elderly. Tolerance and dependence occur with the narcotics.	Pain is a subjective symptom, and its causes have to be explored. Whenever possible, interventions that decrease or alleviate the pain experience should be used. Such interventions include correct handling of injured tissues, positioning for comfort, use of thermal applications, relief of pressure, relief of anxiety, and relaxation techniques. When narcotics are used, the patients' respiratory rate should be monitored. Analgesics are generally administered at intervals determined by the individual's response, preferably when the pain begins and before it becomes too severe. Safety precautions must be exercised with the elderly, who may experience dizziness with narcotic administration.
	Narcotic analgesics are valuable for the elderly experiencing acute pain but should be used cautiously and in small doses. Alcohol potentiates central nervous system depressant effects when given with the following narcotics: hydromorphone (Dilaudid), meperidine (Demerol), morphine, and propoxyphene (Darvon). Research has found increased impairment of motor activities due to synergistic effects of alcohol and morphine; no similar results appear for codeine. The opiates and propoxyphene have been reported to be involved frequently in deaths due to alcohol-drug combinations (FDA, 1979a).	

DRUG (Trade Name)	CHARACTERISTICS	ADVERSE EFFECTS/TOXICITY	NURSING IMPLICATIONS
Salicylates Aspirin 300–600 mg q 3–4 hr orally; not more than 3 g in 24 hr	Salicylates are used for their analgesic, anti-pyretic, anti-inflammatory, and antirheumatic actions. Aspirin interferes with platelet aggregation and prolongs bleeding time. Therefore, aspirin may be used at times for prophylaxis in patients prone to thromboembolic episodes, particularly for the prevention of coronary and cerebral thrombosis (Flower, Moncada, and Vane, 1980).	With low dosages, aspirin causes few ill effects. The larger doses used in chronic rheumatoid arthritis cause gastrointestinal discomfort and toxicity. Gastric bleeding is fairly common, generally being discovered only when iron deficiency anemia develops. More overt bleeding is uncommon but occurs in patients with a history of peptic ulcer, atrophic gastritis, or esophagitis. Salicylates should be avoided in patients with such a history.	Aspirin is available as a nonprescription drug, and individuals should be taught to avoid excessive use. Patients may need to be advised to see a physician when adverse symptoms persist. Aspirin is irritating to gastric mucosa and even with small doses can cause gastrointestinal discomfort. This distress can be avoided by administering it with food (e.g., milk or crackers), after meals, or with an antacid. Aspirin taken with alcohol increases distress.
Other antirheumatic agents Phenylbutazone (Butazolidin) 100–200 mg usually tid; individually adjusted with meals or milk Oxyphenbutazone (Tandearil) Dose should be reduced to minimum for maintenance 100 mg daily in divided doses – orally	These drugs are chemically related and may be used for acute and short term treatment of rheumatic disorders when other agents are ineffective.	Side effects and serious risks are increased with age. These risks are dose and time related. Side effects include gastrointestinal upset, hemorrhage, peptic ulcer, possible severe blood dyscrasias, and edema as a result of drug-induced fluid retention. Davison (1978) suggests that these drugs be avoided in the elderly, especially those with hypertension and incipient cardiac failure.	Administer with meals or milk to minimize gastric distress. Patients need to be monitored by the physician during drug use. Frequent blood counts may be indicated. If edema occurs, the physician may prescribe a limited sodium intake.
Ibuprofen (Motrin) 300–400 mg tid or qid orally Fenoprofen (Nalfon) 600 mg qid orally 30 min before or 2 hr after meals Naproxen (Naprosyn) 250 mg bid orally Sulindac (Clinoril) 150–200 mg bid orally with food Tolmetin (Tolectin) 600–1800 mg in divided doses	These are fairly recent antirheumatic agents used in the treatment of rheumatoid arthritis, osteoarthritis, and other joint inflammations. Present studies have not proved these drugs to be more effective than the salicylates in the relief of rheumatoid arthritis. These newer drugs are more expensive than aspirin.	In usual dosages, all of these drugs cause fewer gastrointestinal complaints than aspirin, estimated at 50% less; however, gastrointestinal discomforts occur, and the ulcerogenic potential is present. Other side effects include drowsiness and blurred vision when given naproxen and fenoprofen. Naproxen and sulindac produce prolonged anti-inflammatory activity.	See aspirin. All of these drugs are contraindicated in patients who are hypersensitive to aspirin. Special effects of these drugs in the elderly are not available at this time.

HYPOGLYCEMIC AGENTS

There is an appreciable incidence of maturity onset diabetes with increasing age. The majority of those affected are obese, and a suitable diet may be all that is required to control the condition. Diabetic ketoacidosis is not common in the older age group. Danger in the treatment of maturity onset diabetes lies in overtreatment since hypoglycemia can be a greater danger for the elderly, leading to permanent cerebral damage (Cape, 1978; Davison, 1978).

SULFONYLUREA DRUGS

Acetohexamide (Dymelor) 250–500 mg qd to qid orally
Duration of action: 12–24 hr

Chlorpropamide (Diabinese) 100–250 mg qd
Duration of action: 24 hr plus

Tolazamide (Tolinase)
Duration of action: 6–10 hr
Individual adjusted dose

Tolbutamide (Orinase)
Duration of action: 3–5 hr
0.5–3 g orally

The sulfonylurea drugs are the drugs used in the treatment of maturity onset diabetes. There is much controversy regarding their use. The University Group Diabetes Program (1970) reported that diabetics receiving tolbutamide or biguanide had a higher mortality rate from cardiovascular disease than patients treated with diet alone, insulin, or placebos. The validity of this study has been severely criticized, and the FDA has not withdrawn tolbutamide at this time. Biguanide has been withdrawn from the U.S. market based on its relationship to development of lactic acidosis, a frequently fatal metabolic disorder.

Chlorpropamide, unlike other drugs in the group, is excreted in unchanged form by the kidneys over a prolonged period of time.

Hypoglycemia is the major adverse effect of sulfonylureas. Many elderly do not manifest classic hypoglycemic symptoms, and diagnosis may not be made until the blood sugar drop is severe. This is further compounded by poor dietary habits, loss of appetite, or inadequate resources of the elderly person.

Chlorpropamide, because of its longer half-life and the possibility of drug accumulation, is associated with severe hypoglycemic reactions in the elderly. Even after correcting the hypoglycemia and stopping the drug, the hypoglycemia may recur because of the prolonged time necessary to excrete the drug (Davison, 1978). Periods of mild hypoglycemia occurring over weeks can cause considerable permanent damage. Patients receiving the longer acting drugs need to be monitored closely.

The second most common side effect of the sulfonylureas involves skin reactions. These reactions may not appear until 6–24 months after therapy is started. Hypersensitivity reactions may be manifested in the skin, bone marrow, and liver.

The patient should be taught the nature of the illness; the importance of diet, exercise, weight control, and personal hygiene; and the role of drugs.

Attention is given to monitoring progress by testing for blood glucose levels.

Patients also need to know causes, symptoms, prevention, and treatment of hypo- and hyperglycemia.

Drug therapy is long term and demands regular follow-up care by the physician.

Drug interactions occur with the sulfonylureas and must be considered. Sulfonamides, propranolol, salicylates, phenylbutazone, probenecid, monoamine oxidase inhibitors, dicumarol, and alcohol increase the risk of hypoglycemia. When combined with alcohol, the sulfonylureas produce a reaction similar to that seen with disulfiram (Antabuse). This is marked by discomfort such as throbbing headache, nausea and vomiting, breathing difficulty, and heart palpitation. Antagonism to the activity of the sulfonylureas has been noted with the use of steroids, diuretics, and high doses of nicotinic acid (Larner, 1980).

DRUG (Trade Name)	CHARACTERISTICS	ADVERSE EFFECTS/TOXICITY	NURSING IMPLICATIONS
INSULIN Dosage always individualized *Quick acting* Insulin injection (regular) Duration of action: 6–8 hr Insulin zinc suspension (Semilente) Duration of action: 12–18 hr *Intermediate acting* Globin insulin with zinc Duration of action: 24–28 hr Insulin isophane suspension (NPH) Duration of action: 24–48 hr Insulin zinc suspension (Lente Iletin) Duration of action: 24–28 hr *Long acting* Insulin zinc suspension, extended (Ultralente) Duration of action: 24–36 hr Insulin protamine zinc suspension (Protamine, Zinc and Iletin) Duration of action: 24–36 hr	The University Group Diabetes Program (1970) results have provoked some physicians to prescribe insulin for the maturity onset diabetic patient whose condition cannot be controlled by diet because as many as 40% may not respond adequately to sulfonlurea drug therapy. Insulin is always indicated for patients with juvenile onset diabetes mellitus as well as for adults who have pancreatic beta cell failure.	The major adverse effect of insulin therapy is hypoglycemia. Hypoglycemic reactions are seen more with the longer acting insulin preparations. Many elderly do not manifest classic symptoms of hypoglycemia; therefore, careful monitoring of insulin therapy becomes most important. Classic symptoms of hypoglycemia include: early symptoms – nervousness, tremors, clammy perspiration, hunger, faintness, and ashen color; later – psychic disturbances, emotional and mental disorder, and complete disorientation; fully developed hypoglycemia – unconsciousness, convulsions, coma, and rarely death. The following drug interactions can occur. With monoamine oxidase inhibitors, insulin action is enhanced; with propanolol, hypoglycemic action is increased; alcohol can cause marked hypoglycemia in some patients.	The older diabetic patient on insulin therapy requires the same basic principles of management used in other age groups (see discussion of sulfonylurea drugs). The elderly person's ability to administer the insulin properly must be carefully assessed. Motor abilities which allow handling of a syringe and vial need to be determined. Age-related visual impairments must be evaluated to assure that dosage calibrations on the syringe can be read. Adequate color perception is also needed to read urine testing results. Patients should be advised to carry a card stating that they are diabetic and what to do in case of emergency (such as hypoglycemic reaction).

ANTIBIOTICS AND ANTI-INFECTIVES

Infections in the elerly are often severe and difficult to treat. The presence of degenerative disease and concomitant therapies present problems of drug interactions with the antimicrobials. Even when overt disease is not present, age-related physiological decrements can affect the treatment of infections. Decrements in renal function reduce the elimination of many antimicrobials, leading to increased serum drug levels and the possibility of toxicity and drug interactions. Older patients are known to experience a greater incidence of nephrotoxic, hepatotoxic, and hypersensitivity reactions to the antimicrobials (Moellering, 1978; Smith and Wiener, 1978; see references at end of chapter for more complete discussions of these drugs).

It is recommended that antibiotics likely to be used systemically in the future should not be applied to the skin. Skin sensitization reactions have occurred in the elderly after topical application of antibiotics to varicose and decubitus ulcers. When these antibiotics were subsequently given systemically, a flare-up of the skin problem occurred. Exfoliative dermatitis is possible, but rare (Davison, 1978).

Drug	Description	Adverse Reactions	Nursing Considerations
Penicillins (various penicillin preparations) Administered orally and parenterally Dosage individualized	Generally speaking, penicillins are of low toxicity in the elderly. Elevated plasma half-life is seen in the elderly; however, the penicillins have a wide margin of safety to balance this increase.	Sensitivity reactions occur to all drugs in this group. With prolonged penicillin therapy in debilitated elderly, superinfections with *Proteus, Pseudomonas,* or *Candida* species are risks. When given in large doses, ampicillin, a synthetic penicillin with broad spectrum activity, may cause pruritic multifor rash in the elderly (Davison, 1978).	Initial antibiotic doses are generally withheld until specimens for culture/sensitivity are sent to the laboratory. Verify that the patient has no history of allergies or idiosyncratic reactions to the antibiotic. If no such history exists, observe for signs and symptoms which may indicate such during therapy. Health practices that support the body's ability to overcome the infection should be promoted. Adequate rest and proper nutrition are most important. To decrease the emergence of resistance to antibiotics, drugs should be given for a prescribed period of time and should not be discontinued before that time. To maintain adequate serum levels of antibiotics, the drugs should be administered over a 24-hr period of time.
Tetracyclines Same as above	This group of broad spectrum antibiotics is considered generally safe in the elderly (Davison, 1978). The kidney is the primary route of elimination for most of the tetracyclines; therefore, these drugs are never given to the elderly with renal failure. In elderly with decrements in renal function, the drug of choice is doxycycline (Vibramycin). This preparation has a long half-life, allowing for a once daily dosage. Side effects are the same as those of other tetracyclines.	The tetracyclines may cause some nausea and diarrhea. Photosensitivity occurs with all the tetracycline preparations, and the elderly are especially at risk. Superinfections similar to those from penicillin are possible. Adverse reactions have been reported in patients ingesting outdated and degraded tetracyclines. Iron preparations and products containing aluminum, magnesium, or calcium ions (antacids, milk, and milk products) will decrease absorption of tetracyclines when taken concurrently.	Superinfections should be suspected if the patient experiences a sore throat, diarrhea, vaginal itching or discharge, or reappearance of fever. When potentially toxic antibiotics are given, monitor the patient's serum drug levels as well as laboratory tests indicative of liver or kidney function. In some individuals, combination of aminoglycoside therapy with cephalosporin, viomycin, polymyxin, colistin, and vancomycin may provide added nephrotoxic potential.
Aminoglycosides Amikacin sulfate (Amikin) Streptomycin sulfate Gentamicin sulfate (Garamycin) Kanamycin sulfate (Kantrex) Tobramycin (Nebcin) Doses are individualized	The aminoglycosides are essentially broad-spectrum antibiotics which must be administered parenterally to treat systemic infections. Their use is limited only by their toxicity.	The aminoglycosides all have the potential for ototoxicity, nephrotoxicity, and neurotoxicity. The elderly, especially those over 70 years of age with decrements in renal function, are at greater risk for these adverse effects (Smith and Wiener, 1978). Evaluation of renal function and audiometric testing are recommended in the elderly prior to and during therapy. Blood aminoglycoside levels provide a useful method of determining therapeutic efficacy. Renal clearance levels of the aminoglycosides vary greatly from patient to patient. Careful monitoring of therapy is essential.	

DRUG (Trade Name)	CHARACTERISTICS	ADVERSE EFFECTS/TOXICITY	NURSING IMPLICATIONS
Other antibiotics Vancomycin hydrochloride (Vancocin) 500 mg qid may be given IV Colistin sulfate/sodium (Coly-Mycin, Coly-Mycin M, Polymyxin E) 100–150 mg daily IM or IV	These are potentially toxic antibiotics which are excreted relatively unchanged by the kidneys and must be used cautiously in the elderly.	Vancomycin can cause severe ototoxicity and nephrotoxicity. Colistin may cause nephrotoxicity as well as neurotoxicity.	See discussion of aminoglycosides for implications.
Isoniazid 50–200 mg tid or bid orally	Isoniazid is one of the important drugs in the treatment of all types of tuberculosis. It must be used in combination with other agents in the treatment of active disease but is used alone for prophylaxis.	Because of possible hepatotoxicity, routine prophylaxis in the elderly with a positive tuberculin skin test should be avoided (Moellering, 1978). The older patient with a clear chest x-ray and no additional risk factors is at low risk of developing tuberculosis and less likely to benefit from isoniazid. Age is the most important factor in increasing the risk of hepatotoxicity.	
GASTROINTESTINAL DRUGS *Gastric antacids* (various preparations, available over the counter/non-prescription)	"As a result of irresponsible advertising, the general public has come to believe that man is constantly fighting a battle against acidity and that every belch or upper gastro-intestinal upset calls for an antacid" (Harvey, 1980a).	Antacids vary in their ability to neutralize stomach acids as well as their potential for producing adverse effects. Antacids can produce constipation as well as diarrhea. With long term use, these drugs may lead to alkalosis, kidney stones, hypermagnesemia, and possible complications of existing disease. The presence of calcium, magnesium, and aluminum ions in antacids tends to interfere with the absorption of tetracyclines, iron salts, warfarin, other weakly acidic drugs such as sulfonamides, and several other agents used in the treatment of urinary tract infections.	The easy availability of antacids without prescription gives rise to frequent misuse. Antacids, when indicated, can be of value. Many available preparations are combined mixtures to increase effectiveness and decrease side effects. Patients receiving antacids as prescribed therapeutically should be monitored to prevent adverse effects. Spacing other medications, which may be prescribed at the same time, is important to decrease drug interactions.

Laxatives	There is no evidence that constipation is related to age, yet constipation is a frequent complaint of the elderly in the Western world.	Constipation is a symptom, and the patient's complaint of chronic constipation should be evaluated to determine the cause.
Dioctyl sodium sulfosuccinate (Colace, Doxinate, and others) 60–250 mg hs and prn orally	Dioctyl sodium sulfosuccinate is a stool softener which is well tolerated. It produces its effects in 24–48 hr. When indicated, it is considered the laxative of choice for the elderly.	A variety of factors can be associated with constipation: a diet lacking in adequate fluids and bulk; insufficient exercise; a preconceived belief that a daily bowel movement is essential; and the therapeutic need for drugs which promote constipation, such as the anti-cholinergic drugs, diuretics, and sedatives. Attractive advertisement of laxatives and their easy availability lead to their use and misuse.
Dioctyl calcium sulfosuccinate (Surfak) 50–240 mg hs or prn orally	Dioctyl calcium sulfosuccinate is similar to dioctyl sodium sulfosuccinate.	This preparation occasionally causes abdominal cramping.
Mineral oil 15–20 ml orally	Mineral oil should be discouraged, especially for long term use.	Mineral oil may interfere with the absorption of fat-soluble substances. In addition, seepage of oil around the anal sphincter may occur. Whenever possible, the elderly should be encouraged to promote bowel elimination without the use of laxatives and enemas.
		Not only is this annoying, but it may lead to occasional pruritus ani (Fingl, 1980).

older adults. The following are basic and essential data in administering and monitoring medications of older individuals:

1. The patient's *health history* should include a biosocial, psychological, and economic profile.
2. *Social resources* available to the individual must be reviewed. Patients living alone without much social stimulus or encouragement were shown in one study to be noncompliant (Komaroff, 1976).
3. *Economic resources* must always be considered with drug therapy. This is especially important for elderly who are on fixed incomes.
4. A *physiological profile,* also viewed as the pharmacokinetic profile, is necessary.
5. A *drug profile* — a complete and updated history of *all* medications that an individual is receiving — should be part of the health record.
6. *Compliance* to the medical (drug) regimen is probably the biggest problem and most difficult to monitor and research. The following are key factors in compliance:

   • The patient's understanding of the illness and of the need for therapy is a particular challenge, at least in patients with asymptomatic disease.
   • The capability of the individual to perform necessary treatments must be considered. Child-resistant drug containers may prove to be adult-resistant containers also! Hands crippled with arthritis may not be capable of applying ophthalmic ointments or manipulating an aerosol container.
   • The number of drugs, as well as the complexity of the regimen, must be taken into account. As these increase, there is a decrease in compliance (Hulka, 1976).
   • Patient response to drug therapy must be monitored. To monitor this response, one must know specific drug action and effects.
   • Side effects, of course, will affect compliance (Warren, 1979). The patient

may not take the drug simply because he was not told to expect certain side effects. This author recalls an elderly woman who did not take her blood pressure pill (a diuretic) because it made her go to the bathroom too much and limited her daytime social activities.

A knowledge of pharmacology, and in particular geriatric pharmacology, is a required foundation in decisions related to drug therapy in the elderly. A therapeutic relationship with the patient is more apt to promote patient adherence to a medical regimen (Barofsky, 1977; Komaroff, 1976). Health care providers must communicate their concern with helping the individual.

Only licensed nurses are allowed to administer drugs, and state laws will define the legal responsibilities of this task. In general, the nurse is expected to have knowledge and skills in the administration of medication. These include incorporating the five Rs of drug administration: right drug, right dose, right route, right time, and right patient.

REFERENCES

Barofsky, I. (Ed.). *Medication Compliance: A Behavioral Management Approach.* Thorofare, N.J., Charles B. Slack, 1977.

Bianchine, J.R. Drugs for Parkinson's disease. In Gilman, A.G., Goodman, L.S., and Gilman, A. (Eds.) *The Pharmacological Basis of Therapeutics* (6th ed.). New York: Macmillan, 1980, pp. 475–493.

Blaschke, T.F. and Melman, K.L. Antihypertensive agents and the drug therapy of hypertension. In Gilman, A.G., Goodman, L.S., and Gilman, A. (Eds.) *The Pharmacological Basis of Therapeutics* (6th ed.). New York: Macmillan, 1980, pp. 793–818.

Butler, R.N. *Medicine and Aging: An Assessment of Opportunities and Neglect.* Testimony before the U.S. Senate Special Committee on Aging, October 13, 1976.

Caird, F.I. and Dall, J.L.C. The cardiovascular system. In Brocklehurst, J.C. (Ed.) *Textbook of Geriatric Medicine and Gerontology* (2nd ed.). New York: Churchill Livingstone, 1978, pp. 125–157.

Cape, R. *Aging: Its Complex Management.* New York: Harper & Row, 1978.

Caranasos, G.J., Steward, R.B., and Cluff, L.E. Drug induced illness leading to hospitalization. *Journal of the American Medical Association* **228**(6):713 (1974).

Colman, R. Guidelines for evaluating and treating hypertension. *Geriatrics* **34**(7):43 (1979).

Community Advisory Committee on Aging and Addiction. *Aging and Addiction in Arizona.* Phoenix, Ariz.: 1979.

Davison, W. The hazards of drug treatment in old age. In Brocklehurst, J.C. (Ed.) *Textbook of Geriatric Medicine and Gerontology* (2nd ed.). New York: Churchill Livingstone, 1978, pp. 651–669.

DeVeaugh-Geiss, J. Neuroleptic drugs: how to reduce the risk of tardive dyskinesia. *Geriatrics* **34**(7):59 (1979).

Exton-Smith, A.N. and Windsor, A.C.M. Principles of drug treatment in the aged. In Rossman, I. (Ed.) *Clinical Geriatrics* (2nd ed.). Philadelphia: J.B. Lippincott, 1979, pp. 132–138.

Fingl, E. Laxatives and cathartics. In Gilman, A.G., Goodman, L.S., and Gilman, A (Eds.) *The Pharmacological Basis of Therapeutics* (6th ed.). New York: Macmillan, 1980, pp. 1002–1012.

Flower, R., Moncada, S., and Vane, J.R. Analgesic-antipyretics and anti-inflammatory agents. In Gilman, A.G., Goodman, L.S., and Gilman, A. (Eds.) *The Pharmacological Basis of Therapeutics* (6th ed.). New York: Macmillan, 1980, pp. 682–723.

Food and Drug Administration. Alcohol-drug interactions. *FDA Drug Bulletin* **9**(2):10 (1979). (a)

Food and Drug Administration. Update on sedative-hypnotics. *FDA Drug Bulletin* **9**(3):16 (1979). (b)

Food and Drug Administration. New angina drugs. *FDA Drug Bulletin* **12**(1):1 (1982).

Gollub, J. Psychoactive drug misuse among the elderly. In Kayne, R.C. (Ed.) *Drugs and the Elderly.* Los Angeles: University of California Press, 1978, pp. 84–102.

Gotz, B. and Gotz, V. Drugs and the elderly. *American Journal of Nursing* **78**(8):1347 (1978).

Gresh, C. Parkinson's disease. *Nursing '80* **10**(1):26 (1980).

Hall, J. Quote from page on thoughts. *Forbes.* July 20, 1981.

Harvey, S.C. Gastric antacids and digestants. In Gilman, A.G., Goodman, L.S., and Gilman, A. (Eds.) *The Pharmacological Basis of Therapeutics* (6th ed.). New York: Macmillan, 1980, pp. 988–1001. (a)

Harvey S.C. Hypnotics and sedatives. In Gilman, A.G., Goodman, L.S., and Gilman, A. (Eds.) *The Pharmacological Basis of Therapeutics* (6th ed.). New York: Macmillan, 1980, pp. 339–375. (b)

Hoehn, M.M. Bromocriptine and its use in parkinsonism. *Journal of the American Gerontological Society* 251–256 (June 1981).

Hulka, B.S., Cassel, J.C., Kupper, L.L., and Burdette, J.A. "Communication, Compliance and Concordance Between Physician and Patients with Prescribed Medications," *American Journal of Public Health,* **66**(9):847 (1976).

Ivey, M. Drug use. In Carnevali, D.L. and Patrick, M. (Eds.) *Nursing Management for the Elderly.* Philadelphia: J.B. Lippincott, 1979, pp. 169–179.

Kayne, R.C., Drugs and the Aged. In Burnside, I.M. (Ed.) *Nursing and the Aged.* New York: McGraw Hill Book Co., 1976.

Komaroff, A. The practitioner and the compliant patient. *American Journal of Public Health* **66**(9): 833 (1976).

Lamy, P.R. and Vestal, R.E. Drug prescribing for the elderly. In Reichel, W. (Ed.) *The Geriatric Patient.* New York: H.P. Publishing, 1978, pp. 1–8.

Larner, J. Insulin and oral hypoglycemic drugs: glucagon. In Gilman, A.G., Goodman, L.S., and Gilman, A. (Eds.) *The Pharmacological Basis of Therapeutics* (6th ed.). New York: Macmillan, 1980, pp. 1497–1523.

Meissner, J.E. and Gever, L.N. Reducing the risks of digitalis toxicity. *Nursing '80* **10**(9):32 (1980).

Moellering, R.C. Factors influencing the clinical use of antimicrobial agents in elderly patients. *Geriatrics* **33**(2):83 (1978).

Moser, M. Hypertension in the elderly. In Rossman, I. (Ed.) *Clinical Geriatrics* (2nd ed.). Philadelphia: J.B. Lippincott, 1979, pp. 606–617.

Moser, M. Hypertension, how therapy works. *American Journal of Nursing* **80**(5):937 (1980).

Parkinson's Disease Foundation. *Newsletter.* New York: January 1982, p. 2.

Payne, B. Community responsibility for drug use by the elderly. In Petersen, D.M., Whittington, F.J., and Payne, B. (Eds.) *Drugs and the Elderly, Social and Pharmacological Issues.* Springfield: Charles C. Thomas Publishers, 1979, pp. 178–189.

Petersen, D.M. and Thomas, C.W. Acute drug reactions among the elderly. In Petersen, D.M., Whittington, F.J., and Payne, B. (Eds.) *Drugs and the Elderly, Social and Pharmacological Issues.* Springfield, Ill.: Charles C. Thomas, 1979, pp. 41–52.

Pfeiffer, E. Use of drugs which influence behavior in the elderly. In Kayne, R.C. (Ed.) *Drugs and the Elderly.* Los Angeles: University of Southern California Press, 1978, pp. 44–66.

Psychotropic drugs (a series of articles). *American Journal of Nursing* **81**(7):1303 (1981).

Rifkin, H., Ross, H., and Shapiro, H.C. Diabetes in the elderly. In Rossman, I. (Ed.) *Clinical Geriatrics* (2nd ed.). Philadelphia: J.B. Lippincott, 1979, pp. 592–605.

Rodstein, M. Heart disease in the aged. In Rossman, I. (Ed.) *Clinical Geriatrics* (2nd ed.). Philadelphia: J.B. Lippincott, 1979, pp. 181–203.

Rosal-Greif, V.L.F. Drug induced dyskinesias. *American Journal of Nursing* **82**(1):66 (1982).

Schmidt, J.P. A behavioral approach to patient compliance. *Postgraduate Medicine* **65**(5):219 (1979).

Schwartz, D. Safe self medication for elderly outpatients. *American Journal of Nursing* **75**(10):1801 (1975).

Sheridan, E., Patterson, H.R., and Gustafson, E. *Fal-*

coner's the Drug, the Nurse, the Patient (7th ed.). Philadelphia: W.B. Saunders, 1982.

Smith, J.K. and Wiener, S.L. Aging, immunity and antibiotics. *Drug Therapy* 3(4):19 (1978).

Stimmel, G.L. Issues in psychotropic drug misuse. In Kayne, R.C., (Ed.) *Drugs and the Elderly.* University of Southern California Press, 1978, pp. 67–74.

Thompson, J.F. and Floyd, R. Effect of Aging in Pharmacokinetics. In Kayne, R.C., (Ed.) *Drugs and the Elderly.* University of Southern California Press, 1978, pp. 143-156.

Todd, B. Beta blockers and calcium channel blockers. *Geriatric Nursing* 3(4):228–229 (1982).

U.S. Department of Health, Education and Welfare, Public Health Service. *Out of Pocket Cost and Acquisition of Prescribed Medicines.* Rockville, Md.: National Center of Health Statistics, June 1977.

U.S. Public Health Service, Office of Long Term Care. *Physician's Drug Prescribing Patterns in Skilled Nursing Facilities.* Washington, D.C.: U.S. Government Printing Office, 1976.

U.S. Public Health Service, Office of Nursing Home Affairs. *Long Term Care Facility Improvement Study: Introductory Report.* Washington, D.C.: U.S. Government Printing Office, 1975.

University Group Diabetes Program. A study of the effects of hypoglycemic effects on vascular complications in patients with adult onset diabetes. *Diabetes* 19(2):474–830 (1970).

Vancura, E.J. Guard against unpredictable drug responses in the aging. *Geriatrics* 34(4):83 (1979).

Warren, F. Self medication problems among the elderly. In Petersen, D.M., Whittington, F.J., and Payne, B. (Eds.) *Drugs and the Elderly, Social and Pharmacological Issues.* Springfield, Ill.: Charles C. Thomas, 1979, pp. 105–125.

Weg, R.B. Drug interactions with the changing physiology of the aged: practice and potential. In Kayne, R.C. (Ed) *Drugs and the Elderly.* Los Angeles: University of Southern California Press, 1978, pp. 103–142.

Whittington, F.J. and Petersen, D.M. Drugs and the elderly. In Petersen, D.M., Whittington, F.J., and Payne, B. (Eds.) *Drugs and the Elderly, Social and Pharmacological Issues.* Springfield, Ill.: Charles C. Thomas, 1979, pp. 14–27.

Ziance, R.J. Side effects of drugs in the elderly. In Petersen, D.M., Whittington, F.J., and Payne, B. (Eds.) *Drugs and the Elderly, Social and Pharmacological Issues.* Springfield, Ill.: Charles C. Thomas, 1979, pp. 53–79.

Zimberg, S. Alcohol and the elderly. In Petersen, D.M., Whittington, F.J., and Payne, B. (Eds.) *Drugs and the Elderly, Social and Pharmacological Issues.* Springfield, Ill.: Charles C. Thomas, 1979, pp. 28–40.

35
Ethnic and Cultural Considerations

Veronica Evaneshko

I have found no differences that are absolute between Eastern and Western life except in the attitude toward age. In China one of the first questions a person asks another on an official call is: "What is your glorious age?" If the respondent says, apologetically, 23 or 28, the other offers comfort by saying that he or she still has a glorious future, and may one day become old. Enthusiasm grows in proportion as the individual is able to report a higher and higher age, and if that is anywhere over 50, the inquirer drops his voice in humility and respect. People actually look forward to the celebration of their 51st birthday.

Lin Yutang (1937)

Ethnicity is increasingly recognized in the biological, psychological, and sociological aspects of aging. Slowly but significantly, ethnic factors are being addressed in research, service delivery models, and curricula of health care professionals. This chapter addresses the interaction of ethnicity and aging, the biopsychosociocultural aspects of aging, and specific ethnic characteristics of aging with implications for nursing in four major groups: black Americans, Mexican Americans, native Americans, and Asian Americans.

Concerns of humanism and caring are hallmarks of the nursing profession. To care for the aged ethnic person, nurses must be able to understand his view of his cultural world (Mayeroff, 1971, p. 42). (Aged ethnic people are more likely to be dependent upon traditional lifeways, and it is their right to adhere to cultural preferences and customs.) This concern for humanism is universally applicable but especially relevant for nursing care of the ethnic aged in the United States. The aged ethnic person's need for nursing care, the likelihood that the health care provider will not share his cul-

tural world view, the concern for maintaining dignity at a time of powerlessness and possibly hopelessness, the type and extent of loneliness, dependency conflicts, the desire to affirm the value of life, and the loss of social support as the aged ethnic person outlives his cohorts — all require a compassionate, ethnically humanistic, caring approach.

INTERACTIONS OF ETHNICITY AND AGING

Ethnic groups are defined by ancestry, self-assessment, and behavior. The term *ethnic group* is frequently used interchangeably with minority group, racial group, and cultural group. Each of these terms emphasizes a different feature of group involvement. Features of ethnic groups include: a group whose membership is largely biologically self-perpetuating and whose members share a cultural system, communicate and interact more often within the group than outside the group, and identify themselves and are identified by others as belonging to the group (Narroll, 1964).

Unfortunately, in this country, aged members of ethnic groups are often placed in what has been called double, triple, and even multiple jeopardy (Barrow and Smith, 1979; Bengston, 1979; Comfort, 1976; Dowd and Bengston, 1978; National Urban League, 1964). These jeopardy situations include age, ethnic discrimination, poverty, and for women, sex, all of which result in a less satisfactory quality of life.

The following factors contribute to the ethnic aged's multiple jeopardy. First, each ethnic group has had its unique history of confrontation with the dominant society, resulting in a subordinate status. Second, differences in language, appearance, and customs have been used to keep ethnic people out of the better paying jobs. The resulting ridicule and accusations of laziness and lack of ambition fostered further discrimination. Third, most ethnic groups have been alienated to a greater or lesser extent from their own cultural heritage, while at the same time they were isolated from the dominant society's social institutions. Finally, the ethnic aged today are frequently isolated even within their own particular group, because experiences that molded their outlook are quite different from the experiences of the younger members of their ethnic group (Benitez, 1976).

As a result of these and other factors, most ethnic aged, by comparison with many members of the dominant culture, "are less educated, have less income, suffer more illnesses and earlier death, have poorer quality housing and less choice as to where they live and where they work . . ." (U.S. Senate Special Committee on Aging, 1971). Problems identified by the 1971 White House Conference on Aging (1973) as common to all aged in this country are even more severe for the ethnic aged. These problems, which persist in 1984, are transportation, income, health, housing, nutrition, loneliness, and inability to cope with bureaucratic systems.

Despite the many negative aspects of ethnicity in this country, aged ethnic groups do have strengths and resources which health care professionals should utilize when planning and providing assistance for them. Genuine feelings of pride and self-confidence that come from surviving prejudice and discrimination are an asset to the aged ethnic person. Identification with the group also provides a source of support, as does the very essence of ethnicity itself since cultural traditions provide structure and continuity. A traditionally featured resource for the ethnic aged is the tendency of ethnic groups to maintain and use stronger extended social networks.

BIOPSYCHOSOCIOCULTURAL ASPECTS OF AGING

Ethnically distinct groups experience the phenomenon of aging differently with respect to biological, psychological, sociological, and cultural factors.

Biological Factors

Since ethnic groups are largely biologically self-perpetuating, they share a common gene pool. Each gene pool tends to evolve different biological responses to the challenge of life and the aging process itself. For example, some ethnic groups' members appear to age later, to live longer, and to have fewer physical problems (Beaubier, 1980; Benet, 1974; Leaf, 1973; Medvedev, 1974).

Psychological Factors

Psychological aspects of aging among ethnic groups include variation in the quantity and quality of mental disorders and emotional satisfactions (Hollingshead and Redlich, 1958; King, 1962; Leighton and Hughes, 1961; Opler, 1959; Stenger-Castro, 1978). Many psychological studies of the ethnic aged in this country feature the effect of prejudice and discrimination on their mental health (Barrow and Smith, 1979; Butler and Lewis, 1981; Carter, 1972; Carter, 1978; Morales, 1976). Life satisfaction and optimism vary as a result of the ethnic aged's experiences as a lifelong member of an ethnic group (Dowd and Bengston, 1978).

Sociological Factors

The major sociological factors for the ethnic aged are socioeconomic status and social support systems. They have lower socioeconomic status and share in the following low socioeconomic status-associated aspects of aging: a more negative view of aging, a greater likelihood of viewing oneself as old, a tendency to see old age as beginning earlier, and a lower life satisfaction (Bengston, Kasschau, Ragan, 1977). The extent of, and reliance on, social support systems are frequently discussed issues in ethnic aging, with emphasis on the family and extended family's role in providing support for all family members, including the aged (Canton, 1979; Dowd and Bengston, 1978; Keefe, 1979; Mindel and Habenstein, 1976; Siemaszko, 1980; Valle and Mendoza, 1978).

Cultural Factors

Various ethnic groups assign different expectations to the aging process. An excellent example of the arbitrariness of cultural expectations associated with aging is provided by Fischer (1978) in *Growing Old in America* in which he traces changes in the American culture's attitudes toward aging over a 270-year span. In the early developmental years of this country, the aged were respected, held in awe, and venerated, although not necessarily loved. Today, the glorification of youth has produced gerontophobia and a concomitant disrespect toward, and a disvaluing of, the aged.

Negative or positive attributes are arbitrarily assigned to the aging process by different ethnic groups. An ethnic group that perceives the aging phenomenon as a pathological condition is already predisposed to view elements associated with aging in a negative light. Thus, aging can be dreaded and perceived as a burden, having no redeeming value, attended by decay and ugliness, and involving a steady decline and a fall from grace. On the other hand, an ethnic group that perceives aging as a natural condition may view aging as a condition of life to be cherished or at least accepted with equanimity. It can be a challenge ("the best is yet to be"), a time for consolidating gains, a time to garner the rewards of a lifetime of hard labor, to think, to appreciate one's family and friends, to relax, and to be free from the working world's incessant competition and strivings. From this viewpoint, old age can be a goal toward which one aspires.

Ethnic groups vary in the characteristics they feature as representative of old age and in the meaning attached to these characteristics. Thus, ethnic people who have to rely on hard physical labor will select and pay attention to aging characteristics that influence their ability to provide for their family. For them, gray hair will be a less important sign of old age than loss of physical strength or diminished eyesight.

Every society has designated behavior that is appropriate for the aged. The aged are expected "to act their age" (Fischer, 1978), to step down and step aside, and to take on new tasks that do not require the physical strength and stamina of youth. The nature of these roles and the prestige attached to them vary among ethnic groups. In one ethnic group, the aged may be assigned low prestige tasks such as baby-sitting, house tending, or animal herding, while in another, they become spiritual or moral leaders, dispensing wisdom and being revered for the knowledge and skills acquired over a long lifetime.

Feelings about death and the treatment of the dead are also learned cultural patterns. The dominant culture in this country perceives death as an end, whereas various ethnic groups see death as the continuation of a life cycle that repeats itself (Myerhoff, 1978). Aspects of death and dying that vary among ethnic groups include: the extent and type of contact with the dying and with death; the belief that the dying person should be told he is dying and who should tell; the willingness to express grief openly in public or only in private; the reliance on family members during times of crises; acceptable times to remarry, stop wearing black, resume work, and start going out socially; the fear of death and frequency of death thoughts; feelings of mysticism associated with death; reasons for not wanting to die; preferences of where to die; and preparation for the funeral (Bengston, Cuellar, and Ragan, 1979; Kalish and Reynolds, 1976; Schulz, 1980).

MAJOR ETHNIC GROUPS

The essential knowledge base for providing culturally relevant health care to the many distinct groups in this country is still being developed (see Bauwens, 1978; Branch and Paxton, 1976; Brink, 1976; Bullough and Bullough, 1972; Leininger, 1978; Lynch, 1969; Martinez, 1978; National League for Nursing, 1976). The specific cultural knowledge and information needed to understand and work with the ethnic aged in this country are not well documented, although a few books and articles have been published (Dukepoo, 1979; Fry, 1980; Gelfand and Kutzik, 1979; Hendricks and Hendricks, 1979; Stanford, 1978; Valle and Mendoza, 1978; Watson and Maxwell, 1977).

The ethnic groups for whom the most information has been published are black Americans, Mexican Americans, native Americans, and Asian Americans. These will be the primary focus for the remainder of this chapter. While it is true that the total population of ethnic peoples is small in comparison with the dominant society, the National Institute on Aging (1980) reports that in the 1980s almost 40% of the entire U.S. population over age 65 will belong to an ethnically distinct group.

According to the Federal Council on Aging (1979), commonalities shared by aged of the four ethnic groups discussed in this chapter are:

- A lower life expectancy than their white counterparts
- Bilingual, bicultural barriers to services
- Fewer median school years completed than the total elderly population
- Low paying, blue collar jobs (many without Social Security or retirement benefits)
- Inadequate benefits from federal income supplement programs
- Fewer opportunities for training and employment for those on income maintenance programs
- A struggle against skyrocketing inflation, high taxes, and increasing energy costs
- Poor housing conditions, reflective of a federal housing policy unresponsive to minority needs
- A fear of the increasing incidence of crime committed against their age group
- Insufficient social and health care services, both mental and physical
- An underrepresentation of members of their ethnic groups on federal, state, and local policy-making bodies
- An emotional and mental attachment to their ethnic communities (i.e., natural support networks)
- A fear of being removed from their cultural surroundings and placed into institutions such as nursing homes or other long term care facilities
- An underrepresentation of the number and socioeconomic characteristics of each of their ethnic groups by census.

Despite the extent of common characteristics shared by the aged of the four ethnic groups, there is greater diversity than similarity among them. Each ethnic group is made up of subgroups based on such factors as differences in social class, geographic location, degree of adherence to traditional cultural practices, type and extent of historical experiences, type and area of the country from which immigration occurred, length of time in the United States, and for native Americans, the tribal group with which one identifies. These characteristics, which result in diversity, have significant relevance for health care needs and health care-seeking behavior. The health care professional who fails to consider the extent of diversity inherent among the ethnic aged will be unable to provide sensitive nursing care to subgroups.

Specific information that professionals should seek to provide ethnically sensitive nursing care include: historical factors affecting the aged today; traditional health/illness beliefs and practices still being followed; cognition of aging, death, and mourning patterns; and resources relied upon and available to the ethnic aged.

Black Americans

Although black Americans as a group are distinct and unique, variations in behavior, values, beliefs, attitudes, and knowledge exist among group members. This variation is dependent upon such factors as geographic location, economic level, educational attainment, occupation, social exposure, and cultural upbringing. Thus, general statements on black Americans as a group must be accepted within the range of this known diversity.

Historical Factors. Most blacks in this country are the descendents of African peoples who were abducted and sold into slavery during the seventeenth and eighteenth century. Family and tribal ties were systematically disrupted to reduce the possibility of tribal uprisings. Traditional languages were forbidden and a special version of Christianity "enforced." It consisted of a religion of enduring hope which encouraged blacks to expect their rewards in heaven. Old age was (hopefully) the time of release from hard labor.

With emancipation, black Americans traded slavery for second class citizenship. The systematic deprivation of education and work opportunities resulted in a high level of role integration within the black family (Greathouse and Miller, 1981). A strong female role evolved as well as a continuation of esteem for, and recognition of, grandparents' contribution to the strength and unity of the family.

Traditional Health System. The black American's folk medical system is a "composite of classical medicine of an earlier day, European folklore regarding the natural world, rare African traits, and selected beliefs derived from modern scientific medicine . . . inextricably blended with the tenets of fundamentalist Christianity, elements from the Voodoo religion of the West Indies, and the added spice of sympathetic magic" (Show, 1974, p. 82). Illness, which is divided into natural and unnatural categories, represents disharmony and conflict in some area of the individual's life. Causes of natural illness include environmental hazards, divine punishment, and impaired social relationships. Unnatural illnesses are caused by evil influences and witchcraft (Jackson, 1976; Snow, 1974).

Traditional healers are ranked in terms of the amount of God-given power they have. The lowest rank with the least power consists of those who learn their craft from others, such as the physician and the chiropractor. Individuals who "receive" the gift of healing through a religious experience have more power than those who learn their craft. The person born with the gift of healing has the greatest amount of power (Snow, 1974); see Figure 35-1.

Historically, a black slave was only allowed to be sick when unable to function, and illness today is often perceived as a condition in which one is unable to labor productively. Given this perception of illness, early signs and symptoms of disease processes may be ignored (Greathouse and Miller, 1981). Health for many blacks is classed as a form of good luck, much as success, money, a good job, and a peaceful home are good luck (Jacques, 1976; Snow, 1974).

Good health is attained and maintained by avoiding excesses and "looking after yourself." This includes proper diet, extensive use of laxatives to "keep the system open," ingestion of cod-liver oil to prevent colds, rubbing a sulfur and molasses preparation on the back to prevent illness, wearing copper and silver bracelets to relieve pain, and wearing herbs around the neck to prevent catching contagious diseases (Snow, 1974; Spector, 1979).

Cognitions of Aging. Black Americans are less likely than whites to deny their advanced age and more likely to perceive old age as a reward in itself (Dancy, 1977; Messer, 1968). Despite financial and health problems, life is still bearable, with many blacks maintaining a serene and optimistic outlook (Swanson and Harter, 1971). Appearance of age is not a criterion to many blacks; rather, the ability to function mentally and physically is far more important. The more active the aged black is, the less he feels he is getting old. Once one is

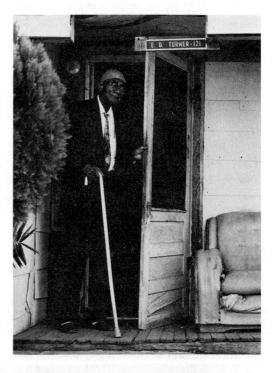

Figure 35-1. Reverend Turner was a self-educated minister who instilled dignity, hope, and optimism through his ministry, from his little old tumbling home, till age 92. (Photo by Jeff Stanton.)

no longer active and intimately involved with family, neighborhood, and personal activities, old age is acknowledged (Stanford, 1978). Although work is valued as an indicator of usefulness, this should not be taken to mean the aged black wants to remain in a wage job. He has earned his rest and looks forward to it (Jackson and Walls, 1978).

In a study on death and ethnicity, Kalish and Reynolds (1976) interviewed 109 black Americans in Los Angeles County, with a mean age of 46 years. Japanese Americans, Mexican Americans, and whites were also included in this study. The black Americans reported having more contact with death but did not report thinking or dreaming about their own death more than the other groups. Visits with the dying were not uncommon among the black sample, and a majority believed the dying should be informed of their condition, preferably by the physician. Very few blacks in the study acknowledged fear of death, but they were concerned about what their death would mean in terms of no longer being able to care for dependents, causing grief to relatives and friends, and the possibility of pain during the dying process. A majority of the blacks felt they would tend to accept death peacefully when it came. Many said they were not likely to encourage family members to spend time with them during their terminal stages if it would be inconvenient. While family members could be relied upon during the dying process, many blacks said they would also utilize friends, church members, neighbors, and other nonrelatives.

Resources. After a lifetime of bitter experiences, aged blacks have learned not to expect a high level of service from public agencies (Dancy, 1977). Racism still pervades the health care system (Spector, 1979, p. 241), and black Americans have devised a number of coping mechanisms to deal with this racism, such as testing behaviors to assess the degree of racism; suspicion of, and caution in using, health care facilities; and avoidance of health care facilities altogether (Greathouse and Miller, 1981). Aged blacks are forced to rely on personal resources to a large extent.

An aged Black's primary personal resource is likely to be his family, which tends to have more family and nonfamily members living together than do whites. Closely knit family ties have resulted from economic hardships. Within the black family, extended kinship network roles are flexible and interchangeable (Dancy, 1977). Thus, a variety of people may head a black family including a young mother, a father, an aunt, a grandparent, or a male relative. The strength of the black family rests on the nature of interpersonal relationships in which everyone pitches in to ward off the hostile world. In such situations, aged family members are especially valued for the important, active, contributing roles they play, as well as for the fact of their survival in the face of hardship and suffering.

Dancy (1977) has identified these strengths in aged blacks: an accumulation of wisdom, knowledge, and common sense about life that comes not only from age but from the experience of hardship and suffering; a creative genius in doing much with little; the ability to accept aging; and a sense of hope and optimism for a better day. Richard Pryor, the black comedian, identifies the aged black's strength when he states, "You don't get old being no fool" (Anderson, 1980). In order to survive, aged blacks have had to learn methods of stress reduction which can serve them well in old age (Anderson, 1980).

Ethnic Characteristics with Implications for Nursing. Some characteristics of aged blacks which can have important consequences for nursing are:

- Some may prefer to be called Negro, a respected and acceptable term that was used for a significant number of years.
- Others may prefer to be called black American if they identify with the more current term and its activist connotations.
- They are likely to prefer being called by a title of respect, such as "Mr." or "Mrs." along with their surname.
- They may identify themselves first as Negro or black, and second as American.
- They probably grew up having great respect for their elders and expected to inherit that respect as they aged.

- They should not be called "boy" or "Aunt . . .," since such terms symbolize years of degradation, subjugation, and little or no respect for age, experience, and personal worth.
- They may be geographically removed from the services that are available to them and may view travel outside their own community as a trip into a hostile world.
- They are likely to resent being patted on the head or patronized in any way.
- They may adopt patterns of accommodation that mask hostility and resentment.
- They may respond with "yes, sir" or "no, ma'am" because of years of deference; they may act servile and placating, adopting a pattern of hanging head, drooping shoulders, speaking slowly as if knowing little, hoping to stay out of trouble, as part of a coping pattern to the hostility experienced in their lifetimes.
- They are likely not to fully understand "patients' rights" and the current encouragement of inclusion of self-determination in health matters because of having lived many years with a sense of powerlessness.
- They are likely to have strong religious beliefs, may cite the Bible and Christian tenets as an explanation for life occurrences, and may seek support and advice from their religious leaders.
- They may have strong beliefs in, and continue to use, folk medicine and home remedies.
- They may be significant members of an extended family network, with a valued role as an adviser, child caretaker, economic contributor, or the focal point of the family's cohesion.
- They may reflect a common characteristic of black Americans in having compassion for others and showing a significant interest in public services which attend to the elderly's social, environmental, and cultural needs.
- They will vary in their identification of, and preference for, soul food — with some refusing traditional foods because of their connotations of poverty and being unable to afford any thing else.

- They may be uncomfortable with the strength of black ethnic identity expressed by younger group members because of having experienced so much reprisal in their lifetimes.
- They will vary in the extent to which they declare their ethnic identity, cross-cutting all strata so that an aged, upper class, northern, urban black may have a stronger identification with black culture than an aged, poor, southern, rural black.
- They are likely to have difficulty coping with lifelong sex stereotypes: aged black males may be refused admittance into nursing homes because of fear of their stereotyped sexual excesses, while many aged black women live in fear of being abused and at the mercy of those in power.

These characteristics suggest intervention strategies for nurses, beginning with attention to preference for terms of address and the patient's historical experiences. Placating behavior should be met with compassionate understanding and showing the aged individual respect for his personal worth as a human being. Knowing that aged blacks have devised testing mechanisms to measure the friendliness and concern of clinic staff, extent of preferential treatment, and potential risk of being made to feel inferior reveals the kinds of concerns blacks must overcome in using health care facilities. Health care providers also must assess their own potential negative ethnocentric and racial attitudes. Hair care, skin care, and shaving problems of aged blacks are other concerns with which many health care providers are unfamiliar and which they must learn how to handle (Greathouse and Miller, 1981). The aged black should be asked about food preferences; it should not be assumed that all aged blacks desire soul food.

On the other hand, the aged black's strengths can be used as resources by health care providers. Many programs for aged blacks inadvertently promote dependence for people who have had to be resourcefully independent most of their lives (Anderson, 1980). The aged black's character and forebearance can be used as the framework for respect and dignity within which to relate and provide assistance, as opposed to perceiving aged blacks as worthless or treating them with condescension. The importance of the aged black's close social network dictates that family members be included in the planning and implementation of health care (Greathouse and Miller, 1981). Aged blacks may need help from health care providers in learning how to become their own advocates for better health care.

Mexican Americans

Diversity within the Mexican American category includes three subgroups existing in large numbers in the Southwest: (1) Spanish Americans, who are descendants of eighteenth century Spanish colonists; (2) Mexican Americans, who were born in Mexico and immigrated to this country, and their native-born descendants; and (3) Mexicans, some of whom are recent immigrants planning to stay permanently, while others will remain only temporarily. Individuals from other Hispanic countries are also frequently categorized with Mexican Americans: these include people from Cuba, Puerto Rico, Spain, and countries in Central and South America. Each of these groups has subdivisions within it adding even more diversity. When speaking of these diverse ethnic groups from different countries where the predominant language is Spanish, the term Hispanic is frequently used. The following material is representative of those Hispanics or Spanish-speaking people with cultural roots in Mexico.

Historical Factors. Spanish-speaking people from Mexico occupied American soil in what is now New Mexico almost two decades before the first permanent English colonists arrived in New England. As such, they are second only to native Americans in the length of time they have occupied American soil (Schaefer, 1979). This lengthy association with their lands is a source of pride as well as source of irritation when whites ignore the Mexican Americans' priority claims.

After Mexico's War of Independence from Spain in 1821, the Southwest experienced a large influx of white settlers. In a bewildering turn of events, Mexican Americans already living in the Southwest became a minority in their own homeland, as whites in overwhelming numbers took over and attempted to force the native Mexican Americans to acculturate. When the Mexican Americans resisted, preferring to keep to their cultural ways and language, they were ridiculed and reduced to second class citizenship (Moquin and Van Doren, 1971).

Later immigrants from Mexico who came in search of jobs, primarily in the Southwest's agricultural industry, were added to the original native Mexican American group and inherited the same second class citizenship. In addition to these two groups, there are thousands, if not several million, Mexicans who have entered this country illegally. This latter group presents special problems, especially for health care providers, as it represents a potential drain on tax-supported health care facilities. The legal status of these individuals presents unique problems, including all the ramifications stemming from fear of disclosure.

Traditional Health System. The Mexican American medical folklore system is a blend of ancient Mexican folk medicine, native American medicine, European medieval medicine, and African folk medical practices (Guerra, 1976; Kay, 1977; Twaddle and Hessler, 1977). Mexican American medical folklore features the need for a balance between the natural and supernatural worlds. Loss of this equilibrium causes emotional, physical, or mental illness. Illnesses have been classified into four traditional folk categories: (1) diseases of hot and cold imbalance, (2) dislocations of internal organs, (3) illnesses of magical origin, and (4) illnesses of emotional origin. Standard scientific diseases originating in the dominant culture's practices have been added to these traditional folk illness categories (Clark, 1959).

The hot and cold contrast has received the most attention in Mexican American folklore literature and is a belief stemming from a Spanish version of medieval medicine. The belief identifies illness, medicines, food, and many natural objects as being either hot or cold, with an imbalance resulting if there is an excess of either the hot or the cold element. The studies on which the categories of medical folklore have been based were conducted more than 30 years ago. A more recent study by Kay (1977) reveals that the hot/cold contrast is not known by Mexican American women under 30 years of age. Another significant finding in the Kay study is that there has been a shift in the meaning of many medical folklore terms. For example, *susto,* a term which used to mean a great emotional shock attended by illness, is now considered to be an unpleasant surprise. *Envidia,* a term which used to mean a form of witchcraft unconsciously inflicted on the sufferer, is now synonymous with jealousy. *Aire* used to indicate a volitional wind causing disease but now is thought of as "gas," an ailment responsive to Alka-Seltzer.

Changes in the traditional health system are more likely to be reflected among younger Mexican Americans, while many aged Mexican Americans are likely to be following the "old ways." Traditional healing techniques still in use and likely to be preferred by aged Mexican Americans include herbs and/or food taken internally or applied topically, massages and manipulation of the body, and religious or magical objects and symbols used in propitiation activities. Traditional health care practitioners likely to be used by aged Mexican Americans include *curranderos* (*curranderas* = women), who have considerable empirical knowledge as well as charismatic qualities associated with the more spiritual aspects of healing; *señoras* (older women), who have acquired empirical healing knowledge from life experiences; *sobadoras,* who specialize in manipulating muscles and bones and giving massages; *parteras,* who are midwives; *espiritualistas,* who have the ability to analyze dreams, premonitions, cards, etc.; and *brujos* (*brujas* = women), who control malevolent and benevolent techniques of witchcraft (Bullough and Bullough, 1972; Dorsey and Jackson, 1976; Martinez and Martin, 1978; Schreiber and Homiak, 1981).

For many Mexican Americans, health means being free of pain. Health is associated with the ability to work, is seen as one's condition as of today, and is perceived as a matter of chance. As a gift from God, health is a reward for good behavior, one not to be taken for granted. A healthy person is well fleshed, with a full face

and rosy complexion. If one is thin, he is not healthy. Thus, a robust person with tuberculosis may not be regarded as ill. Good health is closely tied to being in accord with God, who punishes evil deeds and moral indiscretions with illness. By behaving correctly, eating the right foods, and working the proper amount of time, good health can be achieved and maintained (Baca, 1969; Gonzales, 1976; Spector, 1979).

Cognitions of Aging. Little has been written on how Mexican Americans view aging, but there is evidence to suggest it is accepted as inevitable and undesirable. One study revealed that Mexican Americans perceived old age to begin at or below 60. For many in the study, old age began at 50 or 55, with such subjective criteria of aging as inability to work, a feeling of being old and useless, a breakdown in health, and a need for help to live (Crouch, 1972). Mexican Americans in other studies had negative evaluations of the quality of their own lives, such as greater sadness and worry, feelings that life was not worth living, and a belief that things get worse as one gets older (Bengston et al., 1977; Cuellar, 1978). These attitudes toward aging are different from traditional views which have been reported.

Traditionally, old age was a time of repose and rest from hard labors, an accomplishment, even an honor. The elderly could expect to be cared for by a wide variety of relatives who would continue to look to them for advice and assistance. The aged person's role as adviser might include such activities as spokesperson for the extended family in crisis; judging the extent to which family members performed their responsibilities with regard to religion, child rearing, etc.; and providing counsel with regard to interpersonal relations, medical advice, matrimony, and other family affairs. Such usefulness has been conceived as a horizontal and intergenerational link between members of the extended Mexican American family (Leonard, 1967). However, traditional norms are eroding in the Mexican American family, and recent changes include the shifting of responsibility for the aged's care from the family to the state (Cuellar, 1978). Many aged Mexican Americans feel that their offspring "have enough problems already" and should not have to assume a major responsibility for their care (Crouch, 1972, p. 526).

Death is considered to be the will of God *(la voluntad de Dios)* and is generally announced by omens such as owls hooting and dogs howling at night, mirrors breaking, pictures falling off walls, and doors mysteriously opening and closing. Religion is an extremely important aspect of Mexican American culture, especially for the dying. The last rites of the Catholic Church, which are actually an anointing of the sick, are generally accepted as preparation for dying, but may be perceived as a sign that all hope is gone. At times, therefore, these rites may be delayed as long as possible by the family so as not to appear to have given up hope too soon. Still, the rites bring comfort to the family in the knowledge that their loved one has been properly prepared for death and entry into heaven (Busto, 1978).

Impending death brings a "flood" of caring and concerned family members, for this is a time of reconciliation and forgiveness. Death is often followed by very emotional outbursts of crying and clinging to the dead person. Such outbursts are an accepted expression of grief and are supported by the Mexican American community (Busto, 1978). More traditional families sometimes engage professional weepers — older women of the community — who weep loudly and speak highly of the deceased (Herrera and Wagner, 1977). Respect and homage toward parents and grandparents continue after death (see Figure 35-2).

In their study *Death and Ethnicity,* Kalish and Reynolds (1976) interviewed 114 Mexican Americans in Los Angeles County, with a mean age of 47 years. Approximately equal numbers of black Americans, Japanese Americans, and whites were included in the study. Of all the groups, Mexican Americans were the least likely to think the dying should be told of their condition, believing this made it harder on everyone concerned. By comparison with the other groups, more Mexican Americans were willing to die in a hospital (although this represented only 34%). The Mexican American group was also much more likely to encourage

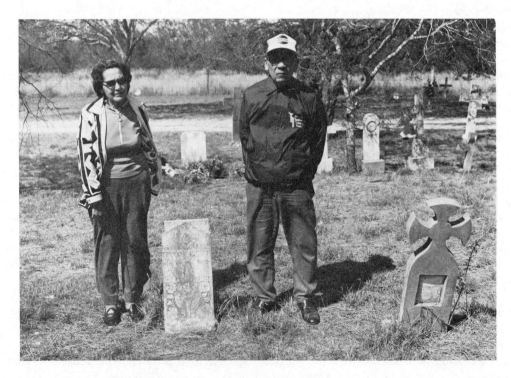

Figure 35-2. Respect for parents continues after death for many Mexican Americans. This man, a grandfather himself, still makes annual trips of over 1000 miles to visit his father's grave. (Photo copyright © 1980 by Robert C. Buitrón.)

their families to spend time with them when dying, even if this caused some inconvenience for family members. Generally speaking, death was perceived by Mexican Americans as an event that should take place in the presence of the entire family.

Resources. As previously noted, the family may no longer be considered the primary and/or sole support for aged Mexican Americans. Traditional family practices which are still prevalent for some Mexican Americans include having the aged parent(s) live with married children; having one or more offspring delegated to live with the aged person or couple; and having the aged live alone, but with children contributing to their support and maintenance (Crouch, 1972). Whereas two studies cite a weakening of the importance of the extended family among Mexican Americans (Cuellar, 1978; Grebler, Moore, and Guzman, 1970). One study finds Mexican Americans to have more kin in town, more frequent interaction with nearby relatives, and more exchange of mutual aid with kin than did whites (Keefe, 1979). Familial support for aged Mexican Americans has also been cited by Valle and Mendoza (1978), and Maldonado (1979).

Other resources for the aged Mexican American may be the church and the government. The church is perceived by many aged Mexican Americans as failing to do as much as it should or could. More is expected of the church than spiritual guidance alone (Crouch, 1972). While the government is also perceived by many aged Mexican Americans as a potential resource that should be used, (Cuellar, 1978), many aged are not specifically clear on exactly what it is the government should be doing for them (Crouch, 1972). The underutilization of nursing home facilities by Mexican Americans has been identified as being due to their unavailability in areas where Mexican Americans live, the preference for living at home with relatives, and a conceptualization of nursing homes as "a last resort" (Eribes and Bradley-Rawls, 1978).

Ethnic Characteristics with Implications for Nursing. Some characteristics of aged Mexican Americans which can have important consequences for nursing are:

- They are likely to prefer being called Latin American or Latino if from Texas; Spanish American if from New Mexico; Mexican American if from California; or Chicano if activists. Currently, Hispanic is preferred by some professionals.
- They may prefer being called by a title of respect along with their surname, such as Mrs. Ortiz, and may perceive terms like "gramps" or "grandpa" as signs of disrespect.
- They may be content with being rather than becoming; with things as they are rather than what might be; with interpersonal values as opposed to achievement, success, and materialism.
- They are likely not to fully understand "patients' rights" and the current encouragement of inclusion and self-determination in health matters.
- They may have strong beliefs in, and continue to use, folk medicine and home remedies.
- They are likely to be significant members of an extended family network, with valued roles as advisers and consultants.
- They may be modest by comparison with whites — having a reluctance to discuss the private functions of urinating, defecating, bathing, and sexual activity, or to expose private parts of the body.
- They may perceive and use time differently from whites, being oriented to the present, which may result in their being labeled irresponsible, lazy, and undependable.
- They are likely to respond to illness as a family affair, expecting and encouraging extensive numbers of family members to be involved.
- They may have a low expectation of self as a nonpaying client in public health agency programs, resulting in a passivity which keeps them from asking for medications, complaining of poor care, requesting simple wants and needs, etc.
- They are likely to speak English as a second language, if at all.
- They will vary in the extent to which they adhere to their traditional culture and such things as food preferences.

Astute and caring health professionals should respect the aged Mexican American person's concern for interpersonal relations, and should carefully avoid imposing their own value system of achievement and materialism on their evaluation of the person's worth. The health care provider should learn what home health care remedies have been used by the aged Mexican American patient to determine compatibility with other treatments. As long as the folk practice does not pose a problem of incompatibility, it should be supported. Each aged Mexican American's degree of modesty and need for personal privacy should be ascertained and respected. Methods of ensuring that the aged Mexican American understands medical and nursing care directions must be developed, and careful attention should be given to whether the aged person has concerns about which he may not feel free to speak.

Native Americans

The native American category has the most diversity of all ethnic cultures because of the large number of tribal groups in this country. The Bureau of Indian Affairs provides federal assistance to more than 263 Indian tribes, bands, villages, pueblos, and groups (Bureau of Indian Affairs, 1970). This number does not include Alaska's native population or a number of other Indian groups who, for a variety of reasons, do not receive federal aid. Each Indian group has its own system of customs and traditions distinct from any other tribal group, its own historical confrontation with the dominant society, and its own accommodation to the dominant society.

Intermarriages between members of different Indian tribes and non-Indians have produced some confusion in defining who is Indian. To qualify for federal assistance, an individual usually must have a minimum of one-quarter Indian blood. To qualify for tribal assistance, an individual must be a registered member of the tribe. Membership requirements vary among the different tribes so that someone with less than 10% Indian blood whose mother was tribally registered may be a tribal member, whereas an individual with 50% Indian blood

whose mother was not tribally registered may not be a tribal member. Anthropologists recognize a category of "Sociological Indian" for those who may not meet a required blood quantum or who may not be tribally registered, but who identify themselves as Indian and are recognized by their community as Indian.

Historical Factors. Prior to European contact, Indians lived dispersed throughout this country, having adapted their life-styles to the environment in a highly efficient manner. Each group had its own distinct language or dialect and cultural patterns. After contact with the Europeans, most Indian survivors were moved to reservations, a system designed to limit Indian control of vast land holdings and to "guarantee" the Indians' rights to what little land was left in their possession. By virtue of their prior claim to the land, Indian tribes were considered sovereign nations having the inherent right to make treaty agreements with the emergent federal government. Various treaty agreements over the years have resulted in the federal government's becoming the trustee of Indian property and providing certain health, education, and welfare services to Indian tribes. As a consequence of the Indians' trustee relationship with the federal government, many tribal groups bypass local and state agencies, preferring to work through area agencies which represent a direct contact with the federal government.

The relative isolation of most Indian reservations has permitted native Americans to retain more of their cultural traditions than most other ethnic groups. Also involved in their cultural integrity is the fact that Indians are not immigrants who left a prior homeland. As residents of their native soil, many have chosen to actively resist the acculturation demands of the dominant culture which has instituted many programs in an attempt to force Indians to become (dark) carbon copies of the white man. Today, faced with the reality that their economic survival is inextricably interwoven with the dominant society, native Americans are judiciously selecting those aspects of the dominant society they want and/or need in order to survive.

Traditional Health System. The native American healing system, which is still adhered to by some aged Indians, is both pragmatic and spiritual, reflecting a sacred relationship between man and nature. Diseases, in the traditional folklore system, can be caused by human agency, supernatural agency, or natural causes. Examples of causal agents include taboo violation, disease-object intrusion, spirit intrusion, and soul loss. Sorcery encompasses the use of power for evil purposes. Taboo violations occur when one fails to adhere to certain behavioral prescriptions. An animal or inanimate object enters the body to cause disease-object intrusion, while spirits symbolic of animals or even humans cause spirit intrusion. Soul loss occurs during dreams when the soul is thought to leave the body (Twaddle and Hessler, 1977).

Some basic techniques employed to achieve healing, which many aged Indians continue to use, include drugs, mechanical intervention, and religious or spiritual actions. Artifacts used during the healing rites include pipe and tobacco, sacred masks, effigies, rattles, medicine bowls, sucking cups and tubes, drums, and medicine lodges. Dancing is a frequent component of healing rites, as are songs and prayers. Health care specialists include the herbalist who is skilled with medicines, the diagnostician who divines the cause of illness, and the medicine man who has the skill or power to effect a cure through specific healing rites.

Cognitions of Aging. Few studies have delineated the concepts of aging among native Americans. In traditional times, old age began for women after their reproductive years and for men after their hunting and warring years. Anthropological literature indicates that the aged were treated with respect and assigned meaningful roles that kept them intimately involved with the rest of society's members. The aged Indian was perceived as a leader, steeped in wisdom, able to educate and advise the young — a possessor of practical, religious, or medicinal knowledge (Levy, 1967; Williams, 1980); see Figure 35-3.

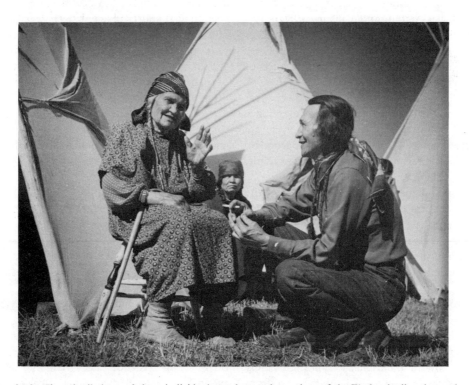

Figure 35-3. Though all three of these individuals are honored members of the Flathead tribe, the aged woman is most venerated for her wisdom. (Photo courtesy of Henry Eide.)

Many aged Indians are still respected today for the wisdom they have attained from the experiences of a lifetime. This respect is shown to aged Indians by listening to and following their advice. "Youngsters" of 45 will be told, "You were born yesterday. You don't know anything yet." The highest credential for authority to speak at gatherings is the acknowledgment of old age. An older person who arises and states, "Listen to me. I am an old man," will receive attention and expects to have his advice followed (Bryde, 1971, p. 20).

In traditional times, old people were respected because guidelines for survival and self-fulfillment were contained in the advice they gave. However, young Indians today often feel that their elders' advice is not relevant to the modern world in which they find themselves (Williams, 1980). The behavior valued by the aged Indian can be seen in this comment by an older Indian about a younger man, "He's a good man. When you talk to him, he listens, all over" (Bryde, 1971, p. 20).

The concept of age was defined within the parameters of productivity, as opposed to a chronological definition (Williams, 1980). Traditionally, tasks continued to be performed as long as the individual was capable, and one was not considered old until the performance of tasks declined (Goodwin, 1942).

Traditionally, native Americans did not fear death for they looked upon it as the entrance into a life after this one. While Indians are perceived as being stoic, there are appropriate times for expressions of emotion, for example, during the grieving process. Upon death, the family may prepare the deceased one's favorite food as a form of honor. Special rituals, such as burying the dead's possessions with him or entreating the dead to depart without taking any family members, are performed to ensure the deceased will not return in spirit form.

Resources. The extended family kinship network is still available to many native Americans, although its support is eroding as many youngsters leave the reservation to find work. Token gestures toward traditionally important family relationships have evolved as Indians confront the reality of high unemployment, lack of jobs on reservations, and loss of traditional economic supports and self-sufficiency. While the mother and grandmother's homemaker role may still provide role-modeling opportunities for young female family members, the father and grandfather's lack of marketable wage-earning job skills leave little for young male family members to emulate. Among some Indian families, young males tend to turn to their brothers or peers for support and as role models (Farris and Farris, 1981).

Despite this apparent breakdown in the extended family, there remains among many native Americans a commitment to the family, especially its aged members. Many an Indian college student has returned home when called upon to help an ailing grandparent or other aged relative. Evidence for the strength of family bonds comes from the fact that to this day, Indian people call one another by their relational name (e.g., brother, cousin) as opposed to their proper name (Bryde, 1971).

Whatever emotional support the native American's extended family can provide its aged members must, however, be coupled with economic support (Block, 1979). In all probability, economic support for aged native Americans must come from the federal government and should include such needs as hospital care, outpatient care, in-home services, communications, nutrition, income, nursing homes, housing, fuel, senior citizen's centers, day care centers, transportation, homemaker services, and legal assistance (National Tribal Chairmen's Association, 1976).

Like aged black Americans, aged native Americans are survivors. As such, they have probably developed personal resources that will stand them in good stead during their later years. The exigencies of a hard life and extreme social changes during their lifetimes have probably forced aged native Americans to develop methods of stress reduction. Furthermore, traditional Indian values can be viewed as resources for the aged.

Many aged native Americans have a reverence for God (or the Great Creator) that pervades their total existence. They believe God is everywhere and in everything, that he takes care of them, is personal to them, has mercy on them, and will respond to sincere prayers (Bryde, 1971). Among Indians, people are valued for what they are and not for what they have. Thus, aged native Americans can acquire a measure of dignity and respect by sharing what they have and helping when they are needed. Riches are measured in terms of the quality of interpersonal relationships and not in terms of material possessions.

Ethnic Characteristics with Implications for Nursing. Some characteristics of aged native Americans which can have important consequences for nursing are:

- They may prefer to be called native Americans, yet may be amenable to being called American Indian or just Indian.
- They will prefer to be identified with their tribal groups and are likely to resent being categorized with all Indians, which implies greater similarity than actually exists and ignores differences among tribes that are important to the individual.
- They may take considerable time to respond to questions as they think over appropriate responses carefully and thoughtfully.
- They are likely to judge people by what is inside them and not by what they have or appear to be.
- They may feel it is important to understand things to their own satisfaction and may not feel their understanding has to be explained to someone else.
- They may be grateful for health care services, not in the sense of receiving a gratuity, but because the health care professional is following the right order of things in sharing with, and providing for, others as all human beings should do. Thus, thank yous may not be extended since such behavior is what is expected of people.
- They are likely to value people before things, to give to others even when they are in dire need, and to refrain from making decisions for others or speaking for others.

- They are likely to be exceptionally quiet and nontalkative when something is bothering them because problem solving is accomplished alone and within the individual.
- They may resist advice if they feel they are being pushed into a decision, but they are likely to respond if ideas are provided that might help them to decide what is best for them.
- They are likely to have some ethnic food preferences. Ethnic food may be very important to some individuals.
- They are likely to have departed from a native diet and to consume considerable amounts of sugar and starch, reflected in obesity and a high rate of diabetes in some tribes.
- They may appear unemotional when facing threatening situations, which is often mistaken for lack of feeling rather than for its real purpose which is to remain calm and in control of the situation.
- They are likely to prefer talking, visiting, and contemplating nature than frenetic activity and work.
- They are likely to have learned English as a second language, if at all, and are most appreciative when non-Indians attempt to learn a few words of their native language.
- They may have strong beliefs in, and continue to use, folk medicine and home remedies, and may rely on traditional ceremonies before coming to the clinic.
- They are likely not to fully understand "patients' rights" and the current encouragement of inclusion and self-determination in health matters, at least as these are defined by whites.

These ethnic characteristics of aged native Americans suggest a number of intervention strategies for nurses. Health care providers working with aged native Americans will have to learn to respect the Indians' concept of autonomy, independence, and individuality. Every Indian individual has control over his own "decision rights," as these relate to possessions and actions, which should not be infringed upon by others. Thus, for example, to directly ask someone for assistance prevents the person from freely exercising his right to refuse since to do so would place him in an embarrassing situation. The preferred method is to make one's needs known so that the individual has the freedom to offer his help if he truly wishes to do so (Lamphere, 1977).

One's control over his own decision rights prevents an individual from speaking for another or giving an opinion on how another thinks since such speculation infringes on the person's decision rights. Thus, a nurse who wants to know how someone is will have to ask that person, otherwise she will receive the standard response, "I don't know, ask him" (Lamphere, 1977).

Native American autonomy and individuality require an egalitarian, rather than a hierarchical, authority since hierarchical authority recognizes the right of a leader to make binding decisions for others (Lamphere, 1977). The significance of this for nurses is that decision making among native Americans should include everyone concerned since no one individual can speak for another.

Other areas in which nurses must develop sensitivity include care in approaching aged native Americans in a quiet and unobtrusive manner, giving them time to think and formulate questions without being overwhelmed with meaningless chatter; identification of appropriate authority figures and inclusion of them in health care decision making; use of interpreters as needed; support of traditional health practices; and assistance in helping aged native Americans to participate in their own health care as patient advocates.

Asian Americans

The Asian American category includes such diverse ethnic groups as Japanese, Chinese, Korean, Vietnamese, Filipinos, East Indians, Thais, Burmese, Indonesians, Laotians, Malaysians, and Cambodians. Major diversities within each group revolve around the area of their country from which they emigrated, the period of their emigration, their age at emigration, and the American-born descendants of these immigrants. Thus, for example, Chinese immigrants

have come from the rich plains of the south and the barren hills of the north, as well as from the commercial and cultural capitals of China (Kalish and Yuen, 1971). Some immigration waves occurred as long as 130 years ago, featuring able-bodied adult workers, while some are occurring presently and include many elderly or the very young.

A complexity inherent among immigrant groups is the difference among generations. For example, first generation Japanese (Issei) were born and raised in Japan; their immediate descendants (Nisei) were born and raised in the United States; some of their United States born offspring (Kibei) were sent back to Japan to live with grandparents for the purpose of education, while their other offspring (Sansei) remained in the United States; both groups (Kibei and Sansei) are beginning to bear and raise another generation of Japanese Americans (Yonsei). Contrasting experiences among these generations are significant. A component aspect of this complexity consists of the young immigrants now entering this country, who bring with them a fresh reservoir of cultural traditions, creating the phenomenon of older ethnic group members with less traditional cultural practices than younger ethnic group members.

The literature concerning elderly Asian Americans is sparse to the point of being virtually nonexistent (Kalish and Moriwaki, 1979). What little is available features Chinese Americans and Japanese Americans; these two ethnic groups will be discussed here.

Historical Factors. Chinese began emigrating to the United States as early as 1788; immigration reached a peak between 1850 and 1880 when their numbers increased from 1,000 to over 100,000 as a response to the 1848 California gold rush and the building of the transcontinental railroad. When white men denied them their gold mining claims and even places to work, the Chinese took over the least competitive (and most undesirable) jobs such as cooking and laundering. Most Chinese immigrants were young, single, male sojourners, who came for economic gain and planned to return to their homeland with their fortunes to raise their families. For many years, the Chinese in this country were a bachelor population, and at one time there were 2000 males per 100 females (Char, 1981).

Open hostility on the part of whites toward the Chinese resulted in the Chinese "withdrawing" and settling in ghetto areas of large cities. Isolated by language and tradition, and surrounded by hostile neighbors, the Chinese began the development of what became Chinatowns across the country. Such enclaves helped to preserve traditional ways, which today's aged Chinese Americans are likely to continue to value. It was not until after World War II, with the relaxation of immigration laws, that a more equitable ratio of Chinese women to men was produced. Thus, an unusually large percentage of aged Chinese Americans is male.

The first concerted emigration of Japanese to the United States began in 1866 with "certain classes of [Japanese] citizens and students who wished to pursue their education abroad" (Sodetani-Shibata, 1981, p. 98). With a change in emigration policy by the Japanese government in 1884, the character of Japanese immigrants changed to young, male sojourners who, like the Chinese, came to seek a fortune and then planned to return to their homelands to raise families. For a number of reasons, most Japanese immigrants stayed in the United States, sending for "picture brides" (prearranged marriages with potential spouses selected from photographs). By the time they married, the men were likely to be middle aged, while their spouses were considerably younger. Because of the age difference, elderly Japanese Americans who survive today are apt to be women (Kalish and Moriwaki, 1973). Many immigrant Japanese became, and still are, gardeners and farmers. A major historical event that significantly affected today's aged Japanese Americans was World War II. With internment in relocation camps, Japanese lost property, savings, businesses, status, and authority. When finally released from their lengthy incarceration, many Japanese had lost their status as respected authority figures and often were "reduced" to a level of equality or even subordination within their family units (Kalish and Moriwaki, 1979). While aged Japanese Americans are less likely to have

lived their adult years in sections of cities as ethnically dense as Chinatowns, they tend to have lived an insular existence (Kalish and Moriwaki, 1979). Thus, some of their traditional ways have been preserved despite the tremendous pressure for acculturation in this country.

Traditional Health System. Asian American literature on folk medical practices features the Chinese folk medical system almost to the exclusion of any other. The principles of yin and yang underlie the Chinese medical system. As opposing forces of the universe, yin and yang regulate the flow of the vital energy force within the body. Yin, the "female" force, stands for such "negative" elements as darkness, death, cold, and emptiness. Yang, the "male" force, stands for such "positive" elements as light, creation of life, heat, and fullness.

The human body is divided into yin and yang parts. The interior of the body, the front of the body, and solid organs are all yin forces. External surfaces, the back of the body, and hollow organs are all yang forces. Interestingly, the Chinese view the body as a gift given them by their parents and forebears. As such, the body is not the person's individual property but a gift to be cared for and well maintained so that at the end of life the physical body will be whole and sound.

Disrupted harmonies between the body's yin and yang forces are the sole cause of disease. This disruption comes not only from within but also from without. Thus, external forces affect the balance of the body's internal yin and yang properties. These external forces operate on the same yin and yang principles, with excesses of either one creating an imbalance and causing problems. For example, excess heat (from the weather or other sources) can be injurious to the heart; excess cold can be injurious to the lungs. Prolonged sitting can be harmful to the flesh and spine, and prolonged lying down can be harmful to the lungs (Campbell and Chang, 1975; Chow, 1976; Spector, 1979; Wang, 1976).

Prevention is the primary focus of the Chinese folk medical system. The Chinese have developed a large number of practices that are designed to prevent illness (as opposed to

Western medicine's large number of practices that are designed to treat illness once it has occurred). These Chinese preventive measures, in the order of their importance as preventive concepts, are philosophy, meditation, nutrition, martial arts (such as kung fu and tai chi chuan), herbology, acumassage, acupressure, moxibustion (therapeutic treatment with heat), acupuncture, and spiritual healing (Chow, 1976). Traditionally, the Chinese, rather than wait for an imbalance to occur, went to their physician for a "tune-up" to keep well by having their energy balanced. The physician's prescription might include proper nutrition, an exercise, ritual, meditation practice, herbs, or acupuncture. Treatment was free if the physician failed to keep a patient healthy (Chow, 1976)!

Cognitions of Aging. Traditionally the aged were venerated in China and Japan. Old age was a time when the grandparents presided over a large group of kin, commanding considerable power. Children were expected, even required, to take care of their aged parents. Failure of parents to produce a son who would look after them in old age and in the afterlife, was one of the greatest misfortunes a Chinese person could suffer. In Japan, the eldest son and his wife were given the responsibility of providing and caring for his aging parents (Char, 1981; Ikels, 1980; Montero, 1979; Sodetani-Shibata, 1981).

Growing old was perceived as a blessing because of the opportunity to relax and enjoy the fruits of a lifetime of labor. The aged could expect to have their advice sought and followed, and to participate in important family decisions that had to be made. There was great freedom during old age to express impulses which formerly had been restricted, to tell off-color jokes, and to be foolish (Kalish and Moriwaki, 1979; Palmore, 1975).

Unfortunately for the immigrant Chinese and Japanese, the theme of filial piety did not fit in well with such dominant U.S. themes as independence, self-reliance, and mastery of one's fate. Thus, Chinese and Japanese Americans — who had been taught to expect to be rewarded in old age for what they had accomplished over a lifetime of honorable labor —

found themselves ignored and forgotten in a country which valued future potential more than past achievement (Kalish and Moriwaki, 1979; Kitano and Sue, 1973).

In Kalish and Reynolds' (1976) study *Death and Ethnicity,* 110 Japanese Americans in Los Angeles County, with a mean age of 49 years, were interviewed on a variety of death-related topics. Approximately equal numbers of black Americans, Mexican Americans, and whites were included in the study; of these groups, the Japanese Americans were the most likely to be living with elderly individuals. The Japanese Americans were also more likely than the other groups to carry out their spouse's last wishes even if these seemed senseless and caused some inconvenience. The traditional Japanese emphasis on control of expressions of all kinds that might upset others extends to death, where grief is kept in check. About half the Japanese American sample felt a dying person should be told he is dying, while close to 80% wanted to be told themselves. As a group, more Japanese Americans (72%) preferred to die at home than any other group in the study.

Resources. Many aged Chinese Americans are men without families or whose families remain in China. Even those with families in this country are poor, have little education, and tend to be isolated in the ghetto. Thus, the family can offer little in the way of material or informational assistance. Even the traditional extended kinship network and "family association" systems for aged Chinese Americans are becoming inadequate sources of support (Carp and Kataoka, 1976). Among aged Japanese Americans are many individuals with few or no relatives in this country. Many are women who married older men and now find themselves alone — their husbands dead, their children married and gone. Traditional kinship ties along with filial piety have eroded so that many of the aged are not automatically cared and provided for by an eldest son and daughter-in-law.

Formal support from government programs is limited because of the relatively small number of Chinese and Japanese Americans in general and because many of these do not qualify for benefits such as Social Security. The programs that are provided must take into consideration the facts that few aged Chinese and Japanese Americans have transportation, and that significant language and cultural barriers exist. In Los Angeles, Keiro, a convalescent day care facility, meets the language, dietary, and cultural needs of aged Japanese Americans (Moriwaki, 1981). In San Francisco's Chinatown, On Lok Senior Day Care and Health Services Center provides culturally relevant day care programs, as does Hawaii's Kuakini Home Day Care Center (Kalish and Moriwaki, 1979); see Figure 35-4.

Like so many other survivors, aged Chinese and Japanese Americans have personal resources upon which they can draw, many which reflect cultural values. Kiefer (1974) identified four factors — companionship, authority and autonomy, productivity, and acceptance of death — as contributing to a comfortable old age for Japanese Americans. For example, the Chinese and Japanese Americans' small numbers, traditional reserve, and language barriers, which prohibit much social intercourse with the dominant society, tend to keep them in tightly knit, small groups that can provide a satisfying social resource. The traditional belief that aged parents could expect to be repaid by their children for their life's work placed the aged in positions of authority and autonomy. While this belief was eroded, remnants of the value remain, and many aged Chinese and Japanese Americans perceive themselves to have autonomy, if not authority. Another traditional value reflects the contribution that aged Chinese and Japanese Americans can make even if they are not productive, because they are seen as continuing to be needed and worthwhile members in a spiritual and philosophical sense after death (Piovesanna, 1979). Finally, since death is viewed as an inevitable, natural event, it is philosophically accepted as the natural order of things. Thus, death need not be feared by many aged Chinese and Japanese American.

Ethnic Characteristics with Implications for Nursing. Some characteristics of aged Chinese Americans and Japanese Americans which can have important consequences for nursing are:

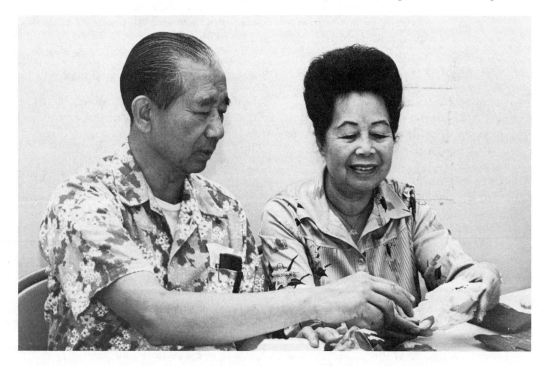

Figure 35-4. These Chinese grandparents enjoy participating in activities at a culturally relevant Day Care Center in Phoenix, Arizona. (Photo by Veronica Evaneshko)

- They are likely to have a strong sense of pride which may result in a sense of failure and shame if they have to accept welfare.
- They may not seek or ask for help, but they may respond to an "outreach" program.
- They are likely to be "caught" between their traditional values of expecting filial piety (including financial support, personal care, even virtual devotion) and such values of their adopted homeland as not being a burden to their children, having the privacy and independence of one's own home, and not sacrificing the needs of offspring (such as education) for the care of aged parents.
- They will prefer to be addressed formally and with respect. The young may drop their voice with humility and respect for their elders.
- They may have adult offspring who are experiencing shame and guilt because of being perceived by the family or community as not providing the appropriate amount of filial piety to their parents.
- They may refuse needed surgery because it is seen as intrusive and destructive, preventing the body from remaining whole.
- They are likely to be wary of governmental authorities and may not seek help until the situation is desperate.
- They may prefer traditional foods prepared in a traditional way and eaten in a traditional manner (i.e., aged Chinese Americans may prefer to have rice every day, eaten with chopsticks, along with Chinese tea prepared in the Chinese style).
- They may not share the philosophical framework of Western medicine (i.e., aged Chinese Americans may not understand why so many diagnostic tests are necessary, and may be especially upset with blood tests since blood is seen as the source of life for the entire body and is believed not to be regenerated).
- They may not speak English and, in the case of Chinese Americans, may speak one of 300 different Chinese dialects.

- They are likely to have high regard or respect for professional health care providers because of their educational attainment and may not ask for needed clarification because it may be perceived as rude, disrespectful behavior.

An awareness of the differences between Western medicine and the Asiatic approach to health care should help to alert health care providers to potential areas of conflict, misunderstanding, or "lack of fit" between the two systems. The small, close-knit community with its high Asian American density can be activated for help. Using family members as "go betweens" who can explain the services to the aged and assist in administering them may be a solution for those aged Chinese and Japanese Americans who are wary of governmental authorities. Should the health care provider's advice or directions conflict with traditional beliefs and practices, the aged Chinese or Japanese American may not indicate the conflict, preferring to remain quiet and noncommunicative so as not to reveal his "disobedience" to an authority figure. Again, sensitivity to potential conflict between medical systems and tactful inquiry are necessary.

Shared Characteristics of Ethnic Groups

Aged members of the minority groups discussed in this chapter, with traditions that are distinct from the dominant society, share many common cultural characteristics that have implications for health care providers:

- These individuals often lack full knowledge or understanding of the services and benefits to which they are entitled.
- They are likely not to understand and to be bewildered by bureaucratic jargon, yet may appear to agree with authorities so as to avoid embarrassment and frustration.
- They are likely to seek emotional support primarily from their kinship network, and secondarily from friends, neighbors, co-workers, and other groups.
- They may see more than one health care specialist (i.e., herbalist, traditional healer,

medical doctor, chiropractor) for an illness, and may be taking herbs and other combinations of medication.

- They may have traditional food preferences and be more comfortable with a native language.
- They may be accustomed to relying on one dose of a medication for a cure and may not understand the need for a number of pills over an extended period of time.
- They may be accustomed to taking traditional medications at various times and for numerous ailments, tending to borrow and lend them at will. They may attempt to do the same thing with medications recommended by the physician.
- They often say little, comply with most requests, rarely complain, and in general exhibit exemplary behavior which may mask communication problems and cultural barriers.
- They need not follow all the traditional practices of their culture and may not reveal the extent of their commitment to traditional ways from external appearances.
- They are likely not to fully understand "patients' rights" and the current encouragement of inclusion and self-determination in health matters.
- They may be under pressure from family members who are in conflict with each other regarding the use of Western medical practices or traditional folk remedies.

RECOMMENDATIONS

The interaction between the health care provider and aged ethnic people sets the stage for potential misunderstanding, miscommunication, discord, and distrust. Imagine the patient — homesick, lonely, and fearful; disliking and unable to eat peculiar food; not understanding why only two relatives may visit; loathed by the brusk, unfriendly, unsmiling health care providers; appalled at their insensitivity and lack of modesty; unable to speak English; knowing that hospitals are places of death; desperate for someone to stop in the headlong

rush in all directions and offer a gentle touch or just sit for awhile in quietude. Imagine the nurse — comfortable in her surroundings; proud and confident in her nursing expertise; knowing what is best for the patient; annoyed that so many relatives in the patient's room keep her from maintaining her schedule; pleased at how quiet and undemanding the patient is; wondering why the patient is so "picky" about his food; frustrated in her attempts to communicate with someone who does not speak English; repulsed by the smell of the amulet around the patient's neck; angry at the number of times the patient's relatives ring his call bell. How does one break through these cultural barriers?

The overriding recommendation is for ethnic humanism *with* regard to race, color, and creed. Without it, safe and effective health care is not possible (Branch, 1976, p. 5). Inherent in the concept of ethnic humanism is the belief that aged ethnic people have the right to adhere to their cultural preferences and customs.

The health care provider should become acquainted with the culture concept to become *aware* of the variety inherent within and among all cultural groups. Becoming aware of the concept of culture permits health care providers to develop sensitivity to potential differences between what aged members of an ethnic group might believe, know, prefer, or perform versus their own beliefs and approaches.

Ethnic humanism includes respect for another's culturally different ways and precludes ethnocentrism in which one assumes one's own way of looking at or doing things is the only and best way. This means that when appropriate, the health care provider should support the aged ethnic client's decision to utilize traditional healing resources and should seek to work within the traditional folk medical system to the extent possible and compatible with Western medicine's practices.

Another ethnically humanistic effort is an attempt to learn the aged ethnic person's language, even if only a few words or phrases. This helps to develop rapport. Sincere human involvement is demonstrated by the care giver who accepts a proffered cup of tea and who sits down, visits for awhile, inquires about the family's health, and in general indicates an interest in the client as a human being and a person first, and as an ethnic member second. Thus, he becomes Mr. Wolfsong, the native American, not the native American Mr. Wolfsong.

Learning something about the aged ethnic person's cultural background indicates a willingness to understand his view of his cultural world and is the hallmark of real caring (Mayeroff, 1971). Participation in cultural activities that are acceptable for "outsiders" indicates an even stronger commitment to meeting the aged ethnic person halfway.

Those who accept the challenge and try to provide ethnically humanistic care are likely to receive more in return than they give. Not only will they understand their aged ethnic clients better, but they will gain new insights into their own cultural behavior. Such insights may help to lay the foundation for some much needed changes in this country's attitudes toward aging.

REFERENCES

Anderson, E.F. *Program innovation for new and meaningful roles for minority elderly persons.* Paper presented at the 7th National Institute on Minority Aging, San Diego, California, February 7, 1980.

Baca, J.E. Some health beliefs of the Spanish speaking. *American Journal of Nursing* 69(10):2172–2176 (1969).

Barrow, G.M. and Smith, P.A. *Aging, Ageism and Society.* St. Paul: West Publishing Company, 1979.

Bauwens, E.E. (Ed.). *The Anthropology of Health.* St. Louis: C.V. Mosby, 1978.

Beaubier, J. Biological factors in aging. In Fry, C.L. (Ed.). *Aging in Culture and Society: Comparative Viewpoints and Strategies.* Brooklyn: J.F. Bergin Publishers, 1980, pp. 21–41.

Benet, S. *Abkhasians: The Long-living People of the Caucasus.* New York: Holt, Rinehart and Winston, 1974.

Bengston, V.L., Ethnicity and aging: problems and issues in current social science inquiry. In Gelfand, D.E. and Kutzik, A.J. (Eds.) *Ethnicity and Aging: Theory, Research, and Policy.* New York: Springer, 1979, pp. 9–31.

Bengston, V.L., Cuellar, J.B., and Ragan, R.K. Stratum contrasts and similarities in attitudes toward death. In Hendricks, J. and Hendricks, C.D. (Eds.) *Dimensions of Aging: Readings.* Cambridge, Mass.: Winthrop Publishers, 1979, pp. 244–259.

Bengston, V.L., Kasschau, P.L., and Ragan, P.K. The impact of social structure on aging individuals. In

Birren, J.E. and Schaie, K.W. (Eds.) *Handbook of the Psychology of Aging.* New York: Van Nostrand Reinhold, 1977.

Benitez, R. Ethnicity, social policy, and aging. In Davis, R. (Ed.) *Aging: Prospects and Issues.* Los Angeles: Ethel Percy Andrus Gerontology Center, 1976, pp. 164–177.

Block, M.R. Exiled Americans: the plight of indian aged in the United States. In Gelfand, D.E. and Kutzik, A.J. (Eds.). *Ethnicity and Aging: Theory, Research, and Policy.* New York: Springer Publishing Company, 1979, pp. 184–192.

Branch, M.F. New approaches in nursing: Ethnic humanism views. In Branch, M.F. and Paxton, P.P. (Eds.). *Providing Safe Nursing Care for Ethnic People of Color.* New York: Appleton-Century-Crofts, 1976, pp. 3–19.

Brink, P.J. (Ed.). *Transcultural Nursing: A Book of Readings.* Englewood Cliffs, N.J.: Prentice-Hall, 1976.

Bryde, J.F. *Indian Students and Guidance.* Boston: Houghton Mifflin, 1971.

Bullough, B. and Bullough, V.L. *Poverty, Ethnic Identity and Health Care.* New York: Appleton-Century-Crofts, 1972.

Bureau of Indian Affairs. *Answers to Your Questions About American Indians.* Washington, D.C.: U.S. Government Printing Office, 1970.

Busto, C. Understanding death and dying in the Mexican-American culture. Unpublished manuscript, Phoenix: Grand Canyon College (1978).

Butler, R.N. and Lewis, M.I. *Aging and Mental Health* 3rd Ed. St Louis: C.V. Mosby, 1981.

Campbell, T. and Chang, B. Health care of the Chinese in America. In Spradley, B.W. (Ed.) *Contemporary Community Nursing.* Boston: Little, Brown, 1975, pp. 189–197.

Cantor, M.H. The informal support system of New York's inner city elderly: is ethnicity a factor? In Gelfand, D.E. and Kutzik, A.J. (Eds.) *Ethnicity and Aging: Theory, Research, and Policy.* New York: Springer, 1979, pp. 153–174.

Carp, F.M. and Kataoka, E. Health care problems of the elderly in San Francisco's Chinatown. *The Gerontologist* 16(1):30–38 (1976).

Carter, J.H. The black aged: a strategy for future mental health services. *Journal of the American Geriatrics Society* 26(12):553–556 (1978).

Carter, J.H. Psychiatry, racism, and aging. *Journal of the American Geriatrics Society* 20:343–346 (1972).

Char, E.L. The Chinese American. In Clark, A.L. (Ed.) *Culture and Childrearing.* Philadelphia: F.A. Davis, 1981, pp. 140–164.

Chow, E. Cultural health traditions: Asian perspectives. In Branch, M.F. and Paxton, P.P. (Eds.) *Providing Safe Nursing Care for Ethnic People of Color.* New York: Appleton-Century-Crofts, 1976, pp. 99–114.

Clark, M. *Health in the Mexican-American Culture.* Berkeley: University of California Press, 1959.

Comfort, A. Age prejudice in America. *Social Policy* 7(3):3–8 (1976).

Crouch, B.M. Age and institutional support: perceptions of older Mexican Americans. *Journal of Gerontology* 27(4):524–529 (1972).

Cuellar, J. El senior citizens club: the older Mexican-American in the voluntary association. In Myerhoff, B.G., and Simić, A. (Eds.) *Life's Career – Aging: Cultural Variations on Growing Old.* Beverly Hills: Sage Publications, 1978, pp. 207–230.

Dancy, J., Jr. *The Black Elderly: A Guide for Practitioners.* Ann Arbor: University of Michigan, 1977.

Dorsey, P.R. and Jackson, H.Q. Cultural health traditions: the Latino/Chicano perspective. In Branch, M.F. and Paxton, P.P. (Eds.) *Providing Safe Nursing Care for Ethnic People of Color.* New York: Appleton-Century-Crofts, 1976, pp. 41–80.

Dowd, J.J. and Bengtson, V.L. Aging in minority populations: an examination of the double jeopardy hypothesis. *Journal of Gerontology* 33(3):427–436 (1978).

Dukepoo, F. *The Elder American Indian.* San Diego: The Campanile Press, 1979.

Eribes, R.A. and Bradley-Rawls, M. The underutilization of nursing home facilities by Mexican-American elderly in the Southwest. *The Gerontologist* 18(4): 363–371 (1978).

Farris, C.E. and Farris, L.S. The American Indian. In Clark, A.L. (Ed.) *Culture and Childrearing.* Philadelphia: F.A. Davis, 1981, pp. 56–67.

Federal Council on Aging. *Policy Issues Concerning the Elderly Minorities* (DHHS Publication No. OHDS 80-20670). Washington, D.C.: 1979.

Fischer, D.H. *Growing Old In America.* Oxford: Oxford University Press, 1978.

Fry, C.L. (Ed.) *Aging in Culture and Society: Comparative Viewpoints and Strategies.* Brooklyn: J.F. Bergin Publishers, 1980.

Gelfand, D.E. and Kutzik, A.J. (Eds.). *Ethnicity and Aging: Theory, Research, and Policy.* New York: Springer, 1979.

Gonzales, H.H. Health care needs for the Mexican-American. In *Ethnicity and Health Care.* New York: National League for Nursing, 1976.

Goodwin, C. *The Social Organization of the Western Apache.* Chicago: University of Chicago Press, 1942.

Greathouse, B. and Miller, V.G. The black American. In Clark, A.L. (Ed.) *Culture and Childrearing.* Philadelphia: F.A. Davis, 1981, pp. 68–95.

Grebler, L., Moore, J.W., and Guzman, R.C. *The Mexican American People: The Nation's Second Largest Minority.* New York: The Free Press, 1970.

Guerra, F. Medical folklore in Spanish America. In Hand, W.D. (Ed.) *American Folk Medicine: A Symposium.* Berkeley: University of California Press, 1976, pp. 169–174.

Hendricks, J. and Hendricks, C.D. (Eds.). *Dimensions of Aging: Readings.* Cambridge: Winthrop Publishers, 1979.

Herrera, T. and Wagner, N.N. Behavioral approaches to delivering health services in a Chicano community. In Reinhardt, A.M. and Quinn, M.D. (Eds.) *Current Practice in Family-Centered Community Nursing,* Vol. 1. St. Louis: C.V. Mosby, 1977, pp. 68–80.

Hollingshead, A. and Redlich, F. *Social Class and Mental Illness: A Community Study.* New York: Wiley, 1958.

Ikels, D. The coming of age in Chinese society: traditional patterns and contemporary Hong Kong. In Fry, C.L. (Ed.) *Aging in Culture and Society: Comparative Viewpoints and Strategies.* Brooklyn: J.F. Bergin Publishers, 1980, pp. 80–100.

Jackson, B. The other kind of doctor: conjure and magic in black American folk medicine. In Hand, W.D. (Ed.) *American Folk Medicine: A symposium.* Berkeley: University of California Press, 1976, pp. 259–272.

Jackson, J.J. and Walls, B.E. Myths and realities about aged blacks. In Brown, M. (Ed.) *Readings in Gerontology.* St. Louis: C.V. Mosby, 1978, pp. 95–113.

Jacques, G. Cultural health traditions: a black perspective. In Branch, M.F. and Paxton, P.P. (Eds.) *Providing Safe Nursing Care for Ethnic People of Color.* New York: Appleton-Century-Crofts, 1976, pp. 115–124.

Kalish, R.A. and Moriwaki, S. The world of the elderly Asian American. *Journal of Social Issues* 29(2): 187–209 (1973).

Kalish, R.A. and Moriwaki, S. The world of the elderly Asian American. In Hendricks, J. and Hendricks, C.D. (Eds.) *Dimensions of Aging: Readings.* Cambridge, Mass.: Winthrop Publishers, 1979, pp. 264–277.

Kalish, R.A. and Reynolds, D.K. *Death and Ethnicity: A Psychocultural Study.* Los Angeles: University of Southern California Press, 1976.

Kalish, R.A. and Yuen, S. Americans of East Asian ancestry: aging and the aged. *The Gerontologist* Spring, Part II:36–47 (1971).

Kay, M.A. Health and illness in the Mexican American barrio. In Spicer, E.H. (Ed.) *Ethnic Medicine in the Southwest.* Tucson: University of Arizona Press, 1977, pp. 99–166.

Keefe, S.E. Urbanization, acculturation, and extended family ties: Mexican Americans in cities. *American Ethnologist* 6(2):349–365 (1979).

Kiefer, C. Lessons from the Issei. In Gubrium, J.F. (Ed.) *Late Life Communities and Environmental Policy.* Springfield, Ill.: Charles C. Thomas, 1974.

King, S.H. *Perceptions of Illness and Medical Practice.* New York: Russell Sage Foundation, 1962.

Kitano, H. and Sue, S. The model minorities. *Journal of Social Issues* 29:1–9 (1973).

Lamphere, L. *To Run after Them: Cultural and Social Bases of Cooperation in a Navajo Community.* Tucson: University of Arizona Press, 1977.

Leaf, A. Everyday is a gift when you are over 100. *National Geographic* **143**(1):93–119 (1973).

Leighton, A.H. and Hughes, J.H. *Cultures as Causative of Mental Disorder.* Cambridge, Mass.: Milbank Memorial Fund, 1961.

Leininger, M. (Ed.). *Transcultural Nursing: Concepts, Theories, and Practices.* New York: Wiley, 1978.

Leonard, O.E. The older rural Spanish-speaking people of the Southwest. In Youmans, E.G. (Ed.) *Older Rural Americans.* Lexington: University of Kentucky Press, 1967, pp. 239–261.

Levy, J.E. The older American Indian. In Youmans, E.G. (Ed.) *Older Rural Americans.* Lexington: University of Kentucky Press, 1967, pp. 221–238.

Lynch, L.R. (Ed.). *The Cross-Cultural Approach to Health Behavior.* Cranbury, N.J.: Associated University Presses, 1969.

Maldonado, D. Aging in the Chicano context. In Gelfand, D.E., and Kutzik, A.J. (Eds.). *Ethnicity and Aging: Theory, Research, and Policy.* New York: Springer Publishing Company, 1979, pp. 175–183.

Martinez, C. and Martin, H.W. Folk diseases among urban Mexican-Americans. In Martinez, R.A. (Ed.) *Hispanic Culture and Health Care: Fact, Fiction, Folklore.* St. Louis: C.V. Mosby, 1978, pp. 131–137.

Martinez, R.A. (Ed.). *Hispanic Culture and Health Care: Fact, Fiction, Folklore.* St. Louis: C.V. Mosby, 1978.

Mayeroff, M. *On Caring.* New York: Harper & Row, 1971.

Medvedev, Z.A. Caucasus and Altay longevity: a biological or social problem? *The Gerontologist* **14**(5):381–387 (1974).

Messer, M. Race Differences in selected attitudinal dimensions of the elderly. *The Gerontologist* **8**(4): 245–249 (1968).

Mindel, C.H. and Habenstein, R.W. *Ethnic Families in America.* New York: Elsevier Scientific Publication, 1976.

Montero, D. Disengagement and aging among the issei. In Gelfand, D.E., and Kutzik, A.J. (Eds.) *Ethnicity and Aging: Theory, Research, and Policy.* New York: Springer Publishing Company, 1979, pp. 193–205.

Moquin, W. and Van Doren, C. (Eds.). *A Documentary History of the Mexican Americans.* New York: Praeger, 1971.

Morales, A. The impact of class discrimination and white racism on the mental health of Mexican-Americans. In Hernandez, C.A., Haug, M.J., and Wagner, N.N. (Eds.) *Chicanos: Social and Psychological Perspectives.* St. Louis: C.V. Mosby, 1976, pp. 211–216.

Moriwaki, S.Y. Ethnicity and aging. In Burnside, I.M. (Ed.) *Nursing and the Aged.* New York: McGraw-Hill, 1981, pp. 612–629.

Myerhoff, B. Aging and the aged in other cultures: an anthropological perspective. In Bauwens, E.E. (Ed.) *The Anthropology of Health.* St. Louis: C.V. Mosby, 1978, pp. 151–166.

Narroll, R. Ethnic unit classification. *Current Anthropology* **5**(4):283–312 (1964).

National Institute on Aging. *Age Page.* Washington, D.C.: U.S. Government Printing Office, August 1980.

National League for Nursing. *Ethnicity and Health Care* (Publication No. 14-1625). New York: 1976.

National Tribal Chairmen's Association, Inc. *Summary report.* National Indian Conference on Aging, Phoenix, Arizona, June 15–17, 1976.

National Urban League. *Double Jeopardy – the Older Negro in American Today.* New York: 1964.

Opler, M.K. (Ed.). *Culture and Mental Health: Cross-Cultural Studies.* New York: Macmillan, 1959.

Palmore, E. *The Honorable Elders: A Cross-Cultural Analysis of Aging in Japan.* Durham, N.C.: Duke University Press, 1975.

Piovesanna, G.K. The aged in Chinese and Japanese cultures. In Hendricks, J. and Hendricks, C.D. (Eds.). *Dimensions of Aging: Readings.* Cambridge, Mass.: Winthrop Publishers, 1979, pp. 13–20.

Schaefer, R.T. *Racial and Ethnic Groups.* Boston: Little, Brown, 1979.

Schreiber, J.M. and Homiak, J.P. Mexican Americans. In Harwood, A. (Ed.). *Ethnicity and Medical Care.* Cambridge, Mass.: Harvard University Press, 1981, pp. 264–336.

Schulz, C.M. Age, sex and death anxiety in a middle-class American community. In Fry, C.L. (Ed.) *Aging in Culture and Society: Comparative Viewpoints and Strategies.* Brooklyn: J.F. Bergin Publishers, 1980, pp. 239–252.

Siemaszko, M. Kin relations of the aged: possible consequences to social service planning. In Fry, C.L. (Ed.) *Aging in Culture and Society: Comparative Viewpoints and Strategies.* Brooklyn: J.F. Bergin Publishers, 1980, pp. 253–271.

Snow, L.F. Folk medical beliefs and their implications for care of patients: a review based on studies among black Americans. *Annals of Internal Medicine* **81**:82–96 (1974).

Sodetani-Shibata, A.E. The Japanese American. In Clark, A.L. (Ed.) *Culture and Childrearing.* Philadelphia: F.A. Davis, 1981, pp. 96–138.

Spector, R.E. *Cultural Diversity in Health and Illness.* New York: Appleton-Century-Crofts, 1979.

Stanford, E.P. *The Elder Black.* San Diego: The Campanile Press, 1978.

Stenger-Castro, E.M. The Mexican-American: how his culture affects his mental health. In Martinez, R.A. (Ed.) *Hispanic Culture and Health Care: Fact, Fiction, Folklore.* St. Louis: C.V. Mosby, 1978, pp. 19–32.

Swanson, W.C. and Harter, C.L. How do elderly blacks cope in New Orleans? *Aging and Human Development* **2**(3):210–216 (1971).

Twaddle, A.C. and Hessler, R.M. *A Sociology of Health*. St. Louis: C.V. Mosby, 1977.

U.S. Senate Special Committee on Aging. *The Multiple Hazards of Age and Race: The Situation of Aged Blacks in the U.S*. Washington, D.C.: U.S. Government Printing Office, 1971.

Valle, R. and Mendoza, L. *The Elder Latino*. San Diego: The Campanile Press, 1978.

Wang, R.M. Chinese Americans and health care. In *Ethnicity and Health Care*. New York: National League for Nursing, 1976, pp. 9–19.

Watson, W.H. and Maxwell, R.J. *Human Aging and Dying: A study in Sociocultural Gerontology*. New York: St. Martin's Press, 1977.

White House Conference on Aging. *Toward a national policy on aging*. Proceedings of the second conference on aging. 1971 Washington, D.C.: U.S. Government Printing Office, 1973.

Williams, G.C. Warriors no more: a study of the American Indian elderly. In Fry, C.L. (Ed.) *Aging in Culture and Society: Comparative Viewpoints and Strategies*. Brooklyn: J.F. Bergin Publishers, 1980, pp. 101–111.

Yutang, L. *The Importance of Living*. New York: Day, 1937.

36
Sexuality and Aging

Bernita M. Steffl

The most important sex organ is the brain.

L.E. Lamb (1973)

FEARS, MYTHS, AND REALITIES

This chapter is devoted to issues and problems that confront health professionals who work with older adults in community settings, acute hospitals, and long term care facilities. Though we have made progress in the past five years, there are still those of us who need to be better educated about human sexuality across the life span and to examine your own feelings and attitudes toward sexuality in the aged.

There are still professionals among us who do not understand that the "dirty old man" and the "shameless old lady" may be the healthiest old people. Instead we go about locking the feelings, hopes, dreams, and fantasies of these individuals in the cage of age. What's more, we may be locking ourselves in that cage via a self-fulfilling prophecy. We can liberate them and ourselves. "They are us" (Eisdorfer, 1977).

In our society we have developed a rather negative attitude to the whole process of aging and toward the aged, so it is not strange that we have rather stereotyped notions about sex in old age. Some of these (Butler and Lewis, 1981) are:

- Old people do not have sexual desires.
- They could not make love if they wanted to.
- They are too fragile physically and it might hurt them.
- They are physically unattractive and, therefore, sexually undesirable.
- The whole notion is shameful and decidedly perverse.

Even though most of us *could not* as children, and cannot now (very well), conceive the notion that our parents are interested or indulge in sex, we are learning that the same hopes, dreams, feelings, desires, and passions we had in youth remain with us! The same "me" of 10, 20, and 30 years ago is still locked in this body, with some of the same desires of yesteryear, and old age is always in the distant future. Even when we are 60 and 70, old age is ten years hence!

In working with older people, it is becoming increasingly clear that sex is a major concern in later life. In my experience with older people, I have noticed much more preoccupation with sex and sexuality since I have become more aware of their basic human needs and since I have sharpened my listening and assessment skills. Fear about loss of sexual prowess is a common preoccupation of the older man and can reach devastating proportions, and "old ladies do not sit on park benches just to watch the children play...they dream of their lovers and their lover's lovers" (anonymous).

The fears and myths common among older adults are:

- Fear of heart attacks and stroke
- Fear that sex shortens life
- Fear of social criticism for sexual behavior and attitudes
- Taboos on masturbation and homosexuality
- Cultural stigma on women who socialize with younger men (though it is quite acceptable for men to select and/or pursue women 10–20 years younger than themselves)

*Parts of this chapter have appeared in *Aging and Sexuality,* edited by R.L. Solnick, published by Andrus Gerontology Center, University of Southern California, Los Angeles, California, and in *Educational Gerontology, an International Quarterly* **4**(4):377–388 (1979).

RESEARCH FINDINGS

Participants ranging in age from 60 to 91 years, with 45% over age 70, in one of the largest surveys conducted in the United States revealed an enormous potential for sexuality in old age as well as a wide acceptance of nudity, positive self-consciousness about aging bodies, and little anxiety about a decline in sexuality with years. Older women, married, widowed and single, expressed a willingness to consider alternatives to genital intercourse including oral sex, masturbation, sharing of men, lesbianism, and taking younger men. Most of the respondents described their ideal lover as someone within ten years of their own age. Only 6%, primarily men, indicated a considerably younger lover as ideal (Aging International, 1980). While this survey should not be used to generalize about all elderly, it provides evidence to dispel common myths.

Birren and Schaie (1977) document the following facts: (1) the frequency of sexual activity declines for both sexes, with the sharpest drop occurring earlier for women (late sixties) than for men (late seventies); (2) men maintain higher levels of interest and activity than women at all ages up to the ninth decade; (3) aging men exhibit a relatively large discrepancy between expressed interest and actual sexual performance; (4) marital status affects the frequency of sexual interest and activity for women, but is less significant for men. The most significant finding in current literature is that amounts of past sexual activity and enjoyment are excellent predictors of sexual activity and enjoyment in old age.

There is universal agreement among researchers that healthy males and females are usually interested in, and capable of, sexual activity, including intercourse, well into the seventh decade and often into the eighth and ninth decade (Pfeiffer, 1972; White and Doyle, 1979).

A very comprehensive and thorough review of the literature in regard to activity and sex drive reveals (in summary) a substantial body of literature which indicates that both sexual interest and sexual behavior decline among healthy aging individuals. It is also increasingly apparent that a significant proportion of this decline may be attributed to social, cultural, and psychological factors which adversely affect sexual expression and the sex drive, such as living arrangements and available partners, especially for the older female (Birren and Schaie, 1977).

Attitudes and incentives are important deciding factors in the sexual behavior of older persons. Even when it is possible to make conducive environmental changes, there are indications that older persons tend to be less self-accepting of unconventional behaviors such as remarriage or cohabitation. For example, single women over 65 far exceed the number of men available as sex partners, and many of these women adopt an attitude of declining interest in sexual activity (Birren and Schaie, 1977). Because women usually cope with involutional problems at a younger age than men, they may have greater adaptational capacity which might apply to losses regarding their sex role.

Adrian Verwoerdt (1976) points out that loss of any capacity including sexual function may give rise to a grief reaction. Other behavioral reactions which may occur include the following: (1) the individual who tries to deny sexual decline may appear to be hypersexual; (2) the decline of sexual function may lead to fears concerning loss of love or hold on spouse; (3) a person may take protective retreat; (4) there may be avoidance for fear of failure, with ensuing withdrawal from one's partner which can lead to further problems (e.g., if sex has to be all or nothing, then options are limited); (5) embarrassment and shame about the aged body are troublesome feelings that orginate in many ways; so when older folks are told to relax, not worry about guilt and inhibitions, and enjoy sex as younger people do (as if age made no difference), a false stereotype is created; (6) personal identity is closely related to one's self-concept as a man or woman, and decline in sexual function affects the person's sense of identity; thus earlier psychological problems dating back to childhood or adolescence are frequently reactivated.

Decline in sexual behavior and interest in sex is not an isolated psychological phenomenon, but is related to lifetime psychosocial situations. Many older persons are involved in deteriorating marriages with long term, deep-seated psychological factors causing withdrawal of incentive for sexual activity (Birren and Schaie, 1977).

As implied earlier, the elderly themselves have some sexual prejudices. A study of romance in SROs (single room occupancy residents of a downtown hotel) revealed that 60-year-old men did not want women their own age. They preferred young prostitutes who arrived at the hotel on the first of each month when Social Security checks came. These men preferred short contacts with prostitutes to involvement with women of their own age because older women expected men friends to do too many things for them. They considered this exploitation (Stephens, 1974).

SEX AND THE AGING FEMALE

The biggest myth is about menopause. Actually, menopause causes no decrease in sexual ability (if other health is good). Desire may increase because of reduced fear of pregnancy. Women do commonly suffer from gradual steroid (hormonal) insufficiency that causes a thinning of vaginal walls, and cracking, bleeding, and dryness of the mucous membranes. The parched vagina itches, and the problem is compounded by scratching; hormone creams and water-soluble lubricants are helpful. The overzealous supernurse may tend to add to the problem by cleansing with very soapy water and friction or by application of aseptic lotions. It is also important to interpret to paraprofessionals that the patient did not necessarily cause the condition by scratching (the dirty-old-lady syndrome). Many older women and men use Vaseline. The petroleum or chemical base of Vaseline prevents it from really being therapeutic; water-soluble lubricants are better.

Bartholin's glands which lubricate the vagina decrease somewhat in secretion. This tends to happen less in women who are stimulated on a regular basis from youth on. In other words, use it or lose it can be true about sex. This decrease in secretion is indication for the use of lubricant (other than Vaseline).

The urethra and bladder become more subject to irritation as they are less cushioned because of atrophied vaginal walls, and there can be burning and/or itching and frequency of urination for several days after sex.

The loss of steroids also reduces the length and diameter of the vagina and may shrink the major labia. The clitoris reduces in size, and stimulation tends to be slower. The vagina loses some of its expansive ability, and the tissue becomes more pink in color. The vaginal barrel loses its corrugated appearance.

Dyspareunia, painful intercourse, sometimes occurs after menopause. This is the result of steroid imbalance, and contractions of the uterus which take place during orgasm at all age levels now become painful. Penile penetration and friction may become too painful for women with this condition. Dyspareunia is usually reversed by treatment with hormones.

Treatment with estrogens seems to have been very helpful in reducing osteoporosis, backache, dowager's hump, and vaginitis. It must be pointed out that there are currently some very strong admonitions about overestrogenizing the middle-aged and older woman because of the association with endometrial carcinoma (Smith, Prentice, Thompson, and Herrman, 1975; Ziel and Finkle, 1975).

One must not overlook the fact that many women who have never been happy about sex during most of their lives find in menopause a respectable reason for ending a duty that has always been distasteful to them. On the positive side, however, expansive ability of the vagina does return with sexual expression, for example, for widows who have been sexually inactive. Libido increases with menopause because there is no fear of becoming pregnant. Orgasm may take longer, but there is no problem. Menopause is not the end of vitality, vibrance, attractiveness, usefulness, sexual ability, or desire, but the availability of men is a problem for older women.

SEX AND THE OLDER MAN

Is there a male menopause? Professionals should be prepared to answer this question.

According to the literature and to clinical studies, there certainly is no valid physical measure of a climacteric among males. We do see a gradual decrease in testosterone and sometimes great variation in this. Men do seem to go through a "pause that perplexes" in their middle years, and often in this period, there are problems related to sexuality, among other things.

In their clinical work with older men, Masters and Johnson (1970) found six general categories of factors which were responsible for loss of sexual responsiveness during the later years:

1. Monotony of a repetitious sexual relationship (boredom with his wife)
2. Preoccupation with career or economic pursuits
3. Mental or physical fatigue
4. Overindulgence in food or drink
5. Physical infirmities of either partner
6. The fear of failure

Sexual boredom is more likely to take place if the couple, like most persons in our society, has restricted themselves to a mechanical and repetitious sex life. One writer says that from middle age on, the wife or husband better take steps to jolt his or her partner out of their rut.

The following physical changes take place in the male:

- The penis and testes become flaccid. This is normal and not an impairment to satisfactory sexual function.
- There are fewer sperm, though viable sperm are found to the tenth decade of life.
- Testicular tubules that store and carry sperm become lined by more and more layers of cells so that the diameters of openings become smaller.
- There is loss of fatty tissue and cushioning in the genital area and around the scrotum and testes.

- The prostate gland grows larger with age. Some clinicians believe this may be due to holding back at a younger age.
- There is a decline in the sex hormone testosterone, as mentioned earlier.

The older man ordinarily takes longer to obtain erection. The reactive quality of the scrotum and testes diminishes. There is a decrease in efficiency of ejaculatory response. Masters and Johnson (1970) say that an advantage of this is that control of ejaculatory demand is far better at age 50–75 than at age 10–40. This means that an older man can maintain an erection and make lover longer before coming to orgasm. Masters and Johnson point out that older men also have the advantage of love-making experience.

Older men experience a reduction in volume of seminal fluid which explains the decrease in pressure to ejaculate. Orgasm begins to be experienced in a shorter one-stage period in contrast to the two stage response in early life. After age 50, the extended refractory period (meaning capacity for erection) following ejaculation takes longer than in young men (12–24 hours). Shumaker (1974) states that sexual feelings are always present in a man and he may still have erections about every 80 minutes while asleep.

Most men over 60 are satisfied with one to two ejaculations per week and are capable of more. A consistent pattern helps maintain sexuality. Both sex partners should also keep in mind that longer and more intense stimulation may be necessary.

The man worries about the inability to always ejaculate; then the female partner worries about not being able to bring the male to ejaculation with her contractions. So one says to the other, "It really doesn't matter, but next time you see a doctor...," and this is the kiss of death! Just as the older female need not have an orgasm with each intercourse, neither does the male need to have an ejaculation each time to derive sexual pleasure. There is no such thing as an uninvolved sex problem says Dr. Edward Adelson (1974). About 50–80% of all couples have some sex problems. Most are not physical: about 95% are psychological.

SEX AND MEDICAL-SURGICAL CHRONIC PHYSICAL CONDITIONS

Sex complicates things for doctors. Sex histories on medical records are usually nonexistent. A good medical history and physical should include a sex history. Not all the blame for avoiding this topic belongs to doctors, though they are guilty and are probably still perceived as the most significant source of help by patients. Psychologists and psychiatrists have paid the most attention to this problem. Nurses, social workers, and other professionals should not avoid the topic just because the medical doctor has.

Arthritis

In chronic conditions, sex can be both therapeutic and preventive. For example there is some evidence that sex activity helps arthritis, even in severly arthritic patients, probably because of the adrenal gland production of cortisone and because the sexual act itself is a form of physical activity. Also, emotional stress can result from sexual dissatisfaction, and stress worsens arthritis so sexual activity can be helpful in maintaining function (Butler and Lewis, 1980).

Sex after Hysterectomy

To many women the uterus is not only a child-bearing organ, but also a sexual organ, a cleansing instrument, a regulator of general body health and well-being, and a source of strength, youth, and feminine attractiveness. So counseling for posthysterectomy sexuality is apt to be much more involved than sometimes anticipated. For example, we often hear women complain about weight gain, feelings of weakness, fragility, and vulnerability. They use phases such as, "I feel an emptiness, a space here in my stomach," or "Something is missing and I eat so much to try to fill up the emptiness" (Drellich, 1967).

There should be no problem having sex after hysterectomy. The outer vagina and vaginal barrel are intact, and there is ample room for penile penetration. Numerous studies have shown that loss of ovarian hormone has virtually no effect on sexual desire, sexual performance, or sexual response. When disturbances do occur, the physician is best equipped to handle problems (or should be if he is interested). These disturbances to sex life are not uniform but are related in most instances to irrational fears and psychological effects of surgery in the genital area (Drellich, 1967).

Common Gynecological Problems of Older Women

A persistent theme in geriatric medicine has been the reticence of many elderly patients to complain about serious physical problems. This is especially true in relation to gynecological problems in the female and prostate problems in the male. Because early detection has a direct relationship to recovery, everyone should have regular physical examinations, and direct questions should be asked by doctors and nurses. The following section deal with a few of the most prevalent gynecological problems.

Senile Vaginitis, Vulvitis, and Peritoneal Pruritis. Senile vaginitis, vulvitis, and peritoneal pruritis are low grade inflammations which cause a great deal of discomfort and itching. They are caused by hormonal deficiencies, vitamin deficiency, sugar in the urine, poor hygiene, allergies, or invasion of organisms from the rectum or outside the body (from equipment or clothing). Symptomatic treatment with cleansing douches, cornstarch, and topical medications is most helpful. These conditions are very persistent and require strict routine care, and the very old and disoriented patient may need special attention (and understanding). As stated earlier, hormonal creams and water-soluble lubricants may be helpful.

Uterine Prolapse. Prolapse of the uterus means a downward displacement. It is measured by degrees. In a third degree prolapse, the uterus descends to the point of hanging out of the vagina. It is suspended by stretched uterine ligaments. A prolapsed uterus can be manipulated into place, but it descends again as soon as the patient stands up. Surgery is the treatment of choice but may be contraindicated by the patient's age or general condition. In older patients, a Gellhorn or doughnut-type pessary may be inserted to hold the uterus in the pelvis. These pessaries must be replaced frequently; they require extreme cleanliness, and care must be taken that they do not cause ulceration or become misplaced (Durbin, 1968). Because older women are too fearful, too embarrassed, or too senile to complain, we unfortunately see more of these conditions than we should in large custodial care settings. We can do something about them, and should consider counseling and educating the families of aged patients about them.

Cystocele and Rectocele. Cystocele and rectocele are prolapses of the bladder and the rectum which, when severe, can cause problems in voiding and bowel elimination. With a cystocele or a urethrocele the patient may dribble urine, compounding the problem. In most cases, surgical intervention alleviates the problem; however, again these are conditions that elderly women hesitate to report until they are major problems.

Finally, the everlasting catheters that are so commonly used for incontinent patients in nursing homes are a major vehicle for introducing bladder infections, sometimes leading to serious problems. First, the writer believes that too often an indwelling catheter is the simple solution, and we get lax about taking them out because bladder retraining for the elderly is not easy. Secondly, most extended care facilities claim they do not have the help to keep patients dry when they are totally incontinent. I can only say that I believe that a catheter should be used only as a last resort.

Prostatectomy

Prostate problems and prostatectomy are so prevalent that we must spend some time on them. In may own experience, I have learned that there are an appalling number of misconceptions about them. Although the operation is widespread, many men and their wives have only a hazy idea of the prostate's function and why its strategic location can

cause distress. The prostate is made up of muscular and glandular tissue, and is located just below the urinary bladder. The urethra, the tube that empties the bladder, passes through it. The sole function of the prostate is to produce a lubricating fluid to transport sperm cells during sex relations.

As men grow older, the urethral glands that lie inside the prostate often grow bigger. The enlarged prostate can then press on the urethral tube and block the outlet of the bladder. This leads to stoppage of urine and, sometimes, serious consequences to the kidneys. Usually surgery is recommended when a man has a diminished stream of urine and/or when he has difficulty starting the stream.

There are several methods of surgery; the urologist will select the best method for the particular patient and his problem. I have found the following problems:

1. Patients are rarely counseled by the doctor about sex life after prostatectomy. When they are, it is not very thorough. These seem to be two alternatives: (a) "You'll soon be good as new." (b) "Well, George, what do you expect at your age?"
2. The surgery is usually worse than the patient expected. The tubes, the blood in the urine, and the general discomfort are much worse and more complicated than he was led to believe.
3. Sexual dysfunction may take place but does not necessarily have to be permanent. Patients need to be educated about what to expect and encouraged to anticipate a return of sexual function.

Procedures commonly used in prostate surgery do not disturb the innervation of the erectile system and only rarely result in impotence (about 5%). In most patients, postoperative impotence is of psychogenic origin, particularly in the case of older men who are convinced that the need for the operation confirms their senescence. Though the procedure does not interfere with erection and ejaculatory sensation, it does often produce sterility. This is obviously important for the young man or the older man who is married to a younger wife and plans to have children (Basso, 1977). Because of the removal of obstructive portions of the prostate, the basic structure of the bladder neck is changed, and usually after surgery the semen is not discharged forward through the penis, but backward into the bladder. The sensation and climax (orgasm) of intercourse are the same, and no harm is done in this "retrograde ejaculation." It must be emphasized that this has nothing to do with obtaining the erection (Daut, 1974).

Nurses are in a strategic position to supplement or initiate this kind of patient education and should be prepared to do so. If they are uncomfortable in doing so, they should still be able to assess the situation and seek out other members of the health team to assist them.

Impotence

Impotency and sterility are often used interchangeably by clients. They may need help in understanding that impotence does not imply sterility. Impotence may be complete or partial, temporary or permanent. A male may be completely impotent with one woman and not another. Potency depends upon two sets of factors — one organic and the other psychic. Therefore, it has been classified as primary impotence when the etiology deals with the psychic mechanism, and secondary impotence when it is due to the existence of an organic fault in the genital tract, the central nervous system, or the endocrine glands. It is important to stress here that nurses and health professionals should understand the physiology of penile erection or seek help in doing so (Finkle and Thompson, 1972).

Myths of childhood about diseases have strong influence over older males in regard to impotence, and these beliefs can become self-fulfilling prophecies. Also, the ego of the aging male is especially vulnerable to rejection, either real or illusional.

Doctors Finkle and Thompson (1972) reported encouraging success in counseling 84 psychogenically impotent males. They suggest that for many of these patients, pragmatic counseling rather than extended psychotherapy will achieve renewal of satisfactory sexual func-

tion. Dr. Finkle also emphasizes the great importance of the physician's attitude, interest, and hope. With the positive and optimistic attitude of the physicians involved, 53% of the patients (N = 84) responded satisfactorily to four or less visits.

Prosthetic splints for the penis have become an established alternative of therapy for both the organically and the psychogenically impotent male. A common type splint consisting of a rigid plastic shaft to which slightly splayed ends of softer plastic material are welded are available through urologists. The splint is inserted, preferably under complete anesthesia, and is quickly and readily accomplished without hemorrhage or shock. At ease, the penis is pendulous as usual; at intercourse, the male manually elevates the penis for insertion. Neither he nor his sex partner experiences pain. However a prospective client for prosthetic device should be adequately counseled about the procedure for implantation as well as the need for patience, practice support of a willing and able partner (Busso, 1977). An inflatable penis prosthesis is also available. It is a hydraulic device. When erection is desired, the patient manipulates a subcutaneous pump and fluid is released into two cylindrical prostheses inside the corpora cavernosa (of the penis) producing an erection. There have been no reported deaths associated with the implantation of more than 6000 devices. A report on 175 inflatable penile prosthesis implanted at the Mayo Clinic in Rochester, Minnesota indicated a functional success rate of 90–95% (Furlow, 1979).

A rubber doughnut ("cockring" sold in "sex" shops for about $5.00) can be helpful in maintaining an erection. This hard rubber device is slipped over the partially erect penis (it does not work in absolute impotence). It fits tightly at the base and retains blood in the penis necessary for erection. A leading marriage counselor once pointed out that a simple strong rubber band may serve the same purpose, be less expensive, and be less objectionable. So, I tell my students, "If you see a dirty old man with a rubber band around his penis, know there may be some 'method in his madness'".

There are some local genital disorders that are often misunderstood and cause not only problems but a great deal of guilt and fear. One such condition in males is Peyronie's disease. Peyronie's disease in men can interfere with performance. Hard tumors form in the body of the penis and interfere with intercourse; the penis angles to the right or left. It's etiology is unknown, and it often disappears by itself in about four years. There are a variety of treatments. Peyronie's disease is thought to be rare, but it may be more common than we thought; it could certainly cause psychological problems (Butler and Lewis, 1981).

Cardiovascular Conditions

Cerebrovascular accidents and coronary attacks are among the greatest fears surrounding intercourse in old age. Some fear that sexual activity may bring on an attack, cause a recurrence, or even lead to death. Attacks and death have occurred during sexual intercourse; however, good and conclusive data and statistics have not been documented. We do know that oxygen consumption in sexual intercourse is equal to climbing stairs or walking briskly, and that the heartbeat increases to 90–150 beats per minute (average = 120).

Death during sex occurs much less often than people fear and probably somewhat more than reported (due to reluctance to report). A conservative estimate is that this accounts for 1% of sudden coronary death. It occurs more often when intercourse is with an extra marital partner. I can validate this from my personal experience in working with older adults. Women have confided about how this happened to their husbands and the problems they have had with their guilt. Most of them indicate they would have liked more postcoronary counseling about sex.

Generalized findings of researchers indicate that with any type of heart disease, the patient who can comfortably climb one or two flights of stairs or take a brisk walk around the block is ready to resume sexual activity, usually 4–5 weeks after heart attack, providing there are no complications. Researchers believe that sexual intercourse should be denied only for those patients in severe congestive heart failure; even for these, other sexual activities involving stroking, touching, and embracing are possible (Scheingold and Wagner, 1974).

Strokes. Strokes (cerebrovascular accidents) do not necessitate cessation of sexual activity. It is very unlikely that further strokes can be produced through sexual intercourse. If paralysis occurs after a stroke, adaptations in sexual positions may be necessary to compensate for weaknesses (Butler and Lewis, 1981).

Parkinson's Disease

Parkinsonism or paralysis agitans is commonly known as the shaking palsy. It is a progressively debilitating disease, with characteristic tremors, shuffling gait, masked expression, and depression. The disease affects twice as many men as women and has a late onset. Working with and communicating with the Parkinson's disease patient is very difficult for most of us. Perhaps it is because of our own helplessness regarding any ability to reverse what we see happening, because these patients often maintain cognitive function. The patient's lack of affect and difficulty in communicating foster alienation by nurses. Assessing his sexual needs is very unlikely. However, we should be aware that fostering social and sexual interest may be helpful. Levodopa (Bendopa, Dopar), the medication often used in treatment of parkinsonism, is one of the few medications that crosses the blood-brain barrier, and studies have demonstrated that in addition to lessening tremors and relieving depression, it may enhance libido and activate provocative sexual behavior in a small number of patients. Nurses working with these patients should be aware of opportunities to counsel and assist them and their spouses regarding sexual intimacy when and if possible (Costello, 1975). Staff may need help in understanding so that the patient is not punished for normal feelings.

WAYS TO RESUME SEXUAL ACTIVITY AFTER ILLNESS

The person who is in good physical condition and who engages in regular exercise will be in better condition, physically and emotionally, to resume and enjoy sexual activity after cardiac problems or any illness. Masturbation, for those who find it acceptable, is a good way to ease back to normal sexual activity. The cardiac cost is substantially less for both men and women than in sexual intercourse. The person can find out if he is still sexually responsive and thus gain confidence when sexual activity with a partner is resumed.

Increasing sanction is given to masturbation these days as professionals are working out their hang-ups and acceptance. However, they may forget to take the patient through this stage. For example, a very attractive and spunky older widow participating in a discussion on this subject said, "Our sexuality is talked about, written about; they wonder — do we? And they say what is bad and what is good for us, widows like me. Masturbation always comes up, but nobody tells us exactly what is is, how you do it, or where you do it!"

There are very specific suggestions and precautions for postcoronary patients, which also apply to other conditions. Warning signs of heart strain include rapid heart and respiratory rate persisting 20–30 minutes after intercourse, chest pain during or after intercourse, sleeplessness following sexual activity, and extreme fatigue on the day following intercourse (Okoniewski, 1977).

When to Avoid Relations

Immediately after a large meal or drinking alcohol, a three-hour wait is advised before sexual relations. If environmental temperatures are extremely cold or hot, especially when the weather is hot and humid, sexual activity should be avoided because of the physiologic demands necessary to maintain body temperatures. If the situation is anxiety provoking or if negative feelings of anger or resentment exist between partners, sex should not be engaged in. Refraining from intercourse is also advisable if strenuous activity is anticipated afterwards.

Variation in Positions for Intercourse

Intercourse may be less stressful if the coronary patient assumes the on-bottom position. Al-though current research shows some measurements of physical exertion are not significantly different in the on-bottom and on-top positions, the increased isometric muscular activity in the arms and shoulders and the increased peripheral resistance occurring in the on-top position are thought to be more demanding on the heart. Because findings are inconclusive, a more passive sexual position is recommended for the coronary patient. The patient is advised to lie on his back during intercourse with his partner kneeling so that he does not bear weight.

An alternate position is to sit on an armless chair with his partner sitting on his lap facing him. The chair must be low enough so that both partners touch the floor with their feet. A side-lying position is also recommended and may work very well for some (Puksta, 1977).

ORGANIC BRAIN SYNDROME

Because of their impaired cognitive functioning, with its consequent poor judgment and poor impulse control, patients with organic brain deterioration may exhibit sexual behavior that is inappropriate with regard to time, place, and social context. Examples are exhibitionism, masturbation in public, and pedophilia. These behavior manifestations of dementia may occur among geriatric patients in long term care facilities and are usually very upsetting to personnel, patients, and families (Verwoerdt, 1976). Nurses, other health professionals, and paraprofessionals often do not realize that they provoke the very behavior that upsets them. That is, they often provoke behavior by saying, "How's my boyfriend today? Are we going out tonight?" Then, when the patient — with assumptions based on a false relationship — makes familiar advances, he is chastised and the nurse becomes upset. This can be very traumatizing and confusing to the disoriented patient. This does not imply that we should not be warm and friendly with these patients — they desperately need our touch, love, and affection. However, we must give it in such a way that the confused patient is aware of the limits and knows where he stands. Working with this kind of patient requires a fixed routine and consistent reality orientation to time, place, and person with a pattern of redundancy cues to help him remain oriented, e.g. It is time to go to bed, it is 9 o'clock, it is dark outdoors, the next meal is breakfast.

Sexual Acting-Out

Patients may express hostile or rebellious tendencies through provocative sex acts such as exposing genitalia. Patients also learn through some sort of conditioning that certain behaviors (such as wiggling out of bedclothes, soiling self, or attacking others) bring about the opportunity to be touched. Disturbing sexual behavior may be a manifestation of confusion, anger, loneliness, or boredom. Too often a patient like this is punished instead of being loved and is then pushed further into his well of loneliness and depression.

APHRODISIACS

One cannot discuss this subject without touching on man's (and woman's) search for eternal youth. The search and various remedies have existed for centuries. Even today, intelligent men and women, young and old, attempt to enhance sex, their sexual conquests, and their sexual abilities with "hallucinogenic drugs" and "aphrodisiacs." Males tend to engage in this search more for the reasons just discussed.

Older individuals are not as apt to try hallucinogenic drugs as they are foods and other so-called aphrodisiacs such as "Spanish fly" (cantharides) and amyl nitrate. All men should be cautioned that these are not really aphrodisiacs, but they are truly dangerous. With Spanish fly, the action actually irritates the lining of the genitourinary tract as it is being excreted; the irritations may produce sensations resembling sexual arousal that bring about genital urge and a reflex erection. However, this is a powerful corrosive poison and can cause tissue destruction.

More recently, amyl nitrate has gained popularity. Aficionados claim that this substance enhances the intensity and pleasure of orgasm. This drug is a vasodilator which is sometimes used to relieve angina pectoris pain. Theoretically, the drug (which is an ampule "popped" during the height of sexual arousal) may act by increasing the vascular response of the genital organs. There are no scientific data to prove that it is an aphrodisiac in this way, but *it is* medically dangerous. Coronary occlusions, some resulting in death, have been reported to follow the use of amyl nitrate during intercourse (Kaplan, 1974). Reports from students in my classes have confirmed that popping amyl nitrate is not uncommon currently among the young, both hetero- and homosexuals.

There is not room here to discuss the aphrodisiac properties attributed to many foods and vitamins. My personal philosophy is: If a substance is not harmful and the individual feels that it helps, why not use it?

DRUGS AND SEXUALITY

Drugs and alcohol are usually more inhibitory than aphrodisiacal. In small doses, they may temporarily liberate behavior from inhibition, but large amounts depress all human behavior including sex, and chronic abuse of sedatives seems to generally diminish human sexuality (Kaplan, 1974). It is important to discuss these effects here because the older population consumes a tremendous number of prescription and over-the-counter drugs.

Drugs may affect various aspects of sexual behavior. Some alter the libido or the intensity of sexual interest and pleasure, while others affect only the physiological response of the genitals: erection, orgasm, and ejaculation. Unfortunately, most drugs or substances which influence human sexuality diminish, rather than enhance, erotic pleasure.

Assessment of drug effects is complicated because drug action is complex and depends on so many variables. In general, the effects of drugs on male sexuality are far better documented and understood than is their influence on the responses of females. This is partly due to the fact that the male response is more visible and quantifiable; for example, erection is easier to assess and study than orgasm. To list and discuss the effects of the various categories of drugs which may affect sexuality would be impossible here, but these three points will serve as a basic guide:

1. There is no drug without some possible side effect.

2. Professionals should include questions and information on drugs when taking a sex history.
3. Clients should be sure to report what drugs they are taking or have taken.

SEXERCISE

To my knowledge, Bonnie Prudden (1961) was the first to set forth in print fundamental exercises that every normal man and woman can practice in order to enjoy a full, happy, and vital sex life. She states that we can do specific exercises to stay physically fit for sex well into late maturity, just as athletes do certain exercises to remain fit for tennis or football. Since sex takes physical expression along with mental and spiritual expression, it seems logical that we keep the necessary muscles in shape.

Sexercises will also improve the appearance of the body. An attractive body is only one of the prerequisites for more pleasurable and meaningful lovemaking. Another is the ability to make that body function as it can and should. "If you set out to develop your sex muscles with exercise, you can for the most part keep them in shape with daily sports. If, however, you don't care for sports, but do like to make love, then it's the exercises ten minutes a day for the rest of your life" (Prudden, 1961).

Space here does not permit me to describe and diagram the sexercises that Prudden recommends. I would suggest that professionals in counseling roles purchase her book *How to Keep Slender and Fit after Thirty* and recommend it to clients who are interested in, and apt to follow up on, physical fitness routines. The following is a list of specific sexercises which are described and pictured in the book:

Gluteal exercise
Pelvic tilt: standing, sitting, supine, etc.
Pelvic tilt, walking
Seat lift
Hip swing
Stretch outs
Circle tilts
Leg lifts, weighted leg lifts
Head to instep exercise
Crotch stretch

It should be noted that very little goes on in life without benefit of the pelvis. Every exercise for the pelvis also improves posture and guards against backaches. "There is no question but that the best lover is the one with whom we are in love. But how much better it is if the partner has a highly trained body. A Beethoven sonata will always sound better on a concert piano than a kazoo" (Prudden, 1961).

In late years, many women develop weakened pelvic muscles which make them feel that the vagina is losing its ability to grip the penis. The Kegel exercises for women are specific for this problem. The Kegel exercises consist of 20–30 contractions of the muscles of the pelvic floor, as though holding back from urinating and defecating at the same time. These exercises should be performed several times daily and can be done while working, sitting, or standing. Contractions are held only a few seconds, and the process must be repeated at least 100 times a day to be truly effective. The Kegel exercises also help to maintain support of the pelvic structure, uterus, bladder, and rectum (Butler and Lewis, 1980). The *Sana Session* (Treber, 1976) also contains sexercises.

WHAT TO TEACH OLD PEOPLE

We can start with the second language of sex which is making it last. It is more than emotional and communicative. It is learned rather than instinctive and can be developed by anyone willing to try. Love and sex are always there to be rediscovered. Older people have time and experience counts! Sex does not merely exist after 60, it holds the possibility of becoming greater. It can be joyful, creative, and a happy, healthy giving. It is morally right and virtuous. It unites human beings (Butler and Lewis, 1980).

Anxiety about coital performance can be lessened if we teach old people that there are a variety of ways besides direct genital contact by which the partner can gain satisfaction, such as digital manipulation of pressure points, oral stimulation, and masturbation. Most older people are not ignorant or unaware of the depth of human sexuality. However, they are often naive about terminology, and may harbor misconceptions and taboos acquired in their early training from which we can help to liberate them. Contrary to expectations, older individuals are not hesitant to discuss sexuality, particularly their own. It is usually the professional who has problems approaching the subject.

I have found that older individuals respond when I use a very factual, professional approach, with a little humor sometimes to ease anxiety. They seem to expect me to be informed, and they respect my opinions and/or advice. I always express my own belief — that sex is a very personal and private affair — but this does not make it a taboo topic. I also like to emphasize the fact that expressing our sexuality helps us maintain a sense of self, a sense of identity, and provides a means of self-assertion that feels good.

In counseling and in health care, it is important to take a sex history (McCarthy, 1979). Most health or medical histories do not include a sex history, or it is ignored. West (1975) reported how this omission was corrected after an elderly client pointed out that the doctor had not asked him about sex and he did have some questions. Subsequently sexual history was included, and he learned that most of the women expressed a desire for sex if available within their moral values and that about half of the men were still interested, although many did not have the opportunity to test their ability (West, 1975). Masters and Johnson (1970) suggest a list of topics to cover. During interviews or in care settings, the nurse (or other professionals in the helping role) should observe for messages from body language and listen for feelings: listen with the third ear for what the patient did not say. Books on general physical fitness and *Sex after Sixty* by Butler and Lewis (1976) and *Joy of Sex* by Comfort, 1972 should be recommended to patients. These books can be especially helpful to couples when the therapist goes over questions with them after the reading.

Dianna Shomaker, a nurse educator experienced in sex education of the elderly, reports success of forums for older individuals that start with basic facts of anatomical and physiological changes and a review of male and female responses (this writer agrees with this need).

Two major responses in these forums have been (1) the demand for more knowledge and (2) the demand for more forums that offer the opportunity to openly share ideas and values about sexuality (Shomaker, 1980).

SEXUALITY AND THE INSTITUTIONALIZED ELDERLY

Everything said here should apply to nursing home patients as well as to elderly persons in the community. Yet because nursing homes are geared more to the needs and desires of families and to smooth institutional operation than to the desires of the patient, and because most nursing home patients are usually without spouses and are somewhat or totally immobile, any kind of socialization represents a challenge — especially the opportunity for sexual expression.

A study of 84 male and 185 female residents of 15 nursing homes revealed that the institutions' social climate did affect the reate of sexual activity. The more supportive the environment, the more likely was the possibility of sexual activity among the residents. The residents' health, unless greatly debilitating, was not a limiting factor in sexual activity or the desire for it, except for the fact that the necessity for institutionalization itself is limiting. The mean ages were 81 for males and 83 for females. All were extensively interviewed by trained interviewers and in complete privacy. Seventy-five percent of those asked participated. Respondents indicated that 91% had been sexually inactive in the past year: 17% of those would be interested if a partner were available; 8% were sexually interested and active. Two were sexually active but not interested (White and Doyle, 1979).

It has been pointed out that the way in which nursing homes ordinarily restrict contact between sexes to lounges so that behavior can be supervised implies that those who supervise believe that sexual behavior is possible. This paradox is illustrated in the following example:

Mrs. S., a widow, and Mr. F., a widower, are often seen in the lounge holding hands. They find comfort in sitting in chairs close to each other. Many comments are made by the personal care attendants of the nursing home — "senile old man — better watch him. Don't let him go into one of the rooms with her — there's no telling what he'll do." (Falk and Falk, 1980)

Prevention of sexual expression in nursing homes is achieved in three ways: (1) it is condemned by society outside of nursing homes; (2) it is enforced in nursing homes by lack of privacy; and (3) it is internalized by the elderly themselves, since they feel they are no longer sexually attractive and that sexual activity is apt to give them a label such as "dirty old man" or "dirty old woman" (Falk and Falk, 1980).

However, since sexuality includes much more than intercourse, there are many opportunities for the alert, sensitive, and motivated professional to provide enhancement of basic human needs for nursing home patients. The following are some question which can serve as guidelines for improving the plight of nursing home patients concerning sexuality:

- If there is a problem related to sex, ask with whom the problem exists: Patient? Staff? Family? What can I do about it?
- Are physical problems related to sexuality well taken care of in your institution, e.g., senile vaginitis, catheters, etc.?
- Are you helping staff examine the meaning of the behavior of "the dirty old man" and "the shameless old woman?"
- Are you aware of the isolation and sensory deprivation of the immobile patient?
- Can you provide more touch, hugging, kissing, hand holding, and intimacy such as back rubs and body massage?
- Can you build sexuality into (rather than separate it from) the spiritual and emotional well-being of your patients?
- Are you able to accept and allow masturbation, and help your staff deal with it?
- Can you provide more touching and feeling things to handle, fondle, and hold, such as yarn balls, prayer beads, and stuffed animals?
- Can live pets be brought into your setting and patients allowed to feel and cuddle them?

- Can more music — romantic, sentimental, sensuous, and erotic — be provided?
- Do you encourage opportunities for sexes to meet, mingle, and spend time together (e.g., small television rooms), without structuring a "trysting time or place" too rigidly?
- Can double beds be provided for married couples?
- Do you counsel families, particularly the adult children of patients, about the sexual needs of older people?
- Can you manipulate the environment to make your facility a therapeutic milieu?
- Do staff and patients laugh (and maybe cry) together?
- Do you have a bill of rights for sexual freedom in your facility?

COUNSELING GUIDELINES FOR PROFESSIONALS

Old people do seek counseling on sexuality and sexual concerns, but we don't always hear them and most of us are not well enough prepared to help them (Glover, 1977). Successful and continuing sexual activity is but one, though possibly the most significant, sign of healthy aging. The following are some pointers and guidelines to assist those working with older individuals who may need sexual counseling.

I. Communication Skills
   1. Examine awareness of your own beliefs, values, and attitudes toward aging, the aged, and sexuality.
   2. Assess interpersonal skills necessary to:
      a) Initiate communication with the elderly
      b) Create an atmosphere conducive to discussion of sexual concerns
      c) Listen for nonverbal cues of sexual concerns
      d) Elicit verbalization of underlying concerns
   3. Review knowledge of sexual physiology and functioning.
   4. Assess client's perception of his/her sexual concerns.
   5. Ask yourself, "What kind of nonverbal messages am I sending?"
II. Helps in Assessing the Problem
   1. Is the problem a request for information about anatomy and physiology?
   2. Is the need a specific sexual problem?

3. Is the problem a clinical situation directly or indirectly related to sexual functioning?
4. Is the problem organic or situational, requiring alterations in preferred mode of functioning?
5. Is it a crisis or a long term problem?
6. Is the person trying to live up to some preconceived performance expectations and creating his/her guilt for failure? The "inner ball game" may be interfering with the real game.
7. Assess for physical illness or disorders and medications.
8. Always look at what is left not what is gone.

III. Points of Departure for Initiating Discussion of Sexuality with Older Persons
1. Consider or find out the client's early orientation to sexual behavior.
2. Look for feelings (residual) about masturbation as a child, which may still be present unconsciously.
3. The "first time" seems to have great significance so consider it as a point of departure in discussion.
4. The "second time around" is often described as being better, so one might use that as a point of departure for discussion.
5. Tie sexual behavior and history in with other social activities and with religion; remember, it may take time to come around to the topic, questions, or problems.
6. Listen for a double message: "I don't think about that." "I would if I fell in love."
7. Remember, there may be increased preoccupation (conscious or unconscious) with sexuality in old age, particularly in certain settings.
8. Keep approach "confidential, private, personal."
9. You don't have to know all the answers to counsel, you just have to help old people find their own answers; sometimes they have them, but they need your sanction and/or support.
10. Avoid avoidance of the subject.

IV. How Do You Limit Overt Sexual Exposure and Improper Advances?
1. Look at circumstances: night, fantasy, etc.
2. Examine precipitating events.
3. Look for need to prove masculinity or sexuality.
4. Assess for sensory deprivation.
5. Look for health in the situation, e.g., is man trying to prove something?
6. Recognize needs.
7. Recognize ability and need to live and function as man or woman.
8. Direct to a healthy outlet in an appropriate place.
9. Do not punish.

V. How Do you Handle the "Dirty Old Man"?
Consider how you handle your own peers. Young women may encourage similar behavior from a 6-foot tall football player and not expect to go to bed with him, but what makes it so "dirty" when an 80-year-old, 100-pound man stares at her from the feet up or reaches for her bosom? Anxieties like these are not easy to handle. They are the result of conflicts in a departure from our culture, our life-style, and our comfortable cohort group. We may need help in handling them. Unfortunately, this help is usually sought after the fact. Nevertheless, it helps to share experiences and to problem solve as a team.

VI. How Should You Deal with Masturbation?
1. Recognize it as acceptable and healthy.
2. Examine your own attitudes.
3. Certain aspects of sex are private, so is masturbation; therefore, encourage a proper time and place.
4. Do not punish or ridicule.

CONCLUSION

In conclusion, I am pleased to share the experience of a nurse. I do not know her but hope that you and I will do as well in our work as she has.

Two weeks ago as I made my hospital rounds, Mr. C extended his right hand and Mr. C with his left hand showed me his penis and stated, "I love you." I had a mental block and finally spoke to him in an understanding way, "You haven't had sex for a long time and this is a normal feeling." Mr. C slowly covered himself with the top sheet. The next day I visited Mr. C and told him of my concerns about his sexual behavior. I asked him if he would like to go on a pass if his wife could handle him. He answered, "yes." I talked to the physician about Mr. C and she left an order for a pass. The social worker made arrangements with Mrs. C for a pass on Father's Day, via Handicab. Mrs. C was also offered the petting room, which she declined and giggled, remarking, "No, I'll take him home where he can touch me." This initial pass led to another weekend pass, and I hope many more passes. (Caringer, 1976)

REFERENCES

Adelson, E. Frank talk about older sex. *Modern Maturity* 17(1):48 (1974).
Aging International, Information Bulletin of the International Federation of Aging. *Sexual Behavior* 7(2): 13 (1980).

Basso, A. The prostate in the elderly male. *Hospital Practice* 117–123 (October 1977).

Birren, J.E. and Schaie, K.W. (Eds.). *Handbook of the Psychology of Aging.* New York: Van Nostrand Reinhold, 1977.

Butler, R.N. and Lewis, M.I. *Aging and Mental Health.* St. Louis: C.V. Mosby, 1977.

Butler, R.N. and Lewis, M.I. *Sex after Sixty.* New York: Harper & Row, 1976.

Caringer, B. *Sexuality of Aging.* Paper presented at the Maluhia Hospital, Honolulu, Hawaii (1976).

Comfort, A. *The Joy of Sex: A Gourmet Guide to Love Making.* New York: Simon and Schuster, 1972.

Costello, M.K. Sex, intimacy, and aging. *American Journal of Nursing* 75(8):1330–1332 (1975).

Daut, R.V. *So You're Going to Have a Prostatectomy.* Norwich, N.Y.: Eaton Laboratories, 1974.

Drellich, M.G. Sex after hysterectomy. *Medical Aspects of Human Sexuality* 62–64 (November 1967).

Durbin, Sr. M.S. Geriatric gynecology. *Nursing Clinics of North America* 3(2):257–258 (1968).

Eisdorfer, C. *Mental Health and Aging.* Speech presented at the meeting of the Western Gerontological Society, Denver, Colorado, March 1977.

Falk, G. and Falk, U.A. Sexuality and the aged. *Nursing Outlook* 28(1):51–55 (1980).

Finkle, A.L. and Thompson, R. Urologic counseling in male sexual impotence. *Geriatrics* 67–72 (December 1972).

Furlow, W.L. Inflatable Penile Prosthesis: May Clinic Experience with 175 Patients. *Urology* Vol. XIII No. 2, (Feb. 1979) pp. 166–170.

Glover, B.H. Sex counseling of the elderly. *Hospital Practice* 101–113 (June 1977).

Kaplan, H.S. *The New Sex Therapy.* New York: Bruner/Mazel, 1974.

Lamb, L.E. Dear Doctor: It's About Sex. New York: Dell Publishing Company, Inc. 1973, p. 142.

Masters, W.H. and Johnson, V.E. *Human Sexual Inadequacy.* Boston: Little, Brown, 1970.

Masters, W.H. and Johnson, V. Sex and the aging process. *Journal of the American Geriatrics Society* 29(9):385–390 (1981).

McCarthy, P. Geriatric sexuality, capacity, interest, and opportunity. *Journal of Gerontological Nursing* 5(1):20–24 (1979).

Okoniewski, G. Sexual activity following myocardial infarction. *Cardiovascular Nursing* 15(1):1-4 (1977).

Pfeiffer, E. Sex and aging. *Sexual Behavior* 17–21 (1972).

Prudden, B. *How to Keep Slender and Fit after Thirty.* New York: Random House, 1961.

Puksta, N.S. All about sex after a coronary. *American Journal of Nursing* 77(4):602–605 (1977).

Scazi, C.C. Sexual counseling and sexual therapy for patients after myocardial infarction. *Cardio-Vascular Nursing* 18(3):13–17 (1981).

Scheingold, L.D. and Wagner, N.N. *Sound Sex and the Aging Heart.* New York: Human Sciences Press, 1974.

Shomaker, D.M. Integration of physiological and sociological factors as a basis for sex education to the elderly. *Journal of Gerontological Nursing* 6(6):311–318 (1980).

Shumaker, S. Frank talk about older sex. *Modern Maturity* 17(2):48 (1974).

Smith, D.C., Prentice, R., Thompson, D.J., and Herrman, W.L. Association of exogenous estrogen and endometrial carcinoma. *New England Journal of Medicine* 293(23):1164–1167 (1975).

Stephens, J. Romance in the SRO (single room occupancy). *Gerontologist* 14:280 (August 1974).

Treber, G.J. *Sana Session.* New York: Source Publishers, 1976.

Verwoerdt, A. *Clinical Geropsychiatry.* Baltimore: Williams and Wilkins, 1976.

West, N. Sex in geriatrics: myth or miracle. *Journal of the American Geriatrics Society* 23:551–552 (1975).

White, C.B. and Doyle, A. *Mental Health, Physical Health, and Sexuality In the Institutionalized Age.* Paper presented at the annual meeting of the National Gerontological Society, Washington, D.C., November 1979.

Ziel, H. and Finkle, W. Increased risk of endometrial carcinoma among users of conjugated estrogens. *New England Journal of Medicine* 293(23):1167–1170 (1975).

37
Pressure Ulcers: Prevention and Treatment

Gloria Rowell
Bernita Steffl

. . . Help us to be gentle with old people
As we are with infants.
Help us to look past the tic, the tremor,
The gray
Faded flesh the way
We look past the baby's helplessness
To see a unique self. . . .

Elsie Maclay (1977)

Decubitus ulcers or pressure sores are a common and continuing problem in the nursing care of elderly, chronically ill patients. A survey by Norton (1975) showed that 70–80% of those with pressure sores are over 70 years of age.

The appearance of a decubitus ulcer is a frightening and demoralizing event for patients – not only because of the added pain and disruption it brings into their lives, but because, for elderly patients, the ulcer reinforces their feelings of helplessness and loss of control. Sadly, this fear and helplessness also grip the caretaker, nurse, or family member. The very thought of necrosis (i.e., decomposing body tissue) is so dreadful, so repugnant, and so repulsive that a deadly attitude toward decubitus care is often present.

The cost of nursing time for patient care increases 50% with the appearance of a decubitus (Gosnell, 1973). In terms of dollars, the cost estimates for treatment range from $2,000 to $15,000 (Edberg, 1973; Merlino, 1969) depending on the severity of the condition. These estimates are constantly increasing as are most medical costs.

Pressure sores are manifested in several ways. The pressure injury may be likened to a bruise caused by a blow or the appearance of a blister or red mark similar to the damage done by an ill-fitting shoe. On light skin, the color changes of tissue destruction are easily discernible. On dark-skinned individuals, the skin may take on a mahogany-brown or blue-brown appearance (see Table 37-1).

Table 37-1. Stages in Pressure Sore Formation (Mahogany Brown or Blue Brown in Coloration).

STAGE I:	The skin is red, warm, and firm to the touch, but unbroken.
STAGE II:	The skin is red and blistered or broken.
STAGE III:	A full thickness of skin is lost, and a hole is formed in the skin.
STAGE IV:	A full thickness of skin is lost, with invasion of deeper tissues including muscle and bone.

The literature presents a myriad of words used to indicate a decubitus ulcer, such as bedsore, pressure sore, ischemic ulcer, and dermal abrasion. In this chapter, decubitus ulcer and pressure sore are terms which are used synonymously to indicate tissue injury due to pressure. It is suggested that fine discriminations in classifying pressure sores be made using the stages of development indicated in Table 37-1.

THE CAUSE OF PRESSURE SORES

Decubitus ulcers occur when pressure is exerted between bony prominences and supporting tissues. The pressure exerted in lying and sitting is at least greater than the 32 mm Hg of capillary pressure. The prolonged obstruction of this capillary circulation deprives the soft tissue of an adequate blood supply, causing cell destruction and death of tissues. A decubitus is the result of pressure, but how much pressure and for how long a period of time are highly complex questions which require nursing judgment.

It All Happens in the Cells

The cell is the locus of the initial damage leading to pressure sores. Understanding the pathological process at the cellular level is basic to understanding the development of pressure ulcers (decubitis). Increased tissue pressure causes ischemia, a local and temporary anemia, resulting from the obstruction in circulation. Each cell in this location is deprived of the food and oxygen it needs to survive. If the ischemic period is long enough and is repeated often enough, cell death and eventual tissue necrosis occur. It is important to note that it is not the pressure itself which causes cells to die, it is the ischemia induced by the pressure that is the mechanism behind all death and tissue necrosis (Constantian, 1980). The nurse can never prevent the patient from experiencing pressure.

However, it is the uninterrupted obstruction of circulation that does the damage.

A patient who experiences four hours of uninterrupted pressure of 40–100 mm Hg will experience microvascular changes and edema. If the compression lasts longer than eight hours, irreversible microvascular changes are likely to occur. Pressure as low as 11 mm Hg, when experienced for a prolonged period, can result in cellular damage (Constantian, 1980). The human body is a fragile and sensitive organism. In bedfast patients, damage to the microvascular system occurs rapidly. The cellular damage, unfortunately, is not always immediately observable.

Kinds of Pressure that Cause Ulcers

The forces of shearing, friction, and compression are well documented as the primary causes of pressure sores (Bush, 1969; Dinsdale, 1974; Reichel, 1958). An example of shearing force

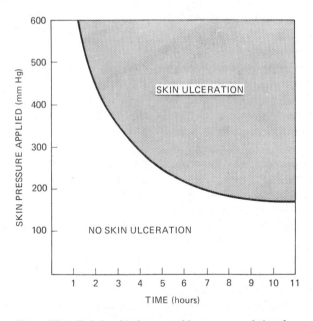

Figure 37-1. Relationship between skin pressure and time for development of skin ulceration. There is an inverse relationship between the amount of pressure exerted and the length of time that pressure can be tolerated without tissue damage. [Adapted from data by Kosiak, M. Etiology of decubitus ulcers. *Archives of Physical Medicine and Rehabilitation* 42:24 (1961) Reprinted with permission of *Archives of Physical Medicine and Rehabilitation.*]

is the friction between the skin and bed sheet which keeps the patient from sliding in bed. The superficial tissues slide over the deep fascia, mechanically impeding the blood flow from one layer of skin to the other. The force of compression is somewhat different. It depends, for its energy, on the force of the body weight pressing on the underlying body surface. The areas under the shoulders, sacrum, and heels are most compressed.

The incidence of pressure sores depends not only on the time period over which the pressure is exerted but also upon the degree of pressure. The results of a study by Kosiak (1961) indicate the relationship between time and pressure in decubitus ulcer formation (Figure 37-1). Thus, if a patient is unable to move from a sitting position in an unpadded chair and experiences a pressure of 300 mm Hg, an ulceration can be expected in 4 to 5 hours. If the same patient is sitting in a padded chair and experiences a pressure of 150 mm Hg, ulceration would be expected in approximately 11 hours.

Factors that effect the energy transfer, perceived by the patient as pressure, are reviewed schematically in Figure 37-2. This simplified cause-and-effect diagram illustrates the most critical influencing factors which nurses should consider in planning patient care.

Critical Variables

The formation of a decubitus ulcer involves a complex interaction between the patient and

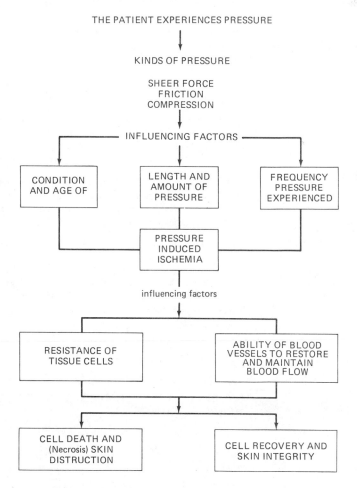

Figure 37-2. Factors that affect pressure sore formation.

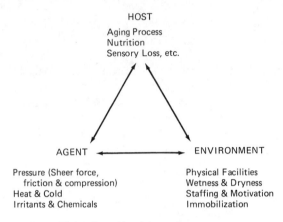

Figure 37-3. The epidemiology of pressure sores.

his environment. An epidemiological model identifying the host (patient), agent (cause), and environmental factors is helpful in determining and defining significant variables which influence the incidence of this common condition. It also assists professionals in a holistic and preventive approach, by enabling them to recognize how these factors interact with one another. Figure 37-3 presents an epidemiological model which serves as a conceptual framework for levels of prevention and intervention.

The Host (Patient).   Berecek (1975) cited five conditions in the patient that contribute to

Table 37-2. Host Factors.

HOST FACTORS	SCIENTIFIC RATIONALE
Malnutrition	Protein is essential for normal growth and healing. Vitamin C depletion contributes to capillary fragility and susceptibility to trauma. Anemia decreases the blood's oxygen-carrying power.
Pathological conditions	A person who is ill or injured loses more protein through tissue breakdown than normal. Protein is needed to maintain positive nitrogen balance. When illness is accompanied by negative nitrogen balance, protein is not available to maintain tissue integrity.
Dehydration	Adequate hydration is necessary to maintain skin turgor and prevent infection.
Metabolic disturbances and vascular deficiencies	Edema extends the distance between cells and capillaries, thereby slowing circulation and waste removal. Arteriosclerosis impedes blood flow. Metabolic disturbances affect healing power.
Skin condition	Any break in the skin predisposes to pressure sore formation, inflammation, and bacterial invasion. Poor hygiene promotes a larger microorganism population and increases the risk of infection.
Incontinence and diaphoresis	Incontinence or diaphoresis causes the patient to be more susceptible to skin maceration. The skin becomes swollen, soft, and irritated, and thus more easily damaged.
Mobility and mental awareness	An altered level of consciousness decreases awareness of discomfort and the need to move.
Age	About 1% of the collagen in skin is lost per year; therefore, the risk of skin damage increases with age.

Table 37-3. Agent Factors.

AGENT FACTORS	SCIENTIFIC RATIONALE
Pressure	Sufficient, sustained pressure will cause ischemia or necrosis. The critical pressure needed to seriously impair cutaneous blood flow in humans has not been definitely established, but it may be as low as 11 mm Hg.
	Hyperemia occurs in tissues rendered ischemic for 5 sec or more – beyond this an inverse relationship exists between the length of time pressure and freedom from pathological changes.
Heat	Heat may originate internally from inflammation or fever or externally. Radiation, electric blankets, hot water bottles, heating pads, and hot drinks are dangerous, especially when there is impaired sensation. Injury from such sources increases the likelihood of a site for decubitus development.
Irritants and chemicals	Maceration and excoriation of the skin produce localized inflammatory response. This is caused by urine or chemicals, even soap.

pressure sore formation: poor nutrition, the aging process, motor paralysis, disturbed autonomic function, and superficial sensory loss with absence of subjective awareness of pain and pressure. Table 37-2 breaks these factors down into smaller units and gives an accompanying scientific rationale for the role they play in pressure sore formation.

The Agent. The agent role in pressure sore formation can be conceptualized as energy forms which, inflicted excessively on the patient, can cause injury. If the nurse can be seen as the user and controller of this energy, it will be easier to assume responsibility for preventing or reducing the "agent" damage in the environment (see Table 37-3).

Environmental Factors. Literally, most prevention and treatment of decubitus require a modification of environmental factors. These factors include the physical (structural), social, psychological, economic, climatic, and geographic parameters within which the care is given and the patient is expected to thrive.

Manipulating the environment has not always been seen as a nursing responsibility, nor have nurses perceived themselves as having the responsibility, power, or option to advocate, intervene, instigate, or facilitate the necessary change. In gerontological nursing, the nurse must assume these responsibilities and an accountability for the patient outcome, and not merely carry out doctors' orders (see Table 37-4).

Table 37-4. Environmental Factors.

ENVIRONMENTAL FACTORS	SCIENTIFIC RATIONALE
Staffing and motivation	It is difficult, if not impossible, to treat pressure ulcers if the pressure cannot be kept off the patient. Patient cooperation is vital. Well-educated, compassionate nursing personnel are required to maintain consistent, attentive wound and skin care.
Physical equipment and facilities	Equipment used to diminish the effect of pressure can increase pressure tolerance. Alternating pressure, allowing relief for 5-min intervals will reduce the amount of skin damage. Sitting humans exert 300 mm Hg on flat chairs with 1 inch of foam rubber. Skin pressure falls to 160 mm Hg when 2 inches of foam are used.
Heat and dryness	Heat increases metabolism and thus increases nutritional requirements and waste products. Heat will produce additional perspiration and increase the growth of bacteria. Excessive dryness robs the skin of moisture and causes it to crack, thus providing a site for skin breakdown.

Although pressure is the cause of decubitus ulcers, their incidence is influenced by predisposing factors which affect tissue resistance. The ulcer is the result of a complex synergistic interaction of maturational, pathological, mechanical, neurological, circulatory, hormonal, cellular, and environmental factors.

PREVENTION OF PRESSURE SORES

Prevention of decubitus ulcers is an ongoing nursing goal for all aged patients. Nurses make judgments based on the use of assessment tools or nursing intuition as to whether or not patients are in jeopardy of injury due to pressure. It is the assessment along with staff response and patient cooperation, however, that results in prevention. The injury to the patient occurs when adequate and aggressive early intervention is not the ongoing response. It does not take long for the damage to occur. In one large study, 70% of the pressure ulcers that developed occurred during the first two weeks of hospitalization (Exton-Smith, 1976).

Assessment — The First Step

The initial nursing action is always assessment. Fortunately, there are well-developed tools, such as the assessment form shown in Figure 37-4, that help with this task. The criteria here are based on factors with which nurses are already familiar and which serve as early warning signs. An advantage of using a standardized assessment form is that it fosters consistency of assessment. Everyone is familiar with the system and those patients in greatest danger are immediately recognized. The assessment form can also follow if the patient is moved to another institution. Familiarity with the rater's guide is readily developed, and it can easily be adapted for use by auxiliary personnel. However, the three categories for skin assessment — appearance, tone, and sensation — will require some practice. Nurses are asked to supply their own descriptive adjectives. The guide recommends that patients skin tone and sensation be evaluated by pinching the skin gently at high risk sites for pressure sores.

A definite protocol for frequency of assessment and documentation should be developed by the health care team, who must keep in mind the fact that the vulnerability to pressure sores in the aged patient may change rapidly from day to day. The nurse may want to examine the lab reports for indications such as the hematocrit and the hemoglobin values as a part of the assessment routine. This type of information gives an indication of the adequacy of cell nourishment and oxygenation. The white blood cell count will alert the nurse to any infectious process present. The pulse and blood pressure are also important in determining circulatory adequacy.

The general health status and the weight of the patient are significant in evaluating the possibility of decubitus formation. Being either underweight or overweight will affect a patient's susceptibility to pressure sores. The medical history is also useful in assessment. Some disease conditions, such as diabetes, vascular diseases, and metabolic conditions, are particularly influential in the precipitation of pressure sores.

Positioning

Some patients confined to beds or wheelchairs can be taught to lift themselves with the help of frames over the bed or pulleys. A rocking motion can be used to shift weight in a chair or in a bed. Isometric exercises can also be useful in relieving pressure and stimulating circulation. If the patient cannot move, then the nurse must do it for the patient. *Although turning every two hours is a generally accepted preventive nursing goal, this frequently is not often enough.*

Since skin is more resistant to pressure than either fat or muscle, it is not enough to depend on the appearance, the reactive hyperemia (redness), to indicate a need for a position change. By the time erythema appears, it is possible that extensive and irreparable damage has already occurred in deep tissues. One study has indicated that if a reddened area remains inflamed for more than five minutes, the turning time schedule should be reduced by a half hour (Taylor, 1980).

McGuire Veterans Administration Medical Center recommends the following routine for

Name _____ Diagnosis _____ Date admitted _____

Age _____ Sex _____ Ht. _____ Wt. _____

Medications _____ Diet _____

DATE OF ASSESSMENT	MENTAL STATUS 1. Unconscious 2. Stuporous 3. Confused 4. Apathetic 5. Alert	CONTINENCE 1. No control 2. Minimally controlled 3. Usually controlled 4. Fully controlled	MOBILITY 1. Immobile 2. Very limited 3. Slightly limited 4. Full	ACTIVITY 1. Bedfast 2. Chairfast 3. Walks with help 4. Walks independently	NUTRITION 1. Poor 2. Fair 3. Good	TOTAL SCORE	SKIN APPEARANCE (dry, oily, wrinkled, scaly, flaccid, etc.)	SKIN TONE loose moderate hard	SKIN SENSATION none slight moderate great

RATER'S GUIDE

MENTAL STATUS response to environment

1. Unconscious: nonresponsive to painful stimuli

2. Stuporous: totally disoriented; no response to name, simple commands, or verbal stimuli

3. Confused: partial and intermittent disorientation to time, person, place; purposeless response to stimuli; restless, aggressive, irritable, or anxious

4. Apathetic: lethargic; passive; drowsy; depressed; can obey simple commands; may be disoriented to time

5. Alert: oriented to time, person, place; responds to all stimuli

CONTINENCE control of urination and defecation

1. No control: incontinent of urine and feces

2. Minimally controlled: often incontinent of urine; occasionally incontinent of feces

3. Usually controlled: incontinent occasionally; or has catheter and is occasionally incontinent of feces

4. Fully controlled: total control of urine and feces

MOBILITY amount and control of body movement

1. Immobile: can't change position without help; dependent on others for movement

2. Very limited: offers minimal help in changing position; may have contractures, paralyses

3. Slightly limited: can control and move extremities, but still needs help changing position

4. Full: can control and move extremities at will; may need device, but can lift, turn, pull, balance, and sit up at will

ACTIVITY ability to walk

1. Bedfast: confined to bed

2. Chairfast: walks only to chair, with help; or confined to wheelchair

3. Walks with help: can walk with help of another, or with crutches, braces; possibly can't handle stairs

4. Walks independently: can rise from bed and walk without help; or with cane or walker can walk without help of another

NUTRITION quality of food intake

1. Poor: rarely eats complete meal; is dehydrated; has minimal fluid intake

2. Fair: occasionally refuses to eat, or leaves large portions of a meal; must be encouraged to take fluids

3. Good: eats some food from each basic food category every day; drinks 6-8 glasses of fluid a day; eats major portions of each meal, or is receiving tube feedings

SKIN APPEARANCE observed skin characteristics

SKIN TONE degree of turgor and tension, determined by pinch at high-risk sites for pressure sores

SKIN SENSATION response to tactile stimuli

COMMENTS:

The Data Collection Sheet for Assessment of Patient's Potential for Pressure Sores was developed by Davina J. Gosnell, RN, PhD. Copyright © 1973. by the American Journal of Nursing Company. Reproduced with permission from NURSING RESEARCH, January/February 1973. vol. 22, no. 1.

ASSESSING A PATIENT'S POTENTIAL FOR PRESSURE SORES

Figure 37-4. Assessing a patient's potential for pressure sores.

turning patients. A pattern of turning should be adjusted so that those areas of greatest risk lateral and posterior to the pelvic girdle are exposed to the least amount of pressure. The procedure would be to turn the patient from his left side to his back, to his right side, to his left side, to his back, and so on. In this way the patient bears weight on his back only one-third of the time (Constantian, 1980).

It is not only the unconscious and paralyzed patient who must be watched for pressure damage. Pain is a frequent cause of immobilization. Patients who find moving uncomfortable are often treated with pain medication and thus are even less likely to be as active as they need to be. Sedated patients, especially the elderly, do not move around in sleep as much as they would normally. Some braces, traction, and other mechanical devices inhibit the patient from moving in bed. Such patients must be observed to determine how often they actually can or are willing to change position. Finally, the elderly, sick patient may not have the will or energy to change positions, or may favor one position or one side. Such patients must be checked frequently and assisted to move about as their skin indicates the need.

Pressure-reducing Devices

There are many devices available for preventing or healing pressure sores, such as water beds, wheelchairs, cushions, sheepskin pads, foam rubber, and rotating frame beds. Kosiak (1961) has indicated from his studies that skin pressure on the hips can be reduced from 300 mm Hg to 160 mm Hg when 2 inches of foam padding are used. Pressure cannot be reduced further, however, even by 6 inches of foam padding.

In a comparison of foam, water, and rocking mattresses on a standard hospital bed, no difference was noted in the amount of tissue ischemia produced (Carpendale, 1974). The important consideration is that nurses not be fooled into believing that such devices have magical properties which prevent or heal tissue destruction. Vigilant nursing remains the most important aspect of decubitus prevention and care. In evaluating a device for possible use in treatment, its effectiveness, ease in nursing care, accep-

tance and comfort for the patient are all relevant factors.

Routine Preventive Skin Care

Good skin care is vital to decubitus prevention. The elderly patients' skin makes them more susceptible to skin breakdown. The outer horny layer of the skin is thinner, and the sebaceous glands are less active. There is less water in the tissues. This causes some older skin to be less pliable, and to appear dry and scaly. Subcutaneous fat in the elderly is often reduced; therefore, the skin is poorly cushioned and more easily traumatized. Dermatitis is more common in the elderly, and skin lesions that develop tend to heal more slowly.

Proper nursing management of the elderly patients' skin provides a preventive barrier to pressure damage. Skin should be kept as soft and pliable as possible. All skin lesions should be watched and treated. Such areas are much more susceptible to the effects of pressure. Incontinence is also damaging to skin, and all-out efforts should be made to control it (see Chapter 29). Maceration of the skin from urine and feces will predispose the patient to accelerated tissue destruction due to pressure.

Sources of Pressure

In addition to body weight, the most obvious sources of pressure are the patient's bed and chair. Both of these pieces of furniture can act as splints, impeding or discouraging movement or a change of position. When a patient is sitting, pressure over the hips is significantly higher when he sits with feet supported rather than hanging free (Bush, 1969). Supporting the feet shifts the patient's weight backwards and puts more pressure on the ischial tuberosities.

Positioning is important in attenuating the effect of pressure in bed or in a chair. Pillows and other devices are used to avoid direct pressure on bony prominences and pressure points illustrated in Figure 37-5. Use care in raising the head of the bed, for even a few inches may increase the shearing force over the sacrum enough to obstruct large areas of skin from receiving an adequate blood supply (Reichel, 1958).

PRESSURE POINTS IN VARIOUS POSITIONS

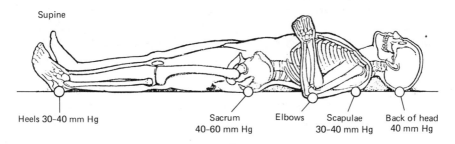

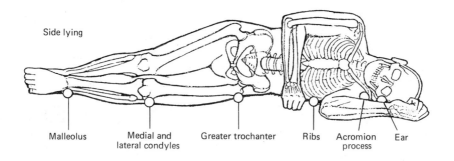

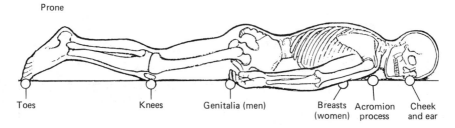

Figure 37-5. Pressure points in various positions.

All kinds of equipment can exert pressure on the patient's skin. Devices such as traction, casts, crutches, and braces are frequent sources of pressure. Wrinkled sheets and foreign objects can also be sources of pressure, and should be matters of concern to the nurse. Once a pressure sore has been formed and healed, that site is always more susceptible to recurrent breakdown.

TREATMENT AND NURSING CARE

Despite intensive effort to prevent pressure sores, the incidence remains high in the immo-
bile, frail elderly. Damage can occur at home, in the operating room, or any place where the patient is forced to experience extended periods of immobilization. On admission, the skin may look normal, even when the tissue underneath it has in fact died. It may take as much as a week before the damage is visible.

Patient cooperation is a necessary part of a pressure sore treatment regime. It is difficult, if not impossible, to treat a pressure sore if pressure cannot be kept off it. This necessarily requires the patient's cooperation. Successful treatment may require the patient to spend time off a favored side or in an awkward position. It may mean sleep disturbances and uncomfortable treatments that are physically draining for the patient and the family. Embarking on a long, monotonous, and expensive program requires patience, understanding, and involvement on the part of the patient and the family. The continuity of care is most important. It is best to begin a pressure record at the first sign of ulcer formation. Such a record should be kept in a Kardex for quick reference by all personnel because healing pressure wounds takes a cooperative effort. All personnel should be aware of the progress and needs of the patient. See Figure 37-6 and Table 37-5 for an example of a decubitus ulcer record.

A wide variety of topical applications, ranging from herbs to chemicals, have been utilized

SKIN CONDITION RECORD
(Decubitus Ulcer Record)

ADMITTED FROM _____

DATE OF ADMISSION _____

DATE OF ONSET _____

DATE PHYSICIAN NOTIFIED _____

LOCATION(S): _____

_____

_____

_____

STAGES:
    I. REDDENED ONLY
    II. REDDENED WITH SKIN BREAK, VESICULATION OR EXCORIATION
    III. FULL THICKNESS LOSS OF SKIN WHICH MAY OR MAY NOT INCLUDE THE SUBCUTANEOUS TISSUE AND WHICH PRODUCES SEROSANGUINOUS DRAINAGE
    IV. FULL THICKNESS LOSS OF SKIN WITH INVASION OF DEEPER TISSUES

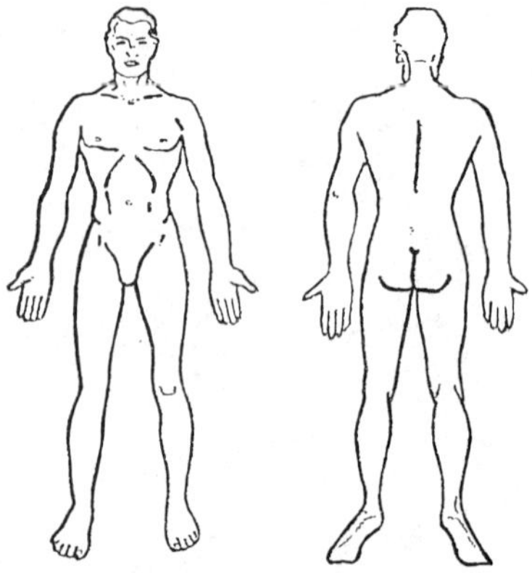

Mark Locations With Ink

DATE							
SIZE							
ODOR							
EXUDATE							
INFLAMMATION							
CRATER CONTENT							
CULTURE							
STAGE							
TREATMENT							
SIGNATURE							

ROOM _____

COMMENTS:

Queen of the Valley Hospital
Napa, California

Figure 37-6. Skin condition record (decubitus ulcer record).

Table 37-5. Nursing Procedure for Skin Condition Record.

SUBJECT: Utilization of the Decubitus Ulcer Record

PURPOSE: To Document Discovery, Stage, Treatment, Progress and Discharge Condition of Decubitus Ulcer(s)

PROCEDURE:

1. Upon discovery of a pressure sore an RN or LVN will initiate the Decubitus Ulcer Record.

2. The record should be stamped with the patient's addressograph plate.

3. All lines must be filled out. If something is not applicable, it should be written as N/A. If more room is needed for documentation, use the other side of the paper.
   a. Refer to the Glossary if necessary.
   b. Measure size of ulcer with measuring guide and record accurately.
   c. Use the extra spaces or area for comments to further describe the area(s) when necessary.
   d. If a culture is done, indicate the date that it was done and organism present.
   e. Utilize the body chart to indicate location of lesion(s).

4. An order from the doctor must be obtained to initiate skin care. If he has a specific order for the procedure to be followed, document it on the record. If no specific order is written (i.e.: Skin Care) the Stomahesive and Karaya procedures will be utilized according to the Stage of the pressure sore.

5. Re-evaluate lesion and document every 3–7 days and upon discharge from the hospital.

   On discharge from the hospital, copy of the record will be made and sent with transfer papers to the extended care facility when appropriate.

Reprinted with permission of Gerry Cameron, B.N., Queen of the Valley Hospital, Napa, California.

to heal pressure sores. Some have been remarkably successful; others have been frightening. The condition of the patient, the individual circumstances surrounding the care, and professional surveillance are all critical determinants in the treatment of pressure sores, including the administration of topical preparations. Table 37-6 provides nursing information on the most current topical treatments.

Wound Care

There are five steps in wound care of pressure sores: (1) assessing and recording the lesion, (2) cleansing the affected area, (3) reducing irritation, (4) providing protection, and (5) relieving the pressure. If any one of these steps is omitted, it can have an untoward effect on the healing process (see Table 37-7).

The type of dressing used for a particular pressure ulcer is a medical decision; however, an open wound should generally be covered. Because the skin is already broken, it should be padded and protected from bacterial contamination. Covering the wound also helps to create a moisture balance and promotes healing.

The rate of wound healing is controlled by many factors, e.g., the amount of tissue damage, infection, the condition of the surrounding skin, and the patient's general physical condition. This complex problem requires multiple levels of intervention. The precise steps of intervention are described in Table 37-7.

Surgical Management of Decubitus Ulcers

Surgical repair of decubitus ulcers is not common in the elderly population, but it should not be automatically ruled out. The gerontological nursing literature offers few references to the care of skin grafts and tissue flaps of surgically treated decubiti. Decisions regarding surgical intervention are generally based on the following considerations:

1. The patient's general physical condition
2. His nutritional status
3. The site of the ulcer
4. Bacterial contamination of the site

The aged and debilitated patient who not only is a poor surgical risk but is also experiencing the latter stages of a depreciating disease condition would not be considered a candidate for the surgical repair of a decubitus ulcer. The nutritional status of an elderly patient is always a critical factor in the advisability of surgery.

It is rarely necessary to operate on pressure ulcers which occur outside the pelvic girdle. Ulcers which are not found on primary weight-bearing areas can be treated by other methods, and are usually smaller in size and depth. It is generally in the sacral, ischial, and trochanteric areas that greater tissue padding is required be-

Table 37-6. A Comparison of Topical Preparations for the Treatment of Pressure Ulcers.

PREPARATION	INDICATIONS	LIMITATIONS	PRECAUTIONS
Antacids	Superficial wounds	Apply frequently	Not reported
Antibiotics Local Systemic	Not useful Systemic infections only	Sensitivity of infecting agent	May destroy normal flora. Watch for superinfection.
Antiseptics Povidone Iodine	Draining infected wounds; clean wounds	Hard necrotic eschar Dress frequently	Watch for allergy to iodine. Protect surrounding skin. Stop if no results in 7 days.
Helafoam	Same as above; severely undermined ulcers	Hard necrotic eschar Dress frequently	Same as above.
Dextran beads (Debrisan)	Draining wounds	Dry ulcers or hard necrotic eschar; possible frequent dressings	Discontinue use when drainage ceases if no further healing is evident. Can cause mild bleeding and burning. Mix with sterile glycerin on shallow ulcers.
Enzymes Collagenase (Santyl)	Soft or hard necrotic tissue; crosshatch first with a surgical blade	Clean healing tissue; dress daily	Manufacturer recommends discontinuation when necrotic tissue is removed. Avoid hexachlorophene, tincture of iodine, Merthiolate, Furacin, and Burow's solution.
Fibrinolysin and deoxyribonuclease (Elase)	Soft necrotic tissue on hard necrosis after deep crosshatching	Clean healing tissue; dress tid	Discontinue when necrotic area is removed. Keep away from skin and granulation tissue.
Gelfoam Powder Sponges	Small to medium size clean wounds; daily to weekly dressing changes	Draining or hard necrotic ulcers; dress q 1–7 d	Debride and clean wound before use. Do not cleanse between applications. Inspect wound daily; if purulent, dedebride and start over.
Gold leaf	Clean wounds only; dress bid	Draining or hard necrotic ulcers; wound edges undermined; wound ringed by scar tissue	Prevent excessive friction; keep hemoglobin above 12 g/100 ml.
Insulin	Superficial wounds; drainage wounds	Deep or hard necrotic ulcers	Watch for hypoglycemia. Apply at mealtimes. Is no better than usual methods.
Op-Site (polythene film)	Superficial ulcers; selected deep, draining, or necrotic ulcers	Skin must be dry; *Pseudomonas aeruginosa* infection; dress q 3–7 d Dress every 3 to 7 days	Remove only the nonadherent portion or skin may tear; cut a hole in the center of Op-Site, clean, and reapply. Film may stick to fingers or patient's skin if not applied carefully.
Sugar Granulated	Clean ulcers	Not reported; dress daily	Therapeutic range is unknown.
Paste	Clean ulcers	Stasis, radiation, or scleroderma-associated ulcers	Improvement should occur within 14 days.
and egg white	None found	Not recommended	Procedure may retard normal healing.
Vegetable gums Karaya Stomahesive	Clean, draining, superficial, and deep ulcers Clean and draining, superficial and deep, hard necrotic ulcers; May be left in place 5–7 days	Hard necrotic eschar; dress daily None reported	Watch for possible skin allergy. Do not remove any karaya left on the wound after gentle irrigation. Reports of use are limited. If seepage or odor develops, remove Stomahesive, clean, and reapply a new piece. Round off edges so they do not cut into skin

NOTE: Used by permission of Mary Cooke Ahmed, published in *Nurse's Drug Alert*, Vol. IV, December Special Report, 1980/No. 15. M.J. Powers and Company, Publishers.

Table 37-7. Specific Nursing Interventions in Pressure Sore Treatment.

NURSING CARE	NURSING CONSIDERATIONS	TREATMENT OPTIONS
Step 1. Assess Lesion and Record a) Degree of tissue damage (*stage*) b) Degree of infection c) Amount and odor of damage	Exact measurement of the lesion in centimeters is helpful in evaluating healing. As new tissue develops in the ulcerated area, caution should be taken to avoid disturbing the newly formed skin. The type of organism and number of bacteria will influence the type of disinfectant and infection control necessary.	Frequency of treatment protocol is based on the degree of damage and environmental factors of mobility and continence. Periodic Polaroid photographs of progress are encouraging to the staff and helpful in medical and nursing evaluation.
Step 2. Cleanse Affected Area Gently a) Bathe b) Disinfect c) Rinse d) Debride (if necrotic tissue is present) e) Apply medication as prescribed by physician	Cellular damage is already present; therefore, massage gently to prevent further tissue damage. Some disinfectants are irritating to tissue, inhibit its development, and must be rinsed off thoroughly. Some cleansing agents have a protective coating that reduces scalding from urine or fecal excretion.	Irrigate open wounds with a syringe. Rinsing with normal saline is compatible with tissue growth. Whirlpool therapy both cleanses and stimulates gently. Disinfectant may be applied in the form of soaks to the area.
Step 3. Reduce Irritation a) Control incontinence b) Increase tissue growth	Unless it was designed for that purpose, avoid getting powder into an open lesion. Avoid abrasive tapes and dressings that create further damage to tissue when removed. Cellular damage is already present; therefore, use heat carefully.	Powders are available that reduce friction and absorb moisture. Skin tougheners are available. Reduce moisture and promote drying with air exposure, heat lamps, hair dryers, and sunlight.
Step 4. Provide Protection	If ulcer is in an area where contact with sheet or clothing will rub — saran wrapping can be substituted for the Telfa dressing.	Skin protection comes in forms that can be washed, sprayed, or painted on ulcer. Prepacked Telfa-like dressings are ready to apply.
Step 5. Relieve Pressure a) Change position of patient as ordered b) Reduce pressure on body surfaces	Pressure from doughnut-shaped pads can increase the pressure of the lesion encircled. The routine for turning patients is usually q 2 hr for prevention of tissue damage — decrease time by 15 min when reddened area occurs. Some patients can be instructed in responsibility to reduce pressure when sitting or lying in bed. Dependence on devices without diligent nursing care often results in tissue damage.	Rotate frame bed position and support with pillows. Use flotation system: bubble pads and mattresses filled with water and gel. Alternate pressure mattresses. Use foam dressings, pads, and splints; sheepskin pads.

cause the scars left by secondary wound healing may not withstand normal pressure. These are the areas most often considered for surgical treatment (Constantian, 1980).

For surgical repair to be considered, the ulcer must be ready. With good nursing management, ulcers of considerable size will frequently contract to more manageable proportions. Primary wound closure is more likely when the bacterial contamination is minimized and when nutritional and vitamin requirements for wound healing are met.

Postoperative Nursing Care.   The surgical procedure is just the beginning of the repair of decubitus ulcers. The new skin flap or graft, as well as the donor site, must receive daily attention. Hematoma is the most frequent complication. Drainage is a frequent occurrence, and catheters should be checked for patency. Turning and positioning are much the same as prior to surgery, except that there may be restriction on weight bearing in the operative area.

Establishment of a stable weight-bearing surface is a cooperation effort of the patient, nurse, and surgeon. The postsurgical care of pressure ulcers and the prevention of recurrence follow the same principles that govern more conservative nonsurgical intervention: (1) no pressure, no ulcer; (2) once an ulcer, always an ulcer.

CURRENT RESEARCH ON PRESSURE SORES

Because pressure sore formation is a complex interaction of multiple factors, the design of research on the subject is not a simple matter. It is encouraging that a few nurses have developed research studies in this area. Most have been concerned with the evaluation of certain treatment modalities or the prevention and healing of pressure sores. Berglas and Sullivan (1980) conducted a nursing care study to determine the effectiveness of collagenase therapy (an enzymatic debriding agent) in the treatment of pressure sores. Conclusions clearly indicated that intensive measures and the use of collagenase contributed greatly to the healing process. Gerber and Van Ort (1979) conducted a study to evaluate topical insulin therapy as a treatment

regimen for decubitus ulcers. They found consistent and significant positive correlations between the number of days of treatment and the rate of healing; they also found that topical insulin can be safely applied at mealtime. An unanswered question was, Why did women who were treated with topical insulin therapy heal significantly more slowly?

David Wastchak, M.S., R.Ph. (1983) of Phoenix, Arizona is conducting a study on hospital and nursing home patients with decubitus ulcers testing a stabilized gel (Dermagel) of the Aloe vera plant (genus barbadenis). He has found that adequate intake of vitamins and trace minerals along with an adequate protein diet will substantially enhance the healing of the ulcerated area. It was noted that patients who were obese and slightly overweight/well nourished responded more favorable to the treatment than did the underweight anorexic patient. Further studies are planned to add controlled amounts of protein such as egg, milk, caesin and spirulina (algae high in protein) along with trace minerals not commonly found in the "average" normal diet, to the diet of anorexic patients. The epithelialization that takes place must be enhanced from within as well as from without with the aloe vera gel.

Steffel, Schenk, and Walker (1979) did a comparison of ten pressure-reducing devices used in the prevention or care of pressure sores. Devices were ranked and rated by subjects and nurses. Some of the factors influencing effectiveness of the devices were whether the device was firm or soft, height of the bed, height and weight of the device, leaking from water devices and linen displacement. It was emphasized that no device is a substitute for turning patients regularly.

There are indications that future research should concern itself with a multivariant analysis of the variables with which the investigator must deal in decubitus ulcer research. Most of these variables are identified in the epidemiological model shown in Figure 37-3. Improved instrumentation is also needed to assess the healing of ulcers in order to increase the precision of ulcer measurement (Gerber and Van Ort, 1979). This will help to increase the validity and reliability of research results.

The investigation of decubitus ulcer formation is of increasing scientific interest, not only in nursing but in other disciplines as well. More research efforts are needed in the study of pressure sores in such diverse areas as surgical intervention, environmental and psychosocial influences, and optimal nursing intervention. It is an interdisciplinary effort that will lead to the control of this debilitating disease process.

A PHILOSOPHY OF CARE

As stated in the beginning of this chapter, the appearance of pressure sores casts a spell of hopelessness, helplessness, and resignation upon patients, families, and professionals. The professional nurse's beliefs (philosophy), attitudes, and actions are powerful in dispelling myths, demonstrating humane care, and instilling hope.

Discovering and rediscovering one's philosophy from time to time constitute an introspective exercise which is as important as research knowledge and technical skills. Nowhere is this needed more than in working with the frail elderly, where deterioration and death are imminent threats to the "healer" image.

The gerontological nurse must seek and keep up with professional preparation, must be committed to a multidisciplinary approach and teamwork, and must demonstrate a secure leadership-manager role — an overwhelming expectation with few rewards! However, there are unrealized rewards and satisfactions to be derived from caring with hope and recognizing others who do so.

L.J. is the nurse in charge of decubitus care at Sunset Lodge. In spite of the many patients with serious deteriorating conditions which foster development of pressure sores, the staff attitudes at Sunset Lodge reflect an unusual optimism. Perhaps this is why: when nurse L.J. gets to Mrs. B. in Room 214 for care of the pressure sore on her back, she asks Mrs. B. if she's ready, makes her comfortable, and then reports what she sees and does to Mrs. B. as she works. She elicits information, feelings, and fears, and feeds back progress and hopeful expectations. Once a week she

holds a bedside conference with other caretakers involved, specifically the paraprofessionals who do much of the bedside care. She demonstrates technical care measures, records the size of the wound, and says, "This is what we will do this week. . . . This is our goal . . . etc." giving everyone, including the patient some responsibility for needs and always recognizing contributions and caring involvement. L.J. points out that caretakers also need anniversaries of acceptance of ourselves when the wound has not been healed.

REFERENCES

Ahmed, M.C. Choosing the best method to manage pressure ulcers. *Nurse's Drug Alert* 4(15) (December 1980).

Berecek, K.H. Ecology of decubitus ulcers. *Nursing Clinics of North America* 10:157-170 (March 1975).

Berglas, C. and Sullivan, O. Decubitus ulcers, a nursing care study. *Journal of Nursing Care* 16–18 (April 1980).

Bush, C.A. Study of pressure under ischial tuberosities and thighs during sitting. *Archives of Physical Medicine and Rehabilitation* 50:207–215 (1969).

Carpendale, M. A comparison of four beds in the prevention of tissue ischemia in paraplegic patients. *Paraplegic* 12:21 (1974).

Constantian, M.B. *Pressure Ulcers: Principles and Techniques of Management.* Boston: Little, Brown, 1980.

Dinsdale, S.M. Decubitus ulcers: role of pressure and friction in causation. *Archives of Physical Medicine and Rehabilitation* 55:147–152 (1974).

Edberg, E.L., Cerney, K., and Staiffer, E.S. Prevention and treatment of pressure sores. *Physical Therapy* 53:246–252 (1973).

Exton-Smith, A.N. Prevention of pressure sores: monitoring of mobility and assessment of clinical condition. In Kenedi, R.M., Cowden, J.M., and Scales, J.T. (Eds.) *Bedsore Biomechanics.* Baltimore: University Park Press, 1976, pp. 133–141.

Gerber, R.M. and Van Ort, S.R. Topical application of insulin in decubitus ulcers. *Nursing Research* 28(1):16–19 (1979).

Gosnell, D. An assessment to identify pressure sores. *Nursing Research* 22:55–59 (1973).

Kosiak, M. Etiology of decubitus ulcers. *Archives of Physical Medicine and Rehabilitation* 42:24 (1961).

Maclay, E. "Green Winter" (poem in *Reader's Digest*). New York: Thomas Y. Crowell, 1977.

Merlino, A.F. Decubitus ulcers: cause, prevention, and treatment. *Geriatrics* 24:119–124 (March 1969).

Norton, D. Research and the problem of pressure sores. *Nursing Mirror* 13:300–303 (February 1975).

Reichel, S.M. Shearing force as a factor in decubitus ulcers in paraplegics. *Journal of the American Medical Association* 166:762–763 (1958).

Steffel, P.E., Schenk, E.A.P., and Walker, S.L. Reducing devices for pressure sores. *Nursing Research* 29(4):228–230 (1979).

Taylor, V. Decubitus prevention through early assessment. *Journal of Gerontological Nursing* 6(7):389–391 (1980).

Wastchak, D., M.S., R.Ph. Decubitus ulcer study. Phoenix: Health Science Lab, 1983 Unpublished (study in progress).

38
Unintentional Injury and Immobility: Hazards and Risks in Old Age

Bernita M. Steffl
Gloria Rowell

Old age is not for sissies.

Anonymous

This chapter addresses special hazards and high risk situations which contribute to the vulnerability, unintentional injury, immobility, and dependency status of older individuals. Many hazards and risks associated with old age have already been discussed in previous chapters. The following require and will receive more specific attention in this chapter: falls, foot problems, dental and oral problems, hypothermia, hyperthermia, choking, abuse and crimes against the elderly, and specific environmental hazards including fires. The hazards of drug abuse and misuse are covered in Chapter 34. Topics discussed here were chosen because they are most common and most devastating, and because nurses in the role of advocates, assessors, intervenors, or researchers can be powerful change agents in prevention.

UNINTENTIONAL INJURY

The concept of unintentional injury is usually expressed in terms of an accident or an unexpected consequence. Follow-up investigations generally prove that the accident could have been prevented; however, most of us still tend to treat the situation as if it had been inevitable. The word "accident" will continue to be used by lay people, but epidemiologists have stopped, by and large, and speak of "injury" and "injury events" (Hogue, 1980). For example, we almost expect old people to fall or have foot problems, even when preventive measures are known. Why? Perhaps because we are dealing with human behavior, our own and that of

patients. Also, the hazards of smoking and obesity are well known but hard to control because they involve a change in human behavior. Control of unintentional injury requires a philosophical commitment, an epidemiological approach, and usually a change in behavior (Price, 1978).

Epidemiology is the study of an occurrence from more perspectives than the disease. It fosters looking at problems from many angles and levels. One must look at causes, inferences, and possible consequences from a physiological, psychological, and sociological aspect, and study the relationships involving the agent (cause), the host (patient), and the environment.

The following situations will be receiving more attention by planners and health care professionals simply because they are costly and because prevention is cheaper than long term treatment and care. A major problem for the elderly is that Medicare provides little, if any, reimbursement for preventive health care and health maintenance versus sick care.

Perhaps a reason for the elderly population's reluctance to seek and utilize preventive care is because of indoctrination from early childhood that health care is synonymous with medical care and is in the hands of the doctor. "I let my doctor worry about that" or "My health is in the hands of a good doctor" are common statements from older individuals. However, this is changing, and trends toward self-help, self-care, and individual preventive health maintenance are emerging rapidly. Books such as *How to be Your Own Doctor Sometimes* by K.W. Sehnert, M.D., 1975 and other books on physical fitness are best-sellers, as emerging cohort groups tune into healthier diets, physical fitness programs, and monitoring their own blood pressure. It is expected that older people themselves, not professionals, will reduce the incidence of the problems discussed herein. However, nurses have a professional role, indeed a professional obligation, to advocate and facilitate the self-help concept.

FALLS

Falls are the second leading cause of accidental death in the United States, and 75% of them involve the elderly. The death rate from falls rises significantly with advancing age. Though the elderly comprise only about 10% of the population, they account for 26% of accidental deaths (Lewis and Windsor, 1974). The aged are more accident prone, and the risk of multiple accidents increases with age (Feist, 1978; Lynn, 1980). The elderly have a higher percentage of hospital falls than members of younger age groups, but most of their falls occur in the home (U.S. Department of Health, Education and Welfare, 1978). The greatest number of accidents in the hospital occurs where there is the highest proportion of acutely ill old people. The stay of old people in the hospital as a result of accidents is longer than the hospitalization period for most diseases.

An early study by Sheldon (1960) is considered classic today because it described so clearly the phenomenon of drop attacks without aura or amnesia, which are so common to the elderly. His study reported 25% of 500 falls as drop attacks. Drop attacks are a sudden loss of muscle tone without specific cause which results in an immediate fall. There is no loss of consciousness, and considerable time may elapse before recovery (Carnevali and Patrick, 1979). Longitudinal studies have shown that there may be a relationship between osteoporosis and fracture rates from falls (Iskrant and Smith, 1969), that fracture incidence is inversely proportional to bone mineral content (Smith, Khairi, and Johnson, 1975), and that there are fewer fractures of the spine among people who live in areas with at least 3 ppm of fluoride in their drinking water (Hegsted, 1968).

Kalchthaler, Bascon, and Quintos (1978), in a study of 190 incident reports of accidents occurring in a nursing home population of 189 residents, selected a random sample of 72 for a retrospective evaluation. The majority were falls — women of advanced age were most likely to be involved in a major fall. The alert wheelchair-bound were at higher risk than those who used assistive devices. The falls were directly related to the number of diagnoses and number medications ordered for each patient. Most incidents occurred at the bedside during evenings and nights, with the greatest frequency during shift change or when the resident was rising or retiring. They also pointed out that the responsibility for prevention rests with the medical director as well as all other staff and administration (Kalchthaler et al., 1978).

Feist (1978), in a survey study of 490 falls in a small home for the aged, found that 13.6% of the falls occurred in the first six weeks after admission and 27.7% in the first six months. The peak time for accidental falls was between 6:00 and 9:00 P.M. Only 3.8% of the falls caused major injuries; however, 14 older persons suffered major disability. Twenty-six percent of the falls happened to well-oriented individuals. Twenty-nine falls involved side rails, and 35% were from wheelchairs. About 79% of those who fell were on drugs either regularly or as needed (Feist, 1978).

A British study reports that only 34% of falls among the aged are accidental and that many are due to environmental hazards (Smith, 1976). Hogue (1980), in an epidemiological report on falls in the elderly, points out the following questions for further study: (1) Why are people injured when they fall? (2) Do characteristics of surfaces struck and distances fallen increase the probability of injury? (3) How soon do injured people get emergency help treatment? The implication to be drawn from this is that there is a need to examine current countermeasures of prevention. For example, most falls involving older people occur in private dwellings, public buildings, or residential institutions — all governed by building codes (Hogue, 1980)!

The reason for more falls by individuals of advanced age is more complex than commonly believed. The acts of walking, maintaining equilibrium, and carrying the body's center of gravity smoothly involve intricate mechanisms that are altered with age and function less efficiently. For example, alterations in gait which occur because of a variety of insidious changes are responsible for many falls.

Review of the incidence and character of falls among the elderly suggests that people over age 75 fall mainly because they have more difficulty maintaining their balance once they trip or start to fall. The older person is inclined to lose equilibrium while hyperextending his neck, sitting up, or rising to a standing position quickly and suddenly turning on the heel. Control is harder to maintain, too, because of the slowing down of the neuromuscular reflexes (Peszczynski, 1965). See Table 38-1 for other factors that make the elderly prone to falls. The following case history typifies, challenges, and almost refutes what we say here.

Case History

Emma King's family attempted to help her remain independent in a small apartment near her son, where she wanted to be after a year of living in a home for the elderly in another city. The apartment was old with high ceilings and steam heat. One day Emma noticed that the cover over an old chimney flue appeared loose. She attempted to climb up to fix it and fell. She hobbled around for two days before she called her son who took her to the hospital emergency room. She had a fractured hip which resulted in hospitalization. Emma was reluctant to give details. Finally, a year later she explained to her daughter how she had climbed from the chair to the table to the top of the refrigerator and tried to stand up to check the flue, when she tumbled and somehow slid to the floor without a more serious or fatal injury.

Nursing Implications

Nurses must be educated in at least the minimum aspects of biological and physiological gerontology and then relate the theory to practice. It can be seen from the example of Emma King that human behavior and psychosocial needs play a significant role in falls of the elderly and

---

Table 38-1. Factors that Make the Elderly More Prone to Falls.

Transient ischemic attacks	Decreased circulation in the brain, causing vertigo, dizziness, and fainting. Mechanical obstruction of vertebral arteries by crushed osteoporotic vertebrae. Arteriosclerotic and orthostatic hypotension.
Muscle weakness	Decrease in mass, strength, and coordination. Loss of balance.
Gait changes	Unsteadiness due to pain, fatigue, arthritic and osteoporotic changes. Interference with balance.
Decreased auditory acuity	Inner ear canal problems.
Decreased visual acuity	Decreased night vision and color vision. Faulty evaluation of spatial relationships (proprioception). Cataracts, glaucoma, presbyopia.
Urinary frequency and urgency	Unsafe maneuvering and toileting.
Foot problems	Improper footwear.
Inadequate venous return	Due to insufficient muscle activity.
Mental confusion and faulty judgments	
Mental depression	Suicidal tendencies.
Improper clothing	
Improper use of wheelchairs, walkers, etc.	Due to lack of or improper patient teaching.
Hostility in response to "trapped" feelings	Due to anxiety and catastrophic reactions.
Medications	Use and improper use.
Environmental hazards	Poor lighting, steps, wet floors.

NOTE: Adapted from Feist (1978) and Witte (1979).

that the cause of most falls is subject to manipulation or management of the environment.

The nursing assessment of falls on a long term care unit may prove more productive and conducive to intervention if approached with the intention of eliminating a variety of contributing causes as well as treating and teaching the patient. It also helps nurses in making inferences beyond what they see.

A paper on the concerns of accidents and the elderly, which was prepared for the 1981 White House Conference on Aging and partially reproduced in *Geriatric Nursing,* supports an epidemiological approach and lists major preventive measures (Cooper, 1981) such as the countermeasures for common hazards given in Table 38-2.

FOOT PROBLEMS

Foot health, foot problems, foot care, and foot comfort have a tremendous impact on immobility and unintentional injury. The American Podiatry Association estimates that about 80% of the population over age 50 has at least one foot condition. Women outnumber men in

Table 38-2. Safety Measures which Need to Be Taught and Reinforced for Elderly Persons Living at Home.

- Illuminated and clutter-free hallways and stairwells; use of night lights
- Rugs, floors, steps kept in good repair; clean but unwaxed floors and anchored floor coverings
- Use of handrails in halls, stairwells, bathrooms
- Use of nonskid tape in bathtub/shower, as well as chair or stool in shower
- Electrical cords and outlets in good condition; avoid stretching cords across areas of traffic
- Use of lightweight pans for cooking; handles not extending over edge of stove
- Placing frequently used items such as utensils and food in easy-to-reach places
- Avoid standing on ladders and chairs since balance may be poor and tremors may be present
- Avoid lifting heavy objects, since compression fracture may result due to osteoporosis
- Periodic eye examination
- Low-heeled, well-fitted walking shoes

NOTE: From Murray, Huelskoetter, and O'Driscoll, 1980.

reported foot problems, 89% to 61%, and only one-third of those seek medical advice (Schank, 1977).

The most common foot problems of the elderly are calluses, bunions, toenail problems, corns, fungus infections, and edema. These problems fall into three main categories: (1) onychial, (2) dermatologic, and (3) mechanical. Most foot problems of older individuals are related to changes in the skin and other medical problems. Arthritis, hypertension, circulatory problems, heart disease, diabetes, and kidney problems are common medical problems reported by well elderly in a foot education and screening program (Schank, 1977). See Table 38-3 for prevalence of foot problems. Diabetes millitus and proper foot care are discussed in Chapter 22.

Silverman (1960) noted years ago that many elderly suffer from problems they feel are not serious enough to warrant medical care. Foot problems fall into this category. However, foot health assumes much more importance when it affects mobility as it often does with increasing age.

In addition, foot care – particularly foot care of the elderly – has not received high priority from health care professionals outside of podiatrists. It has only been in recent years that Medicaid and some health insurance policies have provided for podiatry services. Research on foot care of the elderly, particularly nursing research, has been limited, but reports are beginning to appear. The focus seems to be on the need for foot health education, screening, and assessment skills.

King (1978) has developed and tested (for reliability) a foot assessment tool which has been published in the *Journal of Gerontological Nursing.* This assessment tool facilitates recognition of foot disorders and identifies high risk conditions. King suggests that nurses acquire knowledge of common foot problems and skill in assessing circulation by evaluation and judgment of edema, temperature, color, and pedal pulse (dorsal and posterior tibial). She found that clients living in nursing homes had more foot problems than those in the community and that a large number of them had circulatory impairments which made the problems acute (King, 1978).

Table 38-3. Reported Prevalence of Specified Foot Health Problems — Specific Population Groups versus the Public at Large.

	REPORTED NUMBER OF CASES PER THOUSAND					COMPARABLE FIGURES FOR PUBLIC AT LARGE
	FEMALES	ELDERLY (65+)	UNDER $5000 INCOME	NONWHITES	THOSE WHO LIVE IN THE SOUTH	
Corns and callosities	57	110	68	61	52	42
Bunions	19	44	24	18	16	12
Diseases of the nail	27	52	36	20	32	23
Flatfoot	15	23	23	20	17	16
Clubfoot	0.4	NR*	NR*	0.4	0.6	0.5
Other specified deformities	4	9	6	3	4	4
Totals	122.4	238	157	122.4	121.6	97.5

SOURCE: NCHS Health Interview Surveys 1973-1974 (these numbers are applicable to the civilian, noninstitutionalized population only). National Center for Health Statistics. *The National Ambulatory Medical Care Survey: 1973 Summary, United States, May 1973–April 1974* (DHEW Publication No. HRA 7501772). Washington, D.C.: October 1975.

*NR = Not reported by NCHS: volume of cases too low to be considered reliable.

A survey of 125 well elderly, their foot problems, and needs revealed specific age-related foot problems, as well as the incidence of other medical conditions (Schank, 1977). The survey led to foot examinations and an education program at senior centers in Milwaukee. The educational programs were attended by 487 persons, and 377 of these participated in the foot examination program. The highest percentage of examinees was in the 60–69 year age group (Conrad, 1977).

The findings of these studies and a review of the literature support the following recommendations (Conrad, 1977; Price, 1980; Schank, 1977):

- Periodic foot examinations (screening and assessment)
- Education programs on foot care, foot health, and specific problems
- Publicity and public information regarding the importance of foot care
- Counseling and follow-up care after foot examination
- Increased coverage of cost for foot health service by Medicare and health insurance

Nursing Implications

Nurses are in a key position and have a unique opportunity to advocate, assess, and intervene in regard to foot health problems of the aged. They are equipped to assess for potential difficulties which compound problems of immobility, such as edema, decubitus, footdrop, atrophy, and toenail care. Older individuals need mobility of their feet even in a wheelchair or in bed. Most of the conditions discussed interfere with social functioning and well-being. See Table 38-4 for behavioral and environmental factors which determine foot health and which may assist nurses in their assessments and care plans.

DENTAL AND ORAL PROBLEMS

The state of oral health and dental service to the elderly in this country leaves a lot to be desired and puts many elderly at risk for unintentional injury and illness. One in five

Table 38-4. Behavioral and Environmental Factors which Affect Foot Health in the Elderly.

- Sore and aching feet keep older people from putting on shoes, walking, and standing. These factors relate to immobility, physical fitness, and obesity.
- Sore feet and untreated foot conditions cause older adults to wear tennis shoes, sloppy bedroom slippers, and ill-fitting shoes which add to hazards and risks on the street or in the home, especially on stairs.
- Many older individuals go barefoot because shoes, socks, or stockings are painful or uncomfortable. Also, those who are already handicapped with problems like arthritis may find putting on shoes and stockings such a chore that it is easier to go without. This is extremely hazardous to diabetics and those with vascular problems. Every nurse can relate incidents of cuts, bruises, burns, and broken toes which happened to barefooted clients.
- Many older individuals have been victims of poor foot care or total neglect of foot care because it is not readily available to them or they cannot afford the cost. There are still gaps in Medicare, Medicaid, and health insurance programs in the United States which leave many older persons underserved.
- Older people tend to over- or undertreat their feet with self-care. When a person can no longer safely cut and care for his toenails, has been documented as a significant criterion to measure dependency needs. One in every five white elderly and one in every three black elderly persons have problems with toenails (Shanas, 1980). Poor vision and arthritic hands add to the risk and hazard of trimming corns, calluses, and toenails with sharp instruments and razor blades.
- Language and cultural barriers are not always well addressed in the delivery of health services in this country, particularly to the elderly, many of whom are first generation immigrants.
- Environmental barriers, lack of equipment, and improper use of devices and equipment are common, and demonstrate the need for communication and education.

Americans wears dentures by age 35, and one-half of the population have no natural teeth by age 65. Half of the people over age 65, about 8% of edentulous individuals of all ages, have either an incomplete set of dentures or none at all. Of those with teeth remaining, over 80% have periodontal disease. Over 70% of the elderly have not visited a dentist in five years or more. Even if more effort were made to provide better dental care to older individuals, existing dental manpower would not be adequate. Clearly, this has implications for nursing. Other countries have solved some of this problem by having nurses provide certain types of dental care in selected conditions (Price, 1979).

Oral conditions are discussed in Chapters 18 and 22. Therefore, this chapter deals mainly with risk factors and special hazards. The following factors make the elderly more vulnerable to oral problems:

- There is a lack of sufficient quantity and quality of saliva. A natural decrease occurs with age.
- Dietary problems exist because upper dentures cover part of the taste buds and because biting force is reduced due to muscle weakness. The normal biting force is 300 pounds; some elderly have as little as 50 pounds.
- Mucosal tissue of the mouth becomes more friable and easily injured.
- Alveolar bone resorption of maxilla and mandible occurs with aging. This suggests possible calcium deficiency.
- Inflammatory papillary hyperplasia is common in denture wearers. Therefore, dentures should be removed at night.
- The prevalence of oral cancer increases with age.

Although the survival rate for cancer of the mouth is poor, the number of persons surviving five years or more is doubled if treatment is begun when the lesion is less than 2 cm in diameter. See Table 38-5 for the signs and symptoms of oral cancer.

Nursing Implications

It is recommended that nurses take more responsibility for implementing oral health care. Extended care facilities need the services of a dental hygienist but rarely have them because of the low priority given to dental and oral care. The following are guidelines for patient care and patient education in dental and oral health (Price, 1979):

- Illustrate the proper method of brushing teeth (Bass method).
- Toothbrushes should have soft, rounded bristles, all of equal length. Toothpaste should not be too abrasive.
- Label dentures to reduce the problems of lost, misplaced, or switched dentures. Dentures can be sent to a dental laboratory for marking, or marking can be carried out at the nursing home (3-M Company Kit).
- Provide denture storage containers, and see that those who wear dentures remove them on a regular basis for about eight hours. This permits the oral tissues to rest and repair. Dentures should rest in the container with the teeth down.
- Illustrate the proper method of cleaning dentures. Too stiff a brush or too harsh a toothpaste will cause scratching and damage to denture surfaces.
- An inexpensive, safe, and effective denture cleaning solution consists of 1 tablespoon (15 cc) sodium hypochlorite (household bleach), 1 teaspoon (4 cc) Calgon (for detergent action), and 4 ounces (114 cc) water. (The Calgon protects against the corrosive action of the bleach.) After overnight soaking, dentures should be thoroughly brushed and rinsed.
- Do not rinse dentures in hot water; this may warp or discolor them.
- Sonic cleaners are recommended for all long term care facilities but should not be confused with laboratory ultrasonic cleaners. Sonic cleaners employ vibratory

Table 38-5. Signs and Symptoms of Oral Cancer.

- Ulceration of lips, tongue, or other areas that does not heal promptly
- Lesion in the mouth without pain
- White scaly areas in the mouth
- Swelling of lips, gums, or other areas, without pain
- Repeated oral bleeding without apparent cause
- Numbness or loss of feeling in any part of the mouth
- Tumors located on the side of the tongue and the floor of the mouth

NOTE: Adapted from Price (1979) and Ramos (1981).

energy, not ultrasonic energy, to clean dentures.

- Provide education on the potential dangers of do-it-yourself denture reliner kits. FDA regulations require the following warning on the labels of denture reliners: "Warning — for temporary use only. Long-term use of this product may lead to faster bone loss, continuing irritation, sores, and tumors. For use only until a dentist can be seen." Patients should have improperly fitting dentures relined by a dentist.
- Discourage use of dental adhesives such as powders (karaya gum) and viscous adhesive pastes which may malposition the denture against the underlying tissues, causing undue irritation.
- Use lemon glycerin swabs for xerostomia and for cleaning the oral cavity.
- There should be regular examination of the oral cavity for possible lesions.
- Patients with physical problems may need to have their toothbrushes modified: e.g., for arthritis of the hand, a wide elastic band can be taped to the toothbrush handle; for limited arm movement, the handle of the toothbrush can be taped to a rod to lengthen the handle; for central nervous system disorders, the toothbrush handle may need to be enlarged by pushing the handle of the toothbrush through a soft rubber ball (see Figure 38-1).
- Acquire portable dental equipment for those too ill to travel to a private dentist.
- Add a dental record to the regular medical records.
- Educate clients and family about dental quackery. At the U.S. Senate hearings before the Subcommittee on Frauds and Misrepresentations Affecting the Elderly (1976), it was estimated that 20 million dollars yearly was paid to dental quacks.
- Some patients do not want prosthodontic care or are too ill to receive care, but families press for dentures. The family must be educated to realize that this patient is a poor prospect for wearing new dental appliances. The success of dental treatment rests upon three things: patient motivation, patient ability to physically

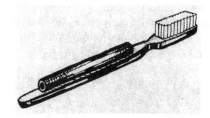

The toothbrush handle can be made easier to grasp by gluing or taping a strip of hard rubber or plastic tubing to it.

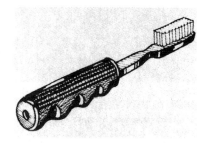

A bicycle handle-bar grip, held in place with a plaster of Paris mix, can also be used over the handle.

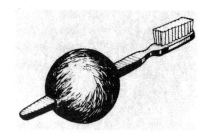

Thrusting the handle into the center of a soft rubber or Styrofoam ball is still another way to make the toothbrush easier to grasp.

Figure 38-1. Toothbrush aids. [Reprinted with permission from Ramos, L.Y. Oral hygiene for the elderly. *American Journal of Nursing* 81(8):1468–1469 (August 1981).]

cooperate, and patient ability to communicate during and after treatment.

Research and Trends in Dental Health of the Elderly

Literature on dental hygiene frequently lists the following as the key measures for intervention in the prevention of dental and oral deterioration in older individuals: (1) plaque control, (2) fluoride, and (3) nutrition (Wilkens, 1976). According to a National Health Survey, oral cleanliness decreases with age, primarily related to calculus accumulation. Periodontal disease has been known for years to be more frequent and severe in older people (U.S. Department of Health, Education and Welfare, 1967). Fluoride in water, diet, toothpaste, or topical application is as important for the elderly as for the young. It tends to counteract tendencies toward cemental caries related to dry mouth (Wilkens, 1976). See Chapter 22 for the impact of nutrition on oral health and Chapter 33 for the nutritional needs of the elderly.

A small pilot study to determine if a relationship exists between dental care and self-esteem in the elderly revealed a significant difference in self-esteem scores between those who are willing to restore their teeth at any cost and those who place an economic limit on oral restoration (Odrich and Dornbush, 1981).

Colonial Manor, in York, Pennsylvania, is a pioneer in providing a dental care program in an extended care facility. The program includes oral examination, dental health charts, referral for dental consultation, emergency dental care, equipped dental room, denture labeling, and oral care instruction. The most common reasons for dental consult in this program are poor retention of dentures due to bone resorption. Loose, unstable dentures are most distressing to wearers. Another reason for frequent dental referrals in peridontoclasia — a loosening of one or more of the permanent teeth. The administration and staff of Colonial Manor say, "Comprehensive dental care can be made accessible in an ECF with minimal expenditures of time, expense, and materials," and they welcome inquiries for further information (Fahs, 1981).

HYPOTHERMIA

Hypothermia is a condition of below normal body temperature, typically 95°F (35°C) or under. Accidental hypothermia may occur when anyone is exposed to severe cold without sufficient protection. However, some older people develop accidental hypothermia after exposure to relatively mild cold. Nearly half of the victims of hypothermia are elderly. At least 10% of the elderly (those over age 65) are considered at risk (National Institute on Aging,

1980). The death rate from hypothermia is 35–40% (Brocklehurst, and Hanley, 1980). The elderly are potential victims because some are unable to afford adequate housing and/or heating, and there are those whose blood vessels fail to respond to cold or to change in position. Also, there are those with postural hypotension who experience vertigo or light-headedness when they change position; they may be taking drugs which produce an adverse effect, such as chlorpromazine or other phenothiazines for anxiety, depression, or nausea, and they may also have hypothyroidism or paralyzing conditions that prevent heat production from muscular contractions. Sometimes those with mobility problems fall and lie on cold floors for hours or days before they are found (Brocklehurst and Hanley, 1980; National Institute on Aging, 1980). Accidental hypothermia has not been studied extensively in the United States, but it is receiving increased attention. Researchers in Great Britain estimate that 10% of the British population is at risk (Green, 1975).

Etiology

The true causes of hypothermia in the elderly are yet unknown, but we do know that the elderly are more vulnerable because their bodies have decreased resistance to stress; they do not adjust to changes in temperature as well as young bodies; they do not shiver readily so the body cannot produce emergency heat; and their blood vessels fail to respond to the change in position when rising from bed or a chair (Hayter, 1980; Wolanin and Phillips, 1981). Alcohol consumption accelerates the loss of heat, and when alcohol is taken along with certain drugs, the risk of hypothermia goes up. Hypothermia has also been associated with hypoproteinemia. Since the elderly are often malnourished, this may add to their vulnerability.

The elderly surgical patient is at high risk. Studies have demonstrated that these patients may have a depressed heat regulatory system due to preoperative medication and the cold operating rooms, cold solutions used, and lack of warm covers. Possible aspiration of vomitus compounds the problem.

Nursing Implications

Signs and symptoms of hypothermia may include pale waxy skin, bloated face, irregular slow pulse, slowed respiration, hypotension, muscle rigidity, diminished reflexes, slurred speech, unilateral trembling, drowsiness, and coma. A special thermometer with a scale that goes below 94°F (34°C) is needed to measure hypothermia (Brocklehurst and Hanley, 1980; National Institute on Aging, 1980). If a special thermometer is not available and a regular thermometer does not register, warm your hands on your own body (chest or abdomen) and compare with the victim's body.

If the body temperature has gone below 90°F (32.2°C), a medical emergency exists. A patient must be hospitalized for slow rewarming and observation. His core temperature is brought back to normal with warmed blankets and warm fluids and, in some cases, with transfusions of warmed blood or peritoneal dialysis (Gröer, 1979). The patient needs to be monitored for cardiac arrhythmia and hypokalemia.

Measures are instituted to prevent aspiration and bronchopneumonia. Intravenous therapy is carefully regulated and may be used to administer medications such as corticosteroids or triiodothyronine. The brain, heart, kidneys, and pancreas may suffer residual damage from the hypothermia. Recovery depends on the degree of hypothermia or body temperature: if above 90°F (32.2°C), the prognosis is good; between 80°F (26.6°C) and 90°F (32.2°C), some residual effects may complicate the recovery; below 80°F (26.6°C), the mortality rate is high (National Institute on Aging, 1980). The body temperature should not be raised more than 1°F (0.6°C) per hour. Too rapid warming causes vasodilation which will lead to hypotension that could be fatal. The temperature should be taken rectally.

The most appropriate intervention is prevention which, in turn, necessitates assessment skills — in this case knowledge of the physical changes of aging. The nurse must be able to recognize subtle clues in the patient so that she can institute an effective care plan and manipulation of the environment. See Table 38-6 for a list of clues to hypothermia. The consequences of

Table 38-6. Clues Indicative of Possible Hypothermia.

- A change in appearance or behavior during cold weather.
- An elderly person may seem to be unaware of the cold, while others shiver and put on sweaters. The older individual may not shiver and may insist that he or she is comfortable.
- Family and friends may notice that a person is not thinking clearly or is not acting as usual.
- Uncontrollable shivering, lack of shivering, or stiff muscles.
- Low indoor temperatures and other signs that the victim has been in an unusually cold room.
- Slow — and sometimes irregular — heartbeat; shallow, very slowed breathing.
- Weak pulse; low blood pressure.
- Confusion, disorientation, or drowsiness.
- Skin feels waxy and cool to touch, even the abdomen which is usually warm.
- Restlessness.
- Slurred speech.
- Shallow respirations.
- Muscular rigidity.

hypothermia are so serious that all nurses should be able to intervene appropriately and to instruct patients and their families about this hazard.

Need for Assessment and Education. Margaret and Augie are in their 80s. He is quite proud of his physical fitness. She is also very self-sufficient but frequently complains of being cold. Augie tells her that she needs to stay active and quit babying herself. He refuses to turn up the heat. Margaret has fallen twice in the past year. In neither situation was there a notable environmental reason. One might wonder if these falls were related to a hypotension from the hypothermia.

Many elderly have low temperatures bordering on hypothermia. They may appear "chilly," listless, and apathetic. It is at this marginal state that nurses may see the first signs of confusion and disorientation if the person cannot respond by shivering (Wolanin and Phillips, 1981). It is also at this stage that patients may be misdiagnosed and treated prematurely as "senile." Wolanin and Phillips (1981) devote considerable space to these disorders (hypo- and hyperthermia) in their text on confusion, and give detailed guidelines for nursing assessment and intervention.

HYPERTHERMIA

There is no single specific definition of hyperthermia, but it is usually considered to be a core body temperature of 100°F. It has two main causes: (1) infection and (2) ambient temperature above the body's heat. Also, the loss of sweat glands in older individuals deprives the body of evaporative cooling.

The signs and symptoms of hyperthermia vary with the degree of fever. The core temperature must be measured by rectal thermometer for both hypo- and hyperthermia. Urinary tract infections, circulatory problems, and dehydration add to the risk for the elderly (Wolanin and Phillips, 1981).

During periods of very high environmental temperatures, the elderly, especially those with specific medical problems, may build up body heat; this can lead to heat stroke, heat syncope, or heat exhaustion.

Heat Stroke

Heat stroke or collapse is a medical emergency requiring immediate attention and treatment by a doctor. The symptoms of heat stroke include faintness, dizziness, staggering, headache, nausea, loss of consciousness, high body temperature (104°F/40°C or higher measured rectally), strong rapid pulse, and flushed skin. Because body heat can continue to build up for days after a heat wave ends, those who care for the frail elderly or the ill elderly should monitor rectal body temperatures closely during and after periods of extreme heat.

Heat Syncope

Heat syncope is marked by dizziness, fatigue, and sudden faintness after exercising in the heat. In contrast to heat stroke, the victim of heat syncope recovers when removed from direct exposure to the heat. The symptoms of heat syncope are cool, sweaty, pale skin; weak pulse; fall-ing blood pressure; and faintness. It results from a lack of acclimatization to the hot weather. Treatment involves resting (it is best to lie or sit down with the head lowered), cooling off, and drinking extra nonalcoholic liquids.

Heat Exhaustion

This is the most common form of illness due to hot weather. This condition takes longer to develop and results from a loss of body fluids and salts. The symptoms of heat exhaustion are thirst, fatigue, giddiness, elevated body temperature, and in severe instances, delirium. When both body water and salt are depleted, muscle cramps may also be present.

Heat exhaustion is treated by resting in bed away from the heat, restoring body water by drinking cool fluids, and lowering body temperature by giving sponge baths or applying wet towels to the body.

Nursing Implications

Slight hyperthermia may yield to cool drinks and rest, lightweight clothing, lightweight bedding, and tepid sponging as comfort measures. If the core temperature is 103°F (39.4°C), body cooling should be instituted with cold packs to the head and back of the neck and sponging with alcohol solution (half water–half alcohol). If the patient begins to shiver, the cooling process is stopped because shivering will raise the temperature. Aspirin may be helpful but should be given with caution.

An analysis of morbidity and mortality related to the heat wave in the southeastern and southwestern United States in the summer of 1980 confirmed earlier studies indicating that heat waves most severely affect those of extreme ages — the very young (infants) and the very old. The highest number of deaths occurred among those over age 65, from inner city neighborhoods and census tracts with a median income below $14,835 per household. The researchers concluded that these findings have implications for community planners as well as for health professionals (Brasfield, Williams, and Applegate, 1981).

CHOKING

Choking and difficulty with swallowing are common among the frail elderly for a number of reasons such as paralysis due to a pathological physical condition, disturbances caused by medications (dyskinesia), overmedication, improper posture and positioning during feeding, poorly fitting dentures, and unintentional aspiration of food or fluid.

Choking on a piece of food causes about ten deaths every day in the United States. These deaths can be avoided if a simple rescue technique is applied as soon as distress is noticed. The main treatment modalities of course are prevention and having staff prepared in first aid measures when choking occurs.

The safest and easiest first aid procedure for choking is the Heimlich maneuver which was devised by Dr. Henry J. Heimlich. All staff in long term care work should learn and practice this procedure, which is illustrated in Figure 38-2. It should be part of all job orientations. The technique, which is easily learned, seems to work because there is always some residual air in the lungs, and pressure below the diaphragm compresses and forces the lodged food upward. The debris pops out "like a champagne cork."

There are a number of "choke saver" devices on the market, but research and literature about them seem nonexistent. The authors have had very limited exposure to them but are of the opinion that (1) users of these devices need very careful training, (2) there may be considerable risk and possible injury if the devices are not properly used or if the user is not well informed about the anatomy and physiology of the mouth and throat and the respiratory mechanisms of the body.

It is important to recognize a person who is choking. The most obvious and important symptom is that the victim cannot speak. He will turn pale, then blue or black, and will collapse if unaided. A person who is choking alone should try anything that applies force just below the diaphragm. Pressing against the edge of a table or chair or using your own fist might compress the abdomen enough to "pop" the obstruction loose (see Figure 38-2).

The following film may also be helpful in teaching health care professionals and paraprofessionals preventive measures for choking victims: *To Save a Life* (16-mm color, 12 minutes long), available from Encyclopedia Britannica Education Corporation, 425 North Michigan Avenue, Chicago, IL 60611.

ENVIRONMENTAL CAUSES OF UNINTENTIONAL INJURY

Nurses have never been seriously involved in the evaluation or manipulation of the environment or physical space of long term care facilities in terms of interface with patients' needs. A good environment should accommodate the disabilities of aged patients and should provide impetus and assistance to retain or regain a functional outlook; there is need for a professional group that is equipped to evaluate those environments created for the aged. A Cornell University study of the physical environment of aged patients in eight nursing homes established that spaces and objects within spaces are determinants of behavior. This and testimonal statements by architects before the U.S. Special Committee on Aging hearings on "A Barrier-Free Environment of Aging and Handicapped" point the way for nursing involvement in assessment and research by (1) interviewing patients regarding their needs and including physical environment in the nursing care plan for the patient, (2) behavioral mapping, (3) photographic studies, and (4) microethnography (Koncelik, 1971, 1972).

The aged patient will be influenced by three major factors in his relationship with space: (1) his own abilities and disabilities, (2) staff concepts of room use and patient capabilities, and (3) the physical features of the design (Koncelik and Snyder, 1971).

Examples of Manipulating the Environment

Mrs. Barnes unendeared herself to the staff at Green Valley Rest Home shortly after her admission by giving the nursing assistant a black eye while in the shower stall. The entire staff were involved and finally succeeded in getting Mrs. Barnes showered. The routine is for all patients to be showered at least two times a week. Mrs.

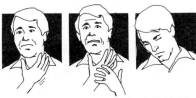

1. CAN'T SPEAK OR BREATHE   2. TURNS BLUE   3. COLLAPSES

CHOKING— HOW TO HELP

THE HEIMLICH MANEUVER
(Causes Lodged Food to Pop Out of The Windpipe)

STANDING POSITION

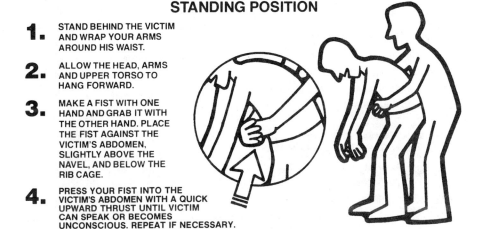

1. STAND BEHIND THE VICTIM AND WRAP YOUR ARMS AROUND HIS WAIST.

2. ALLOW THE HEAD, ARMS AND UPPER TORSO TO HANG FORWARD.

3. MAKE A FIST WITH ONE HAND AND GRAB IT WITH THE OTHER HAND. PLACE THE FIST AGAINST THE VICTIM'S ABDOMEN, SLIGHTLY ABOVE THE NAVEL, AND BELOW THE RIB CAGE.

4. PRESS YOUR FIST INTO THE VICTIM'S ABDOMEN WITH A QUICK UPWARD THRUST UNTIL VICTIM CAN SPEAK OR BECOMES UNCONSCIOUS. REPEAT IF NECESSARY.

PRONE POSITION

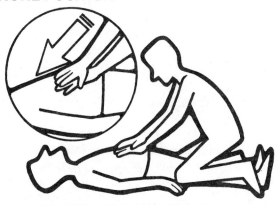

1. PLACE THE VICTIM ON HIS BACK.

2. KNEEL ASTRIDE HIS HIPS WITH ONE HAND ON TOP OF THE OTHER.

3. PLACE THE HEEL OF THE BOTTOM HAND ON THE VICTIM'S ABDOMEN, SLIGHTLY ABOVE THE NAVEL AND BELOW THE RIB CAGE.

4. PRESS INTO THE VICTIM'S ABDOMEN WITH A QUICK UPWARD THRUST. REPEAT IF NECESSARY.

 COMPLIMENTS OF THE ARIZONA DEPARTMENT OF HEALTH SERVICES

Figure 38-2.

Barnes is 83 years old and quite disoriented. Upon her daughter's arrival, it was learned that Mrs. Barnes had never had a shower in her life! Would knowing this have made a difference? Would the routine have been changed? Was the alternative of a tub bath available? If not, why not?

Some years ago one of the authors helped take care of a friend who was terminally ill and died in a nursing home. Carmen shared a tiny room with a patient who was blind and aphasic. When both had company, there was room for only one chair for each; when we gave a bath or changed the bed, we often backed in and out of the limited work space. Our backs ached from the low bed and the unhandy placement of the beds in relation to the sink and toilet. Many months after Carmen's demise, it occurred to me that I had complained a great deal but had never made a serious effort to manipulate that environment!

THE ELDERLY AS VICTIMS OF CRIME AND ABUSE

In June 1975, the first National Conference on Crime against the Elderly was held in Washington, D.C., by the College of Public Affairs of American University. It was funded by the Administration on Aging. Special Committees on Aging of the U.S. House and Senate are now holding periodic hearings and investigations on crime and abuse regarding the elderly. These have assisted in defining the problems more specifically so as to develop preventive counter-measures and educate the vulnerable public.

Consistent and accurate data on aged abuse nationally are not available at this time. However, four types of abuse have been identified: violation of rights, material abuse, physical abuse, and psychological abuse. (1) Violation of rights includes the right to basic human needs and patients' rights (see Appendix A of this book for a patient's bill of rights). (2) Material abuse consists of theft, misappropriation, and confiscation of an elderly person or elderly patient's money (e.g., the children who come home once a month to cash in mother's Social Security check). (3) Physical abuse includes out-and-out physical beating, as well as withholding personal or medical care; neglect is the most common form of physical abuse. (4) Psychological abuse consists of verbal assaults and threats (Beck and Ferguson, 1981).

Battered Parents

There are several parallels between the battered child and the battered parent: both are independent roles; both are presumed to be protected; and both can be a source of emotional, physical, and financial stress to the caretaker.

The English first labeled the problem "granny bashing" and now refer to it as gram-slamming. England has recognized the problem and dealt with it more effectively than the United States by providing periodic respite care, a service which is just being initiated in the United States.

Battering takes the form of benign neglect in behaviors such as tying elderly individuals into chairs and bed because they can't be watched constantly and excessive use of sleeping medications, tranquilizers, and alcohol. However, there are documented cases of older individuals being slapped, beaten, or forcefully restrained to the point of fracturing bones. This happens in long term care facilities as well as in homes. Unfortunately, these battered parents whose attacks cover a wider range than child abuse often refuse to report abuse or deny it in court because of their fear of retaliation (Steinmetz, 1978).

A survey of 1000 medical and social service professionals and paraprofessionals in Massachusetts revealed that almost every professional included in the study had come in contact with or suspected elder abuse by family members. One hundred and eighty-three respondents reported seeing aged abuse in the prior 18 months. The incidents tended to happen repeatedly to the same person. The 60-and-over and especially the 75-and-older group and the frail elderly who live at home are prime targets for abuse. The abusers are typically experiencing some kind of stress situation such as alcoholism, drug addiction, or financial problems. One of the chief barriers to providing service to these victims is the unwillingness of the victim to admit abuse and accept service or help (U.S. House of Representatives Select Committee on Aging, 1979).

Safety and security officers need special training to understand the possible reduced perceptions and altered sensory responses of older persons, especially the frail elderly. Periodic safety and security surveys are helpful in long term care facilities and housing for older adults, and they can be used to involve residents and total staff.

There are a number of "alert" devices now available to help elderly victims of accidents, illness, and crime. An example is EARS, an Emergency Alarm Response System program developed by Lifeline Systems, Inc., 51 Spring Street, Watertown, ME 02172, (617) 923-4141. Innovative programs such as Teen Escort Services, established in cooperation with police departments, Block Watch, and Neighborhood Protective Networks are proving to be effective, but there are not enough of them, and public apathy tends to prevail.

Nursing Implications

As pointed out throughout this book, nurses have unlimited opportunities to exercise advocacy in support of the basic human needs of the elderly. Their observations are extremely valuable to social workers in protective services and to the police. The ability of nurses to assess for reality orientation and cognitive function can be very useful and helpful to the police. The police can also be very helpful to nurses working with the aged, in both the hospital and the community.

FATAL FIRES

Twenty-five of the 37 residents of the Wayside Inn, a licensed boarding house (dormitory facility) near Farmington, Missouri, died in a fire at the facility on April 2, 1979. There were adequate exits in the building, some single-station, battery-powered smoke detectors, and manually operated evacuation alarm, but the mere presence of these building features was not enough to prevent deaths in this unsprinkled facility. The major factors that led to the deaths were the undivided attic, where the fire began, the lack of a complete fire detection system, and *lack of advanced fire-emergency planning and training for the staff and residents* (italics added). (Peterson, 1979)

On November 11, 1979, 14 people died in a fire at the Coats Rooming House in Pioneer, Ohio. A three-year-old child playing with a cigarette lighter was responsible for a rapidly spreading fire that killed 13 residents and one of the owners of the home. The boarding home provided room and board for eleven elderly private residents and eight mentally retarded residents who had been referred to the boarding home after being released from a state mental health care facility. Two rented apartment units in the building had an additional five occupants. The home was operated by the owners, who also resided in the building. Because of the husband's poor health, *the wife supervised the daily operation*

of the boarding home with the help of one employee (italics added). (Bell, 1980)

On July 14, 1980, at approximately 9:30 P.M., a fire in the Extendicare Skilled Nursing Facility in Mississauga, Ontario, resulted in the deaths of 25 patients, most of them elderly. The area of origin of the accidental fire was a patient room on the top floor of the three-story fire-resistive building.

Significant factors that contributed to the fatalities in this fire were rapid fire development, the failure to extinguish the fire in its incipient stage, failure to keep the door to the room of origin closed, *improper staff actions, and delayed alarm to the fire department* (italics added). (Demers, 1981)

Tragic reports such as these are common occurrences in this country. Fire is the third ranking accidental killer in the United States. It brought sudden death to 8621 persons in the United States in 1978, many of them elderly. Since 1971 the National Fire Protection Administration has been studying these fatal fires, and the statistics accumulated are being used to identify leading aspects in defining problems and corresponding action priorities for a vigorous, well-aimed attack on the problem (Derry, 1979).

A sobering problem identified as a leading factor in all these fatal fires was *lack of advance planning and training of the staff and residents on what to do when a fire occurred.* It is tempting to state that fire drills and environmental protection are an administrative responsibility and that nurses do not have authority in these matters, but that is not true. Nurses do have a responsibility for the safety and protection of their patients. They are not responsible for fire codes, but they certainly share a responsibility for fire drills and emergency evacuation of patients. They are also accountable for activities of the paraprofessionals who work under them, and supervision includes preparation and practice in fire prevention. Fire drills are often treated lightly and as a joke. Don't do this! At the risk of being labeled tyrants, nurses should insist on thorough orientation to fire drill and evacuation procedures for all new staff, as well as periodic, routine in-service education on the topic for everyone. Patients have the right to expect reasonable and prudent protection. Fire departments are a helpful resource for planning and teaching fire prevention.

REFERENCES

Beck, C.M. and Ferguson, D. Aged abuse. *Journal of Gerontological Nursing* 7(6):333–336 (1981).

Bell, J. Fourteen die in Ohio boarding home fire. *Fire Journal* 74(4):28–32 (1980).

Brasfield, L., Williams, M.L., and Applegate, W.B. *Environmental Crises and the High Risk Elderly.* Paper presented at Western Gerontological Society meeting, Seattle, Washington, April 15, 1981.

Brocklehurst, J.C. and Hanley, T. *Geriatric Medicine for Students* (2nd ed.). London: Churchill Livingstone, 1980.

Carnevali, D.L. and Patrick, M. *Nursing Management for the Elderly.* Philadelphia: J.B. Lippincott, 1979, pp. 404–406.

Conrad, D. Foot education and screening programs for the elderly. *Journal of Gerontological Nursing* 3(6):11–15 (1977).

Cooper, S. Common concern: accidents and older adults. *Geriatric Nursing* 2(4):287–290 (1981).

Demers, D.P. Twenty-five die in nursing home. *Fire Journal* 75(1):30–35 (1981).

Derry, L. Fatal fires in America. *Fire Journal* 72(5): 67–79 (1979).

Fahs, D. Accessible dental care in an extended care facility. *Journal of Gerontological Nursing* 7(1): 21–26 (1981).

Feist, R.R. A survey of accidental falls in a small home for the aged. *Journal of Gerontological Nursing* 4(6):15–17 (1978).

Green, M.F. Hypothermia and the elderly. *Queen's Nursing Journal* 214–216 (November 1975).

Gröer, M.E. Response to physical and chemical agents. In Gröer, M.E. and Shekleton, M.E. (Eds.) *Basic Pathophysiology: A Conceptual Approach.* St. Louis: C.V. Mosby, 1979.

Hayter, J. Hypothermia-hyperthermia in older persons. *Journal of Gerontological Nursing* 6(2):65–68 (1980).

Hegsted, D.M. Fluoride and mineral metabolism. *Ann. Dent.* 27:134–143 (1968).

Hogue, C.C. Epidemiology of injury in old age. In Haynes, S.G. and Feinleib, M. (Eds.) *Proceedings of the Second Conference on Epidemiology of Aging* (NIH Publication No. 80-969). Washington, D.C.: National Institutes of Health, July 1980.

Iskrant, A.P. and Smith, R.W. Osteoporosis in women 45 years and over related to subsequent fracture. *Public Health Reports* 87:33–38 (1969).

Kalchthaler, T., Bascon, R.A., and Quintos, V. *Falls in the Institutionalized Elderly.* Paper presented at the 31st Annual Scientific Meeting of the National Gerontology Society, San Francisco, California, 1978.

King, P.A. Foot assessment of the elderly. *Journal of Gerontological Nursing* 4(6):47–52 (1978).

Koncelik, J.A. Architectural barriers and the voiceless consumer. Testimony II. *Human Ecology Forum* 2(2):(1971).

Koncelik, J.A. Design to meet patient needs and enhance longevity of the long term care facility. *Empire State Architect* (March 1971).

Koncelik, J.A. Design to meet patient needs and enhance longevity of the long term care facility. *Empire State Architect* (March 1972).

Lewis, D.J. and Windsor, R.J. *Handle Yourself with Care.* An instructor's guide for an accident prevention course for older Americans. Washington, D.C.: U.S. Department of Health, Education and Welfare, Office of Human Development, Administration on Aging, 1974.

Lynn, F.H. Incidents – need they be accidents? *American Journal of Nursing* 80:1098–1100 (June 1980).

Murray, R., Huelskoetter, M., and O'Driscoll, D. *The Nursing Process in Later Maturity.* Englewood Cliffs, N.J.: Prentice-Hall, 1980.

National Center for Health Statistics. *The National Medical Care Survey: 1973 Summary, United States, May 1973–April 1974* (DHEW Publication No. HRA 7501772). Washington, D.C.: October 1975.

National Institute on Aging. *A Winter Hazard for the Old: Accidental Hypothermia.* Bethesda, Md.: U.S. Department of Health and Human Services, 1980.

Odrich, J. and Dornbush, R.L. Dental care and self esteem in the elderly. *Dental Hygiene* 55(6):29–32 (June 1981).

Peszczynski, M. Why older people fall. *American Journal of Nursing* 65(5):86–87 (1965).

Peterson, C.E. Twenty-five die in boarding house. *Fire Journal* 73(6):26–33 (1979).

Price, J.H. Unintentional injury among the aged. *Journal of Gerontological Nursing* 4(3):36–41 (1978).

Price, J.H. Oral health care for the geriatric patient. *Journal of Gerontological Nursing* 5(2):25–29 (1979).

Price, J.H. Foot problems of the elderly. *Journal of Gerontological Nursing* 6–9 (January 1980).

Ramos, L.Y. Oral hygiene for the elderly. *American Journal of Nursing* 81(8):1468–1469 (1981).

Schank, M.J. A survey of the well-elderly: their foot problems, practices, and needs. *Journal of Gerontological Nursing* 3(6):10–13 (1977).

Sehnert, K.W. How to be Your Own Doctor: Sometimes. New York: Grasset and Dunlap Publishers, 1975.

Shanas, E. Self assessment of physical function: white and black elderly in the United States. In Haynes, S.G. and Feinleib, M. (Eds.) *Proceedings of the Second Conference on Epidemiology of Aging* (NIH Publication No. 80-969). Washington, D.C.: National Institutes of Health, July 1980, pp. 269–281.

Sheldon, J.H. On the natural history of fall in old age. *British Medical Journal* 5214:1685–1690 (1960).

Silverman, B.M. *Positive Health of Older People.* New York: National Health Council, 1960, p. 14.

Smith, C. Accidents and the elderly. *Nursing Times* 72:1872 (December 1976).

Smith, D.M., Khairi, M.R.A., and Johnson, C.C. The loss of bone mineral with aging and its relationship to risk of fractures. *Journal of Clinical Investigation* 56:311–318 (1975).

Steinmetz, S.K. Battered parents. *Society* 54–55 (July-August 1978).

U.S. Department of Health, Education and Welfare. *Facts of Life and Death, 1978.* Washington, D.C.: U.S. Government Printing Office, 1978.

U.S. Department of Health, Education and Welfare, Vital and Health Statistics. *Data from Health Survey, Total Loss of Teeth in Adults, United States 1960–1962* (Public Health Service Publication No. 1000, Series 11, No. 27). Washington, D.C.: October 1967.

U.S. House of Representatives Select Committee on Aging. *Elder Abuse: The Hidden Problem.* Washington, D.C.: U.S. House of Representatives, June 23, 1979.

Wilkens, E.M. *Clinical Practice of Dental Hygienist* (4th ed.). Philadelphia: Lea and Febiger, 1976, pp. 577–595.

Witte, N.S. Why the elderly fall. *American Journal of Nursing* 79(11):1950–1952 (November 1979).

Wolanin, M.O. and Phillips, L.R.F. *Confusion: Prevention and Care.* St. Louis: C.V. Mosby, 1981, pp. 128–134.

39
Long Term Care: Discharge Planning, Home Care, and Alternatives

Bernita M. Steffl
Imogene Eide

The professional nurse is responsible for and accountable to the patient for the quality of nursing care, and as an integral part of that nursing care, every professional nurse has the responsibility to plan for the continuity of care for the patient.

American Nurses' Association (1975)

Long term care is more than institutional care. It is the total network of health and social services provided to the chronically ill and "frail elderly" in institutional settings, day care centers, congregate living arrangements, senior centers, foster homes, and in the private homes of individuals. For too long the whole concept has been suffering from an identity crisis in that the lay public and, unfortunately, many professionals have tended to associate the concept of long term care only with skilled nursing home care (Koff, 1981, Monohan and Greene, 1981).

Brody and Masciocchi (1980) in a distillation and synthesis of several studies regarding provision of a data base for long term care planning, concluded that long term care planning is currently based on skilled nursing facility (SNF) utilization rates and that this limited focus is inappropriate and the data are inconclusive. They said that population-based data, including levels of function, age, and living arrangements of those in need of extended support, would provide a more useful approach.

Long term care is usually precipitated by an episode in an acute care setting. How well patients fare depends on the quality of discharge planning for continuity of care in the most appropriate and desirable setting. This chapter addresses long term care with the philosophy of support via a multidisciplinary teamwork ap-

proach to keep patients in their own homes as long as possible. The three major components described are: (1) discharge planning, (2) home care, and (3) alternatives to home care.

DISCHARGE PLANNING

Discharge planning is the term given to the centralized, coordinated program that has been developed by a health care institution to ensure that each patient has a planned program for needed continuing care (Steffl and Eide, 1978). The American Nurses' Association (ANA) describes discharge planning as "the part of the continuity of care process which is designed to prepare the patient for the next phase of care, and to assist him in making the necessary arrangements for it whether it be self care, care by family, or care by an organized health care provider" (ANA, 1975). McKeehan has defined discharge planning as the process of activities that involve the patient and a team of individuals from various disciplines working together to facilitate the transition of that patient from one environment to another (McKeehan, 1980). Although these three definitions vary in approach, they share a commonality in process for coordinated efforts to assure patients of the necessary care as they move up, down, or out of the health care system.

Purpose and Scope of Discharge Planning

The purpose of discharge planning is to ensure comprehensive, coordinated, continuity of care when patients are discharged from any level of care or facility to another facility or home to self-care. Figure 39-1 represents a conceptual

498

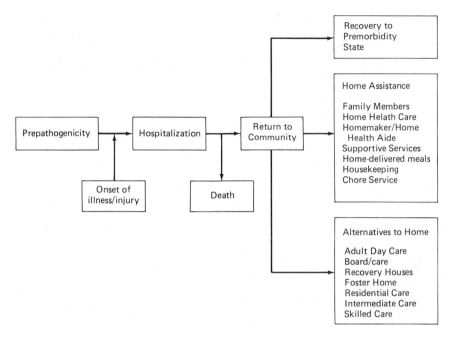

Figure 39-1. Continuity of care.

continuum of patient progression with implications for discharge planning.

The Professional Standards Review Organization was established in 1972 to assure the public that health care would be provided in the most appropriate setting. This federally funded program mandates discharge planning through a utilization review process which attempts to set some limits on expected number of hospital days during the acute phase of various illnesses. The criteria are so limiting that the elderly, in particular, are frequently unable to manage their own care at the time of discharge (Stewart, 1979). The Joint Commission on Accreditation for Hospitals (JCAH) continues to include in its standards a requirement for discharge planning as part of total patient care.

Implementation and Professional Roles

These authors favor a plan which calls for an assigned coordinator and routine discharge planning conferences that include a multidisciplinary team, patient, and family if possible. The size and composition of the team will depend on the patient's diagnosis, prognosis, and constraints of the agency. No one discipline can know all the facts, and the process cannot take place without information sharing among members of the team. In particular, the physician's plan for treatment, expected outcome, and anticipated date of discharge must be known. Table 39-1 is an abbreviated description of roles and functions of discharge planning team members, adapted from more detailed descriptions by Steffl and Eide (1978); David, Hanser, Madden, and Pratt (1973); and Bristow and Stickney (1974).

In a recent survey of 14 hospitals, the most structured model had a discharge planner designated with responsibilities for patient care beyond the hospitalization period. The presence of a discharge planner had a positive effect on interaction between the hospital and referral agencies. This positive feedback supports the value of a specifically assigned discharge planner in establishing helpful community networks (Reichelt and Newcomb, 1980).

Operational Requirements

Implementation of discharge planning will depend on the quality and timeliness of the

Table 39-1. Professional Roles in Discharge Planning.

Coordinator

The coordinator is a program planner who implements, facilitates, and evaluates discharge planning. The coordinator also needs to be an advocate, crusader, mediator, and counselor.

Physician

The physician is a key person. His orders and medical directions are the most essential ingredients in discharge planning. His role is twofold: he informs the patient of his diagnosis and possible risks in treatment, and he predicts outcomes and expected changes in life-style.

Hospital Nurse

Nurses who serve a role in discharge planning are usually head nurses or team leaders on the unit. Nurses have more direct contact with patients than other team members, so they are in a key position to obtain input from the patient and staff for the discharge planning conference.

Social Worker

The social worker assists with the social, emotional, and economic problems related to illness or injury; concentrates on the whole person; and facilitates and counsels about the utilization of community resources. Illness or injury which persists for any length of time may disrupt family functioning, and therapeutic and preventive assistance from a social worker may prevent family breakdown.

Dietitian and/or Nutritionist

Dietitians and nutritionists are assessors, teachers, counselors, and interpreters. They are often researchers and always important team members. The dietitian or nutritionist has a specific role for patients in any setting.

Physical Therapist, Occupational Therapist, and Speech Therapist

The physical, occupational, and speech therapists collect and disseminate information to and from the physician and other members of the discharge planning team, pertinent to a realistic program and plan of discharge for the patient and for posthospital follow-up care.

Community Health Nurse

A community health care nurse, or a visiting nurse from a home care agency, acts as the patient advocate and liaison to provide continuity of care in the patient's home. She is also a planner, facilitator, implementer, evaluator, and personal counselor for the patient and a support person for the family. She may come to the hospital for discharge planning conferences prior to the patient's discharge, make home assessments, and serve as the hospital's (medical) link to the family.

planning conference, the quality and quantity of input from team members (listed on Table 39-1), and the quality and quantity of evaluation. The essential components of discharge planning are philosophical commitment, administrative sanction, support and direction, functional objectives, policies and procedures, sound managerial strategies, and ongoing evaluation. According to Bristow (1974), evaluation should answer the following questions. Is this plan:

realistic → obtainable → economical
functional → efficient → organized
flexible → effective → productive?

Research on Discharge Planning

Though still limited, more research and publications on discharge planning are appearing; several monographs, books, and a number of journal articles by nurses have appeared since 1973. Most have been referred to in this chapter and are available at libraries.

Health care planners and hospital administrators, spurred by the need for cost containment, have produced the most literature and research on discharge planning. Johnson and Pachano (1981) recently developed a tool to survey a selected population in a 220-bed community hospital to more clearly define present discharge planning efforts and to assess whether patients were satisfied with education received prior to discharge. A summary of the study which included nurses and patients indicated that the discharge planning was satisfactory even though not initiated until the final stage of the patient's hospital stay.

A new quarterly called *Discharge Planning Update: An Interdisciplinary Perspective for Health Professionals,* edited by Suzanne Z. Deutsch, M.S.W. and Mary Ross, R.N., M.S., and published by the American Hospital Association, promises to provide readers with current trends, literature, and legislation on discharge planning.

Nursing Implications

Nurses have more and closer contacts with patients than most members of the health team.

Their education and clinical practice provide specific skills in biopsychosocial assessment, particularly in assessment of physical status, self-care ability, pain tolerance and control, and medication regimes and compliance. See Table 39-2 for a description of the different factors that nurses assess for discharge planning.

Nursing education overlaps with that of social workers and other disciplines so the roles and functions of other team members will overlap with nursing roles. Nurses are in a unique position to recognize overlapping. They have the opportunity to point out that some aspects of overlap may be advantageous and to promote a positive dovetailing of roles, functions, and responsibilities (Steffl and Eide, 1981; Tulga, 1981).

Nurses involved in discharge planning and community practice are expected to have some knowledge, understanding, and sensitivity to cultures and ethnic values. The following case history illustrates cultural influence and a nurse's reaction:

A 90-year-old Yaqui Indian (native American) presented herself at the emergency room with a fractured arm and lacerations about the face. Sutures placated the lacerations, and a cast was applied to the arm. The patient was instructed to return the following day for a cast inspection. An astute nurse in her assessment of the patient realized that this patient might not return and immediately made a telephone referral to the community health nurse. A day later the community health nurse arrived at the patient's home and found the patient with cast removed and arm heavily coated with a thick grease. The sutures had been removed and replaced with a poultice of herbs. The community health nurse did not alter the treatment, but observed for pain and infection, and kept the emergency room staff aware of the patient's progress.

More crises in patient care occur at discharge than at admission, yet Reichelt and Newcomb (1981) found in their study that staff nurses in particular are uncertain about how to accomplish discharge planning.

Table 39-2. What Does the Nurse Assess for Discharge Planning and Home Care?

PHYSICAL AND BIOLOGICAL STATUS	PSYCHOLOGICAL STATUS	SOCIOECONOMIC STATUS
Day-to-day physical changes	Sensory alterations and deficits	General financial status, eligibilities
Vital signs, integument, hydration, nutritional behavior, and cultural differences	Vision and hearing	Relationships
	Cognitive functioning	Significant others
	Confusion and disorientation	Family
Bowel and bladder continence	Communication abilities	Widow/widower
Elimination patterns	Coping capacities and strategies, past and present	Support systems
Mobility, level of mastery of self-care	Health teaching needs	Available
		Accessible
Activities of daily living	Knowledge and understanding of condition	Home assessment
Supplies for treatment and care	Family needs – problems	Environmental
Adaptive equipment needed	Counseling needs	Economic
Durable medical equipment needed		Transportation needs
Pain, tolerance and control		
Medication regime		
Compliance		
Therapeutic response		
Contraindications		
Adverse reactions		
Rest and sleep patterns		

RESOURCES AND REFERRALS NEEDED, PRESENT AND FUTURE

NOTE: Some of these assessments are unique to nursing, but most will dovetail with assessments of other professional team members. Reprinted with permission from *Discharge Planning Update* 1(2):4 (1981).

A Philosophy of Teamwork*

To be part of a team means one must be extremely well prepared in his own field, that he must see himself in relation to the contributions of others; that he must sense the constantly changing needs of the individuals whom he and the group are serving; that he must accept the corresponding changes in his contributions and the contribution of the other team members to those needs; that he must have the courage to say what he can do and why he feels that he can do one thing better than another; that he must have the grace to give up what he likes to do if another one can do it better. It means further, that he must learn to do things which do not come too easily, if they can be done best by him for the good of all. It means the will to pull with others and the integrity to withdraw from those parts of an undertaking which are not his. It means the enduring belief that together we can do things which no one of us individually could do alone, and that the togetherness makes possible a concept of the job which is greater than the sum of the individual parts. It functions well or ill depending on the success with which the team has consciously accepted its teamship.

Anonymous

HOME CARE

Home care is that component of comprehensive health care whereby services are provided to individuals and families in their places of residence for the purpose of promoting, maintaining, or restoring health, or minimizing the effects of illness and disability. Services appropriate to the needs of the individual patient and family are planned, coordinated, and made available by an agency/institution or unit of an agency/institution organized for the delivery of health care through the use of employed staff, contractual arrangements, or a combination of administrative patterns.

Home care services are provided under a plan of care that includes, but is not limited to, appropriate service components such as medical

*Reprinted with permission from Steffl, B.M. and Eide, I. *Discharge Planning Handbook.* Thorofare, N.J.: C.B. Slack, 1978.

care, dental care, nursing, physical therapy, respiratory therapy, speech therapy, occupational therapy, social work, nutrition, homemaker/home health aide, transportation, laboratory services, and medical equipment and supplies (National Association of Home Health Agencies, 1980). This definition has been accepted by a wide variety of professionals representing national agencies and organizations.

Traditionally, health care professionals have tended to refer to home health care as an alternative to institutional care. These authors believe that this thinking needs to be turned around: there should be a stronger commitment to keeping patients in their own home as long as possible, and other settings should be considered as alternatives to home care (Eide, 1980). Consumers and health care providers are sharing a marked revival of interest in home health care for economic and humanitarian reasons. For example, more people are opting to die at home now than in the past several decades (Stewart, 1979). Philip Brickner, M.D., Director of the New York Chelsea Village Home Care Program, states that a successful home health care program achieves two major purposes: (1) it helps to keep older people in their home, and (2) it meets the needs of society at large through cost effectiveness (Brickner, 1978).

Most of us would choose to remain in our own homes rather than being placed in a long term care facility. Why then are people placed in institutions when they could be maintained at home? The status of the elderly in our country, ageism, and our youth-oriented society are all reasons why we "put old people away." However, the overriding reason is financial. Medicare (Title XVIII) and Medicaid (Title XIX) support the cost of nursing home care but not home care for chronically disabled older people (Brickner, 1978). This has become a national issue because of the current concern with skyrocketing health care costs and national efforts toward cost containment. (Haltiwanger, 1982)

As of August 1981, there were approximately 3000 home health agencies in the United States, all of which were struggling for survival. Most were located in urban areas, leaving rural areas underserved. Almost half were government operated. We hope that voting consumers, specifically those over age 60 and their families, will demand more support and training services for home care from legislators and professionals, particularly physicians. Though quality home care costs money, home health care is cost effective when targeted to groups most in need. (Brickner, 1981; Government Accounting Office, 1977) (Skellie, Mobley and Coan 1982)

There are many successful models of home care projects throughout the country. Most share a common philosophy with the following basic principles (Sklar and Zawadski, 1981):

- Dependent adults want, and should be allowed, to remain in their own homes and community as long as it is medically, socially, and economically feasible.
- The problems facing the long term care, needy adult are multiple and interrelated; social isolation and malnutrition have a direct impact on health.
- An adequate response must consider the whole individual.
- Coordination of services must include control over their delivery.
- Comprehensive single source funding at the program level is essential for delivery of cost effective long term care.
- Quality long term care is affordable within present day per capita budget restraints.

Specific standards of care and patient's rights have been adapted to home care (see Appendix D).

Types of Patients for Home Care

There are no limitations on the type and age of patients suitable for home health care. The two main criteria used to predict whether or not a patient is a good candidate for home care are (1) an adequate and willing support system and (2) an environment conducive to maximum recovery and rehabilitation. Home care agencies serve (1) patients needing acute short term care, (2) patients with chronic disease who need rehabilitation and/or health maintenance assis-

tance, and (3) terminally ill patients who wish to die at home. The following are examples of each:

1. Mrs. Lopez, age 72, was discharged from the hospital five days postcholecystectomy to her home where she lived alone. She was able to manage her own activities of daily living. Through discharge planning, home health care was requested for the following: (1) daily dressing changes until the wound healed or the patient could manage the necessary care, and (2) diet counseling and assistance with food preparation. Mrs. Lopez received 12 visits over a three-week period, after which she was discharged from home health care. The availability of home care reduced her hospital stay and prevented extended care.

2. Olga Thompson, aged 75, lives alone in her mobile home. She has chronic obstructive pulmonary disease, and has been extremely emphysematous for ten years and on continuous oxygen for the past five years. This lady does her own housework and with a portable O_2 tank drives to the market and to her clinic visits. She receives home care visits once a month except when her condition is exacerbated. She has been hospitalized only for two short periods in the past five years, even though she has had numerous exacerbations including a severe bout with the flu this past year. Olga states, "I would not be here if it weren't for visits from my nurse, the aide, and Tom [respiratory therapist]." This patient's home care services fall in the category of health maintenance and are not reimbursed by Medicare or any third party payer. She is medically indigent, so her care is a public responsibility. It should be evident that this kind of care is costing the taxpayer less than institutionalization, and is helping the patient to remain independent and in her own home (see Figure 39-2).

3. Jacob Blaugh, aged 60, a terminal cancer patient diagnosed as having cancer of the lung with extensive metastases, requested to die at home without heroic measures. He was referred to home care for pain control and optimal maintenance of bodily functions. He lived one month relatively free of pain, nausea, and vomiting. He was rational and in control of his life to

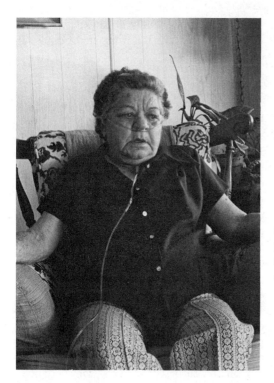

Figure 39-2. Olga Thompson is totally dependent on home health care services to provide continuous oxygen therapy which she has been taught to manage by herself for five years. (Photo courtesy of Maricopa County Health Services.)

the end. He died at home with his wife at his bedside. Approximately 2–3 home visits a week were made by either the nurse, the social worker, or the home health aide. A hospice volunteer, arranged for by the home care team, also assisted the patient and family with visits which continued through the bereavement period.

Home health care nursing visits are often challenging. The following case example illustrates the need for acceptance and understanding of the feelings and behaviors of elderly individuals by the care givers.

Case Example. Mr. Branham, aged 70, has been receiving home oxygen therapy for the past year. He is not always compliant with medical orders. He has been emphysematous for many years and knows that at this time he can sustain only a poor quality of living with almost continuous oxygen. The home health care team, particularly the nurse and the respiratory therapist, assist him in

regulating his oxygen, monitoring medications, and maintaining adequate diet and hydration. His overwhelming helplessness and the hopeless prospects of reversal of his condition are difficult for him to cope with. In addition to episodes of noncompliance, Mr. Branham refuses to quit smoking. His anger often comes out during the nurse's home visits; see Figures 39-3 and 39-4.

Research in Home Health Care

Research in all aspects of home care has been sparse and inadequate. It has been said that studies to date have provided only mixed, partial, and largely indirect findings with respect to the impact of provision of home-based care on rates of institutionalization (Dunlop, 1980; Skellie et al., 1982).

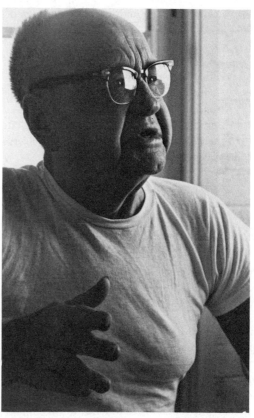

Figure 39-3. Mr. Branham needs almost constant oxygen therapy. He is frequently exasperated and upset because of his immobility and restricted life-style. (Photo courtesy of Maricopa County Health Services.)

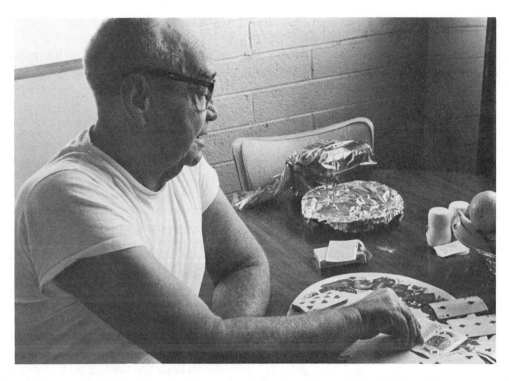

Figure 39-4. By the time the home health nurse leaves, Mr. Branham usually feels better. (Photo courtesy of Maricopa County Health Services.)

In a study of the role of public health nurses in evaluating services needed by the elderly in addition to those which were available, two nurses and 124 individuals over age 65 evaluated the situation. Findings indicated agreement on six of the top ten services most needed. These were ambulance service, hospital service, access to physicians, nursing and custodial homes, services of public health nurses or visiting nurses, and homemaker/home health aide services (Keith, 1976). Interestingly the clients rated the need for more nursing higher than the nurses did.

There have been some research attempts at measuring and projecting the demand for home health care. Professionals perceive a need for expanded home care, but this need must be converted into effective demand. Berry (1980) suggested that individuals be better educated about the benefits, thus influencing home care referrals and decreasing disincentives.

In a study to examine communication services in home health care agencies, the researchers found that although the prevalence and social consequences of communication disorders among the community-based elderly remain unidentified and the public appears to be unaware of this, many home health care programs offer speech, language, and hearing rehabilitation services (Lubinsky and Chapley, 1980).

Nursing Implications

The first implication of course, is that nurses must be educated in the basic principles, knowledge, and skills of community health nursing. Secondly, it would be helpful for nurses to have specific courses in working with, and understanding the feelings and behaviors of, older people and a more firm foundation in rehabilitation and chonic disease than most now receive in their basic education. Thirdly, it appears that nurses need to take a more active role as advocates, assessors, and intervenors for home care. That is, they simply must assume more responsibility for comprehensive, coordinated continuity of care.

Nurses cannot divorce themselves from the scandals frequently reported by the press, which describe the warehousing and neglect of the frail and ill elderly, because they are in key positions to facilitate discharge planning and home care rather than institutionalization when appropriate. They can make unique contributions to the health team, especially in the realm of day-to-day health assessment. See Table 39-2 for a description of what the nurse should be prepared to assess, document, implement, and evaluate on a periodic basis.

ALTERNATIVES TO HOME CARE

Nursing Homes

What is it that we dread so about nursing homes? Perhaps it is the ominous feeling that this is the end of the road which frightens us so, along with fear of being at the mercy of strangers for very personal needs. Dr. Clifford Bennett, who became a patient so he could document what professionals might do better, states that it is the little things which go unnoticed by planners that impinge so forcefully on residents. The following are some of the most painful indignities identified by Bennett (1980), with additions by Steffl and Eide (1981):

- The humiliating shower procedures
- The misery that rational patients (who are the majority) feel when compelled to associate endlessly with irrational and confused persons
- The intimidating effects of huge impersonal places with long corridors
- The small rooms for patients (without room for even two chairs) which preclude bringing the most meaningful possessions from home
- The inhibiting wheelchair
- The lack of privacy
- The limited contact with the outside world (lack of newspapers, radios, and telephones)
- Having to give up most choices regarding food and how it is served
- The interminable noise
- Staff discussion and personal conversations which totally ignore the patient during patient care
- The difficulty of getting to a telephone

The term "nursing home" is a misnomer in many instances. Facilities for provision of institutional long term care range from resident facilities which provide only assistance with personal care to skilled care facilities which are, in a literal sense, the nursing homes. It is extremely important for professionals and the lay public to know the difference between these levels of care because of cost and socialization potential in the placement of clients.

For example, Mrs. B., a professional woman in her 50s, works full time as a teacher and has one child who is in high school left at home. Her mother, aged 80, who has lived with her for years, has in the past two years deteriorated mentally and takes to slipping out of the house in the wee hours of the morning and wandering for miles. She has become increasingly combative and difficult for the family to manage. She is healthy and strong as an athlete, takes no medications, and eats well. With great reluctance, the family has decided that "we can no longer manage mother and we need a nursing home."

This lady does not need skilled nursing home care. She needs only a protective environment, with activities and structured routines befitting her cognitive capabilities. Yet this family almost placed her in a skilled care facility where the rate was the same for all levels. We are very lacking in facilities to individualize care in this country. Instead of facilities meeting the needs of our elderly, the individual case has to fit into the limited categories of care which have been designated in the nursing home regulations promulgated by the various states. However, a trend which is underway nationally is the *Case Management Approach* which attempts to provide comprehensive, coordinated services and care for older individuals in the most appropriate setting and most convenient location for the client.

Nursing Implications. If Vernice Fergeson's* (1981) predictions come true, the nursing home setting will be a location of choice rather than compromise for nursing employment in the future. There are untapped opportunities for leadership, research, and demonstration of specialized bedside nursing care, and the status of gerontological nursing is destined to gain recognition (see Chapter 2 on nursing manpower). The following are some suggestions to assist nurses in advocacy, education, and service in a nursing home setting:

- Become familiar with the *Patients' Bill of Rights* (see Appendix A).
- Become knowledgeable regarding state rules and regulations for long term care facilities in your state.
- Become functionally knowledgeable about Medicare and Medicaid certification coverage and eligibility.
- Become knowledgeable about licensure and requirements of administrators of long term care facilities.
- Assess the long term care facility in regard to staffing and in-service training, individualized nursing care plans, and accountability procedures.
- Prepare to become involved in, and contribute to, nursing input with regard to food service, resident activities, environmental arrangements, and emergency procedures.

The American Hospital Association's Patients' Bill of Rights and other adaptations of patients' rights all recommend certain things a patient should expect, even demand, when hospitalized or institutionalized. Closer examination of these reveals that 75% of the rights involve exchange of information. It behooves the nurse to be prepared in patient education and communication skills (Bille, 1980; see also Chapter 7).

The nurse, particularly the community health nurse, should be prepared to assist clients and families in choosing a nursing

home. The U.S. Department of Health and Human Services (1980) has recently revised an excellent publication *How to Select a Nursing Home* (available from U.S. Superintendent of Documents, U.S. Government Printing Office, Washington, DC 20402). See Table 39-3 for a summary of questions to ask when selecting a long term care facility.

Multiservice Centers

There is a trend to expand service centers and nutrition sites into multiservice centers. Since funding for nutrition programs has changed somewhat in recent years and more funds are coming from Title XX, which mandates inclusion of social services, we are seeing the development of health screening, health maintenance, and health education programs, as well as many support service programs, which all aid in keeping our older citizens in their homes and active in their communities.

One such program is the Minneapolis Age and Opportunity Center (MAO). It exists to solve the problems of seniors, has been the subject of articles in major national publications, and is being observed as a model of health care by the U.S. Senate. It gives seniors the extra help, supportive services, and medical, financial, and moral support that permit them to maintain independence as long as possible and to maximize their quality of life. The services fall into three general categories of need: preventive, rehabilitative, and ongoing supportive. There are many economic and professional advantages to a centralized coordinating system such as MAO. Table 39-4 lists the scope of services offered by a multipurpose senior center (Minneapolis Age and Opportunity Center, 1981); see also Figure 39-5.

Day Care Centers

There are more than 600 day care programs for the elderly in the United States today, and the number is growing. The concept was imported from Great Britain where geriatric day hospitals were developed in the 1950s to provide therapeutic services for outpatients who were

---

*Director of Nursing, Veterans' Administration, Washington, D.C.

Table 39-3. Questions to Ask in Selecting a Long Term Care Facility.

1. Is the home licensed? Ask. If the answer is yes, ask to see the license.
2. Does the administrator have a current state license? Again, if the answer is yes, ask to see it.
3. Is the nursing home Medicare and Medicaid approved?
4. What other insurance plans are accepted?
5. How are residents' medical needs met? Who dispenses medications? What is the policy regarding physicians' visits? Does the nursing home have an arrangement with a nearby hospital to handle emergencies?
6. How often are fire drills held for staff and residents? Are there smoke detectors, fire extinguishers?
7. Are residents allowed to furnish their rooms with their own furniture? Can residents have their own radio or television?
8. Can a husband and wife share the same room? What are the provisions for privacy?
9. Does each resident have his own closet and chest of drawers?
10. Where is the residents' money kept? Are there provisions for personal banking services? Are accurate records kept of residents' financial transactions?
11. Is a phone readily available? Are there restrictions on making or receiving phone calls?
12. What are the visiting hours? Is the resident encouraged to visit friends and relatives outside the nursing home?
13. Are the residents encouraged to leave their rooms when able?
14. What is the capacity of the home? How many residents are presently there?
15. Is there a dining hall or do residents eat in their rooms? Are special diets available for those who need them? Is there a professional dietitian on the staff or available as a consultant? Visit at mealtime. Check the menu.
16. What types of activities are available to residents? Ask to see the schedule of activities.
17. Are there additional charges for personal laundry? Does therapy cost extra? If so, how much?
18. Can residents have alcohol?
19. Can residents smoke in their rooms if they are able to do so unsupervised? Are there other convenient places where smoking is permitted?
20. When was the last state or local inspection? You may want to see the most recent inspection report.
21. Are there environmental adaptations for wheelchairs? Are there hazards or obstacles for the handicapped?
22. Is the location convenient to family and friends; to other services?
23. Are patients' rights posted?
24. Do residents and staff look and act happy?
25. Does the atmosphere fit the life-style of the prospective resident?

NOTE: Adapted and revised from a number of standards and documents from sources such as the Illinois Council for Long Term Care and the U.S. Department of Health and Human Services Publication HCFA-30043-1980.

Table 39-4. Scope of Services of a Model Multipurpose Senior Center.

Home-delivered Meals	Chore Services
Home Care Services	Transportation
Special Health Services	Employment Services
Individual counseling	Legal Services
Therapy groups	Pharmacy
Grief therapy	Food Closet
Alcohol and chemical dependency	Telephone Reassurance Service
Facilitation of Health Services	Police Referral
Assistance with Medicare and Medicaid red tape	Chaplain Service
Dietary Consultation	24-hour Emergency Service
Diet Counseling	Library
Information and Referral Services	Liaison with Community Resources

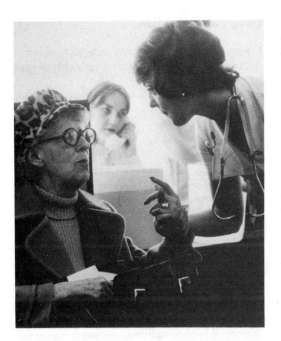

Figure 39-5. Nurses counsel clients by telephone and at the center at the Minneapolis Age and Opportunity Center. (Photo printed with permission of Daphne H. Krause, President of MAO.)

disabled and homebound, and who did not require full-time nursing care (Feingold, 1979).

Generally, day care centers provide supervision and care for older people who cannot be left entirely to their own devices. They offer therapeutic resocialization and companionship. A primary goal is to assist elderly persons in maintaining at least modified independence for as long as possible, to increase independent functioning with handicaps, to enhance abilities and individual uniqueness, to assist families of the frail elderly, and to delay institutionalization for as long as possible.

Most day care centers also offer federally funded nutrition programs at the site. The following are typical services:

Socialization	Recreation
Arts and crafts (individual and group)	Social programs and events
	Counseling
Discussion groups	Educational programs
Activities of daily living sessions	Noon meals and snacks
	Restful relaxation

Current trends in day care indicate an expansion of services in health maintenance programs such as health screening, client education, exercise, and physical fitness programs for preventive health maintenance. Also many centers have found it necessary and effective to increase nursing staff and service for professional assessment and ongoing day-to-day evaluation of the health status of clients.

Two major problems in day care, as seen by the authors, are funding and developing criteria for eligibility. To our knowledge, there is no third party payment allowed for day care in this country. Most are federally funded to some extent. Many have emerged and developed through church and private interest groups. The reader is referred to three unique model programs for creative and innovative ideas: Palmcrest House of Long Beach, California, under the direction of Dr. Julian F. Feingold; On LOK Senior Health Services Center of San Francisco, California, under the direction of Marie-Louise Ansak; and Sirrine Day Care Center of Mesa, Arizona, under the auspices of the Foundation for Senior Adult Living and the direction of Cindy Brennan.

Research on Day Care.   Several studies have addressed the question of cost effectiveness and whether we should be considering day care centers as alternatives to institutionalization. Some suggest we would be more realistic in recommending day care simply as an additional service in the long term care continuum (Wan, Weissert, and Livieratos, 1980; Weissert, Wan, Livieratos, and Katz, 1980). Feingold (1979) states that it is unrealistic and unfair to compare day care with institutions because the average age of today's nursing home patients is over 84: two-thirds of these require assistance with toileting, and fully one-half are incompetent. Many nursing home patients have little awareness of their surroundings and need to be fed, whereas day care clients are in their mid 70s and capable of much self-care and recreational activity. Feingold (1979) has written a magnificent in-depth appraisal of the day care situation in the face of austerity and competition for funding, and has emphasized the role of nonprofit agencies.

The authors found no evidence of nursing research on day care in the literature, but we believe that nurses are perhaps participating in projects and not publishing and/or are unaware of the opportunities for creative nursing leadership roles and research in day care centers for the elderly. A new book *Adult Day Care: A Practical Guide* by Carole O'Brian, published by Wadsworth Publishing Company in 1981, illustrates and analyzes models of day care.

Nursing Implications. The authors recall the early efforts to avoid a medical model and nurses on the staff of day care centers because "nurses will encourage a dependency and sick role with clients." Interestingly, as we predicted, experience has proved that nursing assessments and supervision are essential to providing day care. Most persons using day care centers are in their 70s and will have one or more chronic diseases which are under control but subject to conditional maintenance. Most are not all well or all sick at any one time and, therefore, will frequently need professional assessment. For example, the 70-year-old man who is hypertensive, diabetic, an amputee, and on insulin is a likely candidate for day care; however, his condition is likely to fluctuate with activities from day to day, and establishing a care plan for him requires professional nursing skills on a fairly regular basis.

Day care centers are unique and desirable for placement of student nurses for field practice. They provide excellent experiences in health appraisal, communication, health teaching, and group work.

Foster Home Care

Foster home care for the elderly in terms of a licensed industry is relatively new; however, in truth the old and homeless have lived in foster homes for decades. In most states, foster homes need to be licensed if they take in more than three or four persons. The concept is good, but to date few independent operators have been able to succeed without federal funding or endowments. The advantage, of course, is the family atmosphere and participation of the client in family life.

Co-op Living Arrangements

Co-ops are also a relatively new alternative in living arrangements for older individuals in need of some help and environmental protection. A co-op for the elderly in Phoenix, Arizona, rents small single or double apartments to seniors with the following provisions:

WE	YOU
Serve the main meal	Keep your kitchen privileges
Furnish all groceries	Make your personal list
Do heavy cleaning	Enjoy light housekeeping
Plan activities	Join in – if you wish
Supply nice people	Enjoy their company

FINANCIAL ARRANGEMENTS	
Membership fee	$100.00
Private bedroom	$350.00
(Rates subject to change)	

Multilevel Care Facilities

The most attractive options in long term care are nonprofit and proprietary agencies which offer levels of care in a continuum ranging from apartments, structured room and board (lodge concept), to skilled nursing home care. The facilities are usually in a community grounds area or high rise which features apartments with a 24-hour emergency call system, laundry facilities and service, weekly housekeeping services, a noon or evening meal, recreational facilities, and transportation. The protective environment and security are most reassuring to older couples, widows, and other singles, and provide peace of mind for their children.

Though many of these have been developed to meet the needs of middle-income people, the cost is still prohibitive for many of the elderly. Nursing care, health teaching, and preventive health maintenance are key ingredients in these communities. This type of setting, along with many long term care settings, is finding that nurse practitioners are very helpful members of the care team. Nurses and social workers are the key assessors and intervenors in these settings.

Congregate Living

To date there is not even an estimate available about the number of innovative communal or congregate living arrangements proposed for and by older adults, but we can expect to hear more about them and to see more develop. Elderly widows who try to hold on to and maintain a large home constitute perhaps one of the most vulnerable groups, who might benefit from congregate living in a home versus giving up a home altogether.

A pilot project called Senior Village is underway in Phoenix, Arizona, where seven houses will accommodate 38 persons and a live-in caretaker. Health service programs will be used to assist with home health care, support care, heavy cleaning, yard work, and window washing. This program is for indigent and semi-indigent persons, and is a joint effort of the state of Arizona and Maricopa County.

SUMMARY

In this chapter the authors have attempted to briefly describe long term care needs and services with implications for nursing. In their view (perhaps biased), the major components of quality long term care are (1) discharge planning with a multidisciplinary approach, (2) provision of home health services to keep the elderly client at home as long as possible, and (3) provision of creative and innovative alternatives when the person can no longer remain in his home.

The Federal Council on Aging continues to work on the development of recommendations for a national policy on long term care, particularly with respect to costs and who should bear them from a health and social perspective (Federal Council on Aging, 1979). The American Academy of Nursing (1976) has taken a strong stand in its declaration that by and large, long term care is a neglected area; it proposes that nursing assume major responsibility for health promotion, maintenance, and teaching within the context of its definition of long term care:

Long-term care is the provision of that range of services — physical, psychological, spiritual, and social, including economic — needed to help people attain, maintain, or regain their optimum level of functioning. It includes health maintenance throughout the life span as well as care during acute and protracted

illness and disability. Such care is the legitimate province of nurses who now are making social contributions through health teaching and promotion, prevention of illness, and rehabilitation.

Also, the American Nurses' Association continues to develop its leadership role in promoting and advocating improved long term care for older individuals through the Division of Gerontological Nursing standards of practice and gerontological nurse certifications program (see Appendix B and C). Finally, in November 1981, the White House Conference on Aging in Washington, D.C., addressed long term care and formulated recommendations on a national level.

REFERENCES

American Academy of Nursing, American Nurses' Association. A.N.A. Publication Code No. G-120 2M, p. 3 (April 1976).

American Nurses' Association. *Continuity of care and discharge planning programs in institutions and community agencies.* Publication Code HP-49, **3000**:3 (1975).

American Nurses' Association. *Summary of proceedings of A.N.A. House of Delegates, 49th Convention.* Publication Code G-117-1500 (1975).

American Nurses' Association, Committee on Long Term Care. *Nursing and long-term care: toward quality care for the aging.* Publication Code No. GE-4 3M, pp. 1–87 (April 1975).

Bennett, C. *Nursing Home Life: What It Is and What It Could Be.* New York: Tiresias Press, 1980.

Berry, N.J. Projecting demand for home health care in one health service area. *Home Health Review* **3**(3): 23–27 (September 1980).

Bille, D.A. Educational strategies for teaching the elderly patient. *Nursing and Health Care* **1**:256–260 (December 1980).

Brickner, P.W. Long term home health care for the aged: the program of St. Vincent's Hospital, New York City. *Generations* **5**(3):36–41 (1981).

Bristow, O. and Stickney, C. *Discharge Planning for Continuity of Care.* Richmond, Va.: Virginia Regional Medical Program, 1974, pp. 51–71.

Brody, S.J. and Masciocchi, C. Data for long term care planning. *American Journal of Public Health* **70**(11):1194–1198 (1980).

David, J.H., Hanser, J.E., Madden, B.W., and Pratt, M.K. *Guidelines for Discharge Planning* (rev. ed.). Thorofare, N.J.: Charles B. Slack, 1973, pp. 26–44.

Dunlop, B.D. Expanded home-based care for the impaired elderly: solution or pipe dream. *American Journal of Public Health* **70**(5):514–518 (1980).

Eide, G. Home care for the elderly. In Burnside, I.M. (Ed.) *Psychosocial Nursing Care of the Aged* (2nd ed.). New York: McGraw-Hill, 1980, pp. 87–99.

Federal Council on Aging. *Annual Report.* Washington, D.C.: 1979, p. 25.

Feingold, J. Adult day care. *Nursing Homes* (September–October 1979).

Fergeson, V. Future Directions in Nursing Care of the Aged, Speech presented at International Conference on Nursing Care of the Aged, University of Calif. Extension Division. Biltmore Hotel, Los Angeles, Calif. June 26, 1981.

Government Accounting Office. *Comptroller General's Report to Congress on Home Health Care — The Need for a National Policy to Better Provide for the Elderly* (H.R.D.-78-19). Washington, D.C.: December 30, 1977, pp. 14–19.

Haltiwanger, J.K. Home health services and nursing home care — are they competing factions or unique entities? *Nursing Homes* (January–February 1982).

Johnson, J. and Pachano, A. Planning patient's discharge. *Supervisor Nurse* 12(2):44–50 (1981).

Joint Commission on Accreditation of Hospitals. *Accreditation Manual for Hospitals.* Chicago: 1980, p. XV.

Keith, P.M. A preliminary investigation of the role of the public health nurse in evaluation of services for the aged. *American Journal of Public Health* 66(4): 379–380 (1976).

Koff, T. Long term care. *Generations* 5(3):4 (1981).

Lubinsky, R. and Chapley, R. Communication services in home health care agencies: availability and scope. *American Speech and Hearing Association Journal* 22(11):929–934 (1980).

McKeehan, K.M. (Ed.). *Continuing Care: A Multidisciplinary Approach to Discharge Planning.* St. Louis: C.V. Mosby, 1980.

Minneapolis Age and Opportunity Center, Inc. *Brochure.* Minneapolis, Minn.: 1981.

Monohan, D.J. and Greene, V.L. Long term care: concepts and definitions. *Generations* 5(3):6–9 (1981).

National Association of Home Health Agencies, Policy Statement on Health Care, Washington, D.C.: 1980, p. 1–2.

Reichelt, P.A. and Newcomb, J. Organizational factors in discharge planning. *Journal of Nursing Administration* 10(12):36–42 (1980).

Skellie, F.A., Mobley, G.M., and Coan, R.E. Cost effectiveness of community-based long-term care: current findings of Georgia's alternative health services project. *AJPH* 72(4):353–357 (1982).

Sklar, B.W. and Zawadski, R.T. Comprehensive, coordinated community based care. *Generations* 14–16 (Spring 1981).

Steffl, B. and Eide, I. *Discharge Planning Handbook.* Thorofare, N.J.: Charles B. Slack, 1978, pp. 1, 20.

Steffl, B. and Eide, I. Comprehensive assessment: the heart of discharge planning. *A Nursing Perspective, Discharge Planning Update* 4 (Winter 1981).

Stewart, J.E. *Home Health Care.* St. Louis: C.V. Mosby, 1979.

Tulga, G. Bridging the gap between hospital and home. *Aspen Systems Corporation,* 0160–6379 (1981).

U.S. Department of Health and Human Services. *How to Select a Nursing Home* (Publication No. HCFA-30043). Washington, D.C.: Health Care Financing Administration 1970, 55 pp.

Wan, T., Weissert, W.G., and Livieratos, B.B. Geriatric day care and homemaker services: an experimental study. *Journal of Gerontology* 35(2):256–274 (1980).

Weissert, W., Wan, T., Livieratos, B.B., and Katz, S. Effects and costs of day care services for the chronically ill. *Medical Care* 18(6):567–584 (1980).

40
Research in Gerontological Nursing

Lida F. Thompson
Bernita M. Steffl

I hope most ardently that in nursing we cherish the "poets" among us – the visionaries – those sensitive to universal needs as well as those who are the technically proficient – and I hope that we encourage the research that is most likely, if applied, to result in the greatest good for the greatest number.

Virginia Henderson (1977)

Research on aging has tended to focus on the area of molecular biology. The reasons for this are many, among them the fact that there is great interest in the human time clock and what controls it. Also application of research methodology is less difficult in the natural sciences than in the social and behavioral settings where the interface between the research process and the older person needs to be manipulated.

Considerable progress has been made in the past decade in the broad field of gerontological research as well as in the amount of nursing research report in the literature. Unfortunately, however, research in *gerontological nursing* by nurse researchers has been slow in developing. In this chapter we will review the status of research in gerontological nursing including a discussion of certain deficits and problems which exist in the field. An annotated listing of research by nurses from 1975 through 1981, as well as references to sources listing research of all kinds pertaining to the aged, will offer a broad overview of existing and potential researchable problems. Finally, there is a brief discussion of priority needs to stimulate interest in practice-oriented gerontological nursing research problems.

BACKGROUND

In 1979, Brimmer offered excellent quantitative data documenting an encouragingly steady increase in publications on gerontological subjects devoted to nursing. From only 2 of 379 articles listed in the *International Nursing Index* in 1966, that number had grown to 63 out of 296 in 1971. In 1976, a full 27% of the 416 publications listed were under the heading of gerontological nursing. While this is an encouraging trend, when measured against the total publications of nursing topics gerontological nursing remains an area which calls for increased emphasis (Brimmer, 1979).

In a recent, exceptional report and analysis of gerontological nursing research needs, Kayser-Jones (1981) pinpoints two major issues and goals of gerontological nursing research: (1) to provide a sound basis for the practice of gerontological nursing, and (2) ultimately, to improve the quality of care for the aged. Along with others, she emphasizes the fact that "nursing research studies on aging will not be augmented until there are adequate numbers of nurses prepared to conduct such research." Her analysis of the need for nursing research to investigate the mental health care needs of the aged and of the lack of adequate professional (nurses and doctors) leadership or accountability for the state of care of the aged in this country, offers excellent direction for the interest and talent of nurses that undoubtedly exist in our society (Kayser-Jones, 1981).

DEFICITS AND PROBLEMS IN GERONTOLOGICAL NURSING RESEARCH

Certain recurrent problems and deficits in the body of gerontological nursing research published to date become evident to the reader. These include a lack of consistency in research methodologies, the absence in many cases of identified conceptual models and theoretical

513

frameworks, an imbalance toward samples of institutionalized elderly who constitute a small percentage of the total aged population, the use of samples too small to allow generalization from the data, and a near absence of the replication of studies.

Methodologies

Strumpf (1978) stated succinctly, "Studies of aging ... have been no exception to helter skelter research methods, namely, the gathering and interpretation of data without adequate conceptual models and theoretical frameworks." Robinson (1981) decries the same lack of underlying theoretical framework, pointing out the necessity of such a methodology if the findings are to be related and integrated into a scientific knowledge base for nursing practice. Gunter and Miller (1977) suggest that consistency must emerge in operational definitions and methodologies to offer the potential for comparing as well as replicating studies.

Research Emphasis on Institutionalized Elderly

Review of the gerontological nursing research published to date reveals a severe imbalance toward problems revolving around institutionalization, rather than concern for the more than 90% of our aged population who live in the community. There is, however, an increase in the utilization of samples drawn from senior centers, nutrition programs for the elderly, and the like.

Concern with the skew toward institutionalized patients should not be interpreted as indicating that there is not an acute need for more research among that population. Indeed, there is a crucial need for clinical research which can demonstrate ways to improve nursing care of the frail elderly, in or outside institutional settings.

Research Emphasis on Attitudes

As nursing researchers became more active in the area of gerontological nursing problems, one of the chief concerns which evolved regarded the attitudes of nurses toward aging and the

aged. Indeed, this is and will doubtless remain an area of top priority since attitudes pervade every aspect of improved gerontological nursing care (see Chapter 3). Several questions have been raised recently, however, about these studies as a whole (Strumpf and Mezey, 1980). Are attitude studies reliable? Discussion in the literature give evidence of the need for more refined measurement scales with greater statistical reliability.

Is the quality of nursing care of the aged patient actually affected by the attitudes of the care givers toward the elderly? This assumption has been accepted, but a question can be raised about the validity of using such studies to judge behavioral outcomes. The failure to differentiate between attitudes toward the sick and the well elderly also raises a question regarding how far we can accurately generalize attitude surveys and assume their correlation with the behavioral intentions of care givers.

Problems not well publicized but of increasing interest and concern are the ethical and methodological issues related to the use of the frail elderly as controls in applied research settings. A technical report (1981) on this subject from On Lok Community Care Organization in San Francisco describes the dilemmas and offers some solutions such as building into research proposals and projects some "limited service" components in order to protect the well-being of the vulnerable control group participants. For further information, contact Cathleen Yordi, On Lok Senior Health Service, 1455 Bush St., San Francisco, CA 94109.

Research and Quality Assurance

Current methods to measure quality of care, such as peer review and study of patient outcomes, still need a great deal of refinement. The focus tends to be on benefits of cost effectiveness for the institution rather than the needs of the patient. Because nurses have not been very involved in clinical research, do not perceive themselves as researchers, and frequently lack basic education in gerontological theory and research, they tend to rely on undependable information as a basis for action and to trust (more or less) their intuitive personal values. Intuitive care may in some cases be excellent and very meaningful. However, when intuition fails we must have a design or plan based on tested theory on which we can fall back. In other words, our belief is that nurses who are prepared with a design or tested plan will be able to provide more scientifically based care to more patients all of the time, not just when intuition and experience hold (see Chapter 3).

AN ORGANIZATIONAL FRAMEWORK FOR GERONTOLOGICAL NURSING RESEARCH REPORTS

An invaluable resource for the individual interested in gerontological nursing research is the work of Robinson (1981) in which the author offers a comprehensive survey of the state of the art. Her identification and classification of the substantive areas from which research problems derive offer a workable organizational frame which is a step toward a standard classification. This organizational framework will be followed here with the addition of one category to include a group of studies whose primary concern is with research tools and methodologies.

The absence of a standard identification of substantive areas is revealed readily to the researcher who attempts a computer search for gerontological nursing research reports. The lack of systematic classification has resulted in the absence of descriptors which allow ready access via this timesaving technology.

GERONTOLOGICAL NURSING RESEARCH BY NURSES (1975-1981)

Because this is a handbook and should provide quick reference information as well as a comprehensive view of the topic, and attempt has been made to collect bibliographical information about relevant nursing research which has been reported in the more readily available literature from 1975 through 1981. This has been organized in a format that makes information easy to locate and to decipher (see Table 40-1).

While Robinson (1981) opted to list only research study titles in order to "challenge the reader to pursue the studies at their primary sources," we have chosen to include a brief

annotation (in lieu of an abstract) in Table 40-1 for the same reason. The annotations attempt to highlight that material which might stimulate replication of studies or, at least, encourage the repeated use of tools which require more testing to demonstrate their validity.

RESEARCH AND THE NATIONAL INSTITUTE ON AGING

The National Institute on Aging which came into being in 1976 has been the biggest boon to research in aging. Under the excellent leadership and direction of Dr. Robert N. Butler, it has made tremendous progress in a relatively short time in promoting and supporting highly respected research on biomedical, behavioral, and social aspects of aging and on human services and delivery systems. Excellent summary reports of this research and of research goals for the future have been prepared by learned panels of the National Advisory Council on Aging and published in a series DHEW Publication No. (NIH) 78-1443 through 1446 and DHEW No. 77-1096. The budget for research has increased slowly but significantly in the past 10 years. The National Institute on Aging was funded at $76.091 million for 1981, an increase of $6.091 million over fiscal year 1980 (U.S. Senate Special Committee on Aging, since 1982 unfortunately funding prospects appear to be more limited, 1980).

The National Institute on Aging has announced interest in, and funding of, new studies on sleep patterns in aging, as well as research in gerontological and geriatric dermatology (Murphy and Gastel, 1980). Both of these have direct relevance to nursing and are examples of concerns which the nurse deals with every day. The National Institute on Aging has a nurse researcher on its advisory staff and offers accessibility to research opportunities for nurses.

SUMMARY

Throughout this chapter references have been made to areas of needed research in gerontological nursing. The annotations listed in Table 40-1 suggest many potential subjects as well as much-needed replication. The National Institute on

Table 40-1. Gerontological Research Studies by Nurses (January 1975–December 1981).

AUTHOR(S)	TITLE	SOURCE	ANNOTATION
		I. ATTITUDES	
Brower, H.T.	A Study of Content Needs in Graduate Gerontological Nursing Curriculum	*Journal of Gerontological Nursing* 5:21–28 (September–October 1979)	The study provides an analysis of practicing geriatric nurses' responses to a structured interview regarding the topics of both gerontological and graduate level nursing preparation. Survey was undertaken as part of the developmental process for a master's program in gerontological nursing.
Brower, H.T.	A Study of Graduate Programs in Gerontological Nursing	*Journal of Gerontological Nursing* 3:40–46 (November–December 1977)	Survey of the status of graduate programs in gerontological nursing included comparison of requirements and identification of conceptual models, and defined gerontological courses. Conclusion stated that "graduate preparation in gerontological nursing is . . . at an embryonic state."
Brower, H.T.	Social Organization and Nurses' Attitudes toward Older Persons	*Journal of Gerontological Nursing* 7:293–298 (May 1981)	The broad question raised was whether nurses' attitudes toward aging and the aged are influenced significantly by social organization, age, education level, and amount of time spent with elderly clients. Social organization was found to be a strong determiner of attitudes toward the aged.
Chaisson, G.M.	Life-cycle: A Social-simulation Game to Improve Attitudes and Responses to the Elderly	*Journal of Gerontological Nursing* 6:587–592 (October 1980)	Report evaluated the effectiveness of life-cycle game as an educational strategy for changing stereotyped images of the sick aged held by health care personnel in a nursing home. Findings indicate significantly more positive, accepting attitudes among the experimental group in response to a videotaped situation.
Chamberland, G., Rawls, B., Powell, C., and Roberts, M.	Improving Students' Attitudes toward Aging	*Journal of Gerontological Nursing* 4:44–45 (January–February 1978)	This study administered the Tuckman-Lorge Attitudes about Old People Scale to a population of ADN nursing students as a measure of the success of experimental teaching strategies in improving students' attitudes toward the aged.
Devine, B.A.	Old Age Stereotyping: A Comparison of Nursing Staff Attitudes toward the Elderly	*Journal of Gerontological Nursing* 6:25–31 (January 1980)	An instrument developed by the Ontario Welfare Council to measure opinions of health professionals about the aged was administered to staff in both a government-operated hospital which had instituted a milieu therapy program and a private nursing home planning implementation of such a program. Results did not indicate any statistically significant difference in attitudes toward the elderly. Recommendation was made that future studies change to observation methodology to gain insight into the relationship between attitude and behavior.

Dye, C.A.	Attitude Change among Health Professionals: Implications for Gerontological Nursing	*Journal of Gerontological Nursing* 5:31–35 (September–October 1979)	This study was part of a larger investigation of provider-recipient attitudes in a large metropolitan health facility. Volunteer graduate nursing students were administered the Attitudes toward Old People Scale prior to and following treatment experience, including an attitude discussion group and an attitude experience group. Findings failed to reveal any significant differences either between or among groups and no effect resulting from treatment experience. Recommendations for future research were discussed.
Dye, C. and Sassenvath, D.	Identification of Normal Aging and Disease-related Processes by Health Care Professionals	*Journal of the American Geriatrics Society* 27:472–475 (October 1979)	Study demonstrated a decided tendency of health care professionals to classify conditions included in test as disease processes when they were in fact normal aging processes; indicated need for more content regarding normal changes of aging in health care worker education.
Futrell, M. and Jones, W.	Attitudes of Physicians, Nurses, and Social Workers toward the Elderly and Health Maintenance Services for the Aged: Implications for Health Manpower Policy	*Journal of Gerontological Nursing* 3:42–46 (May–June 1977)	This exploratory-descriptive study compared responses of physicians, nurses, and social workers to a questionnaire designed for this purpose. The tool included Kogan's Attitudes toward Old People Scale. Interpretation of data offers extensive correlational analysis.
Hannon, J.	Effect of a Course on Aging in a Graduate Nursing Curriculum: A Small Descriptive Study	*Journal of Gerontological Nursing* 6:604–615 (October 1980)	Report of an exploratory study indicates that participation of a group of graduate students in nursing in a course on aging resulted in a measurable increase in their "factual knowledge" and "positive changes in their misconceptions and biases toward aging."
Heller, B.R. and Walsh, F.R.	Changing Nursing Students' Attitudes toward the Aged: An Experimental Study	*Journal of Nursing Education* 15:9–17 (January 1976)	This study reports the use of classroom instruction and clinical experience with aged clients as methods of improving nursing students' attitudes toward the elderly.
Kayser, J.S. and Minnigerode, F.A.	Increasing Nursing Students' Interest in Working with Aged Patients	*Nursing Research* 24:23–26 (January–February 1975)	Survey of 311 BSN students regarding preferences for field of specialization revealed minimal interest in nursing home employment, stereotyped view of aged, but increased interest in working with the elderly and increased willingness to work in nursing homes among those with previous experience in such agencies. Study has implication for curriculum content and student clinical experiences.
Meyer, M., Hassanein, R., and Bahr, Sr. R.	A Comparison of Attitudes toward the Aged Held by Professional Nurses	*Image* 12:62–66 (October 1980)	A group of nurses working with elderly clients and a group working with pediatric clients were administered the Tuckman-Lorge Attitude about Old People questionnaire. Results revealed significantly more positive attitude toward elderly held by pediatric nurses. Demographic and environmental variables measured are reported.

Table 40-1. Gerontological Research Studies by Nurses (January 1975–December 1981). (continued)

AUTHOR(S)	TITLE	SOURCE	ANNOTATION
O'Donnell, J., Collins, J., and Schuler, S.	Psychosocial Perceptions of the Nursing Home: A Comparative Analysis of Staff, Resident, and Cross-generational Perspectives	*The Gerontologist* 18:267–271 (June 1978)	Moos' Community Oriented Programs Environment Scale (COPES) was utilized to assess the subjective perception of nursing home living by the residents themselves and by the nursing staff. Results are discussed in terms of possible differential effects of institutionalization and age-wise comparative staff-resident differences in nursing home perception.
Robb, S.S. and Malinzak, M.M.	Knowledge Levels of Personnel in Gerontological Nursing	*Journal of Gerontological Nursing* 7:153–158 (March 1981)	Four hundred and thirty-five providers of direct clinical nursing in a large VA Medical Center were assessed for extent of gerontological nursing knowledge and factors commonly believed to influence levels of knowledge. Findings suggested that education levels and specific course work in gerontological nursing had positive influence on cognitive learning. The study has strong implications for nurse educators.
Taylor, K. and Harned, T.	Attitudes toward Old People: A Study of Nurses Who Care for the Elderly	*Journal of Gerontological Nursing* 4:43–47 (September–October 1978)	Study reports findings of an attitude survey of nurses employed in care of aged clients. Kogan's Attitude toward Old People Scale was utilized and revealed that all respondents scored within the positive to neutral range. Younger nurses and those with fewer years experience all scored more positively than their older, more experienced counterparts.
Thorp, T., Baker, B., and Brower, T.	Nursing Staff Attitudes	*Nursing Research* 28:299–301 (September–October 1979)	Study utilized a semantic differential test to measure nursing staff attitudes toward the geriatric nurse practitioner as an agent of change in a county nursing home. Increasingly positive attitudes were demonstrated in follow-up studies after some changes had been implemented.
Tobiason, S., Knudson, F., Stengel, J., and Giss, M.	Positive Attitudes toward Aging: The Aged Teach the Young	*Journal of Gerontological Nursing* 5:18–23 (June 1979)	Project measured results of an experiment in which baccalaureate nursing students developed a relationship with an elderly client during home visits. Pre- and post-testing revealed development of more positive attitudes by students toward the elderly, changes in perception of the young by the elderly clients, and a view of the nurse as patient advocate as well as care provider.
Wilhite, M. and Johnson, D.	Changes in Nursing Students' Stereotypic Attitudes toward Old People	*Nursing Research* 25:430–432 (November–December 1976)	Study utilized Tuckman-Lorge Attitudes about Old People Scale to test BSN students and faculty before and after an eight-week course. Results revealed a decrease in stereotyping as well as a definite relationship between instructor attitude and effect on students.

II. PATIENT VARIABLES INFLUENCING CARE
A) PATIENT CHARACTERISTICS AS PREDICTORS OF PHENOMENA

Brower, H.T. and Tanner, L.A.	A Study of Older Adults Attending a Program on Human Sexuality: A Pilot Study	*Nursing Research* 28:36–39 (January–February 1979)	An effort was made to measure whether significant changes occurred in older adults' knowledge and attitude regarding human sexuality following a two-session course on human sexuality. Study identified need for personal interview rather than formal testing with older adult subjects and identified sexuality content recommended for nurse practitioner courses.
Bullough, V., Bullough, B., and Mauro, M.	Age and Achievement: A Dissenting View	*The Gerontologist* 18:584–587 (December 1978)	This is a report of an historical investigation of intellectual and creative achievers during two particularly significant periods of history. A significant variable identified was longevity, and creativity tended to be continuous over the whole life span. Study challenges previously held findings that most achievement occurred under age 40.
Copstead, L.	Effects of Touch on Self-appraisal and Interaction Appraisal for Permanently Institutionalized Older Adults	*Journal of Gerontological Nursing* 6:747–752 (December 1980)	Data collected through observation, questionnaire, tape recording of verbal interaction, and administration of the Secord/Jourand Self-Cathexis Scale resulted in conclusion that the nurse can effectively use touch to foster client self-feeling among a group of institutionalized aged.
Edsall, J.O. and Miller, L.A.	Relationship between Loss of Auditory and Visual Acuity and Social Disengagement in an Aged Population	*Nursing Research* 27:296–298 (September–October 1978)	Utilization of the Social Life-space Measure, Perceived Life-space Measure, Role Count Measure, and Total Disengagement Index, in correlation with vision and auditory testing, demonstrated no relationship among the variables in a group of elderly residents from two high rise dwellings.
Gilson, P. and Coats, S.	A Study of Morale in Low Income Blacks	*Journal of Gerontological Nursing* 7:385–388 (July 1980)	This survey of ambulatory elderly subjects participating in a hot lunch program in a low income black community utilized an interview based on selected items from the PGC Morale Scale and the Life Satisfaction Index. Results of the empirical investigation confirmed a previous subjective appraisal that morale among the subjects was positive.
Gioiella, E.	The Relationship between Slowness of Response, State Anxiety, Social Isolation and Self-esteem, and Preferred Personal Space in the Elderly	*Journal of Gerontological Nursing* 4:40–43 (January–February 1978)	Study tested four hypotheses with an all-female population of elderly participants from three senior citizen centers. It includes results revealed by each of five tools used in data collection. This descriptive study explored variables related to personal space in the elderly.
Griev, M.R.	Living Arrangements for the Elderly	*Journal of Gerontological Nursing* 3:19–22 (July–August 1977)	Two descriptive studies measured hospital or visiting nurses' choice and elderly clients' own choice of living arrangements. Process of decision making was studied, with a focus on variables pertinent to choosing between a nursing home and client's own home. Probability ranking for each of seven identified needs and qualitative values assigned to each were measured. Implication was that the choice can be based on outcome probabilities.

Table 40-1. Gerontological Research Studies by Nurses (January 1975–December 1981). (continued)

AUTHOR(S)	TITLE	SOURCE	ANNOTATION
Henthorn, B.S.	Disengagement and Reinforcement in the Elderly	*Research in Nursing and Health* 2:1–8 (January 1979)	A disengagement index was administered to 50 nursing home residents and 50 community registered voters. A Reinforcement Survey Schedule was used to identify positive reinforcers, level of reinforcement, and anticipated reinforcement. A significant correlation was found between disengagement and reinforcement for both groups.
Lolly, M., Black, E., Thornack, M., and Hawkins, J.D.	Older Women in Single Room Occupant (SRO) Hotels: A Seattle Profile	*The Gerontologist* 19:67–73 (February 1979)	Data collected by observation and informal open-ended interview from elderly female women living in downtown Seattle hotels revealed that while the majority express concern over their economic situation, they still maintain optimism about the future. Self-sufficiency and independence are valued highly among the sample who revealed a close identification and strong affect for their fathers and work histories in trades traditionally dominated by men.
Muhlenkamp, A., Gress, L., and Flood, M.	Perception of Life Change Events by the Elderly	*Nursing Research* 24:109–113 (March–April 1975)	Study utilized Social Readjustment Rating Scale (SRRS) to measure perception of the amounts of adjustment necessitated by common life events. Sample consisted of elderly members of a citizen's club who revealed similar rank ordering of events but assigned significantly higher magnitude to them than did the normative control group. This supports belief that change is harder for the elderly.
Swartz, D.	Hamlet Dweller – City Dweller	*Geriatric Nursing* 1:128–132 (July–August 1980)	Report utilized a structured interview with a random sample of chronically ill urban clinic patients and with rural patients under the care of private physicians in a county without hospital facilities. Findings indicate that "fit" between elderly, chronically ill adults and their environment is better among rural population.

B) PATIENT CHARACTERISTICS AS DETERMINANT OF HEALTH CARE NEEDS

AUTHOR(S)	TITLE	SOURCE	ANNOTATION
Baldwin, J.	Knowledge about Hypertension in Affected Elderly Persons	*Journal of Gerontological Nursing* 7:542–551 (September 1981)	Participants were found to possess insufficient knowledge about hypertension. There was little evidence of patients being told much about hypertension. Findings substantiate the fact either that there is very little instructing done of elderly hypertensive clients or that communication of health care providers is deficient.
McGlone, F. and Kick, E.	Health Habits in Relation to Aging	*Journal of the American Geriatrics Society* 26:481–488 (November 1978)	Study of patients over age 80 evaluated their state of health in relation to various factors including health habits. It confirmed premise that good health habits have a positive effect on both quantity and quality of life.

C) RESPONSES OF ELDERLY TO HOSPITALIZATION AND/OR INSTITUTIONALIZATION

Schank, M.J.	A Survey of the Well-elderly: Their Foot Problems, Practices and Needs	*Journal of Gerontological Nursing* 3:12–14 (November–December 1977)	Survey was made to identify health care needs of the well elderly in relation to foot care. Volunteer members of a large urban senior center responded to a semistructured interview regarding foot care management, presence of conditions associated with high incidence of foot problems, ability to manage self-care, and subjects' perception of their foot care needs. Study served as basis for program development (Conrad, 1977).
Chang, B.L.	Generalized Expectancy, Situational Perception, and Morale among Institutionalized Aged	*Nursing Research* 27:316–323 (September–October 1978)	Study was made of the relationship of generalized expectancy of control and perceived situational control to the morale of aged residents in four skilled nursing facilities. Situational Control of Daily Activities (SCDA) interview schedule was developed and utilized in addition to the Self-report Trust Scale (SRT) and the revised Philadelphia Geriatric Center Morale Scale. Results indicate that SCDA may be used to measure residents' perception of locus of control regarding aspects of their ADLs.
Hughes, E.	Institutionalized Older Adults and Their Future Orientation	*Journal of the American Geriatrics Society* 27:130–134 (March 1979)	Findings indicate that residents became less future oriented as length of institutional residence increased; however, this did not limit interaction in the institutional environment as hypothesized. Cottles' Experential Inventory and Pincus's Psychosocial Dimensions were used with residents in six institutions.
Miller, D. and Been, S.	Patterns of Friendship among Patients in a Nursing Home Setting	*The Gerontologist* 17:269–275 (June 1977)	Questionnaire administered to intellectually intact nursing home residents revealed that a significant majority named other residents and staff specifically as "friends." Volunteers were also identified by half the sample. Familial friendships were indicated as the most enduring of preinstitutional relationships.
Munoz, R. and Mesick, B.	Hospitalization of the Elderly Patient for Acute Illness	*Journal of the American Geriatrics Society* 26:415–417 (September 1979)	Survey of characteristics of a large sample of elderly patients admitted to a general hospital for treatment of acute disorders indicated that the typical patient of this group needed minimal assistance from ancillary resources to assure a successful return to the community. Those with limited support systems were those more typically sent to nursing homes.
Rainwater, A.J.	Elderly Loneliness and Its Relation to Residential Care	*Journal of Gerontological Nursing* 6:593–599 (October 1980)	Comparison of frequency and nature of loneliness reported by four women residents from both a "good care" facility and an "insufficient care" facility resulted in the conclusion that while incidence of perceived loneliness was roughly equal, the former group experienced a "normal, possibly situational loneliness" while the second group was more likely "to experience loneliness in a more pathological way." Study used only indirect measurement utilizing factors traditionally indicative of loneliness.

Table 40-1. Gerontological Research Studies by Nurses (January 1975–December 1981). (continued)

Author	Title	Source	Description
Wolanin, M.O.	Relocation of the Elderly	Journal of Gerontological Nursing 4:47–50 (May–June 1978)	A survey and critique of research studies published regarding relocation of elderly individuals, this article discusses demonstrated principles which may prevent increased mortality rates traditionally associated with such moves.

III. DIRECT PATIENT CARE A) INTERVENTIONS FOR SPECIFIC PROBLEMS

Author	Title	Source	Description
Boltes, M. and Zerbe, M.	Independence Training in Nursing Home Residents	The Gerontologist 16:428–432 (October 1976)	An experimental study to change dependency behavior and assist nursing home clients to reacquire and maintain self-feeding skills, it implies that environmental characteristics of the setting contribute and that personnel need training in behavior management skills.
Conrad, D.	Foot Education and Screening Programs for the Elderly	Journal of Gerontological Nursing 3:10–15 (November–December 1977)	Study reports program resulting from recommendations made in 1975 survey by Schank. Additional data relating to age-specific incidence of foot care needs and medical problems by age are identified.
DeWalt, E.M.	Effect of Timed Hygienic Measures on Oral Mucosa in a Group of Elderly Subjects	Nursing Research 24:104–108 (March–April 1975)	Study measured the effect on the oral mucosa of a sample of geriatric patients of the application of oral hygiene at two-, three-, or four-hour intervals during an eight-hour period for ten days. Scores based on nine dependent variables indicated improvement in oral tissue.
Goldberg, W.G. and Fitzpatrick, J.J.	Movement Therapy with the Aged	Nursing Research 29:339–346 (November–December 1980)	Experimental group of institutionalized aged involved in a movement therapy group demonstrated greater improvement in total morale and attitude toward their own aging than a control group.
Heffenin, E. and Hunter, R.	Nursing Observation and Care Planning for the Hospitalized Aged	The Gerontologist 15:57–60 (February 1975)	Study was conducted to explore the effects of using a formal observation tool to facilitate nursing assessment of selected physical function and psychosocial behavior in a chronically ill and aging inpatient population.
Hogstel, M.O.	Use of Reality Orientation with Aging Confused Patients	Nursing Research 28:161–165 (May–June 1979)	The four-cell experimental design was used to evaluate the use of reality orientation with elderly confused patients in a nursing home. A questionnaire was devised for use in a semistructured interview. Findings indicate that the tool would be useful for evaluation of the degree of confusion of elderly patients.
Kolanowski, A. and Gunter, L.	Hypothermia in the Elderly	Geriatric Nursing 2:362–365 (October 1981)	In an elderly population, 3.9% were found to be at risk of accidental hypothermia. Important implications for nursing, such as using low reading thermometers, are described.
Kupfer, D., Spiker, D., Coble, P., and Shaw, D.	Electroencephalographic Sleep Recordings and Depression in the Elderly	Journal of the American Geriatrics Society 26:53–57 (February 1978)	Patients over 60 evaluated for severity of depression by the Hamilton Rating Scale (HRS) were measured with all night EEG recordings after being drug free for two weeks. Findings support EEG sleep recordings as tool for differential diagnosis of depression in the elderly.

AUTHOR(S)	TITLE	SOURCE	ANNOTATION
Lamb, K.	Effect of Positioning of Post-operative Fractured Hip Patients as Related to Comfort	*Nursing Research* 28:291–294 (September–October 1979)	Interview technique was employed with elderly patients who had hip fractures repaired with Richard's compression nail and plate to ascertain preferred position of comfort. Study revealed 50% preferred lying on operative side. Implications exist for presurgery assessment of sleep habits and position information.
Mikhail, S.F., Sonn, M., and Lawton, A.H.	Optimism in the Management of Hip Fracture in Elderly Patients	*Journal of the American Geriatrics Society* 26:39–42 (January 1978)	Study of patients over 70 years of age supports contention that operative reduction and fixation as early as possible have positive results with good prognosis for return to normal activity.
Perry J.	Effectiveness of Teaching in the Rehabilitation of Patients with Chronic Bronchitis and Emphysema	*Nursing Research* 30:219–221 (July–August 1981)	Twenty patients with diagnosed chronic bronchitis and emphysema, who participated in a rehabilitation program that incorporated principles of adult education, reported on their ability to recognize and treat symptoms of their disease. Significant increases in knowledge and skills were found among study subjects.
Voelkel, D.	A Study of Reality Orientation and Resocialization Groups with Confused Elderly	*Journal of Gerontological Nursing* 4:13–18 (May–June 1978)	This comparative study demonstrated greater improvement among moderately to severely mentally impaired residents of a nursing home in a resocialization group than of those in reality orientation groups. Pfeiffer's Short Portable Mental Status Questionnaire (SPMSQ) and Lawson and Brody's Physical Self-Maintenance Scale (PSMS) were utilized both pre- and post-test.
Wichita, C.	Treating and Preventing Constipation in Nursing Home Residents	*Journal of Gerontological Nursing* 3:35–39 (November–December 1977)	Project measured decrease in both incontinence and constipation following the addition of bran, and increased fresh fruits and vegetables, into the diets of nursing home residents. After baseline data gathering, the introduction of the high fiber diet was reported successful particularly among the staff-fed residents.
Williams, M., Holloway, J. Winn, M., Wolanin, M., Lawler, M., Westwick, C., and Chin, M.	Nursing Activities and Acute Confusional States in Elderly Hip-fractured Patients	*Nursing Research* 28:25–35 (January–February 1979)	Study was conducted in seven hospitals, located in five states, to identify predictors of postoperative confusion in elderly patients undergoing surgical repair of hip fractures. Findings imply that environmental factors and nursing care measures are associated with lessened confusion.

B) PROBLEMS CONCERNING MEDICATIONS

AUTHOR(S)	TITLE	SOURCE	ANNOTATION
Battle, E.H. and Hanna, C.E.	Evaluation of a Dietary Regimen for Chronic Constipation: Report of a Pilot Study	*Journal of Gerontological Nursing* 6:527–532 (September 1980)	Experimental study evaluated use of bran cereal as an alternative to laxatives in prevention of chronic constipation in a group of ambulatory chronic and elderly psychiatric patients. Comparison of blood chemistry studies, as well as cost factor for both experimental and control groups, were reported.

Table 40-1. Gerontological Research Studies by Nurses (January 1975–December 1981). (continued)

Brown, M.	Drug-Drug Interactions among Residents in Homes for the Elderly: A Pilot Study	*Nursing Research* **26**:47–52 (January–February 1977)	Epidemiological investigation of clincally significant drug-drug interaction (a subclass of adverse drug reactions) in residents of both an urban and a rural home for the elderly demonstrated significant occurrence of interaction in patients receiving digitalis in combination with thiazide or furosemide.
Dittmar, S.S. and Dulski, T.	Early Evening Administration of Sleep Medications to the Hospitalized Aged: A Consideration in Rehabilitation	*Nursing Research* **26**:299–303 (July–August 1977)	Utilization of a three-part instrument to gather data in areas of demography, positive and negative social behavior, and activities of daily living demonstrated improvement in ADLs but high incidence of negative social behavior resulting from early evening administration of sleep medication.
Garety, F., Barron, J., Barron, P., and Bjork, A.	Efficacy of Nylidrin Hydrochloride in the Treatment of Cognitive Impairment in the Elderly	*Journal of the American Geriatrics Society* **27**:235–236 (May 1979)	A double-blind study compared effects of nylidrin hydrochloride vs placebo in patients with mild to moderate symptoms of chronic brain syndrome. Findings support usefulness of nylidrin hydrochloride in the treatment of a variety of cognitive, affective, and behavioral symptoms in aged patients.
Gerber, R.M. and Rowe Van Ort, S.	Topical Application of Insulin in Decubitus Ulcers	*Nursing Research* **28**:16–19 (January–February 1979)	Report of a project measuring effectiveness of topical insulin application as a treatment for decubitis ulcers with a group of geriatric patients was inconclusive. While it was determined that females healed significantly more slowly than males in the sample and that there was a direct relationship between the number of days of treatment and the rate of healing, the concluding recommendation was for continued study.
Kim, K.K. and Grier, M.R.	Pacing Effects of Medication Instruction for the Elderly	*Journal of Gerontological Nursing* **7**:464–468 (August 1981)	Forty-eight elderly patients divided into three groups were studied to examine the effect of pacing medication instruction on the learning of elderly clients. Results confirmed the importance of slow instruction for the elderly.
Raskind, M., Alvaney, C., and Herlin, S.	Fluphenazine Enanthate in the Outpatient Treatment of Late Paraphrenia	*Journal of the American Geriatrics Society* **27**:459–463 (October 1979)	Experimental study comparing the efficacy of parenteral fluphenazine enanthate with orally administered haloperidol in elderly patients with late paraphrenia. Conclusions suggested superiority of the former was in part attributable to improved compliance with administration.
Raskind, M., Kitchell, M., and Alvaney, C.	Bromide Intoxication in the Elderly	*Journal of the American Geriatrics Society* **26**:222–224 (May 1978)	Four case reports illustrate tendency of elderly patients to manifest CNS toxicity secondary to bromide intoxication, resulting in inaccurate diagnosis of "senility."
Walsh, A.C., Walsh, B., Melaney, C.	Senile-Presenile Dementia: Follow-up Data on an Effective Psychotherapy-Anticoagulant Regime	*Journal of the American Geriatrics Society* **26**:467–475 (October 1978)	Results of a two-year study in which anticoagulants were utilized as therapy for patients presenting with senile dementia are reported. Study establishes brain ischemia as a fundamental factor in many cases with positive improvement demonstrated on Coumadin regimen.
White, P.H.	Psychoactive Medication Non-compliance in a Geropsychiatric Outpatient Clinic	*Journal of Gerontological Nursing* **6**:729–734 (December 1980)	A descriptive study was conducted to determine if there was a relationship between psychoactive medication noncompliance and intellectual impairment as measured by the Short Portable Mental Status Questionnaire (SPMSQ) in a group of noninstitutionalized elderly clients.

AUTHOR(S)	TITLE	SOURCE	ANNOTATION
IV. EVALUATION OF HEALTH CARE PROGRAMS			
Chekryn, J. and Roos, L.	Auditing the Process of Care in a New Geriatric Unit	*Journal of the American Geriatrics Society* **27**:107–111 (March 1979)	Multidisciplinary team audit of charts for over 100 patients evaluated compliance with newly instituted individualized progressive care and POMR. Study included assessment of compliance with criteria and analysis of the relationship between these scores and three outcome indices.
Franck, P.	A Survey of Health Needs of Older Adults in Northwest Johnson County, Iowa	*Nursing Research* **28**:360–364 (November–December 1979)	Replication of survey by Managan et al. (1974) conducted home interviews of older adults utilizing parameters of health condition, physical functioning, accessibility of medical care, social isolation, and health service needs. Nursing needs were documented, and results of previous study were compared to determine whether they could be generalized to a rural setting.
Hain, Sr. M.J. and Chen, S.C.	Health Needs of the Elderly	*Nursing Research* **25**:433–439 (November–December 1976)	Study assessed needs of elderly residents of two high rise apartment complexes. It utilized a 20-item structured questionnaire which was analyzed in relation to health condition, physical functioning, and access to medical care. Implication that nurse practitioner, home health aides, and referral service could be utilized was reported.
Kaiser-Jones, J.	A Comparison of Care in a Scottish and a U.S. Facility	*Geriatric Nursing* **2**:44–50 (January–February 1981)	Comparisons revealed better staffing and higher quality care in the Scottish hospital. Findings illustrated that nurses are a key determinant of the day-to-day care of the elderly; study recommends that all schools of nursing include gerontological nursing in the basic curriculum.
Sullivan, J.A. and Armignacco, F.	Effectiveness of a Comprehensive Health Program for the Well-Elderly	*Nursing Research* **28**:70–75 (March–April 1979)	Study compared effectiveness of three different nursing approaches in provision of health care for a well elderly population living in housing units for the elderly. A structured interview and participant observation scale were utilized along with extensive physical and psychosocial assessment, screening, counseling, and health education sessions.
V. RESEARCH TOOLS AND STRATEGIES			
Brimmer, P.F.	Past, Present, and Future in Gerontological Nursing Research	*Journal of Gerontological Nursing* **5**:27–34 (November–December 1979)	This is a comprehensive overview of the evolution and steady growth of both nonresearch and research publications regarding the aged. It includes a review of the federal, professional, and educational history which contributed to the current state of the art. Present activity and suggestions for future direction for significant research on the aged are thoroughly discussed.

Table 40-1. Gerontological Research Studies by Nurses (January 1975–December 1981). (continued)

Author	Title	Source	Description
Brink, T. L., Belanger, J., Bryant, J., Capri, D., Janakes, C., Jasculca, S., and Olivera, C.	Hypochondriasis in an Institutional Geriatric Population: Construction of a Scale (HSIG)	*Journal of the American Geriatric Society* 26:557–559 (December 1978)	A Hypochondriasis Scale for Institutional Geriatric Patients (HSIG) was constructed and tested among identified hypochondriacal patients in three extended care facilities. It was recommended for use only in confirming staff suspicions of hypochondriasis not as part of clinical intake procedure.
Fitzpatrick, J.J. and Donovan, M.J.	A Follow-up Study of the Reliability and Validity of the Motor Activity Rating Scale	*Nursing Research* 28:179–181 (May–June 1979)	Study compared and extended the evaluation of the validity of the Motor Activity Rating Scale (MARS) for observing and symbolically recording body positions, body movement, and intensity of body movements. Data gathered in testing residents in a home for the aged demonstrated statistically significant correlation between MARS and Actometer scores as well as high interrater reliability.
Friedman, J.S.	Development of a Sexual Knowledge Inventory for Elderly Persons	*Nursing Research* 28:372–374 (November–December 1979)	Study reports development of a questionnaire the "Sexual Knowledge Inventory for Elderly Persons" (SKE) which was administered to volunteer residents in ten independent housing units in the Cincinnati area. Implication is that SKE can be adapted as an assessment tool or as a teaching device for patients or personnel working with aged persons.
Gunter, L.M. and Miller, J.C.	Toward a Nursing Gerontology	*Nursing Research* 26:208–221 (May–June 1977)	This is an overview of studies pertaining to the care of the elderly and a review of psychosocial gerontological nursing research from 1951 to 1976. It includes discussion of methodologic problems and conceptual issues of investigation as well as suggestions for future research.
Robb, S.	Attitudes and Intentions of Baccalaureate Nursing Students toward the Elderly	*Nursing Research* 28:43–50 (January–February 1979)	Primary purpose of this study was to develop instruments which reliably measure belief and behavioral intentions toward the elderly. High reliability was demonstrated when administering a paired comparison-type belief scale and a multiple act behavioral intention scale utilizing the Kogan Old People and Marlowe-Crowe Social Desirability scales as outside criteria.
Stevenson, J.S.	Load Power and Margin in Older Adults	*Geriatric Nursing* 1:52–55 (May–June 1980)	Study reports development of a research instrument for determination of individuals' perception of their own ratio between responsibilities (load) and resources to accomplish the work required (power). Application of instrument to experimental group revealed that older adults in the study perceived themselves as having less load and more power than did the young to middle-aged subjects.

AUTHOR(S)	TITLE	SOURCE	ANNOTATION
Spasoff, R.A., Kraus, A., Beattie, E., Holden, D., Lawson, J., Rosenburg, M., and Woodcock, G.	A Longitudinal Study of Elderly Residents of Long-stay Institutions	*The Gerontologist* 18:281–292 (June 1978)	Structured interviews were held with patients and questionnaires were given to attending physicians both one month and one year following admission. Interview form contained assessment of ADL. Study raises questions regarding appropriate placement and care provided.

D) RESPONSES TO DELIBERATE ENVIRONMENTAL CHANGE

AUTHOR(S)	TITLE	SOURCE	ANNOTATION
Fitzpatrick, J. and Donovan, J.	Temporal Experience and Motor Behavior among the Aging	*Research in Nursing and Health* 1:60–68 (February 1978)	This study identifies differences among an elderly group of individuals based on residential living arrangements and age. Findings identify differences in temporal perspective between institutionalized and non-institutionalized aged with implication for health care providers.
Lester, P. and Boltes, M.	Functional Interdependence of the Social Environment and the Behavior of the Institutionalized Aged	*Journal of Gerontological Nursing* 4:23–27 (March–April 1978)	Based on a theoretical framework of the concept of dependency, this study hypothesized that increased dependent behavior is directly related to positive verbal reinforcers for such action. In the observational study with residents and staff of a skilled nursing home, the findings supported the hypothesis.
Louis, M.	Personal Space Boundary Needs of Elderly Persons: An Empirical Study	*Journal of Gerontological Nursing* 7:345–400 (July 1981)	The purpose of the study was to identify a baseline for personal space of independently functioning elders. Findings suggest several guidelines for nurses working with older persons.
Melillo, K.D.	Informal Activity Involvement and the Perceived Rate of Time Passage for an Older Institutionalized Population	*Journal of Gerontological Nursing* 6:393–397 (July 1980)	Study utilized a series of five tests to measure whether there was a positive relationship between hours of informal activity involvement and perception of time passing swiftly. Findings failed to support the hypothesis.
Miller, Sr. P. and Russell, D.A.	Elements Promoting Satisfaction as Identified by Residents in the Nursing Home	*Journal of Gerontological Nursing* 6:121–129 (March 1980)	An exploratory study conducted among nursing home residents reports specific environmental elements identified by the residents as contributing to their satisfaction or dissatisfaction in the nursing home. Study utilized a modification of the Life Satisfaction Index A and an open-ended questionnaire.
Silverstone, B. and Wynter, L.	The Effects of Introducing a Heterosexual Living Space	*The Gerontologist* 15:83–87 (February 1975)	The Oberleder Attitude Scale (OAS) and the Ward Behavior Inventory (WBI) were utilized to measure the reaction to sexual integration of residents on the same unit of a home for the elderly. Quantitative findings indicated significant improvement in the social behavior of the males and a healthier overall climate.

Aging publications previously cited and *Changes – Research on Aging and the Aged* (U.S. Department of Health, Education and Welfare, 1978) offer an abundance of potentially researchable problems.

Yurick, Robb, Spier, and Ebert (1980) state that research priorities should be given to areas which affect nursing care of the elderly; they list the following five problems as having equal priority:

- Definition of the concept of quality care, development of reliable and valid instruments to measure this concept, and evaluation of nursing practice involving the elderly
- Development of better classification of clients in long term care settings
- Exploration of nonmedical models for delivery of service
- Replication of gerontological nursing studies
- Development of programs and techniques to promote and maintain health and to prevent disease in the elderly

Virginia Henderson (1977) stated a strong case for nursing research in her charmingly titled editorial "We've 'Come a Long Way' but What of the Direction?" In this she urged research into the relevant problems in nursing practice as well as those problems offering the greatest benefits for the greatest number of people. Certainly no single age group has either a higher percentage of health care needs or represents a larger proportion of health care recipients than the elderly. In gerontological nursing research, we have "come a long way," and in this chapter we hope that the reader has been challenged to consider practice-oriented gerontological nursing research which may provide an additional building block toward improved nursing care for older individuals.

REFERENCES

Brimmer, P.F. Past, present and future in gerontological nursing research. *Journal of Gerontological Nursing* 5:27–34 (1979).

Gunter, L.M. and Miller, J.C. Toward a nursing gerontology. *Nursing Research* 26:208–221 (June 1977).

Henderson, V.A. We've "come a long way" but what of the direction? (editorial). *Nursing Research* 26:163–164 (May-June 1977).

International Nursing Index, New York: American Journal of Nursing Co. and National League for Nursing, Vol. 1., 1966; Vol. 6, 1971; Vol. 11, 1976.

Kayser-Jones, J.S. Gerontological nursing research revisited. *Journal of Gerontological Nursing* 7(4): 217–223 (1981).

Murphy, D.G. and Gastel, B. The National Institute of Aging and Dermatologic Research. *Journal of the American Academy of Dermatology* 2(4):341 (1980).

Robinson, L.D. Gerontological nursing research. In Burnside, I.M. (Ed.) *Nursing and the Aged.* San Francisco: McGraw-Hill, 1981.

Strumpf, N. Aging – a progressive phenomenon. *Journal of Gerontological Nursing* 4:17 (March-April 1978).

Strumpf, N. and Mezey, M. A developmental approach to the teaching of aging. *Nursing Outlook* 28:730–734 (December 1980).

U.S. Department of Health, Education and Welfare. *Changes – Research on Aging and the Aged* (Publication No. NIH 78-85). Washington, D.C.: U.S. Government Printing Office, 1978.

U.S. Department of Health, Education and Welfare. *Our Future Selves, Research Summary Reports* (Publication Nos. NIH 78-1443 through 1446). Washington, D.C.: U.S. Government Printing Office, 1978.

U.S. Senate Special Committee on Aging. Memorandum – December 19, 1980. Vol. XII, No. 6, p. 2 (1980).

Yordi, Cathleen, Ph.D. Ethical and Methodological Questions Regarding the Use of Frail Elderly as Controls in Applied Research, Unpublished Technical report presented at the Western Gerontological Society Meeting at San Diego, Calif. March 2, 1982.

Yurick, A.G., Robb, S.S., Spier, B.E., and Ebert, N.J. *The Aged Person and the Nursing Process.* New York: Appleton-Century-Crofts, 1980, pp. 70–76.

Appendices

Appendix A
Patient's Rights for Long Term Care

1. Upon admission, or prior to admission, each patient shall be provided a written contract or agreement specifying all the services the facility is required to provide under R9-10-913, the cost of services, and conditions of termination of the contract or agreement. Responsible parties shall receive at least thirty days prior notice of proposed changes in rates or charges.

2. Upon admission each patient shall receive a copy of patient's rights as evidenced by the patient's or his representative's written acknowledgment. The facility staff shall assure that language barriers or physical handicaps do not prevent the patient from becoming aware of these rights and responsibilities. A copy of the patient's rights and responsibilities shall be posted in a location generally available to patients, their representatives, and responsible parties.

3. Each patient or the patient's representative or the responsible party shall have the right to select his attending physician. If the patient, patient representative or responsible party chooses not to select the attending physician, the name and telephone number of the physician assigned for the patient shall be given to the patient, patient representative or patient's responsible party.

4. Each patient shall receive adequate and appropriate medical, nursing and personal care.

5. Each patient shall receive adequate and appropriate treatment and services to meet his physical, social and emotional needs that enable him to achieve his highest level of functioning or in attaining a peaceful death. Patients shall have prior notice and be afforded the opportunity to refuse treatment, services, or participation in experimental research.

6. Each patient shall be free from medical, psychological, and physical abuse, neglect and negligent treatment.

7. A patient shall be free from restraints unless authorized in writing by a physician to protect the patient from injury to himself or others.

8. Patients shall be afforded the opportunity to participate in the planning of their care and discharge.

9. Patients shall not be transferred within the facility or discharged at the facility's instigation except for medical reasons, nonpayment of appropriate facility charges, or to protect the welfare of patients as documented in the patient's medical record or pursuant to denial, revocation or suspension of the facility's license. For nonmedical reasons a minimum of 14 days notice shall be given to the patient, his representative or responsible party prior to transfer or discharge.

10. Each patient shall have the right to transfer to an appropriate higher or lower level of care or to independent living based on his health needs and capabilities.

11. Patients shall continue to possess and enjoy the personal civil rights of all citizens, and such rights are not limited or terminated by residence in a nursing care institution. Such rights, however, are to be exercised by a patient with due consideration for the rights and interests of other patients. Personal civil rights include, but are not limited to, the rights of free speech, expression and association; legal representation; voting and engaging in political activity outside the facility; privacy; and ownership of property. Patients shall be allowed to voice grievances, and recommend changes to the facility staff and outside representatives of his choice without restraint, interference, coercion, discrimination, or reprisal.

12. Each patient shall be treated with consideration, respect, and full recognition of his dignity and individuality, including privacy in treatment and in personal care.

*From *Proposed Rules and Regulations for Long Term Care Facilities,* Arizona Department of Health Services, June 1980.

13. A patient shall not be required to perform services for the facility except for therapeutic purposes as indicated in the patient care plan.

14. Each patient shall have the right to communicate and associate privately with visitors. The administration or facility staff shall not directly or indirectly interfere, obstruct or hamper in any manner, visits, meetings, discussions, or any other communication between the visitor and the patient. The facility shall grant access to visitors at reasonable and convenient hours which shall be at least 6 hours per day, and shall include evening hours. The specific visiting hours permitted shall be posted at the entrance of the facility. The clergy and family shall be permitted to visit patients at all reasonable hours.

15. The patient shall be permitted to send and receive personal mail unopened.

16. Unless bedside telephones are provided, patients shall have unrestricted access to a telephone with privacy in a common area of the facility. Telephones shall be accessible to all patients, including the handicapped.

17. Each patient shall be permitted to participate in social, religious, educational and other activities both in the facility and in the community to the fullest extent possible. Each patient shall also have the right to refuse participation in such activities.

18. Each patient shall have the right to retain and use his personal clothing and possessions.

19. Each patient shall have the right to manage his or her personal financial affairs, or the facility may accept this responsibility with written delegation.

20. Each patient shall have a clean and safe environment.

21. Each patient shall have the right to use tobacco at his own expense under the facility's safety provisions.

22. Each patient shall have mentally and socially compatible roommates within the capacity of the facility.

23. Each patient shall have the right to consume alcoholic beverages at his own expense unless not medically advisable as documented in his medical record by the attending physician.

24. Each patient shall have the right to retire and rise in accordance with his desires; however, the facility is not required to adjust mealtime schedules to meet individual patient desires.

25. Married spouses shall be assured of privacy for spousal visits and where both spouses are in-patients they shall be permitted to share a room if they so desire.

Appendix B
American Nurses' Association Standards
of Gerontological Nursing Practice

STANDARD I

Data are systematically and continuously collected about the health status of the older adult. The data are accessible, communicated, and recorded.

Rationale. In order to provide comprehensive nursing care for the older adult, the data are collected from a framework that includes the scientific findings and knowledge derived from the fields of gerontology and nursing.

Assessment Factors

1. Health status data includes the older adult's:

   - Normal responses to the aging process.
   - Physiological, psychological, sociological, and ecological status.
   - Modes of communication.
   - Individual patterns of coping.
   - Prior life-style.
   - Independent performance of activities of everyday living.
   - Perception and satisfaction with current health status.
   - Health goals.
   - Available and accessible human and material resources.

2. Health status data are collected from:

   - The older adult, significant others, health care personnel.
   - Other individuals in the immediate environment who are involved in the care of the older adult.
   - Interviews, examination, observation, records, and reports.

3. The data are:

   - Accessible on the older adult's records.
   - Retrievable from record keeping system.

   - Communicated to those responsible for the older adult's care.
   - Accurate.
   - Confidential.

STANDARD II

Nursing diagnoses are derived from the identified normal responses of the individual to aging and the data collected about the health status of the older adult.

Rationale. Each person ages in an individual way. The individual's normal response to aging must be identified before deviations in response requiring nursing actions can be identified.

Assessment Factors

1. The older adult's health status is compared to the norm, and a determination is made regarding deviations from the norm.
2. The older adult's prior life-style, responses to the aging process, and personal goals and objectives are identified.
3. The older adult's strengths and limitations are identified.
4. The nursing diagnosis is related to and congruent with the diagnosis and plan of all other professionals caring for the older adult.

STANDARD III

A plan of nursing care is developed in conjunction with the older adult and/or significant others that includes goals derived from the nursing diagnosis.

Rationale. Goals are a determination of the results to be achieved and are an essential part of planning care. All goals are ultimately directed toward maximizing achievable independence in everyday living.

*Reprinted with permission from the American Nurses' Association Inc., 2420 Pershing Rd., Kansas City, Kansas, 1976.

Assessment Factors

1. Goals are congruent with other planned therapies, are stated in realistic and measurable terms, and are assigned a time period for achievement.
2. Goals determine specific nursing approaches that will promote, maintain, and restore health.
3. Goals are measured by the eventual outcomes of nursing care.
4. The established goals incorporate:

   - Normal developmental processes of aging.
   - Individuality of the older adult.
   - Needs for intimacy and sexual expression.
   - Slowing down.
   - Losses.
   - Adaptability.

STANDARD IV

The plan of nursing care includes priorities and prescribed nursing approaches and measures to achieve the goals derived from the nursing diagnosis.

Rationale. Priorities and approaches are an integral part of the planning process and are necessary to the successful achievement of the goals.

Assessment Factors

1. Physical and psychosocial measures are planned to prevent, ameliorate, or control specific problems of the older adult and are related to the nursing diagnosis and goals of care.
2. Environmental hazards, which may include reducing high frequency sounds, glaring surfaces, and reducing overproduction of stimuli to prevent confusion, are eliminated.
3. Methods of adaptation using concepts of wellness are taught to the older adult.
4. Specific approaches are identified to orient the older adult to new roles and relationships and new surroundings, where applicable, as well as to relevant health resources.

5. Specific approaches are identified to promote the social interactions and effective communication of the older adult.

STANDARD V

The plan of care is implemented, using appropriate nursing actions.

Rationale. Appropriate nursing actions are purposefully directed toward the stated goals.

Assessment Factor

Nursing actions are:

- Consistent with the plan of care that is developed in collaboration with the older adult and with appropriate input from other health disciplines.
- Based on scientific principles.
- Individualized to the specific situation.
- Modified to allow for alternative approaches.
- Used to provide a safe and therapeutic environment.
- Compatible with the physiological, psychological, and social data acquired.
- Task-delegated as deemed appropriate.
- Planned to meet specific criteria as described in protocols.

STANDARD VI

The older adult and/or significant other(s) participate in determining the process attained in the achievement of established goals.

Rationale. The older adult and/or significant other(s) are essential components in the determination of nursing's impact upon the individual's health status.

Assessment Factors

1. Current data are used to measure progress toward goal achievement.
2. Nursing actions are analyzed for effectiveness in goal achievement.
3. The older adult and/or significant others evaluate nursing actions and goal achievement.
4. Plans for the nursing follow-up of the older adult are made to permit for the ongoing assessment of the effects of nursing care.

STANDARD VII

The older adult and/or significant other(s) participate in the ongoing process of assessment, the setting of new goals, the reordering of priorities, the revision of plans for nursing care, and the initiation of new nursing actions.

Rationale. Comprehensive nursing care is dependent upon actively involving the older adult and/or significant other(s) in a continuing, dynamic process.

Assessment Factors

1. Assessment is directed by the level of progress of the older adult in goal achievement.
2. The older adult and/or significant other(s) assist in the identification of new goals and the reordering of priorities.
3. Plans are updated and revised.
4. New nursing actions are appropriately initiated.

Appendix C
American Nurses' Association Requirements for Certification as a Gerontological Nurse and as a Gerontological Nurse Practitioner

The Certification Plan

Certification is a voluntary program established by the American Nurses' Association through its divisions on nursing practice. The purpose is to give tangible acknowledgment of professional achievement in nursing.

Through a peer review system and a specially prepared written examination you are able to quality for certification provided you meet certain criteria prior to taking the test.

Certification recognizes expertise — both in application of current knowledge, and in the ability to consider and initiate new alternatives and strategies in clinical practice.

The certification process also reinforces conscious use of theory in the planning and implementing of nursing care.

Gerontological Nurse

Gerontological nursing is concerned with the health needs of older adults, planning and implementing health care to meet those needs, and evaluating the effectiveness of such care. The primary challenge is to identify and use the strengths of older adults and assist them to use those strengths to maximize their independence. The older adult is actively involved as much as possible in the decision making which influences everyday living.

Special requirement for certification as a gerontological nurse. Two current consecutive years as a registered nurse in the field of gerontological nursing. Practice may include the management of other persons to achieve or help achieve the patient/client goals.

A candidate for certification must provide evidence of 30 contact hours of continuing education relevant to gerontological nursing during the previous two years. These hours may reflect conferences, workshops, institutes, clinical sessions, or courses relating to gerontological nursing.

Submission of documentation of the contact hours completed will be requested after a passing score on the examination has been achieved.

Gerontological Nurse Practitioner

A gerontological nurse practitioner is a registered nurse who has received specialized education that prepares him/her to assume responsibility for delivery of primary health care services to older adults. At present, there are two avenues for preparation as a nurse practitioner — continuing education programs provided under the auspices of an accredited school or department of nursing within an institution of higher education, and master's degree programs. Persons who have successfully completed such a program in gerontological nursing may use the title Gerontological Nurse Practitioner.

An interim plan for certification of gerontological nurse practitioners has been adopted by the Division on Gerontological Nursing Practice.

Special requirements for certification. Submission of evidence of completion of an organized program of study preparing nurse practitioners which meets the published ANA guidelines for short-term programs for adult, family, or gerontological nurse practitioners.

The process requirements entail successful completion of the adult nurse practitioner certification examination and successful completion of the documentation requirements for gerontological nursing.

*Reprinted with permission from *American Nurses' Association Publication,* 2420 Pershing Rd., Kansas City, Kansas, 1980.

Upon completion of the program requirements, the candidate will be certified as a gerontological nurse practitioner.

Dual certification as an adult nurse practitioner and as a gerontological nurse practitioner may be obtained. However, the standard fee for each of the certifications will be assessed.

Nurse practitioners who are currently certified as adult or family nurse practitioners can meet the requirements for this program by completing successfully the documentation part of the process.

Nurse practitioners who are currently certified as gerontological nurses can meet the requirements for this program by completing successfully the written examination for adult nurse practitioners.

The future plan for certification proposes development of an examination for gerontological nurse practitioners. Until this examination is made available, the interim plan described above will remain in effect.

Appendix D
Specific Standards of Care and Patient's Rights for Home Care Patients

These written policies shall be established and be made available to the patient, his family, and the public. Such policies shall ensure that each patient receiving care from the agency shall have the following rights:

STANDARD I

That the patient will receive the care necessary to help regain or maintain his maximum state of health and if necessary cope with death.

STANDARD II

That the agency personnel who care for the patient are qualified through education and experience to perform the services for which they are responsible.

STANDARD III

That the patient will be treated with consideration, respect and full recognition of individuality, including privacy in treatment and in care.

STANDARD IV

That within the limits determined by the physician, the patient and family will be taught about the illness. Within the limits of the agency service policy the patient and family will be instructed in appropriate care techniques.

STANDARD V

That the patient or responsible person will be fully informed of services available in the agency, related charges and complaint procedures.

STANDARD VI

That the patient will be a participant in decisions regarding his/her care plan.

STANDARD VII

That the patient will have the right to refuse treatment to the extent permitted by law and to be informed of the medical consequences of such refusal. The patient will be required to sign a release of responsibility form.

STANDARD VIII

That plans will be made with the patient and family so that continuing services will be available to the patient throughout the period of need. The plans should be timely and involve the use of all appropriate personnel and community resources.

STANDARD IX

That agency personnel will keep adequate records and will treat with confidence all personal matters that relate to the patient.

STANDARD X

That the patient has the right to approve or refuse the release of medical records to any individual outside the agency, except in the case of his transfer to another health facility, or as required by law or third party payment contract.

---

*Adapted from Patient's Rights of the California Association for Health Services at Home and National Association of Home Health Agencies, 659 Cherokee St., Denver, Colorado 80204, 1977, 1979.

Appendix E
Overviews of Literature on Common Problems of the Elderly

Anderson, C.O. Issues in the treatment of psychiatric-geriatric patients: a brief review of the literature. *Journal of Gerontological Nursing* 3(3):32–40 (May–June 1977).

Cath, S. Psychoanalytic viewpoints on aging — an historical survey. In Kent, D.P., Kastenbaum, R., and Sherwood, S. (Eds.) *Research Planning and Action for the Elderly*. New York: Behavioral Publications, 1972.

DeGennaro, D., Hymen, R., Crannell, A.M., and Mansky, P.A. Psychotropic drug therapy: antidepressants, lithium, antipsychotics, EPS and sedative hypnotics. *American Journal of Nursing* 80(7):1303–1329 (1981).

Eisdorfer, C., Cohen, D., and Preston, C. Behavioral and psychological therapies for the older patient with cognitive impairment. In *NIH Conference on Behavior Aspects of Senile Dementia*. Washington, D.C.: December 1978.

Folsom, J.C., Boies, B.L., and Pommerenck, K. Life adjustment techniques for use with the dysfunctional elderly. *Aged Care and Services Review* 1(4):1–12 (1978).

Jeste, D.V. and Wyatt, R.J. Changing epidemiology of tardive dyskinesia: an overview. *American Journal of Psychiatry* 138:297-309 (1981).

McTavish, D.G. Perception of old people: a review of research methodologies and findings. *Gerontologist* 11:90–101 (1971).

Rechtschaffen, A. Psychotherapy with geriatric patients: a review of the literature. *Journal of Gerontology* Vol. 14, 73 (1959).

Schneck, M.K., Reisberg, B., and Ferris, S.H. An overview of current concepts of Alzheimer's disease. *American Journal of Psychiatry* 139 (2):165–173 (1982).

Schulz, R. and Brenner, G. Relocation of the aged: a review and theoretical analysis. *Journal of Gerontology* 32(3):323–333 (1977).

Terry, R.D. Dementia: a brief and selective review. *Archives of Neurology* 33:1–4 (1976).

Appendix F
Health Care Resources and Self Help Groups

ALCOHOLISM AND DRUG ABUSE

Alcoholics Anonymous
468 Park Avenue South
New York, NY 10016

Al-Anon Family Group Headquarters, Inc.
P.O. Box 182
Madison Square Station
New York, NY 10159

ARTHRITIS

The Arthritis Foundation
1314 Spring Street, NW
Atlanta, GA 30309

BLOOD DISORDERS

The Sickle Cell Disease Foundation of Greater
 New York
209 West 125th Street, Room 108
New York, NY 10027
(212) 850-1920

CANCER

American Cancer Society
777 Third Avenue
New York, NY 10017

CARDIAC DISORDERS

American Heart Association
7320 Greenville Avenue
Dallas, TX 75231

Cardiovascular Disease
The American Heart Association
44 East 23rd Street
New York, NY 10010
(617) 732-5609

DIABETES

American Diabetes Association, Inc.
2 Park Avenue
New York, NY 10016

EPILEPSY

Epilepsy Foundation of America
National Headquarters
4351 Garden City Drive
Landover, MD 20785

Epilepsy Foundation of America
Washington D.C. Area Chapter
815 15th Street, N.W., Suite 528
Washington, DC 20005

HEARING

Alexander Graham Bell Association for the
 Deaf
3417 Volta Place, N.W.
Washington, DC 20007
(202) 337-5220

American Humane Society
P.O. Box 1266
Denver, CO
(trains seeing eye dogs)

American Organization for the Education of
 the Hearing Impaired
1537 35th Street, N.W.
Washington, DC 20007

American Speech-Language-Hearing Association
10801 Rockville Pike
Rockville, MD 20852

The Better Hearing Institute
1430 K Street, N.W., Suite 600
Washington, DC 20005
(800) 424-8576 (toll free)

Council of Organizations Serving the Deaf
P.O. Box 894
Columbia, MD 21044

National Association of the Deaf
814 Thayer Avenue
Silver Spring, MD 20910

The National Hearing Aid Society
20361 Middlebelt Road
Livonia, MI 48152
(313) 478-2610

HUNTINGTON'S DISEASE

Committee to Combat Huntington's Disease
250 West 57th Street
New York, NY 10019
(212) 757-0443

KIDNEY

The National Kidney Foundation
116 East 27th Street
New York, NY 10016
(212) 889-2210

LIFE CRISIS

Widow to Widow
25 Huntington Avenue
Boston, MA 02115
(617) 661-6180

LUNG/BREATHING DISORDERS

American Lung Association
1720 Broadway
New York, NY 10019

Emphysema Anonymous, Inc.
P.O. Box 66
Fort Meyers, FL 33902
(813) 334-4266

MENTAL HEALTH

National Association for Mental Health
1800 North Kent Street
Arlington, VA 22209
(703) 528-6405

Recovery, Inc.
116 South Michigan Avenue
Chicago, IL 60603
(312) 263-2292

OSTOMY

United Ostomy Association, Inc.
1111 Wilshire Boulevard
Los Angeles, CA 90017
(213) 481-2811

PARAPLEGIA

National Paraplegia Foundation
33 North Michigan Avenue
Chicago, IL 60601

Paralyzed Veterans of America
7315 Wisconsin Avenue, N.W.
Washington, DC 20014

PARKINSON'S DISEASE

American Parkinson's Disease Association
147 East 50th Street
New York, NY 10022

National Parkinson Foundation
1501 Northwest Ninth Avenue
Miami, FL 33136

Parkinson's Disease Foundation
William Black Medical Research Building
Columbia Presbyterian Medical Center
640 West 168th Street
New York, NY 10032

United Parkinson's Foundation
220 South State Street
Chicago, IL 60604

SPEECH

American Speech-Language-Hearing Association
10801 Rockville Pike
Rockville, MD 20852

STROKE

Stroke Clubs of America
805 12th Street
Galveston, TX 77550

VISION

American Council of the Blind
1211 Connecticut Avenue, N.W.
Washington, DC 20036

American Foundation for the Blind
15 West 16th Street
New York, NY 10011

American Printing House for the Blind
1839 Frankfort Avenue
Louisville, KY 40206

Blind Outdoor Leisure Development
    (BOLD, Inc.)
533 East Main Street
Aspen, CO 81611

Blinded Veterans Association
1735 DeSales Street, N.W.
Washington, DC 20036
(202) 347-4010

Guide Dog Users, Inc.
Box 174, Central Station
Baldwin, NY 11510

Guiding Eyes for the Blind
Yorktown Heights, NY 10599

VISION (continued)

The Library of Congress
Division for the Blind and Physically
    Handicapped
Washington, DC 20542

National Association for Visually Handicapped
    (partially seeing)
3201 Balboa Street
San Francisco, CA 94121

National Foundation for the Blind
218 Randolph Hotel Building
Des Moines, IA 50309
(800) 424-9770

National Retinitis Pigmentosa Foundation
8331 Mindale Circle
Baltimore, MD 21207
(301) 655-1011

National Society for the Prevention of
    Blindness, Inc.
79 Madison Avenue
New York, NY 10801

Appendix G
National Organizations and Programs
Governmental and Voluntary

ADMINISTRATION ON AGING

Department of Health and Human Services
200 Independence Avenue, S.W.
Room 329D
Washington, D.C. 20201
Pat McKelvie
Director of Public Affairs
Lennie Marrie Tolliver, U.S. Commissioner
     on Aging
(202) 472-7257

**AMERICAN ASSOCIATION FOR
GERIATRIC PSYCHIATRY**

230 North Michigan Avenue, Suite 2400
Chicago, IL 60601
Sanford Finkle, MD, Executive Director
(312) 263-2225

**AMERICAN ASSOCIATION OF
RETIRED PERSONS**

National Retired Teachers Association
1909 K Street, N.W.
Washington, D.C. 20049
Cyril F. Brickfield, Executive Director
Paul Kerschner, Associate Director
(202) 872-4700

AMERICAN GERIATRICS SOCIETY

10 Columbus Circle
New York, NY 10019
Kathryn Henderson, Executive Director
(212) 582-1333
(Western Division:
13220-105th Avenue
Sun City, AZ 85351)

**ASSOCIACION NACIONAL POR PERSONAS
MAYORES (NATIONAL ASSOCIATION
FOR SPANISH-SPEAKING ELDERLY)**

1730 W. Olympic Boulevard, Suite 401
Los Angeles, CA 90015
Carmela G. Lacayo
President and Executive Director
(213) 487-1922

**CENTER FOR STUDIES OF THE
MENTAL HEALTH OF THE AGING**

National Institute of Mental Health
Alcohol, Drug Abuse, and Mental Health
     Administration
Parklawn Building
5600 Fishers Lane
Rockville, MD 20857
(301) 443-3673

**DIVISION OF LONG-TERM CARE
EXPERIMENTATION**

Health Care Financing Administration
Oak Meadows Building, Room 1-6-3
6325 Security Boulevard
Baltimore, MD 21207
Linda Hamm, Director
(301) 594-7649

**THE GERONTOLOGICAL SOCIETY
OF AMERICA**

1835 K Street, N.W., Suite 305
Washington, D.C. 20006
Janice Caldwell, Ph.D., Executive Director
(202) 466-6750

GRAY PANTHERS
3635 Chestnut Street
Philadelphia, PA 19104
Maggie Kuhn, Director
(215) 382-3300

HOUSE SELECT COMMITTEE ON AGING
Room 712, House Office Building
Annex No. 1
Washington, D.C. 20515
Charles Edwards, Staff Director
(202) 226-3375

INTERNATIONAL FEDERATION ON AGING
1909 K Street, N.W., Suite 510
Washington, D.C. 20049
Richard E. Johnson, General Secretary
(202) 872-4886

NATIONAL CENTER ON BLACK AGING
1424 K Street, N.W., Suite 500
Washington, D.C. 20005
Samuel Simmons, President
(202) 637-8400

NATIONAL CITIZENS COALITION FOR NURSING HOME REFORM
1424-16th Street, N.W.
Washington, D.C. 20036
Elma Griesel, Executive Director
(202) 797-8227

NATIONAL CLEARINGHOUSE ON AGING
Administration on Aging
330 Independence Avenue, S.W.
Washington, D.C. 20201
Peter Halpin, Eva Nash, Co-directors
(202) 245-1826

NATIONAL COUNCIL ON AGING
600 Maryland Avenue, S.W.
West Wing 100
Washington, D.C. 20024
Arthur Fleming, President
(202) 479-1200

NATIONAL COUNCIL OF SENIOR CITIZENS
925-15th Street, N.W.
Washington, D.C. 20005
William R. Hutton, Executive Director
(202) 347-8800

NATIONAL INDIAN COUNCIL ON AGING
P.O. Box 2088
Albuquerque, NM 87103
Alfred G. Elgin, Jr., Executive Director
(505) 766-2276

NATIONAL INSTITUTE ON AGING
Department of Health and Human Services
Public Health Service
National Institutes of Health
Building 31
Bethesda, MD 20205
T. Franklin Williams, Director
(301) 496-1752

NATIONAL PACIFIC/ASIAN RESOURCE CENTER ON AGING
811 First Avenue
Coleman Building, Suite 210
Seattle, WA 98104
Louise Kamikawa, Executive Director
(206) 622-5124

NATIONAL POLICY CENTER ON HOUSING AND LIVING ARRANGEMENTS FOR OLDER AMERICANS
University of Michigan
2000 Bonisteel Boulevard
Ann Arbor, MI 48109
Leon Pastalan, Ph.D., Dean Robert Metcalf,
  Co-directors
(313) 763-1275

NATIONAL POLICY CENTER ON WOMEN AND AGING
Cole Field House, Room 1150
University of Maryland
College Park, MD 20742
Marilyn Block, Ph.D., Director
(301) 454-6666

SENATE SPECIAL COMMITTEE ON AGING
Room G-233, Dirksen Senate Office Building
Washington, D.C. 20510
John Rother, Staff Director
(202) 224-5364

SENIOR ACTUALIZATION AND GROWTH EXPLORATIONS (SAGE)
2455 Hilgard Avenue
Berkeley, CA 94709

SWING BED CONCEPT IMPLEMENTATION IN SMALL RURAL HOSPITALS

Rural Hospital Program of Extended Care
  Services
P.O. Box 2316
Princeton, NJ 08540

William E. Walch, Assistant Vice President
  Communications
(609) 452-8701
(The Robert W. Johnson Foundation)

STATE AND REGIONAL ORGANIZATIONS AND PROGRAMS

HILLHAVEN FOUNDATION

1900 Powell Street, Suite 400
Emeryville, CA 94662
Sue Roderick, Executive Director
(415) 655-6374

WESTERN GERONTOLOGICAL SOCIETY

833 Market Street, Room 516
San Francisco, CA 94103
Gloria Cavanaugh, Executive Director
(415) 543-2617

PUBLICATIONS

AGING

Administration of Aging
330 Independence Avenue, S.W.
Washington, D.C. 20201
(202) 245-1826

AMERICAN GERIATRICS SOCIETY NEWSLETTER

American Geriatrics Society
10 Columbus Circle
New York, NY 10019
(212) 582-1333

COALITION

National Citizens Coalition for Nursing Home
  Reform
1424-16th Street, N.W.
Washington, D.C. 20036
(202) 797-8227

CURRENT LITERATURE ON AGING

National Council on Aging
Publications Sales Department
600 Maryland Avenue, S.W.
Washington, D.C. 20024
(202) 479-1200

GENERATIONS

Western Gerontological Society
833 Market Street, Room 516
San Francisco, CA 94103
(415) 543-2617

GERIATRIC MEDICINE CURRENTS

Ross Laboratories
Division of Family Medicine
Duke University Medical Center
625 Cleveland Avenue
Columbus, OH 43216
(614) 227-3333

GERIATRIC NURSING, AMERICAN JOURNAL OF CARE FOR THE AGING

American Journal of Nursing Company
555 West 57 Street
New York, NY 10019

THE GERONTOLOGIST

The Gerontological Society of America
1835 K Street, N.W.
Washington, D.C. 20006
(202) 466-6750

GERONTOLOGY TOPICS

Ethel Percy Andrus Gerontology Center
University of Southern California
University Park
Los Angeles, CA 90007
(213) 743-6080

THE INTERNATIONAL JOURNAL OF AGING AND HUMAN DEVELOPMENT

Dr. Robert Kastenbaum, Editor
Adult Development and AGing Program
West Hall
Arizona State University
Tempe, AZ 85287
(Carol Hunter, Managing Editor,
    (602) 965-5093)

JOURNAL OF GERONTOLOGICAL NURSING

Charles B. Slack, Inc.
6900 Grove Road
Thorofare, NJ 08086
(609) 848-1000 Thorofare
(212) 285-9777 New York

JOURNAL OF GERONTOLOGY

Gerontological Society of America
1835 K Street, N.W.
Washington, D.C. 20006
(202) 466-6750

JOURNAL OF HOUSING FOR THE ELDERLY

National Policy Center on Housing and Living
    Arrangements for Older Americans
University of Michigan
2000 Bonisteel Boulevard
Ann Arbor, MI 48109
(313) 763-1275

OMEGA: JOURNAL OF DEATH AND DYING

Dr. Robert Kastenbaum, Editor
Adult Development and Aging Program
West Hall
Arizona State University
Tempe, AZ 85287
(Carol Hunter, Managing Editor,
    (602) 965-5093)

PERSPECTIVE ON AGING

National Council on Aging
Publications Sales Department
600 Maryland Avenue, S.W.
Washington, D.C. 20024
(202) 479-1200

SENIOR CENTER REPORT

National Council on Aging
Publications Sales Department
600 Maryland Avenue, S.W.
Washington, D.C. 20024
(202) 479–1200

THE SENIOR COUNSELOR

Hospital of the Good Samaritan
Social Services Department
616 South Witmer Street
Los Angeles, CA 90017
(213) 977-2121

SENIOR HEALTH UPDATE

Senior Health and Peer Counseling Center
2125 Arizona
Santa Monica, CA 90404
(213) 829-4715

Author Index

Subject Index